BSAVA Manual of Canine and Feline Emergency and Critical Care

Second edition

Editors:

Lesley G. King
MVB DipACVECC DipACVIM
School of Veterinary Medicine, University of Pennsylvania,
3900 Delancey Street, Philadelphia, PA 19104-6010, USA

and

Amanda Boag
MA VetMB DipACVIM DipACVECC FHEA MRCVS
Department of Veterinary Clinical Science, Royal Veterinary College,
Hawkshead Lane, North Mymms, Hertfordshire AL9 7TA

Published by:

British Small Animal Veterinary Association
Woodrow House, 1 Telford Way, Waterwells
Business Park, Quedgeley, Gloucester GL2 2AB

A Company Limited by Guarantee in England.
Registered Company No. 2837793.
Registered as a Charity.

A catalogue record for this book is available from the British Library.

ISBN   978 0 905214 99 3

The publishers and contributors cannot take responsibility for information
provided on dosages and methods of application of drugs mentioned in
this publication. Details of this kind must be verified by individual users
from the appropriate literature.

Printed by: Replika Press Pvt. Ltd, India

Other titles in the BSAVA Manuals series:

For information on these and all BSAVA publications please visit our website: www.bsava.com

Contents

Contributors

Sophie Adamantos BVSc CertVA DipACVECC MRCVS
Department of Veterinary Clinical Science, Royal Veterinary College, Hawkshead Lane, North Mymms, Hertfordshire AL9 7TA

Janet Aldrich DVM DipACVECC
Veterinary Medical Teaching Hospital, University of California – Davis, One Shields Avenue, Davis, CA 95616, USA

Amy J. Alwood DVM
Allegheny Veterinary Emergency, Trauma and Specialty, 4224 Northern Pike, Monroeville, PA 15146, USA

Frances Barr MA VetMB PhD DVR DipECVDI MRCVS
Department of Clinical Veterinary Science, University of Bristol, Langford House, Langford, Bristol BS40 5DU

Amanda Boag MA VetMB DipACVIM DipACVECC FHEA MRCVS
Department of Veterinary Clinical Sciences, Royal Veterinary College, Hawkshead Lane, North Mymms, Hertfordshire AL9 7TA

Adrian Boswood MA VetMB DVC DipECVIM ILTM MRCVS
Department of Veterinary Clinical Sciences, Royal Veterinary College, Hawkshead Lane, North Mymms, Hertfordshire AL9 7TA

Andrew J. Brown MA VetMB DipACVECC MRCVS
Department of Small Animal Clinical Studies, College of Veterinary Medicine, Michigan State University, East Lansing, MI 48824, USA

Dorothy Cimino Brown DVM MSCE DipACVS
School of Veterinary Medicine, University of Pennsylvania, 3900 Delancey Street, Philadelphia, PA 19104-6010, USA

Edward Cooper VMD
Department of Veterinary Clinical Sciences, College of Veterinary Medicine, The Ohio State University, Columbus, OH 43210, USA

Kenneth J. Drobatz DVM DipACVECC DipACVIM
School of Veterinary Medicine, University of Pennsylvania, 3900 Delancey Street, Philadelphia, PA 19104-6010, USA

Gary C.W. England BVetMed PhD DVetMed DVR DVRep DipECAR DipACT ILTM FRCVS
School of Veterinary Medicine and Science, University of Nottingham, College Road, Loughborough LE12 5RD

Gillian R. Gibson VMD DipACVIM MRCVS
Wingrave Veterinary Surgery, 84 Mulgrave Road, Sutton, SM2 6LZ

Reid P. Groman DVM DipACVIM
School of Veterinary Medicine, University of Pennsylvania, 3900 Delancey Street, Philadelphia, PA 19104-6010, USA

Susan G. Hackner BVSc DipACVIM DipACVECC MRCVS
Veterinary Specialty Consulting, Washington, DC 20007, USA

Richard Hammond BSc BVetMed PhD DVA DipECVA MHEA MRCVS
School of Veterinary Medicine and Science, University of Nottingham, College Road, Loughborough LE12 5RD

Daniel Holden BVetMed DVA DipECVA CertSAM MRCVS
The County Veterinary Clinic, 137 Kingston Road, Taunton, Somerset TA2 7SR

David Holt BVSc DipACVS
School of Veterinary Medicine, University of Pennsylvania, 3900 Delancey Street, Philadelphia, PA 19104-6010, USA

Dez Hughes BVSc DipACVECC MRCVS
Department of Veterinary Clinical Sciences, Royal Veterinary College, Hawkshead Lane, North Mymms, Hertfordshire AL9 7TA

Karyl J. Hurley DVM DipACVIM DipECVIM
Waltham Centre for Pet Nutrition, Freeby Lane, Waltham-on-the-Wolds, Leicestershire LE14 4RS

Lesley G. King MVB DipACVECC DipACVIM
School of Veterinary Medicine, University of Pennsylvania, 3900 Delancey Street, Philadelphia, PA 19104-6010, USA

Sorrel J. Langley-Hobbs MA BVetMed DSAS(O) DipECVS MRCVS
Department of Veterinary Medicine, University of Cambridge, Madingley Road, Cambridge CB3 0ES

Sam N. Long BVSc PhD DipECVN MRCVS
School of Veterinary Medicine, University of Pennsylvania, 3900 Delancey Street, Philadelphia, PA 19104-6010, USA

Deborah C. Mandell VMD DipACVECC
School of Veterinary Medicine, University of Pennsylvania, 3900 Delancey Street, Philadelphia, PA 19104-6010, USA

Karol A. Mathews DVM DVSc DipACVECC
University of Guelph, Ontario Veterinary College, Guelph, Ontario, N1G 2W1, Canada

Dawn Merton-Boothe DVM DipACVIM
College of Veterinary Medicine, Auburn University, 109 Greene Hall, Auburn, AL 36849, USA

Kathryn E. Michel DVM MS DipACVN
School of Veterinary Medicine, University of Pennsylvania, 3900 Delancey Street, Philadelphia, PA 19104-6010, USA

William W. Muir DVM PhD DipACVECC
College of Veterinary Medicine, Department of Veterinary Clinical Sciences, 601 Tharp Street, Columbus, OH 43210-1089, USA

Kate Murphy BVSc (Hons) DSAM DipECVIM-CA MRCVS
Department of Clinical Veterinary Science, University of Bristol, Langford, Bristol BS40 5DU

Matthew Pead BVetMed PhD CertSAO ILTM MRCVS
Department of Veterinary Clinical Science, Royal Veterinary College, Hawkshead Lane, North Mymms, Hertfordshire AL9 7TA

Elisa A. Petrollini CVT VTS (ECC)
School of Veterinary Medicine, University of Pennsylvania, 3900 Delancey Street, Philadelphia, PA 19104-6010, USA

Robert H. Poppenga DVM PhD DipABVT
CAHFS Toxicology Laboratory, School of Veterinary Medicine, University of California, West Health Sciences Drive, Davis, CA 95616, USA

Petra J. Roosje DVM PhD DipECVD
Division of Clinical Dermatology, Department of Clinical Veterinary Medicine, Vetsuisse Faculty, University of Berne, Länggassstrasse 128, 3012 Berne, Switzerland

Marco Russo DVM PhD MRCVS
Department of Clinical Science, Section of Clinical Obstetrics, Faculty of Veterinary Medicine, University of Naples, Italy

Emily Savino CVT VTS (ECC)
School of Veterinary Medicine, University of Pennsylvania, 3900 Delancey Street, Philadelphia, PA 19104-6010, USA

Barbara J. Skelly MA VetMB PhD DipACVIM DipECVIM-CA MRCVS
Department of Veterinary Medicine, University of Cambridge, Madingley Road, Cambridge CB3 0ES

Rebecca L. Stepien DVM MS DipACVIM
Section of Veterinary Medicine, University of Wisconsin–Madison, 2015 Linden Drive W., Madison, WI 53706-1102, USA

Charles H. Vite DVM PhD DipACVIM
School of Veterinary Medicine, University of Pennsylvania, 3900 Delancey Street, Philadelphia, PA 19104-6010, USA

Lori S. Waddell DVM DipACVECC
Department of Clinical Sciences, School of Veterinary Medicine, University of Pennsylvania, 3900 Delancey Street, Philadelphia, PA 19104-6010, USA

Sheena M. Warman BSc BVMS DSAM DipECVIM-CA MRCVS
Department of Clinical Veterinary Science, University of Bristol, Langford, Bristol BS40 5DU

Foreword

The Editors have asked me to write a Foreword for this edition of the *BSAVA Manual of Canine and Feline Emergency and Critical Care*. I am happy to do so and feel that it is quite an honour.

For several years now I have been exclusively involved in emergency medicine and critical care and most striking to me is the amount of new knowledge that has accumulated in this area of veterinary medicine. When I was in veterinary school I can remember only two books specifically dedicated to emergency medicine. That has obviously changed, along with the development of the Veterinary Emergency and Critical Care Society, the American College of Veterinary Emergency and Critical Care, the British Association of Veterinary Emergency Care, the European Veterinary Emergency and Critical Care Society, and numerous residencies and internships specifically designed for education in emergency and critical care. It is extremely exciting to be a part of this emerging new specialty.

As with any new specialty, the individuals involved are extremely passionate about what they do and show great willingness to spread the 'Emergency Medicine and Critical Care Gospel'. This book captures that zeal and information in an extremely practical and useful format.

Anyone that valued the last edition will not be disappointed. Those who went without the first version should make this a 'must-have' for their veterinary library. As with the last edition, this book is truly international with an excellent mix of authors from both sides of 'the pond', providing a broad perspective of emergency and critical care that no other book can boast. The credentials of the chapter authors are impressive and Lesley King and Amanda Boag have done a wonderful job in putting together a cohesive and extremely readable and useful manual that you will want to keep readily available for when that next emergency case comes in. You know and I know, it can happen at any time and this book can be there for you in that time of need!

Kenneth J. Drobatz
March 2007

Preface

It is our great pleasure to present the newest edition of the *BSAVA Manual of Small Animal Emergency and Critical Care*. The specialty of emergency and critical care has continued to develop rapidly since publication of the first edition, with this second edition presenting updates, expansions and new illustrations of the material from the first book. Several important new chapters have also been added covering topics vital to the emergency practitioner, such as vascular access, electrolyte and acid–base balance, transfusion therapy, medical approach to gastrointestinal emergencies, analgesia in critical patients, and antibiotic therapy.

This Manual is intended as a quick and easy reference for practitioners who handle emergency and critical cases on a routine or even not-so-routine basis. We hope that the material is accessible and practical, even in a crisis! In addition, the book is intended to act as a useful resource for residents and specialists in the field of emergency and critical care.

The editors would like to express our sincere gratitude to each of the contributing authors. These contributors are truly leaders in their fields, both nationally and internationally. Without their efforts it would not have been possible to put together this Manual, which spans the breadth of our knowledge in this vast field.

We must also acknowledge the incredible contributions of everyone in the BSAVA office, who all worked tirelessly to make this manual as perfect as it can be! In particular, Marion and Sabrina deserve special mention for their persistence, timeliness and attention to detail.

Finally, the editors would like to acknowledge the help and support that we have received from our families and friends, as we worked to bring this project to fruition. Without their constant encouragement and support it would be difficult to achieve any of our goals in life.

We hope that this Manual proves to be useful, helps you to save some lives, and sparks or fuels your interest in the exciting and dynamic field of emergency and critical care.

Sincerely,

Lesley G. King
Amanda Boag
April 2007

Triage of the emergency patient

Andrew J. Brown and Kenneth J. Drobatz

Introduction

Triage can be defined as the evaluation and allocation of treatment to patients according to a system of priorities designed to maximize the number of survivors.

All stages of emergency evaluation are important to the successful management of the critically ill patient: telephone triage, waiting room triage, primary survey and treatment, secondary survey and the emergency plan. Critically ill patients have little physiological reserve to tolerate mistakes of omission or commission. Anticipation and prevention of problems before they occur is one of the cornerstones of optimal emergency and critical care medicine. Always assume the worst and treat for it, while maintaining the philosophy 'above all, do no harm'.

Telephone triage

The initial contact between a client and the veterinary surgery or hospital is often via the telephone. The information obtained from this conversation may assist in triage of the patient, may help in diagnosis, and may provide information regarding first aid treatment for the pet.

The immediate aim of telephone triage is to determine whether the patient needs to be examined by the veterinary surgeon immediately and what the owner should do for the pet before coming to the surgery. The owner should be calmed if necessary, so that concise and accurate information can be obtained. Questions should be directed at determining:

• The nature of the injury
• How the animal is breathing
• The colour of the mucous membranes
• The level of consciousness
• The presence and severity of bleeding
• The presence and severity of wounds
• The ability of the animal to ambulate
• The presence of obvious fractures
• The severity of vomiting and diarrhoea if present
• The ability to urinate
• The degree of abdominal distension
• Whether there is coughing.

Patients with the following should be brought to the hospital without delay:

• Respiratory distress
• Neurological abnormalities
• Protracted vomiting
• Slow or rapid heart rate
• Bleeding from body orifices
• Weakness, pale mucous membranes
• Rapid and progressive abdominal distension
• Inability to urinate
• Severe coughing
• Toxin ingestion
• Collapse
• Extreme pain.

Transport and preparation

Owners often want to administer first aid to their pets. In instances where the problem is clearly determined and relatively simple, advice can often be given over the telephone. Relying on an owner's interpretation of the animal's problems can be risky, however. If there is any doubt about what is occurring, the owner should be advised to bring the pet to the clinic for definitive evaluation.

If trauma has occurred, the patient should be placed on a board or some type of support structure. Fractured limbs can sometimes be stabilized for transport by wrapping a roll of newspaper around the limb or taping or tying a board or piece of cardboard to the leg. The joints above and below the fracture should be stabilized. Splints should be applied with care, since it is often difficult for the owner to determine the location of the fracture. If done incorrectly, splinting has the potential to cause further damage. If doubt exists, the animal should be placed in a confined space or in an area where movement is minimized. Direct pressure or careful application of a tourniquet can control active haemorrhage. Owners should be warned that animals that are in pain, traumatized, neurologically damaged or frightened should be carefully approached and muzzled if possible. Even the friendliest of pets can become aggressive under these circumstances.

Clients may be extremely upset and should be calmed prior to bringing their pet in. Clear directions should be given to the owner for the drive to the clinic, and time of arrival should be estimated. The hospital personnel should be notified about the nature of the emergency and the estimated time of arrival, so that any special preparations may be undertaken if necessary.

Triage and initial assessment

Triage is the sorting out and classification of patients to determine priority of need and the optimal order in which they should be treated. Upon arrival at the veterinary clinic, every animal should be quickly evaluated by a member of the medical team to determine whether it requires immediate treatment or is stable enough to wait if necessary (Figure 1.1). During the triage, a brief history is obtained about the nature of the primary complaint and its progression. Animals that are in containers or blankets should be taken out and examined. Four major organ systems should be assessed:

- Respiratory
- Cardiovascular
- Neurological
- Renal.

Dysfunction in any one of these systems can become life-threatening and should be addressed as rapidly as possible.

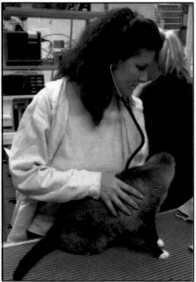

1.1

Following triage evaluation, unstable patients are taken to the treatment area for initial assessment.

Respiratory rate, rhythm and effort should be determined. Signs of respiratory distress include loud airway sounds, increased breathing rate, abducted elbows, extended head and neck, flaring of the nares, open-mouth breathing and paradoxical respiration (see Chapter 7).

Cardiovascular system assessment includes mucous membrane colour, capillary refill time and pulse quality and rhythm. Signs of cardiovascular compromise include pale, grey or hyperaemic mucous membranes, very rapid or prolonged capillary refill time, weak or bounding pulses, very rapid or slow pulse rate and an irregular or asynchronous pulse rhythm.

Immediate neurological assessment should include evaluation of mentation and ability to ambulate. Neurological abnormalities that should be addressed quickly include severe changes in mentation such as stupor, coma, hyperexcitability, delirium and seizures.

Immediate evaluation of the renal system should include assessment of the ability to urinate and palpation of the urinary bladder.

Animals with dysfunction in one of the four major organ systems should be brought immediately to the treatment area for further evaluation and treatment.

Conditions affecting other body systems are generally not immediately life threatening in themselves, but their effects on the four major organ systems can result in death. For example, a fracture of the femur is not life threatening by itself, but the resultant blood loss into the thigh musculature may result in hypovolaemia and cardiovascular compromise. Problems that do not immediately affect the four major organ systems, but require that the animal be immediately brought back to the treatment area, include:

- Recent ingestion of, or topical exposure to, a toxin
- Recent seizures
- Trauma
- Excessive bleeding
- Prolapsed organs
- Snake bite
- Hyperthermia
- Open wounds
- Fractures
- Burns
- Dystocia
- Death.

Also, if an owner is overly concerned, even if the animal appears physiologically stable it should be brought to the treatment area for observation. Emergency assessment of patients conveyed directly to the treatment area then includes the primary survey and the secondary survey.

Primary survey

The primary survey amplifies the information obtained during triage. The purpose of the primary survey is to determine further the stability of the patient and to identify and treat any immediate life-threatening conditions. The primary survey includes evaluation and support of the airway, respiratory system, cardiovascular system (poor tissue perfusion, control of haemorrhage) and central nervous system (level of consciousness). Evaluation of these parameters allows the clinician to classify the patient as stable or unstable. Any patient that cannot be clearly classified into either category should be considered unstable.

The primary survey includes evaluation of the same physical parameters as triage. Evaluation of the respiratory system includes: determination of whether the upper airway is patent; evaluation of mucous membrane colour; and assessment of respiratory rate, rhythm and effort. The trachea and all areas of the thorax should be carefully auscultated. More objective information regarding respiratory function can be obtained from pulse oximetry, arterial blood gas analysis, and end-tidal carbon dioxide measurement. Hypoxaemia can result in pansystemic problems due to poor oxygen delivery to the tissues, and requires immediate correction. Oxygen supplementation (Figure 1.2) should be provided to any emergency patient if respiratory compromise is evident, and definitive treatment for the cause of the respiratory compromise should be provided as soon as possible (see Chapter 7).

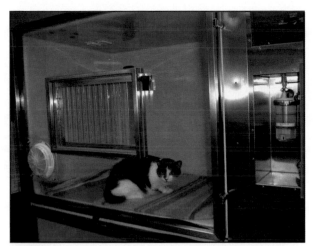

1.2 Critically ill animals have little physiological reserve to tolerate physical examination or medical intervention. Allow dyspnoeic animals to stabilize in oxygen before performing diagnostics and, above all, do no harm.

Assessment of tissue perfusion includes: evaluation of mucous membrane colour; capillary refill time; core body temperature to toe web temperature gradient; auscultation of the heart; and palpation of pulse rate, rhythm and quality. More in-depth and objective evaluation of tissue perfusion could include arterial blood pressure measurement, central venous pressure determination, blood lactate concentration, pulmonary artery catheter placement, and measurement of oxygen delivery and oxygen consumption. Clinical recognition of poor tissue perfusion, such as pale or grey mucous membranes, prolonged or rapid capillary refill time and/or abnormalities of cardiac rate or rhythm, warrants rapid identification of the underlying cause and definitive treatment (see Chapter 3). Prolonged hypoperfusion can cause changes in cellular metabolism that result in intracellular sodium and calcium accumulation, cell swelling, cell membrane damage, lipid peroxidation, release of detrimental oxygen free radicals and cell death.

Extreme changes in the patient's mentation, such as stupor, coma or seizures, require rapid assessment for the underlying cause, and immediate treatment to prevent any irreversible changes from occurring. Prolonged seizures or hypoglycaemia causing CNS dysfunction can result in irreversible changes if not treated rapidly. Similarly, increased intracranial pressure causing stupor or coma may progress, resulting in herniation of the brain through the foramen magnum.

In summary, the primary survey assures identification and immediate treatment of conditions that are life threatening. It also allows identification of unstable patients so that appropriate monitoring can be instituted and potential problems can be anticipated and prevented.

Secondary survey

After the primary survey and stabilization of immediate life-threatening conditions, the secondary survey is performed. This includes a full physical examination, obtaining a detailed history from the owner, assessment of the response to initial therapy and more in-depth diagnostics, including clinical pathology and imaging procedures. It is during this time that a comprehensive diagnostic and therapeutic plan can be made and a cost estimate as well as prognosis can be formulated.

Vascular access

Intravenous access should be obtained in any critically ill patient for administration of intravenous fluids and drugs (Figure 1.3). Peripheral veins, such as the cephalic or lateral saphenous vein, are the most common vessels utilized for intravenous catheterization, mainly due to their accessibility and familiarity to most emergency personnel. Central venous access using the jugular or medial femoral vein allows higher drug concentrations to be achieved in the coronary vessels (important in cardiopulmonary resuscitation) and allows placement of a larger diameter catheter, facilitating more rapid fluid administration. However, central vessels are more difficult to access compared to the peripheral vessels, making them a second choice in an emergency situation when vascular access must be rapid. Jugular venipuncture and catheter placement is contraindicated in patients suspected of having a coagulopathy or raised intracranial pressure. In neonates, the easiest and most expeditious way to obtain vascular access is via intraosseous catheter placement. Absorption of drugs via this route is almost as fast as central venous administration. Vascular access options are discussed in more detail in Chapter 2.

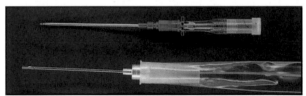

1.3 Intravenous access must be established as quickly as possible in the critical emergency patient. Short 'over-the-needle' catheters (top) placed in peripheral veins are best, as the flow rate is optimal in a short wide-bore catheter. Long 'through-the-needle' catheters (bottom) placed in central veins are ideal for longer periods of hospitalization.

The emergency database

As soon as possible after presentation, blood should be obtained for an emergency database in all critically ill patients. This should include measurement of packed cell volume (PCV) and refractometric total solids (TS) or total protein (TP), glucose and blood urea nitrogen (BUN) and evaluation of a blood smear. Assessment of urine specific gravity prior to fluid therapy, and of serum sodium and potassium levels, can provide valuable information for use in diagnosis and can facilitate appropriate therapy. Blood samples can be collected from the hub of the intravenous catheter as it fills with blood, or obtained from the hub of a 25 gauge needle placed into a peripheral blood vessel (Figure 1.4). The PCV, TP, dipstick glucose, dipstick blood urea nitrogen (BUN) and blood smear can all be obtained from three heparinized microhaematocrit tubes.

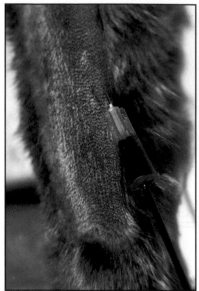

1.4 Blood samples for the emergency database can be obtained by filling a microhaematocrit tube from the hub of a 25 gauge needle placed in a peripheral blood vessel, in this case the cephalic vein.

Packed cell volume and total solids

PCV is used as a good estimate of haemoglobin (Hb) concentration (PCV divided by 3 approximately equals Hb (in g/dl – multiply this by 10 to get g/l)) except when haemoglobin-based oxygen carriers (HBOCs) have been used. In these cases the PCV will give a falsely low estimate of haemoglobin and a haemoglobinometer is required (see Chapter 14). HBOCs lead to changes in serum colour, and care must be taken when interpreting any colorimetric-based tests in these patients. Refractometer measurement of TS allows estimation of serum proteins, which provides a rough indication of plasma colloid osmotic pressure, thereby facilitating decisions about the type of intravenous fluids to be used.

PCV and TS should be interpreted together, and in conjunction with clinical findings. They can provide information regarding hydration status, as well as an estimate of red cell content in the blood. Changes in these two parameters often parallel each other, but an alteration in the normal ratio of PCV to TS gives additional useful information. An increase in both PCV and TS is consistent with dehydration, as total body fluid loss results in concentration of red blood cells and plasma proteins. A decrease in PCV and TS is seen with aggressive fluid therapy or after haemorrhage. The decrease in PCV and TS is not seen immediately following haemorrhage, as it takes time for fluid to shift from the interstitium to the intravascular space and cause dilution. Immediately following an acute loss of blood volume in the dog, splenic contraction causes an influx of erythrocytes into the circulation in an attempt to restore circulating volume and increase oxygen-carrying capacity of the blood, improving tissue oxygen delivery. Thus, following acute blood loss, the initial PCV may be normal or even increased, accompanied by a decreased TS due to interstitial fluid shifts diluting the plasma proteins. When faced with a trauma patient that has a normal PCV but decreased TS, there is a strong possibility that severe haemorrhage has occurred.

A decrease in PCV with a normal TS suggests an increase in destruction or a decrease in production of red blood cells. A decreased PCV with haemolysed or icteric serum suggests haemolytic anaemia, although hepatic and posthepatic causes of icterus cannot be ruled out. Anaemia of chronic disease and bone marrow disorders that cause non-regenerative anaemia are characterized by a decreased PCV with a normal TS.

An alteration in the PCV:TS ratio characterized by an increased PCV but a normal to decreased TS can be seen with severe dehydration accompanied by concurrent protein loss. The most profound example of this occurs in patients with severe haemorrhagic gastroenteritis, who can have a PCV of 70% or higher, but a normal TS. Hypoproteinaemia (low TS) can result from haemorrhage, loss into the pleural or peritoneal spaces (third spacing) or loss from the body through the gastrointestinal tract or kidney. Loss through the kidney (protein-losing nephropathy) results in hypoalbuminaemia, whereas a loss from the gastrointestinal tract (protein-losing enteropathy) results in panhypoproteinaemia. An increase in PCV with a normal TS is seen in patients with polycythaemia, which is relatively rare.

PCV and TS are important in guiding fluid and diuretic therapy. The absolute values determine the choice of fluid (e.g. isotonic crystalloid, colloid, blood products) to be delivered when correcting hypovolaemia or dehydration (see Chapter 4). A change in PCV and TS is expected following aggressive fluid or diuretic therapy, and these parameters should be measured frequently to help monitor response.

Physical appearance of blood samples

Examination of the microhaematocrit tube following centrifugation can provide additional information. A large buffy coat indicates a high white blood cell count. The colour of the serum may provide clues to the disease process; icterus may be due to prehepatic, hepatic or posthepatic problems. Lipaemic serum may be due to pancreatitis, postprandial lipaemia, or may be associated with hyperadrenocorticism. Haemolysed serum may be due to the collection technique or intravascular haemolysis.

Blood glucose

Increased blood glucose may be due to insulin resistance and/or lack of insulin (diabetes mellitus), or acute glycogenolysis. Insulin resistance and glycogenolysis due to stress are seen most commonly in cats, but can also occur in dogs secondary to head trauma, seizures, severe hypovolaemia or hypoxia. The hyperglycaemia in these cases is transient if the underlying problem is corrected (e.g. fluid resuscitation if hypovolaemic). In contrast, although blood glucose levels will decrease slightly following intravenous fluids in a patient with diabetes mellitus, hyperglycaemia will persist in a diabetic unless it receives insulin therapy. Serum or urine ketones should be measured in patients presenting with high blood glucose, especially if they have a metabolic acidosis. Ketones can be demonstrated in the plasma from the microhaematocrit tube using ketone dipsticks, which can detect acetone and acetoacetate but not β-hydroxybutyrate.

Hypoglycaemia is a common finding in the emergency patient. It can be caused by: insulin-secreting tumours; insulin-like growth factor-secreting tumours; sepsis; heatstroke; severe hypothermia; hypoadrenocorticism; juvenile hypoglycaemia; storage diseases; severe hepatic dysfunction; and insulin overdose. Using glucometers or dipsticks, falsely low results are obtained for glucose in whole blood when the PCV is high. This variation differs with each manufacturer, but a more accurate result can be obtained by centrifuging the blood sample and measuring the serum glucose levels.

Blood urea nitrogen

BUN can be estimated using a dipstick. Although this method has limitations, when performed correctly it is a very useful screening test. A low dipstick BUN is accurate, but elevated results should be confirmed by other laboratory methods. Increased BUN may result from prerenal, renal or postrenal causes, while low BUN can occur due to severe liver dysfunction or diuresis.

Blood smear

The red blood cells, white blood cells and platelets should be evaluated using a carefully prepared blood smear. The number and morphology of each cell type should be evaluated and recorded. Examination of the red blood cells is most important in patients with anaemia or if there is a suspicion of blood loss. Signs of regeneration such as polychromasia or anisocytosis help to characterize the anaemia as regenerative or non-regenerative. Cell morphology should be evaluated for the presence of spherocytes (seen in patients with immune-mediated haemolytic anaemia), Heinz bodies (indicating oxidative damage to haemoglobin), schistocytes (suggesting intravascular shear injury) or echinocytes (can be seen after rattlesnake envenomation). Parasites such as *Mycoplasma haemofelis* or *Babesia* spp. may also be seen (see Chapter 13).

The blood smear should be scanned at low power to estimate the number of white blood cells, and then at higher power to assess their morphology. One white blood cell viewed per X40 field at the feathered edge approximates a cell count of $1.5 \times 10^9/l$. The differential count and cell morphology can be assessed using oil immersion. Leucocytosis with a mature neutrophilia suggests a stress response, or an inflammatory or infectious process. Immature neutrophils such as band cells and occasionally metamyelocytes or myelocytes may be released into the circulation, termed a 'left shift', if there is a severe inflammatory or infectious process. The absence of a leucocytosis or a left shift does not rule out inflammation or infection. Leucopenia can be due to decreased production or sequestration of white blood cells. Decreased production can result from viral infections such as parvovirus, or from the administration of immunosuppressive drugs. White blood cell sequestration resulting in leucopenia occurs in patients with severe infections or extensive tissue necrosis, for example those with peritonitis, necrotizing pancreatitis or bite wounds. Transient leucopenia can also be seen in hypothermic patients.

Bleeding patients should be evaluated for adequacy of platelet numbers. The whole slide should be scanned under low power for platelet clumps, since these can result in an artificially low count. In healthy dogs and cats there should be 11–25 platelets per monolayer field under oil immersion. One platelet viewed per oil immersion field (X100) approximates to $15 \times 10^9/l$ (i.e. three platelets per oil immersion field approximates $45 \times 10^9/l$ in the blood). Most patients with spontaneous bleeding due to thrombocytopenia have fewer than two platelets per oil immersion field; animals with four to five platelets per field are unlikely to be bleeding due to thrombocytopenia. Low platelet numbers can result from decreased production, consumption or increased destruction.

Summary

The amount of information obtained from a simple emergency database can be tremendous, and should not be underestimated. This information, combined with a thorough history and physical examination, can often provide a diagnosis as well as a prognosis.

Acid–base and electrolytes

Cage-side blood gas, acid–base and electrolyte monitors are becoming more widely available for veterinarians. Monitors differ, but can provide objective data pertaining to acid–base status, oxygenation, ventilation and electrolytes. Some monitors can also analyse lactate, renal parameters and glucose, whilst newer machines may be equipped with co-oximetry. Analysis typically requires between 0.2 and 0.5 ml of whole blood, which is either inserted directly into the analyser (which contains all the reagents) or is injected into a cartridge that is inserted into the analyser. Different cartridges allow the clinician to choose the parameters to be measured, or the monitor can be programmed to perform selected analyses. Identification of acid–base and electrolyte derangements (see Chapter 5) can expand on the history, physical examination and emergency database, to further develop the problem list and emergency plan.

The emergency plan

The emergency plan depends upon the presenting problem and stability of the patient, and the level of nursing and technical support available. A medical problem list should be generated and the problems prioritized from the most to the least life threatening. The problems should then be addressed in that order, making a diagnostic, therapeutic and monitoring plan for each one. The plans for each problem should be collated and a comprehensive, concise and clearly written hospital order list should be formulated. Categories that should be covered include fluid therapy, medications to be administered, diagnostics to be performed, parameters to be monitored and nursing orders.

Fluid therapy

Fluid therapy orders should include the type of fluid to be administered, the rate of infusion and the route by which the fluid should be given. The frequency of reassessment of the fluid orders depends upon patient stability, and how rapidly the fluid requirements change. In very unstable patients, fluid therapy may require re-evaluation every 30–60 minutes, as the response to therapy is determined. Relatively stable patients, where fluid deficits are being replaced over 24 hours, require less frequent reassessment of fluid orders, perhaps as infrequently as every 12–24 hours. Fluid rate and type are determined not only by cardio-vascular status but also by sodium and potassium concentrations. Type of fluid and rate of infusion become very important with extremes of sodium concentrations, such as severe hyponatraemia or hypernatraemia. In these cases, fluid therapy orders may need to be changed hourly depending upon the desired rate of sodium concentration change and the response to therapy (see Chapter 5). Dextrose, potassium or other electrolytes may need to be added to the fluid bags, but these supplemented fluids should never be administered as a bolus.

Medication

The types of medication and the dose, route, rate and frequency of administration should be clearly written and reviewed with the individual that will be administering the drugs. All drugs that are being administered should be reviewed for incompatibility with each other, as well as potential adverse effects in specific patients or disease processes. If side effects of a certain drug are of particular concern, specific information about the side effects should be noted in the treatment orders, and the parameters to monitor and therapy for adverse reactions should also be included in the record.

Diagnostic plan

The diagnostic plan should be written and tests listed in priority of importance for the emergency care of the patient. The stability of the patient as well as the importance of the information that the test will provide should be considered when requesting a diagnostic test. The question that should be asked for each test should be 'Will the information that I obtain make a difference to what I do on an emergency basis?' If the answer to this question is 'no', then the test should not be done.

Monitoring

Monitoring procedures should be listed and clinician notification criteria should be clearly communicated and reviewed with the nursing personnel. Often, the trend of change in a parameter is more important than the absolute value. Monitoring trends of change allows anticipation of problems before they occur. Monitoring parameters may be divided into physical examination, clinicopathological data and electronic evaluation.

Physical examination parameters should include:

- Mucous membrane colour
- Capillary refill time
- Pulse rate and quality
- Lung sounds
- Respiratory rate and effort
- Neurological function
- Urination
- Defecation
- Vomiting
- Rectal temperature
- Abdominal pain
- Observation of skin and mucous membranes for ecchymoses and petechiations
- Assessment for peripheral oedema.

The most common clinicopathological parameters monitored in the emergency room include:

- PCV
- TP/TS
- Glucose
- Dipstick BUN
- Serum sodium concentration
- Serum potassium concentration
- Blood gas analysis
- Urinalysis
- Blood smear
- Activated clotting times.

Electronic monitoring may include:

- Measurement of central venous pressure
- Continuous electrocardiography
- Blood pressure measurement (Doppler, oscillometric or direct methods)
- Pulse oximetry
- End-tidal capnography
- Cardiac output
- Oxygen delivery
- Oxygen consumption.

Nursing orders

Nursing orders should be tailored to the needs of each individual patient. The specific disease process, the severity of the patient's condition and the level of staffing should all be considered when orders are written. For example, one nurse cannot provide comprehensive nursing care to a comatose, 50 kg large-breed dog that is being mechanically ventilated and receiving peritoneal dialysis.

The emergency plan must take into account the needs of the patient, the client's needs and financial capabilities, the immediate and overall prognosis and the capabilities of the emergency staff and facility (Figure 1.5). If it is recognized that the best emergency plan cannot be accommodated by the facility and staff, referral of the patient to a tertiary facility that can provide optimal care should be considered.

Cardiovascular

Electrocardiogram
Blood pressure monitoring (direct and indirect)
Central venous pressure monitoring
Defibrillator with internal and external paddles
Fluid pumps and syringe drivers
Pressure bags for rapid fluid administration
Selection of intravenous catheters

Respiratory

Means to provide short- and long-term oxygen therapy (e.g. oxygen cage, face masks, etc.)
Means to intubate and ventilate (e.g. laryngoscope, endotracheal tubes, Ambu resuscitation bag)
Pulse oximeter
End-tidal capnograph

Diagnostics

Glucometer (dextrometer)
Means to measure total protein/solids and packed cell volume
Microhaematocrit tubes, centrifuge, refractometer
Microscope, slides, stain (Diff-Quik and Gram) and immersion oil
Electrolyte and blood gas analyser
Lactate analyser
Coagulation analyser
Haemoglobinometer (especially if Oxyglobin™ commonly used)
Snap tests (e.g. feline leukaemia virus, feline immunodeficiency virus, parvovirus)
Osmometer
Colloid oncotic pressure analyser
Urine dipsticks
Dipsticks for BUN and ketones
X-ray machine, processor and view box (or digital radiography)
Ultrasound machine

Surgical

Anaesthetic machine
Surgical gowns and drapes
Surgical sets
Electrocautery
Surgical table and lights
Chest tubes, tracheostomy tubes

Other

Weighing scales
Thermometer
Means of providing warmth
Ophthalmoscope
Otoscope
Pen light
Stomach tubes

1.5 Recommended emergency room equipment.

2

Vascular access

Sophie Adamantos and Amy Alwood

Introduction

The placement and maintenance of intravascular access is one of the most important skills for any veterinary surgeon working in emergency and critical care medicine. Rapid and accurate placement of appropriate intravenous catheters allows administration of fluid and drug therapy, as well as providing an atraumatic means for serial blood sampling. Furthermore, placement of specialized catheters (e.g. arterial or cardiac catheterization) can assist in monitoring intravascular volume status and blood pressure. Familiarization with alternative routes of vascular access can be important in particular situations, for example intraosseus access in collapsed kittens and puppies. This chapter addresses the different types of vascular access (catheter placement and maintenance) and summarizes complications that may occur.

Intravenous access

A number of factors should be considered when choosing the optimal type of intravenous access for each individual patient. These include:

- Vein selection and preparation
- Catheter choice, including material, length and gauge
- Ease of insertion
- Ease of maintenance.

Vein selection
When choosing the site for catheter placement a number of questions should be considered:

- Why am I placing this catheter?
- How long will it remain in place?
- What will I be administering through it?
- Does the patient have any medical or behavioural factors that should be considered?

This latter question may include consideration of the animal's temperament (aggressive animals may prove difficult to manage with a jugular catheter), the presence of coagulopathy (a contraindication for use of the jugular vein) and potential sources of catheter contamination (e.g. local tissue damage, skin infection, presence of vomiting, urination, diarrhoea and excessive salivation). Animals with regional vascular obstruction (e.g. gastric dilatation and volvulus, or cats with saddle thrombus) should have catheters placed in the front legs, i.e. at a site distant to the obstructed vessel.

In emergency patients, the initial catheterization site should be chosen to facilitate rapid and effective catheter placement. Peripheral veins are generally more suitable than the jugular vein. Catheterization via a peripheral vein is adequate for administration of most fluids and medications, and should be the primary site for rapid intravenous access in the majority of emergency patients. There are several suitable peripheral sites in the dog and cat including:

- Cephalic vein and accessory cephalic vein (below the carpus)
- Medial and lateral saphenous vein
- Auricular veins in breeds with large ears, e.g. Basset Hound
- Dorsal common digital vein (over the metatarsal bones).

Most commonly the cephalic vein is used as it is familiar and most animals will tolerate gentle restraint for placement while in sternal recumbency. It is important to be familiar with other readily accessible sites, especially when faced with small patients or those that have suffered trauma to multiple limbs.

Following initial vascular access and fluid resuscitation via a peripheral vein, a decision should be made as to whether the patient is an appropriate candidate for central venous catheterization. Factors that may prompt placement of a central venous catheter include:

- Likely long-term (>5 days) administration of fluids
- Administration of hypertonic fluids or medications
- The need to obtain multiple venous blood samples
- Ability to measure central venous pressure
- Patient factors (e.g. conformation, temperament) suggesting that maintenance of a peripheral catheter may be challenging.

The jugular vein is the most frequently used site for placement of longer central catheters and is easily accessible in most patients. Hyperosmolar fluids (such as >10% glucose infusions or parenteral nutrition (PN)) should always be administered via a central catheter to reduce the risk of thrombophlebitis. Any catheters (or ports of multi-lumen catheters) used for PN should be reserved for that purpose only and strict asepsis should be observed when managing the catheter.

Catheter selection

A large number of catheters is available on the veterinary and human medical market, making selection of catheters difficult and at times confusing. Catheter size, composition and placement method are the predominant characteristics to be considered in catheter selection.

Fluid flow rate through a catheter is related to both the length and radius of the catheter as well as rheological factors. Of these, catheter radius (r) has the greatest effect, flow rate being related to r^4. A reduction in catheter diameter by half results in a 16-fold decrease in flow rate, whereas doubling of the diameter would result in a 16-fold increase in maximum flow. Increasing catheter length also results in decreased flow due to increased resistance. When choosing a catheter for rapid fluid resuscitation the shortest catheter with the biggest radius (gauge) should be utilized.

Catheters are made from a variety of chemically inert materials in order to limit vessel irritation; once they are in the body, however, inflammatory reactions may occur to agents used in the manufacturing process. Silicon and polyurethane are minimally reactive, making these materials ideal for use in long-term catheters. Silicon is particularly desirable due to its additional characteristic of flexibility. In contrast, Teflon® (polytetrafluoroethylene) has intermediate reactivity and is relatively stiff, making it less suitable. Antibiotic-impregnated catheters have been introduced to the human market; however there is currently insufficient data to recommend their use in veterinary patients. Many catheters are rendered radiopaque by the addition of barium or bismuth salts into the plastic.

Catheters can be broadly divided into four categories or types:

- Butterfly or winged-needle catheters
- Over-the-needle catheters
- Through-the-needle catheters
- Over-the-wire catheters (Seldinger technique).

Butterfly catheters (Figure 2.1) are essentially needles with attached wings, which enable them to be secured, and a short extension tube that facilitates attachment of a syringe for collection of blood or administration of intravenous medications. They come in a variety of gauges and lengths. They are not suitable for fluid therapy as the sharp tip will damage the vein if it is left in place for more than a few minutes.

Over-the-needle catheters (Figure 2.2) are the most common catheter type in day-to-day use in veterinary practice. They are suitable for short- to medium-term intravenous access. Insertion is technically easy and associated with few complications. The catheters are inexpensive and there are few contraindications to placement. They comprise a needle (or stylet) with a closely associated catheter fitted over the needle. The stylet is used to penetrate the vessel and guide the tip of the catheter into the vein. The catheter is then slid off the stylet into the lumen of the vein. The catheters are generally made of stiff material (e.g. fluorinated ethylene propylene, FEP®) to prevent damage to the tip as it passes through the vessel wall. A wide variety of gauges and lengths is available making them extremely versatile (Figure 2.3).

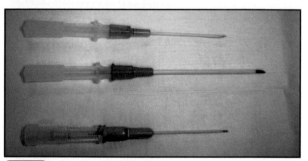

2.2 Over-the-needle catheters are easily placed in peripheral veins and suitable for short- or longer-term administration of drugs or fluid therapy.

Trade name	Company	Composition
Abbocath T	Abbott www.abbott.com	Teflon®
Delta VenT	Delta Med www.deltamedit.com	Teflon®
Surflo	Terumo www.terumomedical.com	Teflon®
Angiocath	Becton Dickinson www.bd.com	FEP® polymer
Jelco	Medex www.smiths-medical.com	FEP® polymer
Optiva	Medex www.smiths-medical.com	Polyurethane
Neo Delta VenT	Delta Med www.deltamedit.com	Polyurethane

2.3 A selection of currently commercially available over-the-needle catheters.

Through-the-needle catheters are classified into two groups depending on their placement method:

- Those in which the needle remains attached to the catheter but is secured within a plastic guard outside the vein
- Those placed using the 'peel-away' technique in which the catheter is inserted though a plastic guide that can then be peeled away and discarded.

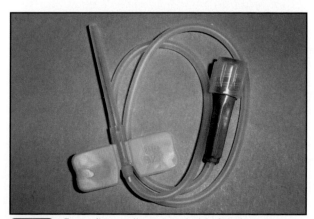

2.1 Butterfly needles are suitable for short-term vascular access to deliver anaesthetic agents or intravenous medications.

Through-the-needle catheters with an attached needle guard (e.g. Centracath, Vygon) (Figure 2.4) are purchased as a unit, with a large-bore needle and attached catheter that is threaded through the needle into the vessel lumen. After successful introduction of the catheter, the needle is withdrawn from the vessel. The needle is then secured within a plastic guard that also partially encompasses the external portion of catheter. This guard prevents inadvertent damage to the catheter or the patient by the needle. These catheters are easy to place and a relatively affordable way of accessing the central venous compartment. However, the presence of the introducer needle and guard makes these catheters difficult to secure and results in bulky dressings.

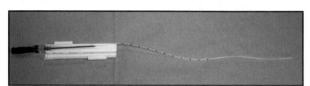

2.4 An example of a through-the-needle catheter with attached introducer and needle guard.

'Peel-away' catheters (Figure 2.5) have a plastic guide (or sheath) which is placed in the lumen of the vessel using an over-the-needle technique. The needle is then removed and the catheter is inserted through the guide. The guide can then be 'peeled away' by pulling gently outwards and upwards on the two tabs of the sheath. The gauge of the catheter is limited to that of the plastic guide.

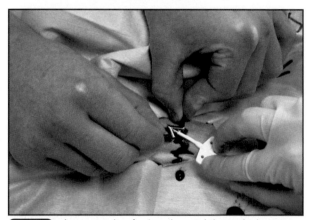

2.5 An example of a 'peel-away' through-the-needle catheter. (Picture courtesy of E. Leece, Animal Health Trust)

Over-the-wire catheters (Seldinger technique) (Figure 2.6) are placed using a wire guide. A needle or introducer catheter is inserted into the vein and a wire is passed through it. The introducer catheter is removed leaving only the wire in place. The catheter is then advanced over the wire into the vessel lumen. Theoretically any gauge of catheter may be placed. This is aided by use of a vessel dilator advanced over the wire prior to catheter placement, which increases the diameter of the subcutaneous tunnel and venous puncture site. These catheters are secured by suturing them to the skin at the entry site via wings. Placement is shown in Figure 2.7.

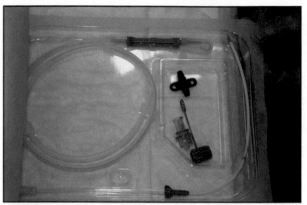

2.6 An example of a catheter kit which utilizes an over-the-wire (Seldinger) placement technique.

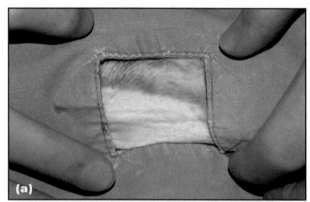

(a)

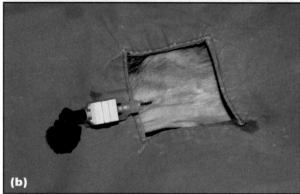

(b)

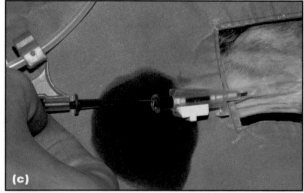

(c)

2.7 Placement of a central line in the jugular vein using the Seldinger (over-the-wire) technique. **(a)** The area is surgically prepared and draped. **(b)** A facilitative skin incision is made and a large introducer needle or catheter placed into the vein. In this case an introducer catheter with flow switch is used. **(c)** A long wire is inserted through the introducer needle/catheter. (continues) ▶

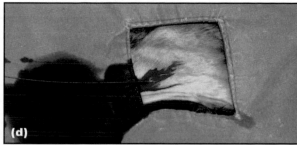

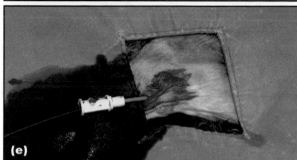

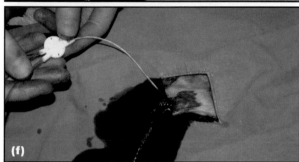

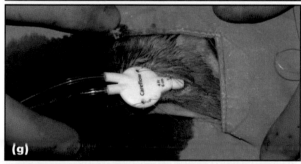

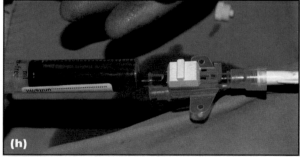

2.7 (continued) Placement of a central line in the jugular vein using the Seldinger (over-the-wire) technique. **(d)** The needle/catheter is removed leaving the wire in place. **(e)** A dilator is passed into the vein over the wire to enlarge the subcutaneous tunnel. The dilator is then removed. **(f)** The catheter is advanced into the vein over the wire. The wire is then removed. **(g)** The catheter is sutured in place. **(h)** Blood is withdrawn from each port of the catheter into a syringe prefilled with heparinized saline to guarantee intravascular placement. The ports are then flushed and the catheter bandaged carefully in place.

A selection of currently available catheters is shown in Figure 2.8. 'Peel-away' and Seldinger technique catheters are available as single or multi-lumen catheters. Multi-lumen catheters have several ports (typically two or three), each running via a separate channel to the tip of the catheter, thus preventing mixing of fluids/drugs until they reach the blood stream. The use of a multi-lumen catheter should be considered if the patient requires a mixture of fluid therapies, drug therapy, parenteral nutrition, central venous pressure monitoring and/or repeated blood sampling (see Chapter 26).

Name	Company	Composition
Centracath	Vygon www.vygon.com	Polyurethane
Hydrocath	Becton Dickinson www.bd.com	Polyurethane
Long-term catheter	MILA international www.milaint.com	Polyurethane
PICC	Arrow www.arrowint.com	Polyurethane
Long-term catheter with peel-away introducer	MILA international www.milaint.com	Polyurethane
Seldinger technique central catheter	Global/Surgivet www.surgivet.com	Polyurethane

2.8 A selection of commercially available central/long-stay catheters.

Catheter insertion

Peripheral veins

A large area of skin surrounding the vein should be clipped before insertion of the catheter. Long hair (feathers) on the caudal aspect of the limb may need to be removed if it will interfere with securing the catheter and to help prevent contamination. In some dogs a complete 360-degree clip of the limb may be necessary. Catheters should be placed aseptically and as distal in the vein as possible to allow subsequent venipuncture at a more proximal site. In the emergency situation there may not be time for full aseptic preparation of the vein. In these circumstances, potentially contaminated catheters should be replaced as soon as practically possible. Peripheral catheter placement is described in Figure 2.9.

A T-port or extension set should be attached and the catheter well secured with conforming non-elastic adhesive tape or sutures. Extension sets are useful as they prevent unnecessary blood loss, provide a method of closure when the catheter is not in use and increase the ease of connection of drip lines and drug administration (Figure 2.10). The catheter should be bandaged in place to prevent contamination. This bandage should comprise a soft primary layer and protective secondary layer.

1. Hands should be washed carefully before placement. Sterile gloves are not necessary for short-term peripheral catheter insertion. The skin overlying the vein should be prepared with an antimicrobial scrub solution and surgical spirit.

2. The vein should be raised by an assistant.

3. The catheter can usually be placed directly through the skin but in some patients, a **small** facilitative skin nick made with a no.11 blade may ease insertion. This is especially useful in dehydrated animals or those with very thick skin, and prevents burring of the catheter tip as it passes through the subcutaneous tissues.

4. The catheter is advanced through the skin into the vein at a 30–40-degree angle with the stylet bevel up.

5. Once blood is visualized in the flash chamber the stylet and catheter are flattened (i.e. the angle between the catheter and limb is reduced). The catheter/stylet unit is then advanced a small distance further into the vein to ensure the catheter lies fully within the lumen.

6. The catheter is advanced off the stylet. The stylet should remain absolutely immobile as the catheter is advanced.

7. Once the catheter has been fully advanced, the stylet is removed and discarded. If problems are encountered whilst advancing the catheter, flushing gently with heparinized saline may help. The catheter should never be pulled back on to the stylet as this may damage the catheter tip or shear off part of the catheter.

8. Once the catheter has been advanced into the vein the assistant can occlude the vessel by applying pressure over the vein at the distal end of the catheter to prevent spillage of blood.

9. A T-port or injection cap should be attached to the catheter and the catheter secured in place with adhesive tape.

2.9 Placement of a peripheral catheter.

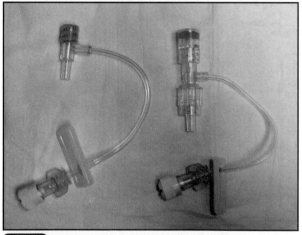

2.10 Examples of T-ports or extension sets.

Central veins

The most commonly used site for central venous access is the jugular vein. As a catheter of any length may be placed using the through-the-needle technique, other sites (e.g. the medial saphenous vein) may also be utilized. Central catheters should be placed using strict aseptic technique. Sterile gloves should be worn and the catheter site should receive full surgical preparation and be draped appropriately before catheter placement. Although central lines may be placed in conscious patients if they are weak or debilitated, sedation or anaesthesia is required in most animals to prevent movement during the procedure. Considering the site and size of needle utilized, it is prudent to check for the presence of coagulopathy or thrombocytopenia before placement. In breeds predisposed to von Willebrand's disease a buccal mucosal bleeding time should also be performed. Central lines may be placed using either the Seldinger (see Figure 2.7), peel-away or through-the-needle (needle guard) technique as described above. These catheters are sutured into place and bandaged securely to prevent contamination and inadvertent removal. Peripherally inserted central catheters (PICC) are useful when access to the jugular vein is limited. In these cases long catheters are inserted through peripheral veins (usually the saphenous) into the caudal vena cava. These catheters can be used in the same way as conventional central catheters.

Catheter maintenance

Maintenance of the catheter is vitally important; the catheter should be examined at least twice daily. The site of insertion should be monitored for signs of heat, erythema, swelling, pain or leakage of fluid. The leg and foot should be checked for swelling above the catheter site (indicating extravasation of fluid) and swelling of the toes (indicating that the bandage or tape is too tight). Jugular catheters should be covered with a light bandage, avoiding application of too much pressure to the neck. Too tight a jugular wrap will rapidly result in swelling of the head or upper airway obstruction. It should be possible to pass a hand comfortably under the bandage after placement. The bandage should be removed and replaced each time the catheter is checked. If signs of phlebitis are present (redness or discharge at the catheter site, thickening along the length of the catheter when it is palpated under the skin) or the animal develops unexplained pyrexia, the catheter should be removed and the tip sent for microbiological culture. Routine use of topical or systemic antibiotic ointments is not recommended.

Catheter patency should be maintained by any fluid running through it. If the catheter is not being used continuously, intermittent flushing with saline or heparinized saline (1IU of heparin per ml of saline) should be performed two or three times a day as well as before and after use. A 'flash' of blood should be observed before flushing the catheter, to ensure the catheter is still in place in the vein. This does not always happen with peripheral or small-gauge catheters. Failure to obtain blood when a central line is aspirated can indicate that a catheter is no longer correctly placed in the vein or that there is a partial obstruction, e.g. thrombus at the tip of the catheter. Some smaller-gauge central catheters, however, function poorly for blood sampling from the outset. Replacement of central catheters should be considered if it is not possible to aspirate blood even if the fluids appear to be flowing well.

Once the catheter is no longer required it should be removed. As long as careful monitoring is performed catheters may be left in place for several days. When a catheter is not in use, sterile injection caps (Figure 2.11) should be used to close access ports;

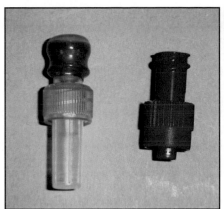

2.11

Examples of injection caps.

ports should never be left open to the air. Disconnection of fluid lines should be avoided and only done when absolutely necessary to reduce contamination of the catheter.

Catheter complications

Catheter displacement/extravasation of fluids or medications
Even with diligent efforts to secure and maintain catheters properly, there is a risk of displacement of any intravenous or arterial catheter. Risk of displacement may be greatest with the use of peripheral over-the-needle catheters. Careful securing and diligent monitoring are the best strategies to limit catheter migration and subsequent extravasation of fluids or medications.

Phlebitis/thrombophlebitis
All patients are at risk for phlebitis or thrombophlebitis by virtue of the inherent endothelial damage and inflammation incited by the presence of any intravenous catheter. Phlebitis may be simply inflammatory, or may be associated with concurrent infection because the catheter entry site and attached fluid administration set represent an important portal for bacterial entry. As discussed above, catheters should be checked regularly and if examination of the catheter insertion site or vessel identifies any redness, swelling, pain, firmness or other signs of inflammation, immediate removal of the catheter should be considered. The presence of phlebitis increases the risk for other more serious catheter-related complications such as endocarditis.

Thrombosis/thromboembolism
Continuous administration of intravenous fluids and/ or regular intermittent flushing decreases the risk of thrombosis but does not completely prevent it. Blood clots may occur within the catheter lumen, obstructing flow, or outside the catheter between it and the vessel wall. Thrombi that form outside the catheter or attached to the tip of the catheter may not obstruct flow through the catheter, but can break off to form a thromboembolism at any time. Patients with underlying diseases predisposing to hypercoagulability (i.e. endocrine disease, cardiac disease, severe inflammation) are considered to be at greater risk for thrombosis and/or thromboembolism. In these patients careful risk–benefit assessment should be performed before placement of a central catheter. Placement of a peripherally inserted central catheter (PICC) via the saphenous vein may be preferred. Septicaemia is considered to be an absolute contraindication to central vein catheterization in human patients due to the increased risk of thrombophlebitis, although this contraindication is not considered absolute in small animal patients and central lines are routinely placed in dogs and cats with sepsis.

Infection
Routine practice of good hygiene and aseptic techniques whenever intravenous catheters are used, combined with daily catheter maintenance, are the best strategies for prevention of catheter-related infections. Catheter contamination will be minimized by limiting the number of disconnections from fluid lines and injection ports.

Dislodgement/catheter embolism
Embolism by a piece of an intravenous catheter is an uncommon but serious complication which may result from inadvertent transection of the catheter with a blade or scissors as bandage or suture material is being removed. Extreme caution should be practised whenever sharp instruments are used near a catheter.

Air embolism
Air embolism may occur with any indwelling venous catheter. The risk of air embolism is thought to be greatest during the placement of central venous catheters. This can be avoided by delaying release of vascular occlusion until the catheter has been connected to the T-port. Air embolism can also occur if fluid administration sets are not flushed properly and air bubbles remain within the line. In most circumstances, when air embolism does occur, small emboli will be contained within the pulmonary vasculature without adverse clinical consequence.

Exsanguination
Blood loss may occur whenever a catheter becomes disconnected from its injection cap, T-port or fluid extension set. The risk of significant blood loss is greatest with arterial catheters as blood can be lost rapidly under arterial pressure. Patients with arterial catheters should always be under direct supervision. Patients with venous catheters can also suffer haemorrhage if their catheter becomes disconnected and a clot does not form, however significant blood loss is rare. All patients with intravenous access should be observed at regular intervals.

Specialized techniques

Cut-down technique for venous access
In some patients, it may not be possible to obtain percutaneous peripheral or central venous access and a surgical cut-down approach will be required. This occurs most commonly in animals with severe peripheral oedema or vascular collapse. The technique may be used for peripheral or central veins and is similar for both. If time allows, strict aseptic technique

should be followed; if not, clipping of the hair and brief wiping with an antiseptic solution will suffice. These 'dirty' catheters should be removed as soon as is practically possible and should never remain in place beyond 24 hours. Drainage of the site may be required after catheter removal.

After skin preparation, the location of the vein is identified using anatomical features and circumferential compression of the leg or neck. The location of the jugular vein can be estimated by drawing an imaginary line from the manubrium to the angle of the jaw. The jugular will lie approximately half way along this line. The skin is pulled laterally so that it no longer overlies the vein and a longitudinal incision is made through the skin to the subcutaneous tissues. The length of the incision will depend partially on the site and partially on the skill of the veterinary surgeon or nurse. The subcutaneous tissues are bluntly dissected away from the vein using the index fingers or sterile curved-tip haemostats. Catheter insertion is facilitated by removal of as much of the fascia from around the vein as possible (Figure 2.12). Once the vein is exposed, catheter placement is accomplished using one of two main techniques. The first technique utilises two loops of suture material passed beneath the vein. The distal loop is used to elevate and partially occlude the vein during placement and the proximal loop can subsequently be used to secure the catheter. This technique requires complete dissection of the vessel from the surrounding tissues. The other technique uses no suture; the catheter is placed in the conventional manner once the vein is directly visualized. Less dissection is required with this latter technique although stabilization of the vessel is more challenging. Once the catheter is in place it should be secured immediately by suturing it to the vessel or surrounding tissues. The skin may then be sutured and the catheter bandaged into place as previously described.

Intraosseous catheters

Intraosseous access is particularly useful in cases where direct intravenous access is not possible but where rapid fluid administration is required, such as with hypovolaemic puppies or kittens, or in animals with severe vascular collapse. This route may be used to provide initial fluid resuscitation and medication as necessary until intravenous access is possible. Most substances that can be given intravenously may be given into the medullary space and absorption into the vasculature is extremely rapid. Although intraosseous needles are considered to access the central compartment, hypertonic and alkaline fluids may cause pain when infused and can lead to lameness. Intraosseous cannulas are commercially available (Figure 2.13); however a spinal or bone marrow aspiration needle may be used. In young animals a regular hypodermic needle may be used as the cortical bone is soft. Ideally the needle should have a central stylet to prevent a core of bone from obstructing the needle.

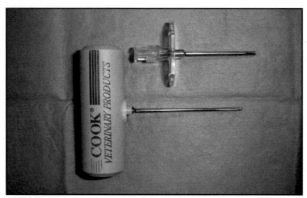

2.13 A commercially available intraosseous cannula.

Placement of an intraosseous catheter is easy and rapid. The technique is described in Figure 2.14. Any site with a good marrow cavity may be used and suitable sites include:

- The medial aspect of the trochanteric fossa of the femur
- The flat medial surface of the proximal tibia, 1–2 cm distal to the tibial tuberosity
- The cranial aspect of the greater tubercle of the humerus
- The wing of the ilium.

The preferred sites are those in the femur and tibia. Damage to the sciatic nerve can be avoided by walking the needle off the medial edge of the greater trochanter. Care should be taken in young animals to avoid damaging the growth plate.

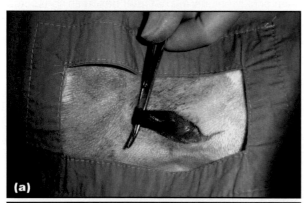

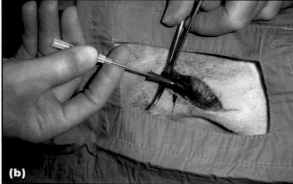

2.12 An illustration of a cut-down technique. **(a)** The jugular is shown dissected free from the subcutaneous tissues. Stabilization of the vein with a pair of artery forceps or suture can aid subsequent catheter placement. **(b)** The catheter is placed into the vein, advanced and secured carefully before use.

1. The skin overlying the chosen area is clipped and surgically prepared.

2. Local anaesthesia is infiltrated down to the level of the periosteum with 1% lidocaine.

3. A no.11 blade is used to make a small skin nick.

4. The needle is inserted into the bone using a firm twisting motion until well seated through the cortex. When properly seated in the medullary cavity the needle will feel secure and movement of the needle will result in movement of the bone.

5. The needle should be flushed with heparinized saline and a T-connector or infusion set attached.

6. The cannula should be secured either with sutures or tape and the entry site covered with a sterile swab and antiseptic ointment. A bulky wrap should be applied to prevent damage to the needle.

2.14 Placement of an intraosseous cannula.

Once in place, fluids can be given rapidly to provide volume resuscitation. Intraosseous catheters and needles may be left in place but are difficult to secure in active animals; their most useful application is therefore in patients during initial stabilization where intravenous access is impossible. Extravasation may occur so the subcutaneous tissues should be monitored. Should this occur the cannula should be removed and a different bone selected for subsequent placement, or efforts made to place an intravenous catheter once initial resuscitation has been performed.

Arterial catheterization

Arterial catheters are placed less commonly than venous catheters in veterinary practice. They are, however, particularly useful for monitoring critically ill patients as they allow direct arterial blood pressure measurement and serial collection of arterial blood gas samples. They require greater technical skill to place than venous catheters, however with practice arterial catheters may be placed in the majority of medium to large-sized dogs. Placement in cats and small dogs is more challenging.

The main sites used for arterial catheterization are the dorsal pedal artery, femoral artery, auricular artery and palmar metacarpal artery. A 20–22 gauge peripheral venous catheter can be placed in most arteries. The site is prepared *gently* with an antimicrobial scrub solution and surgical spirit. Vigorous scrubbing may cause arterial spasm and should be avoided. Use of a small stab incision (no.11 blade) through the skin facilitates placement as it minimizes damage to the catheter tip. The artery is palpated during placement and this is used to guide the catheter tip towards the vessel (Figure 2.15). As the walls of arteries are more muscular than those of veins, entrance of the catheter into the vessel is aided by short, firm, purposeful movements once the catheter tip is in the region of the artery. The flash chamber is watched closely for signs of vessel penetration, and once this has occurred the stylet should be flattened and advanced a little further into the vessel before the catheter is advanced into place. To facilitate feeding of the catheter, it is important that the catheter is

aligned parallel to the artery at all times and approached at a gentle angle (10–30 degrees). The dorsal pedal artery runs at about 30 degrees to the long axis of the limb from medial to lateral. Once in place the catheter is secured firmly, bandaged, and heparinized. It may then be used as required for blood pressure monitoring and collection of samples for blood gas analysis.

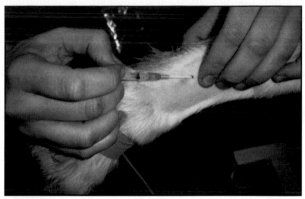

2.15 Placement of an arterial catheter in the dorsal pedal artery. The artery is palpated during insertion and the catheter is aligned with the artery to facilitate feeding.

Arterial catheters may be placed in patients that are thrombocytopenic or coagulopathic, but this should be done with care and only the more distal sites on the limb should be used. There is an increased risk of bleeding in these situations; if this occurs firm pressure should be applied to the site for 10–15 minutes. Arterial catheters should be maintained in a similar way to venous catheters; however they require more frequent flushing (at least every 1–2 hours) as they are prone to occlusion. Alternatively, arterial catheters used for continuous monitoring of direct arterial blood pressure may be connected to a disposable pressure transducer, through which dilute heparinized saline is continuously infused under pressure via microtubing (Figure 2.16). Care must be taken to identify clearly arterial catheters

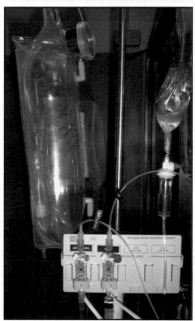

2.16 Constant flushing of an artery via microtubing.

as such, to avoid inadvertent administration of fluids or drugs into the artery. Due to the risk of vascular damage and subsequent tissue necrosis, use of arterial catheters should be restricted to blood sampling and pressure monitoring; they should never be used for administration of drugs or fluids.

The pulmonary artery catheter

Cardiac catheterization is an uncommon catheterization procedure which is generally reserved for the intensive care unit and requires the participation of an experienced specialist. Pulmonary artery (PA) catheters (Swann-Ganz catheters) are specialized multi-lumen catheters equipped with a balloon-tip to facilitate catheterization of the pulmonary artery and subsequent measurement of vascular pressures (wedge pressure). They are also equipped with a thermistor to allow determination of cardiac output and systemic vascular resistance. Select PA catheters may also allow additional monitoring (e.g. oximetry). Indications for the use of a PA catheter include patients that are refractory to routine fluid resuscitation, patients with known cardiac disease that require aggressive fluid therapy and patients with distributive shock. Contraindications for cardiac catheterization include: the presence of bleeding disorders, acquired coagulopathies or severe hypercoagulability; unstable cardiac conditions; and any pre-existing risk for complications (i.e. severe dysrhythmias or predisposition to them).

Placement of the pulmonary artery catheter

A detailed discussion of the available catheter types and their use for advanced cardiac monitoring has been discussed elsewhere and is beyond the scope of this chapter.

Successful and humane cardiac catheterization typically requires either sedation or light anaesthesia (depending upon the severity of disease in the individual patient). For the most part, placement of a PA catheter requires the same basic skills/techniques needed for placement of any central catheter within the jugular vein. It may involve either direct surgical exposure of the vessel or percutaneous placement of an introducer sheath. In the critical care setting, an introducer catheter is most commonly placed via the

Seldinger technique. After placement of the introducer, the PA catheter is inserted through the sheath into the jugular vein. The PA catheter is then advanced from the jugular vein into the cranial vena cava and then the right atrium. Ventral direction and gentle rotation of the catheter as it is passed may encourage entry into the right atrium rather than the azygous vein. Upon successful positioning in the right heart (confirmed via pressure tracings or use of fluoroscopy) the balloon is inflated and further advancement of the catheter allows it to pass through the tricuspid valve into the right ventricle and then into the right ventricular outflow tract and PA. When in position, the most distal lumen of the PA catheter lies within the pulmonary artery, the opening of the second lumen should be in the right ventricle, and the most proximal luminal opening should be in the right atrium. Access for cardiac catheterization via the femoral vein is described but is not advised for most clinical cases.

Specific complications of cardiac catheterization are listed in Figure 2.17.

Dysrhythmias (atrial or ventricular ectopic tachycardia, ventricular fibrillation (rare), right bundle branch block)

Cardiac/vascular injury (perforation, rupture, haemorrhage, tamponade)

Local haemorrhage or haematoma (at site of placement)

Entanglement/enlodgement

Uncommon complications (thrombosis, air embolism, cardiopulmonary arrest)

2.17 Specific complications of cardiac catheterization.

Further reading

Beal M and Hughes D (2000) Vascular access: theory and techniques in the small animal emergency patient. *Clinical Techniques in Small Animal Practice* **15**, 101–109

Mellema M (2001) Cardiac output, wedge pressure and oxygen delivery. *Veterinary Clinics of North America – Small Animal Practice* **31**, 1175–1205

White R (2002) Vascular access techniques in the dog and cat. *In Practice* **24**, 174–192

3

Assessment and diagnosis of shock

Janet Aldrich

Introduction

Shock is a syndrome characterized by the presence of severe clinical signs, including alterations in mental state, mucous membrane colour, capillary refill time, heart rate and pulse quality. It occurs when a global but unequal deficit in tissue perfusion damages cells. In vasoconstrictive shock, profound constriction of some tissue beds damages cells by depriving them of oxygen and other nutrients. In vasodilative shock, inflammatory mediators damage cells. In most cases, elements of both ischaemic and mediator-induced damage are present. Cell damage by these mechanisms impairs cell function and can result in organ failure and death. Treatment of shock aims to prevent more cell damage and to promote healing by optimizing tissue perfusion. Therapeutic endpoints include improvement in clinical signs and normalization of other measured parameters, such as base deficit, blood lactate concentration and urine output.

Classification of shock

Events causing shock do so by decreasing:

- The effective circulating blood volume
- The capacity of blood to deliver oxygen to cells
- The ability of the heart to pump blood
- The ability of the vascular system to maintain appropriate vasomotor tone.

Shock may be classified as primarily hypovolaemic (decreased intravascular volume secondary to salt and water loss or whole blood loss), traumatic, obstructive, cardiogenic or distributive (sepsis or anaphylaxis) (Figure 3.1). Classification schemes, including this one, tend to be oversimplifications because relatively few global, clinically assessable parameters represent a large number of complex, interacting processes occurring at the cellular level.

Hypovolaemic shock

Hypovolaemic shock occurs when loss of circulating blood volume causes a severe decrease in tissue perfusion. Vasoconstriction is the primary compensation for hypovolaemia. Constriction of venous capacitance vessels improves venous return, while arteriolar constriction in non-essential tissues redistributes blood flow to essential circulatory beds (coronary and cerebral). The effect of this vasoconstrictive compensation is perfusion of some vital areas but deprivation of others, particularly the splanchnic circulation. Cells damaged by ischaemia are likely to release inflammatory mediators, potentially causing more cell damage. Vasoconstriction is a short-term solution to a vascular volume problem and is life saving, provided that volume is restored before irreversible cell damage has occurred.

Salt and water loss

Losses outside the body in urine, faeces or vomitus come from the intravascular and interstitial compartments and, reflecting the composition of those

	Hypovolaemic shock		Traumatic shock	Obstructive shock	Cardiogenic shock	Distributive shock	
Causes	Salt and water loss	Blood loss	Trauma	Obstruction of venous return to the heart	Failure of the heart as a pump	Sepsis	Anaphylaxis
Vasomotor tone	Constriction	Constriction	Constriction	Constriction	Constriction	Dilation	Dilation
Cardiac output	Decreased	Decreased	Decreased	Decreased	Decreased	Increased	Increased
Systemic vascular resistance	Increased	Increased	Increased	Increased	Increased	Decreased	Decreased
Initial mechanism of cell damage	Ischaemia	Ischaemia	Ischaemia	Ischaemia	Ischaemia	Inflammatory mediators	Inflammatory mediators

3.1 Classification of shock.

compartments, predominantly contain sodium chloride and water. Losses of this type are distributed across the extracellular space. Decreases in skin turgor as well as changes in the cardiovascular parameters (mental state, mucous membrane colour, capillary refill time, heart rate and pulse quality) are expected. Red blood cells and proteins are concentrated in a smaller volume of plasma, as indicated by an increase in packed cell volume and total solids.

Blood loss

Haemorrhage causes shock by a combination of intravascular volume loss and a decrease in red cell mass, such that oxygen delivery to cells is critically low. Because the lost fluid has the same composition as the remaining blood, no changes in packed cell volume or total solids are initially expected. Over time, redistribution of salt and water from the interstitium replaces a portion of this loss and dilutes the remaining red blood cells and proteins.

Traumatic shock

In trauma, shock is often due to hypovolaemia secondary to bleeding. Extensive tissue trauma can also cause enough capillary damage to result in substantial loss of plasma into the tissues. Additionally, pain can inhibit the vasomotor centre and interfere with the vasoconstrictive response. Extensive tissue damage activates the inflammatory response, causing release of inflammatory mediators from damaged cells.

Obstructive shock

Inadequate tissue perfusion may occur due to an obstruction of blood flow within the vasculature. In order to cause a global deficit in tissue oxygen delivery this obstruction must occur in a vessel close to the heart. Although uncommon in veterinary medicine, obstructive shock may be seen in animals with massive pulmonary thromboemboli or pericardial effusion. Pericardial effusion causes an effective obstruction of blood flow, as the increased intrapericardial pressure reduces flow into the right side of the heart.

Cardiogenic shock

Failure of the pump function of the heart causes cardiogenic shock. Ventricular volumes and central venous pressure may be increased, but forward flow is inadequate. For example, Dobermanns with severe dilated cardiomyopathy may present with pale mucous membranes and weak pulses because of systolic failure. In contrast, cats with cardiogenic shock due to hypertrophic cardiomyopathy are experiencing severe diastolic failure.

Distributive shock

Distributive shock is characterized by non-uniform loss of adequate peripheral vascular resistance. Resistance in specific tissue beds may be increased, decreased or normal, and the clinical picture is that of vasodilation. With adequate volume resuscitation, tissue perfusion increases. Some areas, such as splanchnic tissues, may continue to be perfused ineffectively or, in spite of adequate perfusion, may be unable to use the substrates presented. These vascular and cellular effects largely result from the global release of inflammatory mediators (see 'The systemic inflammatory response syndrome and the multiple organ dysfunction syndrome').

Septic shock

Sepsis is the systemic inflammatory response to severe infection, most commonly caused by bacteria or bacterial toxins. Other causative agents include fungi, protozoans and viruses. When sepsis is combined with clinical signs of shock, septic shock is present.

Anaphylactic shock

Anaphylaxis results from an antigen–antibody reaction occurring immediately after an antigen, to which the patient is sensitized, enters the circulation. Anaphylactic shock is characterized by: venous dilation that increases venous capacitance and decreases venous return; arteriolar dilation that decreases arterial pressure; and increased capillary permeability that results in hypovolaemia due to loss of plasma into tissues. Urticaria, angioedema, laryngeal oedema and bronchospasm may also be present.

Clinical signs and related cardiovascular parameters

The clinical signs of shock and the cardiovascular parameters that these signs represent are shown in Figure 3.2. Correct interpretation of these signs, based on knowledge of their physiology, is of primary importance

Clinical signs	Cardiovascular parameters represented by the clinical signs	Changes in clinical signs due to changes in vasomotor tone	
		Vasoconstriction	Vasodilation
Mental state	Perfusion to the brain	Altered mental state	
Mucous membrane colour	Volume and composition (haemoglobin, oxygen) of capillary blood	Pale to white mucous membranes	Hyperaemic (red, injected) mucous membranes
Capillary refill time	Peripheral vasomotor tone	Slow to absent capillary refill time	Fast capillary refill time
Heart rate	Response to vascular volume	Increased heart rate	Increased heart rate
Pulse quality	Pulse pressure (systolic minus diastolic blood pressure)	Poor pulse quality	Bounding pulse quality
Extremity temperature	Perfusion to the extremities	Cool extremities	Warm extremities

3.2 Clinical signs of shock and related cardiovascular parameters in the dog.

in the initial management of shock patients. The signs serve to identify that a state of shock exists and their resolution or improvement serves as some of the endpoints of resuscitation.

Clinical signs related to intravascular volume

Mental state
Mental state refers to the level of consciousness and the behaviour of the patient. The brain has a high metabolic rate and low energy reserves, making it dependent on a constant supply of oxygen and glucose. Decreases in brain perfusion cause deterioration in the mental state.

Mucous membrane colour
The amount and the composition (haemoglobin, oxygen) of blood in the underlying capillary beds create the normally pink colour of mucous membranes. Either anaemia or severe vasoconstriction can cause mucous membranes to be pale or white. Vasodilation and venous pooling cause mucous membranes to be excessively red, a condition common in sepsis.

Capillary refill time
Digital pressure applied to a mucous membrane pushes blood out of the underlying capillary bed. Capillary refill time is the time it takes, in seconds, for blood to refill the capillary bed after digital pressure is removed. This is usually about 1–1.5 seconds. The rate of refill is determined by the tone of the precapillary arteriolar sphincters. Vasoconstriction lengthens and vasodilation shortens the capillary refill time. Capillary refill time is not a measure of cardiac output; rather, it is a measure of peripheral vasomotor tone.

Heart rate
Increased heart rate is an early and sensitive indicator of vascular volume loss, acting as a compensatory mechanism to increase cardiac output even though stroke volume is diminished. If tachycardia is due to volume loss, restoration of an effective circulating blood volume should cause the heart rate to return to normal. Other causes of tachycardia, such as pain, fever, hypoxaemia or hypercapnia, should be considered. Compared with dogs, cats in shock often have heart rates that are slower than normal, frequently in the 120–150 beats per minute (bpm) range.

Pulse quality
Pulse quality is a subjective impression of the fullness, or amplitude, of the pulse. It is determined by the pulse pressure (difference between systolic and diastolic pressure) and the duration of the pressure waveform. Pulse quality is most indicative of stroke volume and is not well correlated with arterial blood pressure. Vasoconstriction and small stroke volume are the most common causes of poor pulse quality (lack of fullness of the pulse).

Temperature of extremities
Vasoconstriction decreases blood flow to the extremities, causing them to cool. The surface temperature of an extremity can be measured by taping a clinical thermometer between the toes. The rectal to toe-web temperature difference is normally 4°C. Increases in the gradient indicate peripheral vasoconstriction.

Clinical signs related to interstitial volume
Interstitial volume can be assessed by evaluating skin turgor and mucous membrane moistness. Losses of salt and water (as with severe vomiting, diarrhoea or diuresis) cause loss of both interstitial and intravascular volume. Acute blood loss causes a decrease in vascular volume, but, at least in the early stages, may leave the interstitial volume unchanged.

Skin turgor
Skin turgor (skin elasticity) causes skin to return to its normal position after being gently lifted into a tented position. The elasticity of the skin and subcutaneous tissues is a measure of the amount of fluid (salt and water) and fat in the interstitial space. Interstitial dehydration causes the skin to remain tented for several seconds. However, the assessment of skin turgor is subject to a fairly large degree of error. In states of normal hydration, thin patients have decreased skin elasticity due to loss of subcutaneous fat. Because of higher subcutaneous stores of fat and water, young patients usually have more skin elasticity than do older patients.

Mucous membrane moistness
The degree of moistness of the mucous membranes reflects the status of the interstitial space. However, other problems such as nausea or oral disease may cause excessive salivation, which may make the membranes appear moist, even in the face of interstitial volume deficits.

Changes in vasomotor tone
Changes in vasomotor tone characterize the shock state, and form the basis for its recognition and treatment. Vasoconstriction and vasodilation are not uniform across the vascular system or throughout the body. Moreover, changes in the tone of arteries have different effects from changes in the tone of veins. Since shock is a cellular event, impairment of adequate blood flow to the capillaries, where oxygen and nutrient transport to the cells occurs, is of primary concern.

The tone of metarterioles determines most (80%) of the systemic vascular resistance, and changes in metarteriolar tone redistribute blood flow. Some organs, particularly brain, heart and kidney, have an intrinsic ability (autoregulation) to regulate their blood flow in the face of changes in arteriolar tone. The capillary beds comprise the largest area of the vascular system and the site of nutrient exchange between blood and cells. Changes in capillary hydrostatic or oncotic pressure cause changes in fluid movement across capillary membranes, with increases in hydrostatic or decreases in oncotic pressures promoting loss of fluid to the interstitium. In shock, arteriovenous connections allow blood to bypass the capillary bed. The venous system normally contains about 65% of the total blood volume, as veins store large quantities of blood that can be made available to the remainder of the circulation. This capacity is exploited in shock therapy when large volumes of fluid are administered rapidly. Venoconstriction causes an increase in venous return to the heart.

Vasoconstriction

Hypotension initiates a vasoconstrictive response within 30 seconds, as sympathetic reflex responses are mediated through baroreceptors in the thorax and central nervous system receptors. Within 10 minutes, angiotensin and vasopressin begin to contribute to vasoconstriction and to conservation of sodium and water by the kidneys. Over the next few hours, as capillary hydrostatic pressure decreases, reabsorption of interstitial fluid and stimulation of thirst contribute to complete restoration of vascular volume. The vasoconstrictive response supports life in the short term, but puts some organs at risk. Arteriolar vasoconstriction redistributes flow to the cerebral and coronary circulations, which, in combination with intrinsic autoregulation, favours perfusion of the heart and brain. At the same time, it severely decreases flow to splanchnic, muscle and skin vascular beds.

Vasodilation

Infectious agents and/or their toxins, trauma and ischaemia can damage cells. Any severe cellular insult can initiate a systemic inflammatory response in which cells produce mediators that change the extracellular environment. Vasodilation is one sign of the presence of systemic inflammation. Tissue perfusion is compromised and venous return is decreased when blood pools in the capillary beds. Improvement in blood volume can restore tissue perfusion, provided that adequate forward flow is maintained.

Irreversible shock

If the state of shock is sufficiently severe and prolonged, irreversible cell damage occurs and treatment will be unsuccessful. Processes contributing to irreversible shock include:

- Decreased coronary blood flow that damages the myocardium and causes decreased cardiac output, further compromising coronary blood flow
- Decreased blood flow to the vasomotor centres in the brain that impairs the vasoconstrictive response, resulting in further decreases in cerebral and coronary circulation
- Release of inflammatory mediators from cells damaged by shock, promoting the production of more inflammatory mediators and thus causing more cell damage.

Cardiovascular elements of tissue perfusion

Deficits in tissue perfusion have important negative consequences on cell function, including energy deficits and stimulation of systemic inflammation. Restoration and maintenance of tissue perfusion are the primary goals of shock therapy. Figure 3.3 is a schematic representation of the cardiovascular elements that combine to provide adequate blood flow to cells (tissue perfusion). These cardiovascular elements are global parameters taken at one point in time and represent an average measure of multiple, interactive processes.

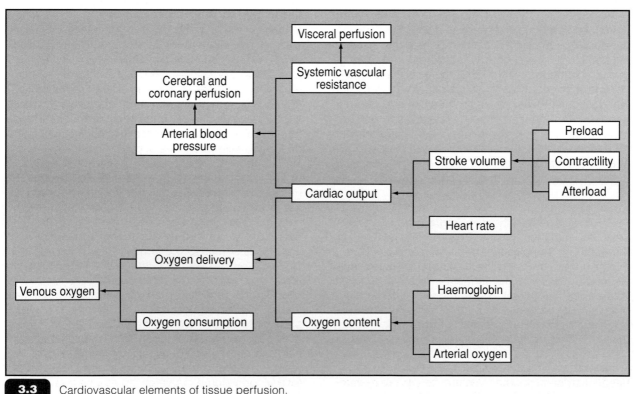

3.3 Cardiovascular elements of tissue perfusion.

Cardiac output

Cardiac output is the volume of blood pumped by the heart each minute, and is the product of heart rate and stroke volume. In the closed cardiovascular system, cardiac output cannot exceed venous return to the right ventricle.

Stroke volume

Stroke volume is the volume of blood ejected per heartbeat. It depends on preload, contractility and afterload.

Heart rate

Increased heart rates usually produce increased cardiac output. However, excessively fast heart rates (greater than 220–240 bpm) allow insufficient time for ventricular filling and can result in decreased cardiac output. When heart rates are slow, cardiac output is partially maintained, because increased time for ventricular filling results in increased stroke volume. Pathologically slow heart rates do not allow sufficient beats per minute to maintain cardiac output.

Preload

Preload refers to the volume of blood in the ventricles at end-diastole. In a physiological sense, it depends on circulating volume, venous tone, atrial contraction and intrathoracic pressure. From a clinician's viewpoint, circulating volume and venous return are usually the most important and the most readily treated components of preload. Venous return depends on the state of the systemic venous circulation. Venoconstriction, induced by sympathetic stimulation, increases venous return and preload. Decreased venous tone (increased venous capacitance) reduces venous return.

Contractility

Contractility, the ability of cardiac myocytes to shorten during systole, reflects the ability of the heart to act as a pump. In shock, decreases in myocardial perfusion, sympathetic activation, acidosis and myocardial depressant factors have deleterious effects on contractility.

Afterload

Afterload refers to the forces that oppose myocardial muscle contraction and thereby ejection of blood from the ventricle.

Systemic vascular resistance

Resistance, the relationship between blood pressure and blood flow, is calculated rather than directly measured. Mean arterial pressure (MAP) is the arterial pressure averaged over time. Central venous pressure (CVP) is the pressure measured at the tip of a catheter placed in a jugular vein, usually positioned so that the tip is close to the heart. It represents right atrial pressure and reflects the filling pressure of the right ventricle. Cardiac output (CO) is the volume of blood pumped by the heart each minute. Systemic vascular resistance (SVR) is calculated as: $(MAP - CVP) \div CO$.

Arterial blood pressure

Cardiac output and systemic vascular resistance create arterial blood pressure. Each left ventricular ejection into the aorta and arterial tree creates a pressure pulse whose highest peak is systolic blood pressure. Cardiac output, systemic vascular resistance and blood viscosity interact in complex ways to affect systolic blood pressure. Normal values for systolic pressure are 110–190 mmHg in dogs, and 120–170 mmHg in cats. Blood ejected during systole is partly stored in the distended arteries that rebound to create diastolic pressure. Duration of diastole, blood volume and arterial elasticity all affect diastolic pressure. Normal values for diastolic pressure are 55–110 mmHg in dogs and 70–120 mmHg in cats. Mean arterial pressure is the integrated mean of pressures throughout the cardiac cycle, and is calculated using the following formula:

$$MAP = \text{diastolic pressure} + \frac{(\text{systolic pressure} - \text{diastolic pressure})}{3}$$

While adequate blood pressure is required for blood flow, the presence of normal arterial blood pressure does not guarantee that adequate flow is occurring. For example, administration of α-adrenergic agonists to support blood pressure can create extreme vasoconstriction in some vascular beds. The resultant increase in overall vascular resistance can create adequate blood pressure but a decreased total systemic perfusion. On the other hand, low blood pressures do not necessarily mean that flow is not occurring, because tissue perfusion is determined by the difference between arterial blood pressure and intra-organ pressure. If intra-organ pressure is low, then adequate flow can be obtained even with lower than normal arterial blood pressures.

Hypotension is an important component of all forms of shock; it can occur early or late in the shock state. In patients presenting with clinical signs of shock, arterial blood pressure can be so low that it is difficult to get an accurate reading before the first resuscitative fluids are delivered, and time should not be wasted trying to get such a measurement. Conversely, in less severely affected shock patients, compensatory processes act to maintain blood pressure, usually at the expense of perfusion to splanchnic and other tissues. Patients with clinical signs of shock should therefore be treated to restore tissue perfusion even if their blood pressure on presentation is normal. Hypertension is unexpected in patients with clinical signs of shock. Possible causes include: renal failure; hyperthyroidism (cats); fever; pain; central neurological disease; drugs; polycythaemia; and fluid overload.

Blood pressure cannot be reliably estimated by digital palpation of the pulse because pulse quality (amplitude) reflects stroke volume and is not well correlated with arterial blood pressure. Palpation of pulses is therefore not a substitute for measuring blood pressure because the pulse pressure is the difference between systolic and diastolic pressure. A large difference creates a high amplitude pulse, but is only weakly correlated with arterial blood pressure. Therefore, blood pressure should be measured as soon as is practical, and monitored frequently during treatment. It is especially important to identify persistent hypotension in patients thought to have been adequately treated for shock, because this might be the only sign of undertreatment and might indicate a need for vasopressors. Systolic pressure <90 mmHg, diastolic pressure <50 mmHg and mean pressure <60 mmHg should be corrected, with consideration of all the components of tissue perfusion as depicted in Figure 3.3. The usual sequence of treatment for hypotension is:

1. Volume restoration.
2. Treatment of oxygenation and ventilation problems.
3. Pain control.
4. Control of bleeding and restoration of adequate haemoglobin.
5. Cardiac support if needed.
6. Vasopressor therapy.

Methods of blood pressure measurement

Arterial blood pressure can be measured by direct and indirect methods. Direct methods require a needle or catheter placed in a systemic artery and connected to a pressure transducer, with the waveform displayed on a patient monitor. Direct blood pressure monitoring is more likely to be used in the continuing management of a critically ill patient than in the emergency treatment of shock. Because they are non-invasive and can be rapidly applied, ultrasonic Doppler and oscillometric methods are the indirect methods usually used for blood pressure monitoring in shock patients. The clinician should choose a system that has been validated for dogs and cats and that has been demonstrated to correlate well with direct blood pressure measurements. (Pedersen *et al.*, 2002; Sawyer *et al.*, 2004).

Cuff selection for indirect methods: For either method of indirect blood pressure measurement, choosing the correct cuff size and applying it properly is essential. The proper cuff width (in centimetres) is 40% of the circumference (in centimetres) of the site where the cuff will be placed. Cuffs that are too wide give falsely low readings, those that are too narrow give falsely high readings. The cuff should be applied snugly enough to only allow insertion of a small finger between the cuff and the leg. If the cuff is applied too tightly, the measurement will be erroneously low because the cuff partly occludes the artery; if too loosely the measurement will be erroneously high because excessive cuff pressure is required to occlude the artery. The cuff must be prevented from moving down the leg or tail when inflated, either by flexing the carpus or tarsus, or by blocking distal movement of the cuff by placing a hand on the appendage, not on the cuff. If the cuff is placed on a limb, that limb must not be weightbearing. Motion interferes with measurements in either method.

Doppler ultrasound: In the ultrasonic Doppler method, an inflatable cuff attached to a manometer (Figure 3.4) occludes an artery, and a piezoelectric crystal placed over the artery distal to the cuff detects

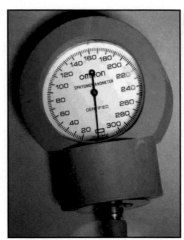

3.4 Manometer used to determine pressure within a cuff positioned to occlude a peripheral artery. When used with a means to determine arterial flow distal to the cuff (e.g. Doppler ultrasound probe), systolic arterial blood pressure can be determined.

flow. Based on the Doppler principle, the re-entry of blood into the artery as the cuff is released causes a frequency change (Doppler shift) in sound waves, which is detected by the piezoelectric crystal and converted to a sound detected by the operator. This method measures systolic pressure.

The measurement site for the transducer is commonly the superficial palmar or plantar arterial arch, or the medial caudal artery of the tail. The area is shaved and adequate coupling gel applied. The transducer is positioned so that the sound of flow is detected and is taped in place with the transducer perpendicular to the artery. The cuff, which is placed proximal to the measurement site, is inflated to a pressure above the expected systolic pressure to occlude the artery, and slowly deflated at a few mmHg/sec until the sound of flow is detected. At this time the cuff pressure is equal to systolic pressure. In patients with very low systolic blood pressure (<70 mmHg) the value obtained may be closer to the mean rather than the systolic pressure.

Oscillometric techniques: The oscillometric technique uses a cuff to occlude the artery, and detects oscillations of the underlying artery when it is partly occluded. This system determines systolic, diastolic and mean arterial pressures. In the oscillometric method, the cuff is snugly placed over the radial artery proximal to the carpus, the saphenous artery proximal to the tarsus, the brachial artery proximal to the elbow, or the median caudal artery at the base of the tail. The cuff is attached to a control unit (Figure 3.5) that continually senses arterial pressure and inflates to a pressure greater than systolic, and then automatically deflates the cuff. The first oscillation is detected when the cuff pressure equals systolic pressure, the largest oscillation at mean pressure, and the oscillations disappear at diastolic pressure. Muscle contractions also create oscillations and are a source of potential error. The heart rate is displayed and the operator must verify that it matches the patient's heart rate. The operator records the values for three to five cycles and reports the averages for systolic, diastolic and mean pressures, verifying that the displayed heart rate corresponds to the patient's heart rate. This method is less accurate in very small patients, patients with low blood pressure and patients with dysrhythmias.

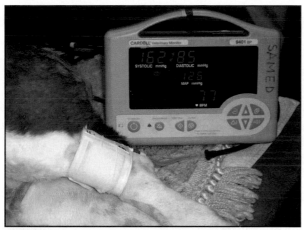

3.5 Automated oscillometric blood pressure monitor; invaluable for both intensive care unit and anaesthesia monitoring. With correct cuff size selection, these instruments provide clinically accurate and repeatable measurements in the majority of patients.

Arterial oxygen content

The purpose of blood circulation is, in large part, to deliver oxygen to the tissues. The amount of oxygen contained in a volume of blood is the total of the oxygen carried bound to haemoglobin and that carried in a dissolved state in plasma. Of the two, by far the largest contribution to arterial oxygen content comes from haemoglobin.

Haemoglobin

Haemoglobin combines reversibly with oxygen. When all of the haemoglobin is combined with oxygen, the blood is fully saturated. The saturation of arterial blood (S_aO_2) depends primarily on the partial pressure of oxygen (P_aO_2). Under normal conditions arterial blood is about 97% saturated, i.e. 97% of the haemoglobin is combined with oxygen.

P_aO_2

P_aO_2 measures the tension of oxygen dissolved in physical solution in plasma, irrespective of the haemoglobin concentration. The P_aO_2 determines the saturation of the haemoglobin molecule with oxygen according to the haemoglobin dissociation curve (see Figure 7.2). P_aO_2 will be normal as long as the respiratory system is working properly. Severely anaemic patients will have a normal P_aO_2 but a severely decreased arterial oxygen content, since there is little haemoglobin with which molecular oxygen can associate.

Energy deficit in shock

Energy production

Shock is a cellular event with life-threatening consequences, many of which are due to a cellular energy deficit. Cellular processes depend on a supply of energy obtained from food and transferred to ATP (adenosine triphosphate). ATP is one of the most important molecules in nature, as it is the common currency of energy exchange. ATP provides energy for ion and metabolite transport, cellular motility, muscle contraction and anabolism. Life depends on its continual production and availability for use.

Aerobic metabolism

In aerobic metabolism, cells extract energy by oxidative combustion of foodstuff molecules, using oxygen as an electron acceptor, in a series of enzymatically controlled steps of oxidation–reduction that are built into the cell. Molecular oxygen is a perfect electron acceptor because it has a high affinity for hydrogen and its electron, thus allowing liberation of the largest amount of free energy. This sequence allows complete oxidation of food and extraction of the maximum amount of energy.

Anaerobic metabolism

In anaerobic metabolism, cells use electron acceptors other than oxygen in the process of extracting energy from foodstuff molecules. Glycolysis is an anaerobic fermentation process that occurs in the cytosol and produces pyruvate or lactate, NADH and ATP. When the oxidative pathways in the mitochondrion have stopped because of lack of oxygen, pyruvate becomes the final electron acceptor and is reduced to lactate. This allows anaerobic glycolysis to proceed, but only 2 mmol of ATP (instead of the potential 36 mmol during aerobic metabolism) are formed from each millimole of glucose.

In pathological states of decreased tissue perfusion, such as shock, global energy production switches from efficient, mitochondrial-based oxidative metabolism to inefficient, oxygen-independent, cytosol based glycolysis. This is a short-term and only partial solution to the problem of inadequate energy production caused by failure of oxygen delivery to cells. Additionally, the increase in lactate production can cause lactic acidosis (see 'Lactic acidosis').

Consequences of an energy deficit

The consequences of an energy deficit include:

- Failure to maintain ionic gradients across cell membranes
- Loss of the transmembrane potential
- Intracellular accumulation of ions and water
- Cell swelling and, eventually, cell death.

Cell membranes are fitted with pumps (e.g. Na^+–K^+–ATPase) that maintain intracellular ionic concentrations and a transmembrane potential. Loss of energy for these pumps allows sodium and water to accumulate intracellularly, while potassium and magnesium are lost to the extracellular space. The transmembrane potential decreases. As sodium and water enter the cells, cell swelling causes changes in microfilament and microtubule function. The energy deficit causes mitochondrial dysfunction and decreased electron transport. As ischaemia persists, mitochondrial swelling worsens and lysosomal breakdown occurs. Terminally, structural integrity of the cell is lost due to breakdown of intracellular structures and the cell membrane.

Metabolic acidosis and base deficit

Metabolic acidosis is common in patients with shock. Adverse effects of a decrease in pH with particular importance in shock patients include:

- Decreased cardiac contractility and heart rate; dysrhythmias
- Arteriolar dilation and venoconstriction
- Increase in rate and depth of respiration (Kussmaul respiration)
- Renal sodium and potassium wasting.

Base deficit is calculated from the blood gas and is an approximation of global tissue acidosis. An increased (i.e. more negative) base deficit is commonly associated with increased blood lactate. Both parameters, base deficit and blood lactate, address the same issue of tissue perfusion and therefore their normalization is an appropriate endpoint of resuscitation.

Lactic acidosis
Increased blood lactate concentration is significant in shock patients because it is a marker of decreased tissue perfusion, and because high levels are correlated with decreased survival. Lactate is produced by anaerobic glycolysis. Lactate and hydrogen ion production can be substantially increased in shock because of the increase in anaerobic glycolysis and ATP hydrolysis. Lactic acid accumulates intracellularly and diffuses out of the cell into the extracellular space where it causes an approximately equimolar decrease in bicarbonate concentration. The resultant acidosis contributes to the metabolic acidosis that is common in shock. There is sometimes a poor correlation between the presence of acidaemia and blood lactate concentration. Simultaneous counteracting processes tending to produce alkalaemia may mask the presence of an acidaemia. Direct measurement of lactate in blood is the best means of detecting lactic acidosis. Limitations of availability and the technical requirements of this test may make this determination difficult to obtain in some circumstances.

The systemic inflammatory response syndrome and the multiple organ dysfunction syndrome

Inflammation is, in general, a beneficial and appropriate response to injury, whether from ischaemia, trauma or infection. The redness, heat, swelling and pain that signal inflammation are caused by vasodilation, increased blood flow, increased capillary permeability and stimulation of nerve endings. These and many other changes are caused by inflammatory mediators that interact with cells to change cell function and intercellular communication. The inflammatory process is normally self-regulating and balanced between pro- and anti-inflammatory processes. It is essential to the control and eventual resolution of tissue damage.

In combination with an appropriately severe insult, tachycardia, tachypnoea, hyper- or hypothermia and leucocytosis or leucopenia indicate the presence of systemic inflammation. This may be an entirely appropriate response and one that is essential to control and resolve the injury. However, if inflammation becomes excessive, or if the balance between pro- and anti-inflammatory processes is lost, cells distant from the original site can be damaged.

Systemic inflammation becomes an amplifying cascade that interferes with the function of various organs, potentially causing their failure. In these circumstances, instead of being the solution, inflammation has become the problem. The same changes that would benefit damaged tissue can, when poorly regulated, cause microvascular injury, cardiac dysfunction, hypotension and shock. Organs distant from the site of original injury then fail – a syndrome that has been named the multiple organ dysfunction syndrome (MODS).

Attempts have been made to define types of systemic inflammation with and without infection. The goal is to recognize the progression of systemic inflammation to multiple organ dysfunction, and to allow grouping of patients with similar disease so as to evaluate various therapies. An abbreviated version of those definitions is:

- Systemic inflammatory response syndrome (SIRS) – the systemic inflammatory response to a severe insult, represented in the patient by two or more of the following: tachycardia, tachypnoea, hyper- or hypothermia, leucocytosis or leucopenia
- Sepsis – SIRS with evidence of infection
- Severe sepsis – sepsis with evidence of organ dysfunction and evidence of hypoperfusion that responds to intravascular volume loading
- Septic shock – severe sepsis that requires both intravascular volume loading and the use of inotropes to restore tissue perfusion
- Non-infectious SIRS – progresses through similar stages to those described above and may be termed severe SIRS or sterile shock.

The clinician concerned with the management of individual patients already recognizes that the sickest patients are the most likely to die. These definitions do not necessarily contribute additional information. However, the concept of the systemic inflammatory response is important in explaining how any severe insult can lead to an amplifying and dysregulated cascade of tissue-damaging events that eventually leads to failure of multiple organs and death.

Mediators of inflammation
The inflammatory cascade is a mediator-driven, complex, overlapping system with a high degree of redundancy. An inflammatory mediator may induce a cell to:

- Elaborate a receptor
- Shed a receptor
- Secrete a mediator
- Adhere to another cell
- Release an enzyme
- Enhance its usual function
- Perform a new function.

Some mediators induce mostly pro-inflammatory activities, others mostly anti-inflammatory activities. Some mediators may elicit different effects at different times, stimulating or suppressing the same cell depending on circumstances. This effect has been likened to that of a toggle switch. Mediators may suppress, stimulate, or have no effect on their own production or on that of other mediators. Cells once stimulated to produce inflammatory mediators may respond to a second insult with much greater production of these mediators. It is beyond the scope of this chapter to discuss any but a few representative examples of inflammatory mediators. The reader is referred to the list of references at the end of this chapter for a more complete discussion of the inflammatory process.

Cytokines
Cytokines are polypeptides produced by macrophages and many other cells in response to cell injury. Tumour necrosis factor (TNF) and interleukin 1 are major pro-inflammatory cytokines that promote cellular proliferation, endothelial adhesion, vascular permeability and intravascular coagulation, as well as producing clinical signs of anorexia, hypotension and fever. Other members of the large family of interleukins, such as interleukin 10, have anti-inflammatory activity. An important effect of cytokines is their ability to induce activity of other inflammatory mediators, such as eicosanoids and nitric oxide.

Eicosanoids
Prostaglandins, thromboxanes and leucotrienes are produced by the metabolism of arachidonic acid. Thromboxanes produce hypotension but increase pulmonary vascular resistance. Some prostaglandins are required for maintenance of normal vascular tone and the anti-thrombotic state of vascular endothelium. Leucotrienes decrease blood pressure and increase vascular permeability. Understanding the widespread effects of eicosanoids is important in making therapeutic decisions. For example, non-steroidal anti-inflammatory drugs (NSAIDs) decrease production of prostaglandins and can adversely alter renal blood flow and gastric mucosal integrity.

Kinins
Bradykinin is a peptide mediator that promotes nitric oxide-induced hypotension. It also causes a change in shape of vascular endothelial cells and increases vascular permeability. These changes are prominent in anaphylaxis.

Complement
The products of the complement cascade increase vascular permeability and decrease systemic vascular resistance.

Other mediators
Platelet-activating factor increases platelet and neutrophil aggregation. Interferon activates B cells, neutrophils and macrophages. Transforming growth factor promotes cell repair.

Adhesion molecules
Intercellular adhesion molecules (ICAM), integrins and selectins mediate the adhesion of endothelial cells and leucocytes. They are important in the delivery of leucocytes to areas of inflammation. However, they can also promote inappropriate aggregation of leucocytes and cause microvascular obstruction.

Nitric oxide
Nitric oxide (NO) is a gas produced by vascular endothelium and is the final mediator of vasodilation and a regulator of normal vasomotor tone. It also inhibits platelet aggregation and contributes to the normal anti-thrombotic property of vascular endothelium. Normally, NO is produced in pulses. Inflammation induces continuous production of large amounts of NO, which can cause excessive vasodilation and vascular hyporeactivity to vasoconstrictors.

Multiple organ dysfunction syndrome
When inflammation becomes systemic, organs, tissues and systems distant from the site of the original insult can be damaged. This is the syndrome of multiple organ dysfunction and has been recently reviewed (Johnson et al., 2004). Organs commonly involved include the vascular endothelium, lungs, kidney, heart, liver and the blood clotting system. The number of organs that are malfunctioning is inversely correlated with survival in critically ill patients. Prevention, when possible, is preferred over waiting until dysfunction is evident and then attempting to revive a failing organ. Following are three representative examples of organ failure caused by ischaemia and systemic inflammation. Specific management of these and other organ failure syndromes common in emergency patients is discussed in more detail in other sections of this text.

Acute lung injury and acute respiratory distress syndrome
Acute lung injury (ALI) is the clinical state of impairment of pulmonary gas exchange that follows acute injury to the alveolar capillary membrane. In its most severe form, it is called the acute respiratory distress syndrome (ARDS). The pathophysiology of ALI/ARDS is inflammatory mediator-related damage to the capillary membrane that allows exudation of fluid from the vascular space and its accumulation in the alveoli. Clinical indications that ARDS is occurring include:

- Thoracic radiographs showing bilaterally symmetrical alveolar filling without evidence of left heart failure
- P_aO_2/F_iO_2 ratio of <200, where F_iO_2 is the fractional concentration of oxygen in inspired gas.

Shock is a major risk factor for the development of ALI. Treatment of the shock state and any underlying cause of shock are of primary importance in the prevention of ALI.

Acute renal failure
Acute renal failure in shock may be caused by ischaemia secondary to decreased renal perfusion (prerenal) or by mediator-related damage to renal cells. Drugs that impair renal perfusion also contribute to renal failure. Catecholamines and NSAIDs are commonly implicated. Adrenaline, particularly in high doses, can cause profound renal vasoconstriction. NSAIDs reduce the synthesis of renal vasodilatory prostaglandins. Prevention of acute renal failure by prompt restoration of renal perfusion is of paramount importance. Urine output is a measure of kidney perfusion and should be closely monitored in all shock patients.

Disseminated intravascular coagulopathy

The normal anti-thrombotic properties of vascular endothelium can be severely impaired by the actions of inflammatory mediators released in shock, especially in septic shock. The mechanisms of haemostatic dysfunction have been recently reviewed (Hopper and Bateman, 2005). Inappropriate and widespread activation of the coagulation cascade results in the formation of microthrombi that obstruct blood flow and further compromise tissue perfusion. Consumption of platelets and coagulation factors can lead to bleeding. Disseminated intravascular coagulopathy (DIC) is always secondary to a primary disease and is common in shock patients. Prompt restoration and maintenance of adequate tissue perfusion and treatment of the underlying cause are the best preventive measures.

Treatment of shock

General considerations

The best outcome is achieved by the application of a therapeutic plan that addresses all aspects of the disease. Treatment is directed toward the underlying cause, as well as the multi-system consequences of the initiating event. In critically ill patients such as shock patients, there are no unimportant problems. Therapy must be directed toward all aspects of the disease, but must be prioritized to manage the most life-threatening aspects first. If the patient is not breathing or the heart is not beating effectively, cardiopulmonary cerebral resuscitation is the first priority (see Chapter 20). If the patient is in shock, but also has life-threatening breathing or airway problems, management of the respiratory emergency takes precedence over intravascular volume restoration (see Chapter 7). Pre-existing problems, especially cardiac disease, may limit the clinician's ability to use volume restoration to improve tissue perfusion. Once initial resuscitation has been achieved, ongoing management and careful monitoring should continue.

Special considerations

Cardiogenic shock

Treatment of cardiogenic shock is directed toward improving myocardial contractility, reducing afterload and/or preload and controlling serious dysrhythmias (see Chapter 6). In some patients, heart disease may not be the primary cause of shock, but may compromise the effectiveness of the heart as a pump and limit the application of volume restoration therapy. This is always a concern when using fluid therapy for shock, because the pre-existing status of the heart is usually not known. However, most dogs and cats presented in shock do not have serious pre-existing heart disease and intravascular volume restoration is the first treatment unless there are specific indications (heart murmur, abnormal lung auscultation, history compatible with chronic cardiac disease) that the patient will be volume intolerant. Careful continuous monitoring of cardiovascular and pulmonary status and appropriate adjustment of therapy are fundamental for all shock patients.

Hypovolaemic, traumatic and distributive shock

Treatment of the underlying cause of these types of shock, while beyond the scope of this chapter, is essential to the long-term outcome and, especially regarding control of bleeding, essential to the short-term outcome as well. Resuscitation from these types of shock is primarily directed toward volume restoration.

Endpoints of resuscitation

The goal of shock therapy is to restore tissue perfusion by increasing intravascular volume and consequently increasing venous return, stroke volume, cardiac output and delivery of oxygen and other nutrients to cells (see Figure 3.3). Therefore, therapeutic goals (endpoints) of resuscitation should be readily available observations or measurements that are relevant to tissue perfusion. An ideal endpoint would be a parameter that unequivocally reflected tissue perfusion at every level, was perfectly correlated with outcome and could be easily measured in the clinical setting. Such an endpoint has not yet been identified. Although not perfect, the following parameters related to cardiovascular status and tissue perfusion are useful.

Clinical signs related to intravascular volume and vasomotor tone (see Figure 3.2):

- Mental state
- Mucous membrane colour
- Capillary refill time
- Heart rate
- Pulse quality
- Extremity temperature.

Parameters related to tissue perfusion:

- Blood lactate
- Urine output
- Base deficit.

There are limits to these parameters, since they are global measurements and can represent a sum of opposing processes. Adequate tissue perfusion at every level may not be achieved even if these global endpoints are met. However, these appear to be the best endpoints available at the current level of knowledge. Other cardiovascular parameters, such as central venous pressure and arterial blood pressure, can also be used as endpoints.

Although not a specific endpoint of resuscitation, treatment of the underlying cause of shock is an essential goal of therapy. Outcome is closely related to the ability of treatment to restore all tissues to normal.

Supranormal oxygen delivery

Some have proposed that one important goal of therapy should be to achieve supranormal oxygen delivery. The justification for this approach is that during the period of shock an oxygen debt accrued, due to mismatch between oxygen delivery and oxygen demand. A period of supranormal oxygen delivery is a means of correcting this debt. This approach resulted in improved survival in some groups of critically ill patients. A meta-analysis of seven studies in this area concluded that there was insufficient evidence to recommend this strategy in a group of unselected patients (Heyland *et al.*, 1996). Overall, it appears that survival may be improved in some groups of patients if supranormal oxygen delivery is achieved by optimizing vascular volume, but not if persistent use of vasopressors is required to achieve this goal.

Gastric intramucosal pH
The perfusion of gut mucosa is likely to be decreased in shock, and decreased splanchnic perfusion often persists after apparently adequate resuscitation to global endpoints. Because gut intramucosal pH (pHi) falls below normal when perfusion is inadequate, a decreased pHi is a potentially valuable tissue-specific marker for perfusion. Published reports have shown variable correlation between pHi (measured by tonometry) and other measures of tissue perfusion. Anecdotal reports indicate that the technique can be moderately difficult to implement in clinical patients. pHi is not commonly measured in veterinary patients at this time.

Endpoints in uncontrolled abdominal bleeding due to trauma
In the special circumstance of uncontrolled abdominal bleeding secondary to penetrating trauma, a delay in volume restoration until bleeding is controlled has been proposed (Bickell *et al.*, 1994). This approach should be used with caution if control of abdominal haemorrhage cannot be achieved in a short time (less than 1 hour). While a decrease in hydrostatic pressure may decrease blood loss, failure to restore tissue perfusion can damage cells and lead to organ failure and death. Moderate resuscitation (rather than no resuscitation) has been recommended (Smail *et al.*, 1998) and is probably the best choice in these patients.

Fluid therapy
Appropriate fluids for resuscitation of shock are isotonic, or nearly isotonic, crystalloids (Na^+ 130–154 mmol/l) with or without the addition of colloids or hypertonic saline (see Chapter 4). If improvement in the endpoints of resuscitation is not achieved at the end of the initial fluid bolus, a repeat bolus of the same amount should be considered. If isotonic crystalloids are used, a decrease in vascular volume is expected following initial resuscitation, as redistribution occurs across the extracellular space. With colloids, a more steady state of vascular volume expansion is expected. Hypertonic saline has only a transitory effect and follow-up therapy with isotonic crystalloid or colloid is usually necessary.

Blood transfusion
Oxygen content and delivery of oxygen to tissues cannot be maintained without adequate haemoglobin concentration. The minimum acceptable packed cell volume (PCV) in shock patients has not been established. If there is no evidence to the contrary, it is safest to assume that the patient is not well adapted to anaemia, and the PCV should be maintained above 18% in cats and above 25% in dogs. It is desirable to administer blood slowly over several hours but a rapid infusion may be needed in unstable patients. The blood transfusion can be administered simultaneously with other fluids, if they are needed to support vascular volume. Blood product use is discussed further in Chapter 14.

The transition plan
When the initial endpoints of resuscitation have been achieved, these parameters may thereafter oscillate within a range of normal, or deteriorate. Initial success in resuscitation cannot be assumed to be a complete resolution of the problem of shock. Tissue perfusion must not only be restored, it must be maintained. Often the initial resuscitation plan, or a modification of it, must be repeated several times before the patient's condition is stabilized. Close monitoring provides for early detection of deterioration of endpoints, so that therapeutic interventions can be made in a timely manner.

Treatment of metabolic acidosis in shock patients
Metabolic acidosis in shock patients is primarily due to decreased tissue perfusion and is best corrected by directing therapy toward restoration of blood flow to all tissues. Bicarbonate therapy may also be used, especially if acidaemia is severe (see Chapter 5). When oxygen delivery is restored, the liver can metabolise lactate. A high blood lactate level, which persists after apparently adequate resuscitation, suggests that tissue perfusion has not been restored. This is a legitimate indicator of a poor prognosis in a shock patient. Blood lactate levels should begin to decline within 15–30 minutes after successful resuscitation.

Urine output
Since renal vasoconstriction (and decreased urine output) is an appropriate response to hypovolaemia, sufficient preload must be established before the adequacy of urine output can be evaluated. A central venous pressure of about 10 cmH$_2$O, mean arterial blood pressure >80 mmHg, and absence of peripheral vasoconstriction indicate that preload is adequate. Under these conditions, and in the absence of any other source of fluid losses, urine output should be only slightly less than fluid input.

Because urine output is such a good indicator of perfusion of a local, and vital, tissue bed (the kidney), the establishment of adequate urine output is an excellent endpoint of resuscitation. Therefore, urine output should be closely monitored in all shock patients. A urinary catheter and closed collection system should be considered if clinically indicated.

Vasoactive therapy
The goal of fluid therapy in shock is to support adequate tissue perfusion without the need for vasoactive therapy. Pulse quality, or amplitude of the pulse, is related to stroke volume and is not well correlated with arterial blood pressure. Therefore, blood pressure cannot be reliably estimated from digital palpation of a peripheral artery. In shock patients, vasoactive drugs are usually not administered unless significant hypotension, determined by direct or indirect blood pressure measurement, persists after adequate volume resuscitation. If such drugs are needed, an agent that

causes minimal peripheral vasoconstriction such as dobutamine (5–15 µg/kg/min) or dopamine (3–10 µg/kg/min) should be used, monitoring the effect with frequent or continuous blood pressure measurement.

Anaphylactic shock

In addition to fluid therapy, treatment with adrenaline is of proven efficacy in anaphylactic shock. For life-threatening reactions, adrenaline should be given intravenously (0.01–0.02 mg/kg).

Antibiotic therapy

Specific indications for antibiotics in shock patients include direct evidence of a bacterial infection, such as sepsis and septic shock, or penetrating trauma. Often the clinician simply has a concern that infection, especially of gut origin, might develop. One of the most important barriers to bacterial translocation from the gut to the systemic circulation is the presence of facultative anaerobes on the mucosal surface. These are quite susceptible to antibiotics and their destruction has been shown to promote bacterial translocation. Because of this effect, antibiotics administered for prophylaxis may increase bacterial translocation, possibly predisposing a patient to infection.

Even in the absence of known infection, intravenous broad-spectrum antibiotic therapy is indicated in shock patients who are febrile, have bloody diarrhoea, or have substantially increased or decreased neutrophil counts. The risks and benefits of antibiotic therapy, in the absence of known infection, are very difficult to define in this patient group.

Prevention of reperfusion injury

The univalent reduction of oxygen forms reactive oxygen intermediates (ROI) such as superoxide ion, hydrogen peroxide and the hydroxyl radical. Under ischaemic conditions, cells accumulate abnormal concentrations of cytosolic calcium and iron. This provides a source of substrate for the generation of superoxide and hydroxyl radicals when cells are reperfused. The significance of these reactive oxygen intermediates is their reactivity. They damage cell membranes, proteins and nucleic acids. Scavengers of oxygen radicals include mannitol, dimethylsulphoxide (DMSO), superoxide dismutase (SOD), vitamin E and 21-amino-steroids. Other treatments include inhibitors of oxygen radical production such as allopurinol (inhibits xanthine oxidase). Ischaemia–reperfusion injury has been recently reviewed (McMichael and Moore, 2004).

Immunoregulatory and mediator-directed therapy

Corticosteroids

Corticosteroids have been extensively studied as therapy for septic shock. Studies in experimental animal models where corticosteroids were given *before* the shock state was induced yielded encouraging results. However, the clinical application of this research data has been disappointing, to say the least. Several randomized controlled clinical trials in human patients have been published. A meta-analysis of these trials (Cronin *et al.*, 1995) concluded that there

was no benefit to the administration of a short course of steroids (<48 hours) in septic patients. Moreover, there was a trend toward increasing mortality in some treated patients. Interest in the use of steroids in septic patients continues. Studies have addressed the dose and timing of administration (low dose, constant rate infusion over 5–10 days) as key issues in finding a place for these agents in the treatment of sepsis and septic shock (Bollaert *et al.*, 1998).

Current studies are addressing the possible usefulness of corticosteroids in veterinary patients with septic shock accompanied by temporary adrenal insufficiency. In this subset of patients, replacement with physiological doses of corticosteroids may prove to be beneficial (Martin and Groman, 2004). In contrast to those patients with temporary hypoadrenocorticism, in other cases tumour necrosis factor and interleukins, generated as part of the inflammatory response in shock, activate the hypothalamic–pituitary–adrenal (HPA) axis and can cause an increased production of corticosteroids. In spite of the increased endogenous levels of corticosteroids, their effect at the cellular level may be diminished by receptor resistance and decreased extraction from the blood.

Corticosteroids are the most important modulator of the host defence response. At the current level of understanding, we do not know enough about the use of these potent agents in shock patients. Corticosteroids suppress arachidonic acid metabolism and reduce the production of prostaglandins, thromboxane and leucotrienes. Adverse effects of corticosteroids include gastrointestinal ulceration and increased risk of infection. Both are major concerns in shock patients. The risk:benefit ratio of these drugs therefore cannot be properly identified without more information. In the absence of adequate data, advice about whether or not to use these drugs is mostly a matter of how each clinician interprets the scientific data. With the exception of using them to counteract a severe allergic reaction in anaphylactic shock, the author's preference is not to use corticosteroids in shock patients.

Mediator-directed therapy

Therapy directed against many of the inflammatory mediators induced by shock states has been studied extensively. The results of clinical trials have been disappointing in that no improvement in survival has been demonstrated when these agents are used. The clinical failures were most likely due to a combination of factors, including:

- Interference with the balance between pro- and anti-inflammatory cytokines
- Selection of patients with heterogeneous disease processes
- Inappropriate endpoint selection (survival may not be the best endpoint for certain therapies)
- Improper dose, route or timing of administration.

A commentary (Vincent, 1998) and two scientific reports (Abraham *et al.*, 1998; van Dissel *et al.*, 1998) illustrate some of the work and challenges in this area of research. Inflammatory mediators cause a wide variety of changes in cell function that are only crudely represented by clinical signs. The inflammatory process and its interconnection with haemostasis is complex, highly integrated and, at present, incompletely understood. It contains both pro- and anti-inflammatory processes, both of which, when properly regulated, are essential to eventual recovery. Due to our incomplete knowledge in this area, it is not possible to determine the need of an individual for external regulation of the inflammatory response. Therefore, it is also not possible to predict whether mediator-directed therapy will be helpful or injurious. It is even possible in individual patients that specific therapies might prove to be helpful at one point in time, and detrimental at another. New therapies, especially for sepsis and septic shock, are under study (Bernard *et al.*, 2001; Fink, 2003).

References and further reading

Abraham E, Anzueto A, Gutierrez G *et al.* (1998) Double-blind randomised controlled trial of monoclonal antibody to human tumour necrosis factor in treatment of septic shock. *Lancet* **351**, 929–933

Astiz ME and Rackow EC (1998) Septic shock. *Lancet* **351**, 1501–1505

Bernard G, Vincent JL, Laterre P *et al.* (2001) Efficacy and safety of recombinant human activated protein C for severe sepsis. *New England Journal of Medicine* **344**, 699–709

Bickell WH, Wall MJ Jr, Pepe PE *et al.* (1994) Immediate versus delayed fluid resuscitation for hypotensive patients with penetrating torso injuries. *New England Journal of Medicine* **331**, 1105–1109

Bishop MH, Shoemaker WC, Appel PL *et al.* (1995) Prospective randomized trial of survivor values of cardiac index, oxygen delivery, and oxygen consumption as resuscitation endpoints in severe trauma. *Journal of Trauma* **38**, 780–787

Bollaert P-E, Charpentier C, Levy B *et al.* (1998) Reversal of late septic shock with supraphysiologic doses of hydrocortisone. *Critical Care Medicine* **26**, 645–650

Cronin L, Cook DJ, Carlet J *et al.* (1995) Corticosteroid treatment for sepsis: a critical appraisal and meta-analysis of the literature. *Critical Care Medicine* **23**, 1430–1439

Dinarello CA (1997) Pro-inflammatory and anti-inflammatory cytokines as mediators in the pathogenesis of septic shock. *Chest* **112**, 321S–329S

Fink MP (2003) Ethyl pyruvate: A novel anti-inflammatory agent. *Critical Care Medicine* **31**, S51–56

Heyland DK, Cook DJ, King D, Kernerman P and Brun-Buisson C (1996) Maximizing oxygen delivery in critically ill patients: a methodologic appraisal of the evidence. *Critical Care Medicine* **24**, 517–524

Hopper K and Bateman S (2005) An updated view of hemostasis: mechanisms of hemostatic dysfunction associated with sepsis. *Journal of Veterinary Emergency and Critical Care* **15**, 83–91

Hoyt DB (1998) Immune regulation with hypertonic saline in trauma patients. Proceedings of the Society of Critical Care Medicine 27th Educational & Scientific Symposium. Postgraduate Review Course, pp. 32–33

Johnson V, Gaynor A, Chan DL *et al.* (2004) Multiple organ dysfunction syndrome in humans and dogs. *Journal of Veterinary Emergency and Critical Care* **14**, 150–166

Martin LG and Groman RP (2004) Relative adrenal insufficiency in critical illness. *Journal of Veterinary Emergency and Critical Care* **14**, 149–157

Members of the American College of Chest Physicians/Society of Critical Care Medicine Consensus Conference Meeting (1992) Definitions for sepsis and organ failure and guidelines for the use of innovative therapies in sepsis. *Critical Care Medicine* **20**, 864–874

McMichael M and Moore RM (2004) Ischemia-reperfusion injury pathophysiology, part I, part II. *Journal of Veterinary Emergency and Critical Care* **14**, 231–252

Pedersen KM, Butler MA, Ersboll AK *et al.* (2002) Evaluation of an oscillometric blood pressure monitor for use in anesthetized cats. *Journal of the American Veterinary Medical Association* **221**, 646–650

Sawyer DC, Guikeme AH and Siegel EM (2004) Evaluation of a new oscillometric blood pressure monitor in isoflurane-anesthetized dogs. *Veterinary Anaesthesia and Analgesia* **31**, 27–39

Smail N, Wang P, Cioffi WG, Bland KI and Chaudry IH (1998) Resuscitation after uncontrolled venous haemorrhage: does increased resuscitation volume improve regional perfusion? *Journal of Trauma* **44**, 701–708

van Dissel JT, van Langevelde P, Westendorp RGJ, Kwappenberg K and Frolich M (1998) Anti-inflammatory cytokine profile and mortality in febrile patients. *Lancet* **351**, 950–953

Vincent JL (1998) Search for effective immunomodulating strategies against sepsis. *Lancet* **351**, 922–923

4

Fluid therapy

Amanda Boag and Dez Hughes

Introduction

Fluid therapy is part of the treatment plan in most critically ill animals. In some patients fluid therapy is used acutely to treat absolute or relative intravascular volume deficits over a period of minutes to hours. Alternatively, fluid therapy may be used on a more chronic basis, during treatment of the haemodynamically stable patient, to re-establish and maintain normal water, electrolyte and acid–base balance over a period of several days. The precise type, rate and total volume of fluid to be administered for optimal management of a patient can be difficult to determine, especially at the beginning of treatment, and fluid therapy plans may need to be altered depending on the patient's response and the progression of their disease. Unfortunately there are no 'recipes' that can be followed that will guarantee a successful outcome. Good fluid management comes from understanding why the patient requires fluid therapy, and considering both the goals of fluid administration in that patient and the advantages and disadvantages of the different fluid types in achieving those goals. In assessing the fluid therapy requirements of an animal, it is extremely important to separate those patients requiring life-saving intravascular volume expansion from those requiring a more gradual correction, or maintenance, of fluid and electrolyte balance. Central to this goal is an appreciation of the difference between hypoperfusion and dehydration.

Hypoperfusion refers to a local or generalized deficit in tissue blood flow, which results in inadequate oxygen and nutrient delivery and failure to remove metabolic by-products from the tissues. Global hypoperfusion can occur due to hypovolaemia (a reduction in the effective circulating intravascular volume), reduced cardiac function or the maldistribution of blood flow seen in the systemic inflammatory response syndrome (SIRS) (see Chapter 3). Hypovolaemia is the most common cause of hypoperfusion. Most animals with SIRS and some animals with cardiogenic shock also have concurrent reductions in effective circulating intravascular volume. Common causes of hypovolaemia include: haemorrhage; extracellular fluid losses in excess of fluid and solute intake, such as vomiting, diarrhoea and polyuria; and internal losses of plasma volume due to exudation or transudation of fluid from the intravascular space ('third spacing').

Dehydration is strictly defined as a net reduction in the free water content of the body; however, in veterinary patients the term is most often used to refer to combined water and solute loss in excess of intake. Dehydration may ultimately lead to hypovolaemia and hypoperfusion depending upon the volume and nature of the fluid which is lost; however, the terms are not synonymous.

Both perfusion and hydration abnormalities are initially evaluated using the physical examination. Unfortunately, the parameters used for assessment of hydration status (moisture of the mucous membranes, skin turgor, presence or absence of retraction of the globe) are often combined with those used to assess perfusion (heart rate, pulse quality, mucous membrane colour and capillary refill time). This combination of hydration and perfusion parameters has compounded the confusion between the terms and should be avoided.

To illustrate the difference, consider a dog hit by a car 1 hour previously, which has suffered a fractured spleen and bled half of its blood volume into its peritoneal cavity. This animal would have no net change in the water content of its body and no physical examination findings suggestive of dehydration; however, it would be severely hypovolaemic. In contrast, the geriatric cat with anorexia, hypodipsia and chronic renal failure, with prolonged net water loss in excess of intake, may be severely dehydrated but often has surprisingly good perfusion status. The former animal would require rapid intravascular volume replacement to re-expand effective blood volume and thereby preserve perfusion to the major body systems. In the latter animal, in which perfusion of major organs is adequate, more conservative fluid therapy would be appropriate with a goal of re-establishing normal fluid and electrolyte balance over 24–48 hours. A clear understanding of the distinction between dehydration and hypovolaemia and the clinical assessment of both conditions is therefore necessary to ensure appropriate fluid therapy.

Extracellular fluid homeostasis

To understand the choice of intravenous fluids, it is necessary to appreciate how fluids are normally distributed within the body and the factors that control movement of fluid between different compartments. Three major fluid compartments make up the total body water: the intracellular fluid; the interstitial fluid between cells; and the intravascular fluid (Figure 4.1). Together the intravascular and interstitial fluids comprise the extracellular fluid compartment. Total body water is approximately 60% of total body weight; however, this may vary depending upon such factors as the species, age of the animal and the body composition (mainly the fat content). Movement of fluid between compartments depends upon the permeability of the relevant barrier and the concentration of molecules contained within each compartment. For example, the capillary membrane is freely permeable to water and electrolytes, whereas the cell membrane is only freely permeable to water. Movement of water across the cell membrane depends upon the relative concentration of solute molecules within cells compared to the concentration around the cell. Net movement of water will occur by osmosis into an area with a higher concentration of solute molecules.

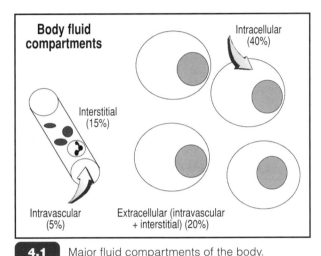

4.1 Major fluid compartments of the body.

Maintenance of intravascular volume – colloid osmotic pressure

Capillaries are freely permeable to water and small solutes, and are relatively (but not completely) impermeable to macromolecules. This means that a protein concentration gradient exists from the vasculature to the interstitium. The higher concentration of impermeant solutes within the capillaries exerts an osmotic pressure (termed the capillary colloid osmotic pressure (COP)) which acts to retain fluid. Fluid exchange between the vasculature and the interstitium is governed by the balance between hydrostatic and osmotic pressure gradients throughout the intravascular compartment and the interstitium. A hydrostatic pressure gradient in excess of the osmotic gradient, at the arterial end of the capillary bed, results in a net transudation of fluid into the interstitium. At the venous end of the capillary bed, plasma proteins exert an osmotic force in excess of the hydrostatic gradient, resulting in a net fluid flux from the interstitium into the vessels. Although the microvascular barrier greatly restricts macromolecular flux, capillaries are slightly permeable to protein. Of the total quantity of albumin

present in the body, 40% is intravascular and 60% is extravascular. Furthermore, all of the albumin present in plasma circulates through the interstitium every 24 hours. The microvascular barrier of skeletal muscle or subcutaneous tissue is relatively impermeable to protein, whereas the pulmonary capillary endothelium is more permeable. Different plasma proteins or artificial colloid molecules will differ in their rate of efflux from a vessel depending upon such factors as their molecular radius, shape and charge. For example, smaller plasma proteins, such as albumin, can pass through with less impedance than larger plasma proteins. In healthy animals, the hydrostatic and osmotic pressure gradients governing transvascular fluid flux and the permeability of the microvascular barrier can vary between different tissues and at different levels of the capillary bed within the same tissue; these may vary even further with different disease states.

By virtue of its relatively high concentration in the vascular space, albumin usually accounts for 60–70% of the plasma COP, with globulins making up the remainder. Variations in COP in healthy dogs are due to differences in globulin concentration rather than albumin. Albumin synthesis, which is unique to the liver, is regulated by the hepatic plasma COP. Equations have been calculated to estimate plasma COP from plasma protein concentrations; however, direct measurement, using a colloid osmometer, is more accurate. Normal COP in dogs is approximately 16–24 mmHg.

Excess fluid in the interstitium (oedema) can have detrimental consequences, the exact nature of which depends on the anatomical site. Three major mechanisms guard against interstitial fluid accumulation. First, extravasation of fluid into a relatively non-distensible interstitium results in an increased interstitial pressure which thereby opposes further extravasation. Second, following extravasation of low-protein fluid, the interstitial COP falls due to dilution and washout of protein, thereby maintaining the COP gradient between the intravascular space and the interstitium. Third, because the interstitium is not compliant, increased interstitial fluid results in an increased driving pressure for lymphatic drainage. These alterations in Starling forces which act to limit interstitial fluid accumulation have been termed the 'tissue safety factors'. Their relative importance varies depending upon the characteristics of the tissue. In a relatively non-distensible tissue such as tendon, a rise in interstitial pressure may be the most important means by which to counteract filtration. In a tissue with moderate distensibility and a relatively impermeable microvascular barrier, such as skin, the fall in interstitial COP assumes more importance in protecting against interstitial fluid accumulation. In a distensible tissue that is quite permeable to protein, such as the lung, increased lymph flow appears to be the most important safeguard against interstitial oedema.

Because of this marked heterogeneity in Starling forces and transvascular fluid dynamics between tissues, it is a potentially dangerous oversimplification to view the body as the homogenous sum of its individual parts. A great deal of emphasis has been placed on the manipulation of individual Starling forces in isolation, such as the intravascular COP with the use of colloid fluids, rather than addressing the system in its entirety. The effects of this manipulation on different tissues and organ systems should be carefully considered, especially if microvascular permeability is likely to be increased. If the increase in microvascular permeability is sufficient to allow significant extravasation of colloid, then administration of colloid may not be an effective way of increasing intravascular COP. If a COP gradient cannot be maintained between the intravascular and interstitial spaces then the capillary hydrostatic pressure becomes the major determinant of fluid extravasation. Smaller rises in capillary hydrostatic pressure will result in much greater fluid extravasation than when the endothelium remains intact. From a clinical standpoint, the differences between transvascular fluid flux in the lungs compared to the systemic circulation are the most important.

Control of extracellular volume and concentration

Extracellular fluid homeostasis in the normal animal is controlled by two distinct, but intertwined, feedback loops. One system acts to maintain the concentration, or osmolality, of the body and one regulates the volume of the extracellular fluid. No distinction is made between intravascular fluid and interstitial fluid because the capillary membrane is extremely permeable to water and small solutes.

Osmolality is controlled by hypothalamic osmoreceptors that stimulate thirst and the release of antidiuretic hormone (ADH) from the neurohypophysis. If net water loss from the body exceeds net water gain, plasma osmolality will rise and hypothalamic osmoreceptors then stimulate thirst and release of ADH. The augmented water intake and increased reabsorption of water by the kidney combine to decrease plasma osmolality towards normal. Fluctuations in plasma osmolality necessary to stimulate thirst and ADH release are very small (approximately 4 mOsm/kg in the dog, i.e. an increase in plasma sodium concentration of only 2 mmol/l).

Extracellular volume is primarily dependent upon total body sodium content controlled by the renin–angiotensin–aldosterone system and modulated by the natriuretic peptides. Sympathetic discharge and decrease in stretch of renal afferent arterioles stimulate renin release from the juxtaglomerular cells. Renin activates angiotensinogen to angiotensin I which is then converted to angiotensin II. Sodium and water reabsorption is increased by angiotensin II in the proximal tubule and angiotensin II-mediated aldosterone release promotes distal tubular sodium reabsorption.

The feedback loops controlling extracellular volume and osmolality overlap as they can both cause ADH release and thirst. The latter is mediated, at least in part, by angiotensin II. During hypovolaemia, the renin–angiotensin–aldosterone system, ADH and thirst act to increase retention of sodium and water and to expand extracellular volume. In summary, the concentration of the extracellular fluid is controlled primarily via modulation of water balance, whereas the volume of the extracellular fluid is regulated by changes in sodium and water balance.

Maintenance of arterial blood pressure

With acute or severe reductions in effective circulating blood volume, the body reacts to maintain arterial blood pressure and effective circulating blood volume to the heart, lungs and brain. With mild to moderate degrees of hypovolaemia, baroreceptor reflexes initiate sympathetic discharge, causing an increase in heart rate and cardiac contractility and, to a lesser degree, vasoconstriction. This is the so-called 'compensatory' or 'hyperdynamic' phase of hypovolaemia, when mean arterial blood pressure is maintained. After moderate reductions in blood volume, cardiac compensatory mechanisms are insufficient but vasoconstriction in the peripheral and splanchnic circulation increases to maintain arterial blood pressure; although there is partial compensation with maintenance of blood flow to vital organs, this stage of moderate hypovolaemia is associated with poor perfusion to some organs notably the gastrointestinal (GI) tract. Ultimately after severe reductions in blood volume, despite a maximum response from counter-regulatory mechanisms, progressively falling blood volume results in a fall in arterial blood pressure, the so-called 'decompensatory' or 'hypodynamic' phase of hypovolaemia.

Pathophysiology of abnormal fluid losses

In a normal animal, fluid is lost in urine and faeces and via evaporation from the respiratory tract. Abnormal losses include: vomiting and diarrhoea; polyuria; increased body temperature and panting; bleeding; wound exudation; loss from chest or abdominal drainage tubes; and loss into the interstitium or body cavities (often called 'third spacing'). The effect of fluid loss on intravascular volume depends upon the magnitude of the loss, and on the water shifts that occur between the extra- and intracellular spaces as a result of changes in extracellular fluid concentration. These water shifts depend upon the tonicity (concentration) of the extracellular fluid lost relative to the intracellular fluid.

Loss of pure water or hypotonic fluid causes the extracellular fluid to become more concentrated compared to the intracellular space. Water moves out of cells thereby supporting extracellular (and therefore intravascular) volume (Figure 4.2). This type of fluid loss is uncommon but occurs for example in animals that produce large volumes of hyposthenuric urine because of diabetes insipidus. The fluid loss is distributed over the total body water and intravascular depletion is a small proportion of the total loss. With loss of isotonic fluid (for example, with bleeding or in animals with surface losses through burn or bite wounds) no water movements occur because there is no change in extracellular concentration to create an osmotic gradient.

With hypertonic fluid loss, the extracellular space becomes hypotonic relative to the intracellular space and water moves into cells, exacerbating the extracellular fluid deficit and hypovolaemia (Figure 4.3). The very acute and severe haemoconcentration and hypovolaemia seen in haemorrhagic gastroenteritis in dogs is an example of hypertonic fluid loss, ostensibly due to a secretory diarrhoea.

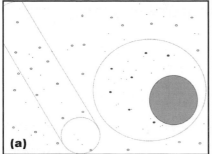
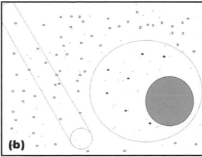
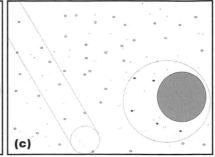

4.2 **(a)** Normal fluid volumes and concentration. The major extracellular cation is sodium (○) and the major intracellular cation is potassium (●). Small dots represent water molecules. **(b)** Hypotonic fluid loss results in a reduced plasma volume and increased concentration of the extracellular fluid. An osmotic gradient exists which favours the movement of water from the intracellular to the extracellular space. **(c)** Water moves out of the cells to buffer the reduction in extracellular fluid, thereby supporting the intravascular volume.

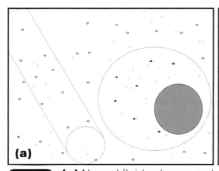
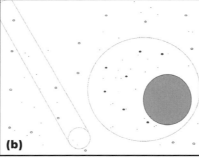
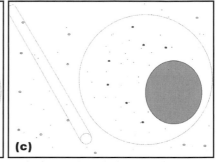

4.3 **(a)** Normal fluid volumes and concentration. **(b)** Hypertonic fluid loss results in a reduced plasma volume and a reduced concentration of the extracellular fluid. An osmotic gradient exists which favours the movement of water into cells from the extracellular space. **(c)** Water movement into the cells exacerbates the reduction in intravascular volume.

To illustrate the effects of fluid loss on intravascular volume status, consider a dog with dehydration due to water restriction alone. Dehydration of 12% of body weight would imply a free water deficit of 120 ml/kg. As water moves freely across cell membranes, this loss would be shared equally between the intravascular, interstitial and intracellular fluid compartments. Assuming that the free water deficit is distributed between these compartments on the basis of their relative size (i.e. 1:3:8 or 5, 15 and 40% of body weight, respectively; see Figure 4.1), one twelfth of the fluid loss would be borne by the intravascular compartment. This would result in a decrease in intravascular volume of approximately 10 ml/kg; an amount comparable to the volume of blood normally removed from a canine blood donor, usually with few or no untoward effects. Conversely, with loss solely from the intravascular space, i.e. haemorrhage, loss of 5% of body weight (i.e. 50 ml/kg or more than 50% of the blood volume) would result in clinical signs of severe hypovolaemia.

Approach to fluid therapy in the clinical patient

The approach to fluid therapy suggested by DiBartola (1992) is helpful when deciding upon a fluid therapy plan.

- Does the animal require fluid therapy?
- What type or types of fluid should be given?
- Which route should be used?
- How much should be given?

- Over what time period should it be administered?
- For how long should therapy be continued?

Careful consideration of the first question with critical evaluation of whether the animal requires fluid therapy to treat hypoperfusion, to treat dehydration, or for maintenance purposes (or some combination of those three) will allow the subsequent questions to be answered and the fluid therapy plan to be tailored to that patient's needs. As hypoperfusion represents an imminently life-threatening situation for the patient, abnormalities of perfusion should *always* be corrected prior to considering the longer-term fluid requirements.

Does the animal require fluid therapy?

Clinical assessment of perfusion status
The perfusion status of the animal should be assessed using: mucous membrane colour; capillary refill time (CRT) and vigour; pulse profile (height and width); heart rate and cardiac auscultation. In uncomplicated hypovolaemia in dogs, the clinical perfusion parameters tend to change in a relatively predictable manner (Figure 4.4). A normal animal should have pink mucous membranes with a vigorous capillary refill which takes 1–1.75 seconds. A 2-second CRT is often prolonged in the setting of a veterinary clinic. Pulses (femoral and metatarsal) should be carefully palpated to allow assessment of both the height or amplitude (to estimate pulse pressure) and the width or duration of the pulse. Assessment of both the height and width of the pulse

Clinical sign	Mild (compensatory)	Moderate	Severe (decompensatory)
Heart rate	130–150 bpm	150–170 bpm	170–220 bpm
Mucous membrane colour	Normal to pinker than normal	Pale pink	White, grey or muddy
Capillary refill	Vigorous, <1 second	Reduced vigour, 2 seconds	>2 seconds or absent
Pulse amplitude	Increase	Moderate decrease	Severe decrease
Pulse duration	Mild decrease	Moderate decrease	Severe decrease
Metatarsal pulse	Easily palpable	Just palpable	Absent

4.4 Guidelines for the clinical assessment of uncomplicated hypovolaemia in the dog.

allows estimation of pulse volume and, with careful palpation, a perceptive clinician can generate a mental image of the pulse profile (Figure 4.5). An awareness of the normal pulse profile facilitates a meaningful assessment of changes in pulse profile in sick patients. A normovolaemic animal which is stressed or in pain will have a slightly taller and narrower pulse profile than a resting animal. The vast majority of unstressed dogs have a heart rate of 80–120 beats per minute (bpm) in the setting of an emergency clinic. The effect of body size on heart rate has been somewhat overemphasized in the veterinary literature.

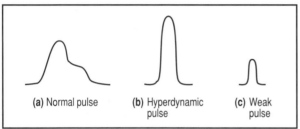

(a) Normal pulse   **(b)** Hyperdynamic pulse   **(c)** Weak pulse

4.5 Pulse profiles from direct arterial pressure measurement. Assessing the height and width of the pulse together allows an estimation of pulse volume.

Clinical assessment of perfusion in cats is more challenging. Normal heart rate in cats usually varies from 170–200 bpm in the veterinary clinic, although this probably represents a moderate tachycardia compared to resting heart rate at home. Mucous membranes in normal cats are significantly paler than in dogs and, although it is possible, it is much more difficult to appreciate the pulse profile in a cat. Critically ill feline patients also tend to develop an inappropriate bradycardia (heart rate in the 130–150 bpm range) despite the presence of hypovolaemic or distributive shock, further complicating their assessment.

In the compensatory stages of uncomplicated hypovolaemia, dogs develop a moderate tachycardia of 130–150 bpm. This increase in rate along with the reduced blood volume and increase in cardiac contractility produces a pulse which is narrower and taller than normal (Figure 4.5b). This pulse will also be narrower than the pulse profile of a normovolaemic dog with tachycardia secondary to stress/exercise or pain. This pulse profile is often referred to as 'bounding' or 'snappy', but these terms often serve to confuse rather than clarify. In compensatory hypovolaemia, metatarsal pulses should still be palpable. Mucous membranes should be pink to pinker than normal with a rapid CRT of less than 1 second duration.

The increases in heart rate seen in dogs with hypovolaemia are surprisingly independent of body weight, such that severe hypovolaemia results in a heart rate of 170–220 regardless of size. Heart rates in excess of this range should raise suspicions of a primary dysrhythmia rather than a physiological sinus tachycardia in response to hypovolaemia. Heart sounds are often quiet when there is severe hypovolaemia. Mucous membranes have little or no red colouration (white, muddy or grey) and the CRT is prolonged or absent. Femoral pulses are extremely weak (Figure 4.5c) (sometimes referred to as 'thready') and metatarsal pulses are not palpable. While clinically assessing perfusion, the findings should be continually cross-referenced. For example, in a recumbent patient with very weak femoral pulses, pale mucous membranes and a prolonged CRT, the heart rate should be approximately 180–220 bpm. An inappropriately low heart rate should prompt a search for the underlying reason, such as hyperkalaemia associated with postrenal, renal or endocrine causes.

Lactate

Tissue hypoperfusion results in increased lactate production and decreased lactate clearance, and blood lactate concentration can be used to assess the severity of hypovolaemia. The reference value for plasma lactate concentration in normal dogs by direct amperometry is <2.5 mmol/l, irrespective of sample site. A blood lactate concentration in the range of 3–4 mmol/l constitutes a mild increase, 4–7 mmol/l is a moderate increase and >7 mmol/l represents a severe increase. Clinical experience suggests that lactate concentration accurately reflects the degree of uncomplicated hypovolaemia in dogs. Furthermore, plasma lactate concentrations almost invariably fall with successful fluid resuscitation and can be used to guide fluid therapy. Failure of plasma lactate concentration to normalize following fluid resuscitation suggests ongoing systemic hypoperfusion or an occult source of lactate production. Lactate can also be used as a prognostic indicator. In one of the landmark studies in people, as lactate concentration increased from 2.1 to 8.0 mmol/l, survival decreased from 90% to 10%. Experimental evidence and clinical experience suggest that similar results will be obtained in canine patients. If plasma lactate concentration fails to fall following an appropriate fluid challenge, or if a significant and sustained rise in plasma lactate concentration occurs, the prognosis for survival appears to be grave.

Clinical assessment of hydration status

The widely accepted method for determining hydration status involves assessing the moisture of the gums and cornea, skin turgor, presence or absence of retraction of the globe, and perfusion parameters (Figure 4.6). Dryness of the mucous membranes alone is said to reflect dehydration equivalent to 5% of the body weight, and >12% dehydration may represent a fluid loss sufficient to cause overt signs of mild to moderate hypovolaemic shock. Interestingly, there is little or no scientific evidence supporting this. When one considers the variable effect on intravascular volume depending upon the tonicity of fluid losses and the compartments from which the loss occurs, it is apparent that this scheme allows only a rough approximation of fluid deficits. Body weight represents the only easily available, reasonably accurate way of assessing the severity of dehydration, but is rarely relevant immediately following admission as few patients have a known accurate body weight from the time immediately before their illness started. Body weight can however be used as a monitoring tool; dehydrated patients should gain weight following appropriate fluid therapy.

The classic scheme will tend to underestimate losses when free water is lost in excess of solute and to overestimate losses of hypertonic fluid. A clinical study performed over 25 years ago (Hardy and Osborne, 1979) found that the clinical signs of dehydration due to free water loss were extremely unpredictable. Of the 20 dogs that were deprived of water for periods ranging from 2–4 days, 10 showed no clinical signs of dehydration and no dogs exhibited dry mucous membranes or dry or sunken eyes. One dog deprived of water for 4 days lost 16% of its body weight, showed no change in skin turgor, had no change in its packed cell volume and a minimal change in total protein concentration.

Despite the limitations of the classic scheme for assessing fluid requirements, it nevertheless provides a tried and tested starting point on which to base fluid replacement therapy. The tendency to underestimate replacement requirements in animals with greater free water loss may actually be appropriate, because these losses tend to be chronic and require more gradual replacement. This scheme should not be used when an animal is showing signs of hypoperfusion; in that situation fluid therapy should be aimed at rapid intravascular volume replacement.

Types of parenteral fluid

Fluids should not be regarded as a single entity; rather, they are a range of pharmacological products each with its own indications and contraindications, much like the choice of antibiotics for different infections or the selection of heart medications for different types of heart disease. Knowledge of the underlying disease processes and assessment of fluid deficits will help to determine the most appropriate fluid. There are three main groups of fluids:

- Crystalloids
- Colloids
- Blood products.

Crystalloids are electrolyte solutions that can pass freely out of the vascular space, whereas colloids contain macromolecules that are retained within the vascular space for a longer time period. Blood products (including haemoglobin solutions) are covered in more detail in Chapter 14.

Crystalloids

Crystalloid fluids can be hypotonic, isotonic or hypertonic (Figure 4.7) compared to extracellular (and therefore intracellular) fluid. The tonicity of the solution will determine its distribution following intravenous infusion (Figure 4.8).

Clinical signs		Dehydration estimate (% of body weight)
Normal		<5%
Dry mucous membranes only		5%
Reduced skin turgor	Mild	6–8%
Increased heart rate	Moderate	8–10%
Weak pulses	Severe	10–12%
Collapse, shock		12–15%

4.6 Guidelines for the clinical assessment of dehydration.

Name of fluid	Description of fluid (*in vivo* tonicity)	Na+ (mmol/l)	K+ (mmol/l)	Cl− (mmol/l)	Ca2+ (mmol/l)	Osmolality (mOsm/l)	pH
Hartmann's (lactated Ringer's) solution	Isotonic replacement	131	5	111	2	272	6.5
NaCl 0.9%	Isotonic replacement	150	0	150	0	308	5
Ringer's solution	Isotonic replacement	147	4	155.5	2.25	310	5.5
NaCl 0.9% + Glucose 5%	Isotonic replacement	150	0	150	0	560	4
NaCl 0.45%	Hypotonic	77	0	77	0	154	
NaCl 0.18% + 4% glucose	Hypotonic	30	0	30	0		
Glucose 5%	Hypotonic	0	0	0	0	252	
NaCl 7.2%	Hypertonic	1232	0	1232	0	~2400	
Plasma-lyte M	Maintenance	40	16	40	2.5		

4.7 Composition of crystalloid fluids for intravenous administration.

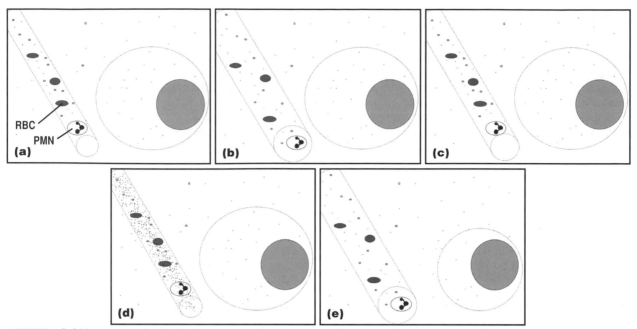

4.8 **(a)** Hypovolaemic shock. Large open dots represent albumin molecules and small dots represent small solutes. **(b)** Intravascular expansion during infusion of isotonic crystalloid. There is no concentration gradient change between the intracellular and extracellular space. **(c)** Intravascular expansion with isotonic crystalloid. Intravascular crystalloid equilibrates with the interstitial space and intravascular volume falls compared to the initial volume of expansion. **(d)** Intravascular expansion following hypertonic crystalloid results in a large increase in intravascular sodium concentration and a large osmotic gradient for water flow into the vasculature. **(e)** Intravascular expansion following hypertonic crystalloid. Water passes into the intravascular space from the interstitial and intracellular compartments, producing a rapid, but transient, expansion of intravascular volume.

Isotonic solutions

Isotonic replacement crystalloid solutions are the most familiar and frequently used fluid group in small animal veterinary medicine. They are tremendously versatile fluids and can be used (at different rates) to treat both hypovolaemia and dehydration, and to support the patient with ongoing losses. The most widely available isotonic replacement fluids are normal (0.9%) saline, Ringer's solution and Hartmann's solution (lactated Ringer's solution). When used to treat hypovolaemia, there is no concentration gradient change between the intracellular and extracellular spaces, therefore water shifts do not occur across the cell membrane (Figure 4.8c). Intravascular crystalloid equilibrates with the interstitial space, with 20–25% of the infused volume remaining within the intravascular space 1 hour following infusion.

Isotonic replacement crystalloids have an electrolyte composition similar to extracellular fluid, with a relatively high sodium and low (or zero) potassium concentration (Figure 4.7). Consequently when used for longer-term fluid therapy, there is a tendency for patients to develop hypokalaemia and have a mild increase in their serum sodium. Whilst the change in sodium is rarely of clinical significance, if the patient has limited intake of potassium from other sources (e.g. is anorexic) the decrease in serum potassium may be significant. Supplementation of the intravenous fluids with potassium should be considered once acute volume deficits have been replaced (see Chapter 5).

Alternatively, isotonic maintenance fluids can be used. These fluids have an electrolyte composition that more closely mimics the electrolytes lost due to insensible causes in a healthy animal. As these fluids have a relatively high potassium concentration (Figure 4.7), they must only be used at slow 'maintenance' rates (e.g. 2 ml/kg/h). Due to their lack of versatility and the small number of patients for which their use is indicated, they are rarely used in veterinary practice.

Hypertonic saline

Hypertonic saline is most commonly supplied at a concentration of 7.2–7.5% which, at 2400 mOsm/l, is more than eight times the concentration of plasma. A dosage of 4–7 ml/kg (dogs) or 2–4 ml/kg (cats) is given over 2–5 minutes, and produces a haemodynamic response similar to that of an isotonic crystalloid dose of 60–90 ml/kg. Intravenous infusion of hypertonic crystalloid creates a large osmotic gradient (Figure 4.8d) and water is drawn from the interstitial and intracellular compartments producing a rapid expansion of intravascular volume (Figure 4.8e).

However, as the sodium rapidly diffuses out of the vasculature, the effects can begin to wane in as little as 30 minutes following infusion. To prolong the duration of effect, hypertonic saline is often constituted with a colloid such as dextran 70 or hetastarch.

Hypertonic solutions have been reported to be safe and effective for the treatment of hypotension in experimental studies in a wide range of species including dogs and cats. When compared with crystalloid solutions alone, many potential benefits have been demonstrated, including:

- A greater, more rapid and sustained restoration of arterial blood pressure
- More rapid, greater and more sustained increment in plasma volume

- Increased cardiac contractility
- Greater and more sustained increment in cardiac output
- Improved oxygen delivery and oxygen consumption
- Improved organ blood flow
- Lower intracranial pressure post resuscitation
- Improved survival in certain studies
- Lower total volumes of resuscitation fluids required
- Reduction in time taken for resuscitation
- Inexpensive.

Indications: Hypertonic saline is extremely useful when rapid intravascular volume expansion is required, such as the occasional case of severe hypovolaemia when death is imminent. It is also useful in large-breed dogs and in hypovolaemic animals in which inappropriately small intravenous catheters have been placed. A combination of hypertonic saline and iso- or hyperoncotic colloid appears to be the most appropriate fluid for intravascular volume expansion in the patient at risk for increased intracranial pressure, such as with head trauma. This combination appears to provide the best compromise between improving the arterial blood pressure and minimizing the increase in intracranial pressure, i.e. optimizing cerebral perfusion pressure.

Contraindications

Dehydration and hyperosmolality: Animals suffering from dehydration do not have a normal reservoir of interstitial and intracellular fluid for mobilization following infusion of hypertonic saline. Some studies have documented a higher mortality with use of this product in dehydrated as opposed to euhydrated animals. Similarly, use of hypertonic saline may be contraindicated in animals with hypernatraemia or other hyperosmolal states.

Volume overload: Hypertonic resuscitation has been referred to as small volume resuscitation. Unfortunately, this has led to the mistaken assumption that the magnitude of volume expansion is also small. Volume expansion with hypertonic saline is a very rapid and aggressive method of fluid resuscitation irrespective of the small volume infused. It should be avoided or used with extreme caution in patients in which aggressive volume expansion would be dangerous, such as patients with heart or lung disease. In the authors' experience, it can also cause ventricular dysrhythmias, especially when given rapidly, therefore an electrocardiogram should be monitored during infusion of hypertonic saline.

Uncontrolled haemorrhage: Experimental evidence and clinical experience support the view that aggressive volume expansion in patients with uncontrolled haemorrhage is associated with a higher mortality rate. This is probably due to an increase in the volume of haemorrhage and loss of red blood cells, platelets and clotting factors following aggressive volume expansion. However, there are also studies documenting increased mortality following hypertonic saline resuscitation, even

after changes in blood pressure and volume of haemorrhage are taken into account. The most common situation in which uncontrolled haemorrhage is encountered in clinical small animal practice is following road traffic accidents. Intra-abdominal haemorrhage and pulmonary contusions are the most common sites of bleeding. Notably, pulmonary bleeding appears to be exquisitely sensitive to volume expansion. Aggressive fluid resuscitation, such as with hypertonic saline, almost always worsens pulmonary bleeding and the authors consider the use of hypertonic saline, or any form of aggressive volume expansion, to be contraindicated in this patient population.

Hypotonic solutions

Hypotonic solutions include:

- 5% glucose (D5W)
- 0.18% NaCl + 4% glucose
- 0.45% NaCl.

Although the osmolality of 5% glucose solution is 252 mOsm/l (and thus in the fluid bag it is close to being isotonic), once administered to the patient, the glucose is rapidly taken up by cells and metabolized. Administering glucose solutions is therefore tantamount to giving free water (i.e. water without associated solute). Free water rapidly passes out of the intravascular space and distributes across the total body water, thus it is an ineffective intravascular volume expander and should not be used for the treatment of hypoperfusion. Furthermore, rapid infusion of hypotonic solutions can cause severe dilution of serum electrolytes, especially sodium, and result in acute cerebral oedema and death. Although there are rare uses for hypotonic fluids (e.g. in patients with severe hypernatraemia), their use is contraindicated in most situations.

Artificial colloids

The basis for the use of colloids for volume expansion, as opposed to crystalloids, is that they are retained in the intravascular space to a greater degree than crystalloids and are therefore more efficient in maintaining intravascular volume. As long as microvascular permeability is normal, colloids will also maintain the intravascular COP and the COP gradient between the intravascular and interstitial spaces, thereby reducing the rate of fluid efflux from the vasculature. There is some evidence that microvascular perfusion may be better following colloid infusion compared to infusion of physiologically equivalent volumes of crystalloid. Despite these advantages, it is very important to maintain perspective when assessing the need for colloid therapy. Colloids are not a panacea; rather, they are one more group of drugs with specific indications, contraindications, benefits and risks. Two meta-analyses (Velanovich, 1989; Schierhout and Roberts, 1998) documented a higher overall mortality in human patients treated with colloids compared to crystalloids. The limitations of meta-analyses notwithstanding, one study demonstrated a 12.3% difference in mortality rate in favour of crystalloid therapy in human trauma patients. Another study showed a

7.8% difference in mortality rate in favour of colloids when data from studies that used human non-trauma patients were pooled. One of the most interesting conclusions was that colloid therapy appeared to be deleterious in patients with sepsis, capillary leak syndrome and adult respiratory distress syndrome following trauma.

There are three common types of artificial colloid: the gelatins, the dextrans and the hydroxyethyl starches (Figure 4.9). Gelatins are produced from mammalian collagen, whereas dextrans are prepared from a macromolecular polysaccharide produced from bacterial fermentation of sucrose. Hydroxyethyl starches are derived from amylopectin (the branched form of plant starch). The parent mixtures of macromolecules are separated into fractions according to molecular weight. Artificial colloids contain a mixture of molecules of varying weights (i.e. are polydisperse), with the hydroxyethyl starches having a much wider range of molecular weights than dextran 70 or the gelatins. Albumin, by comparison, is a monodisperse colloid, with molecules that are all the same size (molecular weight 69 kD, molecular radius 3.5 nm). An average molecular weight of 100–300 kD would seem to be ideal, providing the best compromise between colloid osmotic volume expansion and duration of action. Mean molecular weights of the commonly available colloids are shown in Figure 4.9. In addition to their weight, hydroxyethyl starches are also described by their degree of molar substitution. To reduce intravascular hydrolysis of the hydroxyethyl starch by amylase, the amylopectin may be hydroxyethylated at carbons 2, 3 and 6. The number of hydroxyethyl groups per glucose unit is defined as the molar substitution ratio. The pattern of substitution varies depending upon the synthetic process. Substitution at the carbon 2 position is more effective at reducing intravascular hydrolysis than hydroxyethylation at the other positions. Hydroxyethyl starches can therefore be described on the basis of their average molecular weight, degree of substitution and C2/C6 hydroxyethylation ratio. These factors can be used to predict their intravascular persistence and their potential effect on coagulation (see below).

The effect (both magnitude and duration of action) of colloids may be measured in several ways, including assessment of plasma colloid concentrations, plasma colloid osmotic pressure (COP) and intravascular volume expansion. These parameters do not change in an identical way following infusion of a colloid. The initial volume of intravascular expansion is due to the osmotic pressure of the infused colloid, which is determined by the number of molecules and not their size. Smaller molecules, which are responsible for a large part of the COP and intravascular volume expansion, are excreted or extravasated within hours. The larger molecules remain in circulation and are enzymatically degraded or removed by the monocyte phagocytic system. The rapid initial excretion of small, osmotically active molecules, followed by a gradual elimination of large molecules, results in an exponential decline in intravascular expansion and a narrowing of the distribution of molecular weights. Because the larger molecules persist longer than the smaller ones, the concentration (i.e. the mass per unit volume) will remain high; however, as the total number of molecules decreases very quickly, the COP will decrease more rapidly. In summary, the COP and degree of volume expansion tend to fall faster than the plasma concentration of colloid. Studies that report the pattern of volume expansion are therefore most applicable to the clinical situation.

Many factors influence the volume and duration of intravascular expansion associated with artificial colloids, including the species of animal, the dosage, the specific colloid formulation, the pre-infusion intravascular volume status and the microvascular permeability. It should be apparent that data from an experimental study in normovolaemic human volunteers given twice the usual dose of a low molecular weight form of hydroxyethyl starch may have little bearing on the effects of high molecular weight hetastarch in a dog with SIRS that is in hypodynamic septic shock.

Most studies have been performed using high molecular weight hetastarch or dextran 70. Estimates of the initial plasma volume expansion for hetastarch and dextran 70 vary from 70 to 170% of the infused

Type of colloid	Fluid name	Mean molecular weight (kD)	Degree of molar substitution	COP (mmHg)	Na⁺ (mmol/l)
Gelatin	Haemaccel®	30	–	~30	145
Gelatin	Gelofusin®	35	–	~25	154
Dextran	Dextran 70	70	–	62	150
Hydroxyethyl starch	Hetastarch 6% in 0.9% NaCl	450	0.7	33	154
Hydroxyethyl starch	Pentastarch 6% in 0.9% NaCl	200	0.5	36	154
Hydroxyethyl starch	Tetrastarch Voluven® (6% in 0.9% NaCl)	130	0.4	~30	154
Human serum albumin	Zenalb® (20%)	69	–	>200	50–120
Polymerized haemoglobin	Oxyglobin®	65–500	–	43	

4.9 Description of colloid fluids. It should be noted that Haemaccel also contains calcium and must not be administered with blood products. A 10% solution of Pentastarch (HAES-steril®) is also available.

volume, which falls to approximately 50% of the infused volume after 6 hours. Over the next 12–18 hours, the intravascular expansion seen with hydroxyethyl starch declines gradually from 60 to 40% of the infused volume, whereas with dextran 70, it falls from 40 to 20% of the infused volume. In the authors' experience, the duration of volume expansion using artificial colloids may be even shorter than these estimates, especially when administered to patients with capillary leak syndromes. In one study of dogs with hypoalbuminaemia of varying causes receiving hydroxyethyl starch, COP was not significantly different from baseline 12 hours post infusion (Moore and Garvey, 1996). Gelatins have a shorter duration of action than the other colloids because of their smaller molecular size. Following infusion over a 90-minute period, intravascular expansion with polygeline was only 24% of the infused volume. For comparison, on average 20–25% of the infused volume of crystalloid remains in the intravascular space 1 hour following infusion. As colloids are frequently used in the most critical patients when it may be impossible to predict the degree of effect, it is vital that all patients are monitored to evaluate the clinical effect of the dose and product chosen in that patient.

Indications

Volume expansion: Colloids are a very efficient means of intravascular volume expansion. They are especially useful in disease states that are associated with an increase in microvascular permeability (e.g. SIRS, sepsis), provided that the increase in permeability is not sufficient to allow significant extravasation of colloid. Because the osmotic effect of the colloid macromolecules is due to their number rather than their size, if more than 50% of the molecules leak into the interstitium, then there could theoretically be a net reduction in intravascular volume and a worsening of interstitial oedema as water leaves the intravascular space along with colloid. The dilemma therefore becomes the estimation of the increase in capillary permeability, i.e. the size of the 'gaps' in the microvascular barrier. A growing body of evidence suggests that hydroxyethyl starches can reduce the increases in microvascular permeability seen in several capillary leak states. The optimal molecular weight for this effect appears to be between 100 and 300 kD.

Hypoproteinaemia: Although colloid fluids may be considered for use in hypoproteinaemic patients with the aim of raising COP, the rapidity of onset of the hypoproteinaemia and the clinical consequences in the patient should always be carefully considered. It is extremely important to bear in mind that the effective COP acting to retain fluid within the intravascular space is the net difference between the intravascular and interstitial COP. As intravascular COP falls, fluid with a lower COP will pass from the vasculature and dilute the interstitial protein concentration such that the interstitial COP will also fall. Consequently with chronic disease, the gradient between intravascular and interstitial COP will be preserved. This means that a low plasma COP per se does not necessitate colloid therapy in the absence of clinical signs such as

hypovolaemia or oedema, and as long as crystalloid fluids, which may further decrease COP, are not being administered. Indeed, people with a hereditary form of complete albumin deficiency have a plasma COP which is still half of normal due to elevated globulin levels, and affected individuals exhibit minimal peripheral oedema. There also appear to be no serious clinical signs in an autosomal recessive, hereditary albumin deficiency reported in rats. Interestingly, the affected rats exhibit marked hypercholesterolaemia as is also seen in protein-losing nephropathy with nephrotic syndrome in dogs. In the authors' clinical experience and in experimental studies, animals with severe hypoproteinaemia (COP <11 mmHg) may exhibit peripheral oedema but rarely develop pulmonary oedema. In dogs with hypoalbuminaemia, hydroxyethyl starch has been shown to result in short-term clinical improvement of peripheral oedema or ascites (Smiley and Garvey, 1994). It is more important to diagnose and treat the cause of the hypoproteinaemia, rather than to administer palliative colloid therapy, which is unlikely to be successful for more than a few hours if the underlying cause is not corrected.

Contraindications and side effects

Coagulopathy: Deleterious effects on coagulation can occur when hydroxyethyl starch or dextran are administered at doses above 20 ml/kg/day. The important question is whether these coagulopathies are clinically significant. Some studies suggest that clinically significant haemorrhage does not occur; however, there is also clinical and experimental evidence suggesting occasional serious, potentially life-threatening bleeding. This paradox means simply that the coagulation abnormalities are only clinically significant in some cases. Clinical experience suggests that bleeding complications are relatively uncommon in veterinary patients. The effects on coagulation appear to be directly related to the intravascular concentration of artificial colloid. Higher plasma concentrations of colloid may occur following larger doses, repeated administration or reduced intravascular degradation. Larger colloid molecules have a greater effect on coagulation than small molecules. With repeated administration, the small molecules are constantly excreted and the relative concentration of larger molecules increases. This explains why many studies reporting clinically significant bleeding refer to patients who received repeated administration over a period of days.

The exact mechanism of action by which coagulation is affected is still not fully understood. The most repeatable findings are a reduction in factor VIII and von Willebrand factor (greater than expected by dilution alone) and weakened clot formation. Desmopressin has been shown to increase factor VIII:C activity following hydroxyethyl starch infusion, and should be considered as an adjunct to fresh frozen plasma administration in high-risk patients. Colloid molecules may reduce the action of endothelial adhesion molecules thereby reducing endothelial release of von Willebrand factor as well as affecting other leucocyte– and platelet–endothelial interactions.

Volume overload: Colloids are retained within the vasculature to a greater extent than crystalloids; therefore there is a greater likelihood of volume overload with injudicious administration. Most clinicians are more familiar with crystalloid infusion rates, so a helpful method to ensure a safe colloid infusion rate is to estimate the equivalent crystalloid rate. Approximately 20–25% of crystalloid remains within the intravascular space 1 hour after infusion, compared to approximately 100% of the volume of infused colloid, therefore multiplying the colloid infusion rate by four allows one to conceptualize the volume expanding effects of the colloid in terms of an equivalent crystalloid volume. While this approach can be helpful to limit excessive infusion rates, when using colloids in patients with cardiac or pulmonary disease or oliguria, direct monitoring of central venous pressure is warranted.

Renal failure: The low molecular weight dextrans such as dextran 40 have been reported to cause renal failure. Glomerular filtration of a high concentration of small dextran molecules is postulated to cause blockage of the renal tubules and/or osmotic nephrosis. Because the major route of excretion for all artificial colloids is via the kidneys, they should be used with caution in patients with oliguric or anuric renal failure. In contrast, for those patients with oliguria due to hypovolaemia and hypotension, colloids may provide the most effective means of intravascular volume expansion.

Allergic reactions and reticuloendothelial dysfunction: Anaphylactic or anaphylactoid reactions have been reported for dextrans, hydroxyethyl starches and gelatins; however, the incidence of serious complications is extremely low. Hydroxyethyl starch has been associated with pruritus in up to one third of people treated with long-term infusions. Deposits of hydroxyethyl starch in cutaneous nerves and histiocytic skin infiltrates are thought to be responsible. Interestingly, pruritus has also been reported following infusion of lactated Ringer's solution. Several studies have raised concerns regarding the potential effects of plasma substitutes on reticuloendothelial function. Decreased concentrations of the opsonic plasma factor, fibronectin, have also been reported. These appear to be most significant with the artificial gelatins but have also been noted with hydroxyethyl starch.

Interference with clinical biochemistry: The use of refractometric total solids (TS) as a convenient and cheap way to assess total protein concentrations and estimate COP is no longer valid once an artificial colloid has been administered. High molecular weight hydroxyethyl starch and dextran 70 both yield refractometric TS of 45 g/l. As plasma volume is replaced by artificial colloid, theoretically the measured refractometric TS should tend towards that of the artificial colloid. In clinical patients, administering artificial colloid to an animal with an initial TS >45 g/l will tend to reduce the measured TS despite the fact that it will lead to an increase in COP. However it is rare that administration of artificial colloid will cause a significant increase in TS if the initial TS is <45 g/l. Failure to appreciate the effect of artificial colloid on refractometric TS can lead the clinician to misinterpret a fall in TS as an indication for more colloid. Because assays for serum colloid concentrations are not readily available, therapy with artificial colloids is best monitored by direct measurement of COP using a membrane osmometer.

The intravascular expansion due to colloid infusion results in significant dilutional effects. Packed cell volume, albumin concentration and serum potassium concentration seem to be most affected. Serum amylase may be elevated to 200–250% of normal following administration of hydroxyethyl starch due to complex formation and reduced excretion. Hydroxyethyl starch can also produce predictable but potentially misleading results in blood typing and cross-matching, due to increased rouleaux formation.

Urine specific gravity (USG) should be interpreted with caution following colloid administration. As many of the colloid molecules are excreted through the kidneys and as USG is a measure of the weight of solutes in urine, the USG may increase without representing an increase in osmolality of the urine.

Natural colloids

Until recently, albumin has been administered to small animal patients only in veterinary transfusion products (see Chapter 14). However human serum albumin, obtained from purified human plasma, is available commercially and is now being used increasingly in small animal medicine. Albumin is a monodisperse colloid (i.e. all albumin molecules are the same size) with a molecular weight of approximately 69 kD and a molecular radius of 3.5 nm. In addition to its role in maintaining plasma COP, it also a carrier molecule with a wide range of substances being bound to it in plasma (e.g. bilirubin, fatty acids, metals and other ions, hormones and drugs). Albumin supplementation has been suggested in critically ill people because of its numerous important roles, and because serum albumin concentration has been shown to be an accurate prognostic indicator. The role of albumin in maintaining the selective permeability of the microvascular barrier to macromolecules provides another rationale for the prophylactic use of albumin. However, a recent trial in human medicine comparing resuscitation of critically ill patients with either albumin or saline found no significant differences in outcome between the groups for a number of variables, including 28-day outcome (Finfer *et al.*, 2004). Clinical data in veterinary species is limited at this time; one study reported that administration of human serum albumin to a heterogeneous population of critically ill dogs was associated with an effective increase in plasma albumin and COP with relatively few adverse effects (Chan *et al.*, 2004).

As human albumin is not biochemically identical to canine or feline albumin, patients should not receive multiple doses separated in time, as there is a risk of anaphylaxis. Since the albumin molecule is relatively small, when it is used as a volume expander it equilibrates with the interstitial space more rapidly and to a greater extent than the hydroxyethyl starches. Thus, relatively large volumes must be given to achieve a sustained increase in plasma albumin concentration. The amount of albumin required can be estimated using an equation which corrects for the expected volume of distribution across the intravascular and interstitial spaces:

Albumin deficit (g) = (desired albumin (g/l) − patient albumin (g/l)) x (body weight (kg) x 0.3)

Therefore, to raise the serum albumin from 15 to 25 g/l in a 20 kg dog:

Albumin deficit = (25 − 15) x (20 x 0.3) = 60 g

Commercially available albumin solutions are prepared as 0.2 g/ml (20%) or 0.25 g/ml (25%), therefore this dog would need to receive 240–300 ml of human serum albumin. Alternatively, if canine blood products were to be used instead, this would be equivalent to the amount of albumin in 2 l of plasma or 4 l of fresh whole blood. Typically infusion rates are based on the patient's response, but vary between 1.0 and 1.5 g/kg total dose given as a bolus over several hours, or continuous infusions of 0.2–1.0 ml/kg/h of 20 or 25% human serum albumin solution.

Volume, rate, duration and route of administration of fluid therapy

Acute intravenous fluid therapy to replace absolute or relative plasma volume deficits in a patient with hypoperfusion is a life-saving procedure that must be performed over minutes to hours. In contrast, chronic fluid therapy to re-establish and maintain normal water, electrolyte and acid–base balance, is not usually an emergency response and is planned and re-evaluated on a daily basis. It is vital that one clearly separates the doses and rates used for acute volume expansion from the rates used for chronic fluid therapy to ensure that life-threatening problems are corrected in a timely manner. In many situations there is more than one fluid type that could be used and the clinician must consider the relative indications and contraindications of each fluid in that particular patient.

It is also important to remember that all fluid therapy calculations are based on estimates. Successful fluid therapy relies on monitoring the patient closely to ensure that appropriate goals are being achieved, with adjustment of the plan if necessary. For all patients receiving fluid therapy, the clinician should ask 'What do I want the fluids to achieve in this patient?' and 'Are there contraindications to the use of any fluid groups in this patient?' Once these questions are answered, the clinician makes a decision on the initial type and dose/rate of fluid to be administered and the parameters to be monitored, both to check that the fluids are having the required effect and to ensure that no complications of fluid therapy develop. If the patient is not responding as expected, the clinician should re-evaluate the fluid plan, including both the type and rate of fluids.

Acute fluid therapy for the animal with perfusion abnormalities

To determine the appropriate fluid dosage, abnormalities of perfusion should be graded as to their severity (see Figure 4.4). A dose (ml/kg) of fluid should be chosen with the aim of restoring intravascular volume (and therefore perfusion parameters) to within normal limits. Considering isotonic crystalloids, a full 'shock' dose (bolus) of 60–90 ml/kg (dog) or 40–60 ml/kg (cat) should be given to patients showing signs of severe hypoperfusion. For patients with signs of moderate hypoperfusion, a 30–50 ml/kg bolus should be used (10–20 ml/kg in the cat) and for patients with signs of mild hypoperfusion a smaller bolus of 10–20 ml/kg (5–7 ml/kg in the cat) should be chosen. The fluid dose should be administered over a defined time frame (usually 1 hour), although in dogs with severe hypoperfusion it may be necessary to administer the dose more rapidly. At the end of the dose the patient's perfusion parameters should once again be assessed. If they are within normal limits, fluid therapy should continue to replace ongoing losses, with doses as outlined in the chronic fluid therapy plan described below. In contrast, if perfusion parameters are still abnormal, another fluid bolus should be given.

Prior to administering aggressive fluid therapy, a careful assessment should be made of possible reasons for the hypoperfusion and whether there are any contraindications to rapid fluid therapy. The vast majority of animals with poor perfusion have hypovolaemia, distributive shock (sepsis or other causes of SIRS) or less commonly cardiogenic shock (see Chapter 3). Fluids are essential in the treatment of both hypovolaemic and distributive shock but contraindicated in most animals with cardiogenic shock. Most animals with significant heart disease as a cause of their shock will have a murmur or gallop rhythm on cardiac auscultation. However, in patients with severe hypovolaemia, the heart sounds can be quiet, making it challenging to auscultate concurrent cardiac abnormalities. The major contraindications to aggressive fluid therapy are cardiac, respiratory or brain disease. Although anuric renal failure also warrants careful fluid therapy, it is impossible to confirm this diagnosis without an appropriate fluid challenge.

Fluids for acute intravascular volume replacement should always be given by the intravenous or intraosseous route. Flow rate through a catheter is proportional to the fourth power of the radius of the catheter, thus the largest bore possible should be used (see Chapter 2). It is often helpful to place two intravenous catheters to ensure that an adequate fluid volume can be administered and to provide a back-up if one catheter does not flow or becomes dislodged. In animals with severe hypoperfusion surgical venous cutdowns may be necessary to establish venous access (see Chapter 2).

Animals receiving intravenous fluids for rapid intravascular volume expansion should be constantly monitored to assess the clinical response to therapy. In general, during successful volume replacement, perfusion parameters will gradually and predictably return to normal. Mental status should improve and there should be no deleterious effects on the respiratory system. Given a dog of a certain body weight with a given degree of hypovolaemia, one can estimate the expected clinical response from a given volume and type of intravenous fluid. This enables the clinician to detect an inadequate response to volume resuscitation rapidly and pursue the underlying cause (e.g. ongoing haemorrhage, sepsis/SIRS). The fluid type and rate should be reassessed, as patients with severe ongoing losses may require colloid or blood component therapy.

Although isotonic replacement crystalloids are often the first choice in the fluid resuscitation of patients in shock, colloids, blood products or hypertonic saline may also be chosen. Colloids should be considered if the patient is suspected to have a low COP or exhibits clinical signs of oedema. A colloid dose of 20 ml/kg is considered equivalent to a 60–90 ml/kg dose of isotonic crystalloid, and the dose should be scaled down according to the severity of shock in the same manner as described for crystalloids. Blood products should be considered if the patient has pre-existing anaemia or has experienced severe haemorrhage, but their use is often limited by availability. Fluid resuscitation with asanguineous fluids should rarely if ever be withheld due to concerns about decreased red cell mass. Hypertonic saline should be considered in patients with concurrent hypovolaemia and head trauma or in large patients in severe shock.

Chronic fluid therapy for the patient with normal perfusion parameters

If the patient's perfusion parameters are within normal limits (either at presentation or following correction of shock with acute fluid therapy as described above), a chronic fluid therapy plan should be formulated. For the animal that is dehydrated but not seriously hypovolaemic, it is appropriate to correct fluid, electrolyte and acid–base abnormalities over a period of 24–48 hours. When devising a chronic fluid therapy plan, three components should be considered:

- Pre-existing fluid deficits (replacement of hydration losses)
- Maintenance requirements
- Ongoing losses.

The volume of fluids required for replacement of dehydration is estimated as a percentage of the animal's body weight, based on the clinical signs of hydration status (see Figure 4.6). As discussed previously, this provides only a rough estimate rather than an accurate guide. Because of the need to expand the intravascular and interstitial compartments effectively, an isotonic fluid is used for replacement of pre-existing deficits. Maintenance fluid requirements are simply the water and electrolytes needed on a daily basis in a normal animal. They are estimated empirically at 60 ml/kg/day for small dogs and cats and 40 ml/kg/day for larger dogs. In general, the fluid composition required for maintenance is low in sodium (approximately 0.3–0.45% NaCl) and high in potassium (approximately 20 mmol/l). Ongoing losses should also be estimated, although occasionally they may be measured (e.g. losses via a chest tube by

collecting drainage or losses in diarrhoea by weighing soiled bedding). Increased insensible losses, such as panting (especially with pyrexia), can be significant and should be taken into account when planning daily requirements.

In practice, replacement isotonic crystalloids are used for the chronic fluid therapy plan, as most patients have some degree of replacement needs or ongoing losses. The use of replacement fluids in this situation tends to predispose patients to the development of hypokalaemia. Patients who only have maintenance requirements (e.g. the neurological patient with inability to drink) are rarely encountered. In this situation, although a maintenance fluid may be used, the use of a replacement solution with potassium supplementation is also likely to be successful.

In animals that require potassium supplementation, an empirical dose is usually added to the intravenous fluids (see Figure 5.5). In very small patients or those on rapid fluid rates, the potassium infusion rate should be calculated to double check that the patient is not being overdosed. An empirical maximum infusion rate of 0.5 mmol/kg/h is suggested for potassium. The converse also should be kept in mind: the standard potassium supplementation of fluids may be insufficient to correct plasma potassium concentrations in patients who are receiving relatively low fluid rates. Potassium should not be added to fluids that are likely to be used for rapid intravenous infusion because of the risk of administration of a high dose quickly. Furthermore, inadequate mixing of intravenous fluids after addition of supplementary potassium can result in delivery of fluid with potassium concentrations an order of magnitude higher than expected.

Monitoring fluid therapy

Fluid requirements should be re-evaluated and adjusted regularly. In a patient receiving a bolus for hypovolaemia this may be every 15–30 minutes, whereas in a patient with chronic renal disease it may be on a daily basis. One of the most common mistakes with continued intravenous fluid therapy is failure to readjust fluid rates as the condition of the animal changes. There is a tendency to misconstrue the impressive autoregulatory abilities of the body (and more specifically the kidney) to infer that the choice of intravenous fluids is somewhat academic. Certainly, the normal kidney often compensates admirably for an inappropriate choice of fluid therapy. In animals with renal dysfunction or failure of the body's normal homeostatic mechanisms for water, electrolyte and acid–base balance, failure to select the appropriate fluid and monitor the effects may result in serious and potentially life-threatening complications. The most basic yet useful monitoring technique is the serial physical examination, which should include both assessment of perfusion and hydration parameters as well as evaluation for complications of fluid therapy (increased respiratory rate/effort, development of peripheral oedema). Other techniques discussed below may be used to augment the physical examination.

Body weight

Acute changes in body weight are largely due to changes in the fluid content of the body. When treating dehydrated patients, an increase in body weight is a positive sign that euhydration is being restored. However an increase in body weight in a non-dehydrated patient may be an early indicator that the patient is becoming fluid overloaded.

Serial bloodwork

It is recommended that packed cell volume, total solids (PCV/TS) and electrolytes are monitored frequently (at least daily) in patients on intravenous fluids. As discussed above, hypokalaemia is a common complication of chronic fluid therapy. In a patient with shock receiving aggressive fluid therapy, changes in PCV/TS can be used to guide the clinician as to when fluids such as colloids or blood products may be required.

Arterial blood pressure

Arterial blood pressure is frequently measured in critically ill veterinary patients and reflects the interplay between cardiac output and systemic vascular resistance (see Chapter 3). Arterial hypotension is a late change in shock, as many of the homeostatic mechanisms act to maintain blood pressure. Fluid boluses are therefore often still warranted in patients that are normotensive on presentation, but which are showing signs of compensated shock. Arterial blood pressure monitoring may be used to monitor patients in hypotensive shock which are receiving fluid boluses to restore perfusion. A minimum systolic arterial pressure of 70–80 mmHg or mean arterial pressure of greater than 60 mmHg should be the initial goal. In normotensive patients, although there may be transient increases in arterial blood pressure in response to fluid boluses, arterial blood pressure does not continue to climb with further fluid loading and is thus less useful than central venous pressure for assessment of vascular filling.

Central venous pressure

The central venous pressure (CVP) is a measure of the hydrostatic pressure within the central venous compartment, and as such provides the most accurate assessment of vascular filling. It is typically measured via a catheter, placed percutaneously into the jugular vein (Chapter 2), which has its tip in the cranial vena cava. Catheters placed into the caudal vena cava via the saphenous or femoral veins may also be used but tend to give less predictable and less accurate readings. The CVP is measured by attachment of the central venous catheter to either an electronic pressure transducer or a water manometer. Electronic pressure transducers provide a continuous readout of CVP and allow assessment of the waveform, however the equipment required is not widely available. A water manometer is used to provide intermittent readings of CVP but can be constructed from equipment available in most practices (three lengths of drip tubing, a ruler, a 60 ml syringe and a three-way stopcock; Figure 4.10).

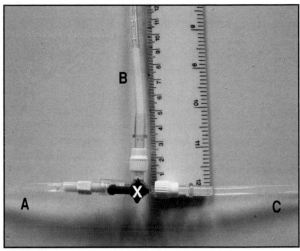

4.10 A water manometer for measurement of central venous pressure (CVP). Tube A is attached to the central line in the patient and the patient is positioned in right lateral recumbency. For an accurate reading it is important that point X is at approximately the same height as the patient's right atrium. The three-way stopcock is closed to the patient. Tube B is filled with saline from a syringe attached to tube C, until the height of the water column is at least 20 cm. The three-way stopcock is then opened so that it allows communication between tubes A and B (i.e. off to tube C). The saline in tube B will run into the patient until the water column reaches a height that is in equilibrium with the patient's CVP. This height is read as the CVP in cmH$_2$O. Repeat measurements can be taken as often as necessary but for reliable interpretation the patient position must be consistent. Note: for the purposes of this illustration, a coloured dye was added to the saline in this manometer.

Normal CVP is 0–5 cmH$_2$O. A low CVP implies inadequate vascular filling whereas a high CVP implies intravascular volume overload, right-sided cardiac dysfunction or increased intrathoracic pressure (e.g. pleural effusion). The change in CVP following a fluid bolus can be a useful guide to the necessity for further fluid loading, especially in patients in which volume overload is a concern, for example patients with possible anuric/oliguric renal failure. If the CVP is low, increases following a fluid bolus but then rapidly returns to pre-bolus levels, then more fluid therapy is warranted. In contrast, if it rises and remains high, this implies that the vascular volume is adequate and hypovolaemia is not the cause of the poor urine output.

Urine output

Urine output represents the balance between glomerular filtration rate (GFR) and tubular fluid reabsorption, and can be affected by a large number of different factors. It is thus impossible to define a 'normal' urine output but only to assess whether the output achieved is appropriate for the animal's clinical state. Assuming postrenal causes have been ruled out, critically ill patients may have a low urine output (<0.5 ml/kg/h) due to poor renal perfusion and low GFR (hypotension), anuric/oliguric renal failure, or high tubular reabsorption rate. The latter, which is associated with a high urine specific gravity, implies that the animal's homeostatic mechanisms are actively conserving water and suggests normal renal function. In all of these instances, the goal should be to increase urine output into the 0.5–2.0ml/kg/h range. In many cases this is achieved by providing the patient with adequate fluid therapy, although in the case of oliguric/anuric renal failure, pharmacological measures may be necessary to restart urine flow (see Chapter 8).

A falling urine output, in a patient that had previously been considered to be volume replete, can be an early indicator that the current fluid therapy plan is not supplying a sufficient volume of fluid. In most critical patients, this occurs because of changing and increased losses from the body, through the GI tract, wounds, or into third spaces. Patients may have an obligatory high urine output (>2 ml/kg/h and in some cases as high as 10–20 ml/kg/h) as a consequence of their underlying disease (e.g. polyuric renal failure, post-obstructive diuresis). In this scenario, accurate monitoring of urine output helps guide the rate of intravenous fluid therapy that the patient requires. The goal in this situation should be to 'match ins with outs'.

Urine output is best measured by placement of an indwelling urinary catheter. Strict aseptic technique should be adhered to whenever handling the urinary catheter to reduce the risk of ascending urinary tract infection. Alternative methods include attempting to catch all the urine passed in ambulatory patients or weighing urine soaked bedding in recumbent patients. Neither of these techniques is as accurate as catheterization.

Conclusion

Fluid therapy is an important part of the treatment of many critically ill veterinary patients. It should be remembered that fluids are a group of drugs just like any other, and have the potential to have adverse effects as well as positive ones. Numerous different fluids are available to veterinary practitioners, all of which can be used at a variety of different rates and doses. Successful fluid therapy comes from understanding why the patient requires fluid therapy and devising a fluid therapy plan for that individual based on both the goals of fluid treatment and an awareness of potential complications (Figure 4.11). Appropriate monitoring and a degree of flexibility with the plan as the patient's status changes are also important elements in achieving a successful outcome.

Patient details
6-month-old, male entire Labrador Retriever, body weight 20 kg, presents with a history of 3 days of vomiting and diarrhoea that has been getting progressively worse. He is unvaccinated and a diagnosis of parvovirus is confirmed.

Physical examination
- Depressed
- Heart rate 170, cardiac auscultation is unremarkable
- Pulse quality weak/moderate
- Mucous membranes pale with a CRT of 2.5 seconds
- Respiratory rate and effort are within normal limits as is auscultation of the lungs
- When raised, the skin over the back of the neck falls back more slowly than normal

Minimum database
- PCV 39% (reference range: 37–55%), TS 50 g/l (reference range: 57–70 g/l)
- Glucose 5.6 mmol/l (reference range: 3.5–5.5 mmol/l)
- Azostix – BUN mildly elevated

Initial assessment
The patient requires fluids. He is showing evidence of both moderate to severe hypoperfusion (tachycardia, abnormal pulse quality, abnormal mucous membranes) and moderate (~8%) dehydration. This is consistent with his history.

Initial plan
The hypoperfusion should be addressed first as it is potentially life-threatening. Plan to administer a fluid bolus of 50 ml/kg isotonic replacement crystalloid over 1 hour, with the aim of normalizing perfusion parameters. 50 x 20 = 1000 ml/h for 1 hour.

Assessment 1 hour later
Perfusion parameters have normalized (HR 120, pulse quality improved, mucous membranes pink with 1.5 second CRT). Consider chronic fluid therapy plan. Need to calculate and sum for 24 hours:

- Replacement of hydration
- Maintenance
- Ongoing losses.

If perfusion parameters had not normalized at the end of the first fluid bolus, a second fluid bolus would have been required. The size of the second bolus and the type of fluid used should be chosen on the basis of the patient's physical examination at that time:

Replacement of hydration
Fluid deficit   = % dehydration x body weight x 10
                         = 8 x 20 x 10
                         = 1600 ml

Maintenance
Maintenance requirement   = 50 ml/kg/day
                         = 50 x 20
                         = 1000 ml/day

4.11 Example of a fluid therapy plan. (continues) ▶

Ongoing losses	
Ongoing losses	= diarrhoea + vomitus
Estimated diarrhoea volume/episode	= 100 ml x 5 episodes/day = 500 ml
Estimated vomitus volume/episode	= 50 ml x 5 episodes/day = 250 ml
Total ongoing losses	= 500 + 250 = 750 ml/day
Daily fluid requirement	= replacement + maintenance + ongoing losses
	= 1600 ml + 1000 ml + 750 ml
	= 3350 ml/day
	= 3350/24 ml/h
	= 140 ml/h

It should be recognized that this fluid rate is a 'best estimate' and may need to be increased or decreased depending on the patient's progression.

4.11 (continued) Example of a fluid therapy plan.

References and further reading

Aukland K and Reed RK (1993) Interstitial-lymphatic mechanisms in the control of extracellular fluid volume. *Physiological Reviews* **73**, 1–78

Boon JC, Jesch F, Ring J *et al.* (1976) Intravascular persistence of hydroxyethyl starch in man. *European Surgical Research* **8**, 497–503

Brown SA, Dusza K and Boehmer J (1994) Comparison of measured and calculated values for colloid osmotic pressure in hospitalized animals. *American Journal of Veterinary Research* **55**, 910–915

Chan DL, Rozanski EA, Freeman LM *et al.* (2004) Retrospective evaluation of human albumin use in critically ill dogs. *Journal of Veterinary Emergency and Critical Care* **14**, S8

Chi OZ, Lu X, Wei HM *et al.* (1996) Hydroxyethyl starch solution attenuates blood-brain barrier disruption caused by intracarotid injection of hyperosmolar mannitol in rats. *Anesthesia and Analgesia* **83**, 336–341

Conroy JM, Fishman RL, Reeves ST *et al.* (1996) The effects of desmopressin and 6% hydroxyethyl starch on factor VIII:C. *Anesthesia and Analgesia* **83**, 804–807

Cope JT, Banks D, Mauney MC *et al.* (1997) Intraoperative hetastarch infusion impairs hemostasis after cardiac operations. *Annals of Thoracic Surgery* **63**, 78–82

Culp AM, Clay ME, Baylor IA *et al.* (1994) Colloid osmotic pressure (COP) and total solids (TS) measurement in normal dogs and cats. Proceedings of the Fourth International Veterinary Emergency and Critical Care Symposium, San Antonio, TX, p. 705

Curry FE, Michel CC and Phillips ME (1987) Effect of albumin on the osmotic pressure exerted by myoglobin across capillary walls in frog mesentery. *Journal of Physiology* **387**, 69–82

DiBartola SP (1992) Introduction to fluid therapy. In: *Fluid Therapy in Small Animal Practice*, ed. SP DiBartola, pp. 321–340. WB Saunders, Philadelphia

Falk JL, Rackow EC and Weil MH (1989) Colloid and crystalloid fluid resuscitation. In: *Textbook of Critical Care*, eds WC Shoemaker and S Ayres, pp. 1055–1073. WB Saunders, Philadelphia

Farrow SP, Hall M and Ricketts CR (1970) Changes in the molecular composition of circulating hydroxyethyl starch. *British Journal of Pharmacology* **38**, 725–730

Finfer S, Bellomo R, Boyce N *et al.* (2004) A comparison of albumin and saline for fluid resuscitation in the intensive care unit. *New England Journal of Medicine* **350**, 2247–2256

Funk W and Baldinger V (1995) Microcirculatory perfusion during volume therapy. A comparative study using crystalloid or colloid in awake animals. *Anesthesiology* **82**, 975–982

Guyton AC and Lindsay NW (1959) Effect of elevated left atrial pressure and decreased plasma protein concentration on the development of pulmonary edema. *Circulation Research* **7**, 649–657

Hardy RM and Osborne CA (1979) Water deprivation test in the dog: Maximal normal values. *Journal of the American Veterinary Medical Association* **174**, 479–483

Jones PA, Tomasic M and Gentry PA (1997) Oncotic, hemodilutional and hemostatic effects of isotonic saline and hydroxyethyl starch solutions in clinically normal ponies. *American Journal of Veterinary Research* **58**, 541–548

Lamke LO and Liljedahl SO (1976) Plasma volume changes after infusion of various plasma expanders. *Resuscitation* **5**, 93–102

Moore LE and Garvey MS (1996) The effect of hetastarch on serum colloid oncotic pressure in hypoalbuminemic dogs. *Journal of Veterinary Internal Medicine* **10**, 300–303

Navar PD and Navar LG (1977) Relationship between colloid osmotic pressure and plasma protein concentration in the dog. *American Journal of Physiology* **233**, H295–H298

Oz MC, FitzPatrick MF and Zikria BA (1995) Attenuation of microvascular permeability dysfunction in postischemic striated muscle by hydroxyethyl starch. *Microvascular Research* **50**, 71–79

Pappenheimer JR, Renkin EM and Borrero LM (1951) Filtration, diffusion and molecular sieving through peripheral capillary membranes. A contribution to the pore theory of capillary permeability. *American Journal of Physiology* **167**, 13–46

Rackow EC, Fein IA and Leppo J (1977) Colloid osmotic pressure as a prognostic indicator of pulmonary edema and mortality in the critically ill. *Chest* **72**, 709–713

Ring J (1985) Anaphylactoid reactions to plasma substitutes. *International Anesthesiology Clinics* **23**, 67–95

Rippe B and Haraldsson B (1998) Transport of macromolecules across microvascular walls: the two pore theory. *Physiological Reviews* **74**, 163–219

Schierhout G and Roberts I (1998) Fluid resuscitation with colloid or crystalloid solutions in critically ill patients: a systematic review of randomised trials. *British Medical Journal* **316**, 961–964

Shoemaker WC (1976) Comparison of the relative effectiveness of whole blood transfusions and various types of fluid therapy in resuscitation. *Critical Care Medicine* **4**, 71–78

Smiley LE and Garvey MS (1994) The use of hetastarch as adjunct therapy in 26 dogs with hypoalbuminemia: a phase two clinical trial. *Journal of Veterinary Internal Medicine* **8**, 195–202

Starling EH (1896) On the absorption of fluid from the connective tissue spaces. *Journal of Physiology (London)* **19**, 312–326

Staub NC and Taylor AE (1984) *Edema*. Raven Press, New York

Taylor AE (1990) The lymphatic edema safety factor: the role of edema dependent lymphatic factors (EDLF). *Lymphology* **23**, 111–123

Thomas LA and Brown SA (1992) Relationship between colloid osmotic pressure and plasma protein concentration in cattle, horses, dogs and cats. *American Journal of Veterinary Research* **53**, 2241–2243

Treib J, Haass A and Pindur G (1997) Coagulation disorders caused by hydroxyethyl starch. *Thrombosis and Haemostasis* **78**, 974–983

Treib J, Haass A, Pindur G *et al.* (1995) HES 200/0.5 is not HES 200/0.5. Influence of the C2/C6 hydroxyethylation ratio of hydroxyethyl starch (HES) on hemorheology, coagulation and elimination kinetics. *Thrombosis and Haemostasis* **74**, 1452–1456

Velanovich V (1989) Crystalloid versus colloid fluid resuscitation: a meta-analysis of mortality. *Surgery* **105**, 65–71

Villarino ME, Gordon SM, Valdon C *et al.* (1992) A cluster of severe postoperative bleeding following open heart surgery. *Infection Control and Hospital Epidemiology* **13**, 282–287

Wareing TH, Gruber MA, Brigham KL *et al.* (1989) Increased plasma oncotic pressure inhibits pulmonary fluid transport when pulmonary pressures are elevated. *Journal of Surgical Research* **46**, 29–34

Weil MH and Afifi AA (1970) Experimental and clinical studies on lactate and pyruvate as indicators of the severity of acute circulatory failure (shock). *Circulation* **41**, 989–1001

Wiig H and Reed RK (1987) Volume–pressure relationship (compliance) of interstitium in dog skin and muscle. *American Journal of Physiology* **253**, H291–H298

Yuan Y, Granger HJ, Zawieja DC *et al.* (1992) Flow modulates coronary venular permeability by a nitric oxide-related mechanism. *American Journal of Physiology* **263**, H641–H646

Zarins CK, Rice CL, Peters RM *et al.* (1978) Lymph and pulmonary response to isobaric reduction in plasma oncotic pressure in baboons. *Circulation Research* **43**, 925–930

Zarins CK, Rice CL, Smith DE *et al.* (1976) Role of lymphatics in preventing hypooncotic pulmonary edema. *Surgical Forum* **27**, 257–259

Zikria BA, Oz MO and Carlson RW (1994) (eds) *Reperfusion Injuries and Clinical Capillary Leak Syndrome*. Futura Publishing Company, Armonk, NY

5

Electrolyte and acid–base balance

Amanda Boag

Introduction

The evaluation of electrolytes and acid–base status in critically ill patients is an important tool, both for helping to achieve a rapid diagnosis and for refining patient management. Electrolyte and acid–base parameters can change over very short time periods with disease progression or treatment, and the ability to measure these parameters in-house is essential. An increasing number of veterinary surgeons have access to 'bench-top' machines such as i-Stat or IRMA blood gas analysers, allowing greater numbers of patients to benefit from the information they provide. For the emergency practitioner, a blood gas machine is arguably more important for acute patient management than an in-house biochemistry machine. Hour-to-hour treatment decisions may be made on the basis of changes in electrolyte and acid–base status, whereas this is rarely the case with clinical biochemistry parameters.

This chapter reviews the relevant physiology and clinical significance of changes in the major electrolytes (sodium, potassium, chloride, calcium and magnesium) as well as providing an introduction to acid–base interpretation.

Sodium

Sodium is the most important osmotically active particle in the extracellular fluid (ECF) and, as such, is a vital determinant of ECF volume. The regulation of sodium concentration and water balance is intimately related. The kidneys are the prime site for sodium and water homeostasis. The endocrine mechanisms for volume regulation (i.e. sodium content) and osmoregulation (i.e. water content) are integrated in the nephron. Volume regulation involves detection of intravascular volume changes at a number of anatomical sites (carotid sinus, aortic arch, glomerular afferent arterioles, cardiac atria) with alterations in the activation of the renin–angiotensin–aldosterone system (RAAS), the sympathetic nervous system (NS) and atrial natriuretic peptide (ANP) being the principal effector mechanisms. The complex actions of these hormones lead to either increased (RAAS, sympathetic NS) or decreased (ANP) sodium retention by the kidneys. Osmoregulation involves detection of changes in osmolality by the hypothalamus with control effected by anti-diuretic hormone (ADH; vasopressin). An increase in ADH leads to increased body water by stimulating thirst and increasing water reabsorption in the distal part of the nephron.

Ultimately, the measured serum sodium concentration reflects the balance between the amount of sodium relative to the amount of water within the ECF compartment, and is not a direct indicator of total body sodium. Patients with hypernatraemia (or hyponatraemia) may therefore have normal, increased or decreased total body sodium in different disease situations. For example, a patient with significant loss of a hypotonic fluid (e.g. osmotic diarrhoea) may have *decreased* total body sodium, but actually be *hyper*natraemic if their loss of water exceeds their loss of sodium. These patients are likely to be hypernatraemic and hypovolaemic. Conversely, a patient with hypernatraemia secondary to excessive intake of salt (impermeant solute gain), which also has had access to water, may be hypernatraemic and hypervolaemic. When evaluating patients with sodium abnormalities it is vitally important to make an assessment of intravascular volume status on the basis of physical examination and history (see Chapter 4). Recognition of the patient's volume status allows refinement of the differential diagnosis list and has important implications for treatment. As the sodium ion is monovalent, 1 mmol/l is equivalent to 1 mEq/l.

Disorders of sodium

Causes

The differential diagnoses for sodium abnormalities, categorized according to the patient's intravascular volume status, are shown in Figure 5.1. Several of the causes (e.g. vomiting and diarrhoea) may cause either hyper- or hyponatraemia depending on the exact nature of the losses (i.e. whether they contain more sodium than water or vice versa) and the ability of the animal to drink and regain free water. The presence and influence of other osmotically active particles in the plasma should also be considered when interpreting serum sodium values. This is clinically most relevant when evaluating diabetic patients. In these patients, the elevated serum glucose acts as an osmotically active particle and draws water into the vasculature, leading to dilution of the serum sodium. It is expected that for every 1 mmol/l increase in glucose, the serum sodium will be reduced by approximately 0.3–0.4 mmol/l. Finally, when assessing patients with hyponatraemia, the possibility of pseudohyponatraemia should be

Hypernatraemia

Hypervolaemia (impermeant solute gain)
    Salt poisoning
    Iatrogenic (hypertonic saline administration)
Normovolaemia (pure water deficit)[a]
    Hyperthermia
    Diabetes insipidus (central/nephrogenic)
    Inadequate access to water
    Primary hypodipsia
Hypovolaemia (loss of water in excess of sodium)
    Renal failure (acute or chronic)
    Vomiting and diarrhoea
    Burn injuries
    Drug induced (furosemide, mannitol)

Hyponatraemia

Hypervolaemia (impaired water excretion)
    Congestive heart failure
    Severe hepatic disease
    Renal disease (nephrotic syndrome)
Normovolaemia
    Syndrome of inappropriate ADH secretion (SIADH)
    Hypotonic fluid administration
    Psychogenic polydipsia
Hypovolaemia (loss of sodium in excess of water)
    Hypoadrenocorticism
    Vomiting and diarrhoea
    Drug induced (diuretics)
    Third-space loss

5.1 Differential diagnosis of serum sodium abnormalities. Diagnoses in italics are those encountered most frequently in clinical practice. [a] It should be noted that although the conditions listed here initially lead to normovolaemic hypernatraemia, in clinical practice, by the time patients with pure water deficit present to a veterinary surgeon they are often exhibiting signs of hypovolaemia.

considered. This is an artefact that occurs when serum sodium is measured by flame photometry methodology (used by most commercial laboratories) in patients with concurrent hyperlipidaemia or hyperproteinaemia. In this situation the true serum sodium is likely to be within normal limits. Pseudohyponatraemia has no negative clinical consequences but it is important that it is recognized so that the low serum sodium is not overinterpreted.

Clinical signs

Mild abnormalities in serum sodium are common and rarely cause clinical signs. If sodium abnormalities are severe and especially if they develop rapidly, clinical signs may ensue. The clinical signs are principally neurological. With hypernatraemia, the increased tonicity of the ECF leads to movement of water out of brain cells, causing cerebral dehydration and development of neurological signs. With hyponatraemia, the decreased ECF tonicity promotes movement of water into the brain, with development of cerebral oedema. The rate of change in sodium is an important determinant of the severity of the clinical signs. If the sodium abnormality develops slowly (i.e. over a period of days to weeks), the brain is able to compensate and clinical signs may not be seen. When hypernatraemia progresses gradually, the brain generates intracellular substances known as idiogenic

osmoles that prevent cerebral fluid loss. With gradual onset of hyponatraemia, the brain is able to adjust by losing osmotically active particles. This has important implications for treatment. Rapid correction of chronic sodium abnormalities may precipitate clinical signs that are more severe than those induced by the sodium abnormality itself.

Treatment

The principles of treatment of both hyper- and hyponatraemia are similar, and generally involve manipulation of the patient's intravenous fluid therapy. For the majority of patients with serum sodium abnormalities, the serum sodium concentration does not need specific treatment but will correct itself as the underlying disease is treated. Patients with clinical signs may, however, require treatment aimed specifically at the sodium abnormality. It is also vital to ensure that treatment for the underlying disease does not lead to rapid changes in sodium, and development of iatrogenic clinical signs.

When the serum sodium abnormality has been gradual in onset, the serum sodium should be corrected slowly, with a maximum change of *0.5 mmol/l sodium per hour* in either direction.

If hypovolaemia is present, initial treatment should be directed at restoration of the patient's intravascular volume with the use of fluid boluses (see Chapter 4). To avoid rapid changes in the patient's serum sodium, the fluid chosen for boluses should have a sodium concentration close to the animal's serum sodium. For the majority of hypernatraemic patients 0.9% NaCl (sodium concentration 150 mmol/l) is suitable, and for hyponatraemic patients, Hartmann's solution (sodium concentration 131 mmol/l) or lactated Ringer's (sodium concentration 134 mmol/l) are the fluids of choice. Once the animal's intravascular volume status is restored, the serum sodium concentration can be returned to normal over a period of 24–48 hours. If possible, hypernatraemic patients should be encouraged to drink and regain their free water by that route. If the patient is vomiting or unable to drink (e.g. with neurological disease), free water must be administered using hypotonic fluids (0.45% NaCl, 5% dextrose in water). The patient's approximate free water deficit can be calculated:

Free water deficit (l) =

$$0.6 \times \text{current weight (kg)} \times \left(\frac{\text{serum sodium concentration (patient)}}{\text{serum sodium concentration (normal)}} - 1 \right)$$

This volume of free water can then be administered gradually over 24 hours. An example calculation is given in Figure 5.2. Frequent monitoring of sodium is recommended (up to every 2–4 hours) to ensure that the sodium is not changing too rapidly. The fluid therapy plan may need to be adjusted frequently during this time period.

For normo- or hypervolaemic, hyponatraemic patients, treatment commonly involves medical therapy directed at the underlying cause of the hyponatraemia (Figure 5.1). If fluid therapy is required in these patients, careful consideration should be given to the underlying disease process and the reason for administration of fluids. In many instances a fluid with a sodium concentration slightly greater than the

6-month-old Staffordshire Bull Terrier with hypodipsia since birth presents with serum sodium of 190 mmol/l. Current body weight is 15 kg

Free water deficit = 0.6 x 15 x $\left(\frac{190-1}{145}\right)$

Free water deficit = 2.8 l

This should be administered over 24 hours

If 5% dextrose in saline is used, this is equivalent to 100% free water, thus the rate of fluid administration would be 2800/24 = 116 ml/h

If 0.45% NaCl is used, this represents 50% free water, thus the rate of fluid administration would be (2800/24) x 2 = 233 ml/h

Any ongoing electrolyte losses should also be taken into consideration, with concurrent administration of isotonic fluids if necessary

5.2 Example of free water deficit calculation.

patient's serum sodium is appropriate. The rate at which the serum sodium will change is very difficult to predict. As with correction of hypernatraemia, frequent monitoring of serum sodium is required with adjustment of the fluid therapy plan as necessary.

Potassium

Potassium is the most abundant intracellular cation. Approximately 95% of total body potassium is found within the cells, and intracellular potassium concentration is approximately 140 mmol/l. Serum potassium is maintained within a much lower and very narrow range (approximately 3.5–5.5 mmol/l); this difference between intracellular and extracellular concentrations is vitally important for determining the resting membrane potential of excitable tissues (including cardiac conduction tissue). Serum concentrations do not reflect whole body potassium levels. Translocation between the extracellular and intracellular compartments can be a cause of potassium abnormalities, or may be utilized during treatment. Potassium intake is principally via the gastrointestinal tract and typically exceeds daily potassium requirements. The excess potassium is excreted mainly via the urinary system, with aldosterone being the principal hormone affecting potassium excretion in the distal tubule. As the potassium ion is monovalent, 1 mmol/l is equivalent to 1 mEq/l.

Hyperkalaemia

Causes

Causes of hyperkalaemia may be divided into those that occur secondary to reduced renal excretion of potassium, and those that involve translocation of potassium from the intracellular to the extracellular compartment. Rarely, increased intake of potassium may lead to hyperkalaemia. The differential diagnoses are shown in Figure 5.3. Artefactual hyperkalaemia can also be caused by improper sample handling, especially the use of blood anticoagulated with EDTA for electrolyte measurement, or haemolysis in some breeds (e.g. Akitas) whose red cells have a high potassium concentration.

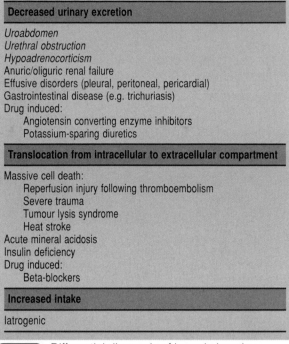

Decreased urinary excretion
Uroabdomen
Urethral obstruction
Hypoadrenocorticism
Anuric/oliguric renal failure
Effusive disorders (pleural, peritoneal, pericardial)
Gastrointestinal disease (e.g. trichuriasis)
Drug induced:
Angiotensin converting enzyme inhibitors
Potassium-sparing diuretics
Translocation from intracellular to extracellular compartment
Massive cell death:
Reperfusion injury following thromboembolism
Severe trauma
Tumour lysis syndrome
Heat stroke
Acute mineral acidosis
Insulin deficiency
Drug induced:
Beta-blockers
Increased intake
Iatrogenic

5.3 Differential diagnosis of hyperkalaemia. Diagnoses in italics are those encountered most frequently in clinical practice.

Clinical signs

The most life-threatening consequence of hyperkalaemia is its effect on myocardial conduction. Clinically this is detected by an inappropriate bradycardia and characteristic electrocardiogram (ECG) changes. As serum potassium increases, initially there is a prolonged PR interval, decreased R wave amplitude and increased T wave amplitude. This progresses to atrial standstill (absent P wave) with widened QRS complexes and bradycardia (see Figure 6.12). A 'sine wave' trace may be seen shortly before asystole. A precise correlation between the magnitude of the hyperkalaemia and the ECG changes does not exist, as other factors (e.g. acid–base status, ionized calcium levels) also affect myocardial conduction. Treatment should therefore be based on the severity of the ECG changes and their clinical effects on the patient, rather than simply on the measured serum potassium level.

Treatment

Emergency treatment of hyperkalaemia is required whenever the patient has high serum potassium and is showing consistent clinical or ECG changes. If serum potassium cannot be measured in-house but the index of suspicion for hyperkalaemia is high (e.g. bradycardia in a patient with urethral obstruction), treatment could still be considered. Specific treatment for hyperkalaemia includes:

- Intravenous calcium gluconate at a dose of 0.5–1.5 ml/kg of a 10% solution. This acts rapidly to counteract the effects of the high potassium on myocardial conduction. Its effects last approximately 20 minutes and the dose can be repeated. It does not lower serum potassium but is the first choice therapy in severely affected animals due to its rapidity of action

- Intravenous regular (soluble) insulin at a dose of 0.25–0.5 IU/kg administered with 2 g dextrose per unit of insulin and followed by addition of 2.5% dextrose to the intravenous fluids. Insulin acts to lower serum potassium by promoting potassium uptake into cells along with glucose. It takes about 20 minutes to have an effect. It is essential that intravenous fluids are supplemented with glucose for 12–24 hours following this treatment to prevent the development of hypoglycaemia
- Intravenous sodium bicarbonate at a dose of 1–2 mEq/kg. This acts to drive potassium intracellularly by changing plasma pH. It is rarely necessary and should only be used if the acid–base status can be monitored.

Most patients also require intravenous fluid therapy with a replacement crystalloid fluid. The fluid should be chosen after consideration of all the patient's electrolyte abnormalities. Although Hartmann's solution contains small amounts of potassium, this small dose is unlikely to have a clinical impact on the patient in comparison to the dilution produced by fluid administration. In a recent study evaluating electrolyte changes in cats with urethral obstruction receiving either 0.9% NaCl or lactated Ringer's solution (LRS), there was no significant difference between fluid groups in the speed of correction of the potassium, but the acid–base status was corrected more rapidly in the patients receiving LRS (Cole and Drobatz, 2003).

Alongside emergency treatment of the hyperkalaemia, it is important to identify and treat the underlying cause. This may include placing a urethral catheter (urethral obstruction; see Chapter 8), surgery (uroabdomen; see Chapter 12) or medical therapy (acute renal failure, hypoadrenocorticism; see Chapters 8 and 16 respectively).

Hypokalaemia

Causes
Hypokalaemia is a common finding in critically ill patients, especially those which are inappetent and on long-term fluid therapy. Causes include decreased intake, increased loss through either the kidneys or gastrointestinal tract, or translocation from the extracellular to the intracellular compartment. The differential diagnoses are summarized in Figure 5.4.

Clinical signs
The physiological consequences of hypokalemia are generally less imminently life threatening than those associated with hyperkalaemia. Signs are typically non-specific and consist of weakness, lethargy, ileus and anorexia. In cats, ventroflexion of the neck may be seen. As these signs may contribute to patient morbidity, correction of even mild hypokalaemia is recommended. Severe hypokalaemia (serum potassium <2.8 mmol/l) can lead to respiratory muscle weakness and hypoventilation, with the potential to progress to respiratory paralysis and death. Potassium depletion also produces abnormalities within the

Increased loss
Gastrointestinal tract
Vomiting
Diarrhoea
Urinary tract
Chronic renal failure (particularly cats)
Postobstructive diuresis
Drug induced:
Diuretics (loop, thiazide)
Penicillins
Mineralocorticoid excess

Translocation from extracellular to intracellular compartment
Insulin/glucose-containing fluids
Alkalaemia
Catecholamine release

Decreased intake
Inappetence/anorexia
Long-term administration of intravenous fluid with low potassium concentration

5.4 Differential diagnosis of hypokalaemia. Diagnoses in italics are those encountered most frequently in clinical practice.

kidney (hypokalaemic nephropathy), a feature of which is impaired responsiveness to ADH. This leads to polyuria and further renal potassium losses.

Treatment
Hypokalaemia is treated with potassium supplementation via the oral or intravenous route. In critically ill patients the intravenous route is used most frequently, by adding potassium chloride to the intravenous fluids. In an anorexic patient receiving an isotonic replacement fluid (e.g. Hartmann's, 0.9% NaCl) at maintenance rates, addition of 14–20 mmol K^+/l is usually sufficient to maintain serum potassium levels. If the patient has pre-existing hypokalaemia higher rates of supplementation may be needed (Figure 5.5). All fluids to which potassium chloride has been added must be well mixed and clearly labelled. These fluids should never be administered as a bolus due to the potential effects of rapid intravenous potassium infusion on cardiac conduction. *Potassium should not be infused at a rate greater than 0.5 mmol/kg/h.* It is recommended that if rates approaching 0.5 mmol/kg/h are used, the patient is monitored continuously with an ECG. If the patient is eating voluntarily or has a

Serum potassium (mmol/l)	KCl (mmol) to add to 1l fluids	Maximum recommended infusion rate for supplemented fluids (ml/kg/h)
3.5–5.0	20	25
3.0–3.5	30	18
2.5–3.0	40	12
2.0–2.5	60	8
<2.0	80	6

5.5 Guidelines for supplementation of intravenous fluids with potassium chloride (KCl) for the treatment of hypokalaemia.

feeding tube in place, enteral potassium supplementation is safe and effective. The dose of enteral potassium required is difficult to predict and monitoring of serum potassium is advised; a suggested initial dose is 0.5–1.0 mmol/kg orally twice daily.

Chloride

Chloride is the major extracellular anion and serum chloride levels generally change in a similar way to those of serum sodium. Treatment of the sodium abnormality generally leads to concurrent resolution of the chloride abnormality. Chloride has an important role in acid–base balance due to its interactions with renal sodium and bicarbonate reabsorption.

Hyperchloraemia

Hyperchloraemia rarely requires specific treatment and is commonly accompanied by hypernatraemia, which is of greater clinical significance. The presence of hyperchloraemia may aid with interpretation of acid–base abnormalities (see Metabolic acid–base disturbances, later). Artefactual hyperchloraemia may be seen in patients receiving potassium bromide therapy for seizures. These patients generally have normal serum sodium.

Hypochloraemia

Hypochloraemia is of clinical relevance principally because of its effects on systemic acid–base balance. Hypochloraemic patients are prone to developing a metabolic alkalosis, especially if they have concurrent hypovolaemia with avid renal retention of sodium. As sodium is reabsorbed, the nephron must also reabsorb or regenerate anions in order to maintain electroneutrality. The anion reabsorbed is principally chloride, but in situations of chloride depletion, bicarbonate (HCO_3^-) is regenerated instead, thus predisposing the patient to the development of alkalaemia. Clinically this is seen in patients with severe vomiting that develop a significant hypochloraemic metabolic alkalosis. Use of 0.9% NaCl as the resuscitative fluid of choice in these patients will aid the restoration of acid–base balance, as the higher chloride concentration allows the kidneys to excrete the bicarbonate whilst continuing active sodium retention.

Calcium

Calcium has many important extracellular and intracellular functions, as well as being a major component of the skeleton. Extracellular calcium consists of three fractions:

- Ionized calcium (iCa^{2+}). This forms about 55% of total calcium and is the physiologically active fraction. As calcium is divalent, 1 mmol/l is equivalent to 2 mEq/l
- Complexed calcium. This forms about 10% of total calcium and consists of calcium complexed to anions such as citrate, lactate and bicarbonate
- Protein-bound calcium. This forms about 35% of total calcium.

The total calcium value reported by most biochemistry laboratories represents all three fractions, whereas blood gas machines more commonly measure the ionized calcium fraction. It is important to know which component has been measured when interpreting calcium abnormalities. Ideally the ionized calcium should be measured, as this is the biologically active component. Although equations have been suggested to predict the ionized calcium concentration from the total calcium value and serum albumin, they are not accurate and are not recommended (Schenk and Chew, 2005).

Calcium intake is principally via the gastrointestinal tract, with excretion via the kidneys. Calcium stored in bone can also be mobilized in response to hypocalcaemia. Three hormone systems are involved principally with calcium homeostasis:

- Parathyroid hormone (PTH). A peptide hormone secreted by the parathyroid gland, PTH leads to increased plasma iCa^{2+} by reducing renal calcium excretion, increasing bone resorption and increasing calcium absorption from the gastrointestinal tract (via calcitriol). Parathyroid hormone-related peptide (PTHrP) is a PTH-like substance that is secreted by some tumours and is often responsible for the humoral hypercalcaemia of malignancy
- Calcitonin. A peptide hormone secreted by the C cells of the thyroid gland leading to decreased iCa^{2+} by inhibiting bone resorption
- Calcitriol (1,25-dihydroxycholecalciferol). A steroid hormone manufactured in the kidneys in response to increased PTH, calcitriol acts to increase iCa^{2+} by increasing gastrointestinal absorption and bone resorption.

Hypercalcaemia

Causes

The causes of hypercalcaemia may be divided into those in which the ionized calcium is elevated (Figure 5.6) and those in which the total calcium is elevated but the ionized calcium is normal. The latter situation may occur due to increases in the protein-bound fraction (increased albumin with dehydration) or increases

Neoplasia:
  Lymphoma
  Anal sac adenocarcinoma
  Multiple myeloma
  Mammary gland adenocarcinoma
Primary hyperparathyroidism
Acute renal failure
Hypoadrenocorticism
Granulomatous disease:
  Infection with *Angiostrongylus vasorum*
  Fungal disease
Vitamin D toxicosis:
  Some rat poisons
  Psoriasis cream
Non-neoplastic disorders of bone
Idiopathic (cats)

5.6 Differential diagnosis for ionized hypercalcaemia. Diagnoses in italics are those encountered most frequently in clinical practice.

in the complexed fraction (e.g. in chronic renal failure because there is an increase in many of the anions with which calcium forms complexes). Young growing animals have a mild physiological ionized hypercalcaemia. Emergency treatment for hypercalcaemia is warranted only if the ionized calcium is increased.

Clinical signs

Clinical signs of hypercalcaemia are often vague and non-specific. Typically patients are inappetent (or anorexic), lethargic and polyuric/polydipsic. Vomiting, constipation, cardiac dysrhythmias and muscle twitching are less common clinical signs. The increased calcium affects the kidney's ability to respond to ADH (a form of nephrogenic diabetes insipidus) therefore patients may have a prerenal azotaemia with relatively dilute urine. If the hypercalcaemia is prolonged, severe and/or associated with a high phosphate, soft tissue mineralization of several organs may occur. Renal mineralization leads to the development of renal failure which is the most serious complication of untreated hypercalcaemia.

Treatment

Treatment should be instituted if the animal has a high iCa^{2+} and/or is showing clinical signs related to the hypercalcaemia. Soft tissue mineralization is more likely to occur if the total calcium (mmol/l) x phosphorus (mmol/l) product is >5 (>60 if these electrolytes are measured in mg/dl, US), and aggressive treatment should be used in these animals to reduce the risk of renal failure. Treatment options include:

- Fluid diuresis with 0.9% NaCl at 4–6 ml/kg/h. The high renal sodium load promotes calciuresis
- Furosemide at 1–2 mg/kg every 6–12 hours to promote renal calcium excretion. This diuretic should only be used after dehydration has been corrected with fluid therapy
- Salmon calcitonin at a dose of 4–7 IU/kg s.c. q6–8h. As salmon calcitonin is a foreign antigen, there is a theoretical risk of anaphylaxis, especially with multiple doses
- Bisphosphonates, which act to reduce bone resorption. The dose depends on the preparation used and is not well defined in small animal species. The author has used clodronate at 10 mg/kg diluted in 0.9% NaCl as a slow infusion over 4–6 hours, with success in reducing iCa^{2+} and minimal apparent side effects
- Peritoneal dialysis or haemodialysis for life-threatening hypercalcaemia
- Glucocorticoids at anti-inflammatory doses. Glucocorticoids act by several mechanisms to reduce serum calcium; however they may also interfere with tests necessary to diagnose the underlying cause, and therefore compromise future treatment options. It is recommended that they are only used once the diagnostic evaluation has been completed.

Saline diuresis and furosemide are successful in controlling hypercalcaemia in the short term in the majority of patients. Long-term treatment relies on identification of the underlying cause with appropriate

specific treatment. Diagnostic tests to be considered include a thorough physical examination (including rectal examination), toxicological history, thoracic and abdominal imaging, aspiration of any masses or enlarged lymph nodes, PTH and PTHrP levels, bone marrow aspirate and tests for infectious diseases as suggested by geographical location. Specific treatment may involve surgery (e.g. to remove a parathyroid tumour), chemotherapy or treatment of infectious disease. The prognosis depends on the underlying disease. Patients that have already developed renal failure secondary to hypercalcaemia have a poorer prognosis. The hypercalcaemia seen with vitamin D toxicosis tends to carry a poor prognosis as it is typically of high magnitude, of long duration and is associated with high serum phosphorus.

Hypocalcaemia

Causes

As with hypercalcaemia, it is important to assess whether hypocalcaemia represents an ionized hypocalcaemia (which may lead to clinical signs) or a total hypocalcaemia related to a low serum albumin concentration. Causes of ionized hypocalcaemia are shown in Figure 5.7. Artefactual hypocalcaemia can be caused by improper sample handling, especially testing using blood anticoagulated with EDTA.

Hypoparathyroidism:
    Primary
    Iatrogenic (post thyroidectomy)
    Nutritional secondary hypoparathyroidism
Chronic renal failure
Eclampsia (puerperal tetany)
Ethylene glycol toxicity
Acute pancreatitis
Severe intestinal malabsorption
Iatrogenic:
    Phosphate enema
    Rapid or massive administration of blood products (citrate toxicity)
    Rapid administration of phosphate-containing fluids
Hypomagnesaemia
Hypovitaminosis D

5.7 Differential diagnosis of ionized hypocalcaemia. Diagnoses in italics are those encountered most frequently in clinical practice.

Clinical signs

Low serum iCa^{2+} leads to increased excitability of neuromuscular tissue. Common clinical signs include muscle tremors, facial rubbing, behavioural change, stiff gait, panting and hyperthermia. If severe, the patient may exhibit tetany, ECG changes (prolonged QT interval) and hypotension. Ultimately severe hypocalcaemia can cause respiratory arrest and death.

Treatment

In the patient presenting with signs of tetany, urgent treatment with intravenous calcium is warranted. Calcium gluconate (10%) is given slowly intravenously to effect. The typical dose is 0.5–1.5 ml/kg administered over 10–20 minutes. Patients should be monitored by ECG during administration, if possible. The infusion should be discontinued if the patient becomes bradycardic or develops a short QT interval. If an ECG is not available, pulse quality and heart rate should be monitored closely. Following resolution of the immediate crisis, supplementation with calcium gluconate can be continued if necessary as an intravenous infusion of 5–15 mg elemental calcium/kg/h. Calcium gluconate can be diluted 1:1 with 0.9% NaCl and administered as a subcutaneous dose, however this is not recommended routinely as there is a risk of localized tissue necrosis/mineralization.

Calcium chloride is an alternative formulation, but it is caustic and should only be administered with extreme care intravenously and never subcutaneously. Calcium gluconate contains 9.3 mg elemental calcium per ml whereas calcium chloride contains 27.2 mg elemental calcium per ml. If the underlying cause of hypocalcaemia cannot be resolved, chronic management with oral vitamin D or calcium supplementation may be required.

Magnesium

Magnesium is measured less frequently than the other electrolytes; however a small number of clinical studies have shown magnesium abnormalities to be present in a high proportion of critically ill dogs and cats (Martin *et al.*, 1994; Toll *et al.*, 2001). In human medicine hypomagnesaemia is one of the most commonly seen electrolyte disturbances in critically ill patients. Magnesium has a role in many intracellular processes including the synthesis and degradation of DNA, oxidative phosphorylation and the production of second messengers (e.g. cAMP). It is also important for normal cardiac and neuromuscular function and is involved with potassium regulation at the level of the kidney (Bateman, 2006). Clinical signs associated with hypomagnesaemia include refractory hypokalaemia, cardiac conduction disturbances and increased neuromuscular excitability. The incidence and clinical importance of these signs has yet to be determined in small animal patients, however normalization of serum magnesium levels is recommended if serum magnesium is low and one or more compatible clinical signs are present. Magnesium sulphate or magnesium chloride should be administered as a slow intravenous infusion at a dose of 0.375–0.5 mmol/kg/day. As the magnesium ion is divalent, 1 mEq is equivalent to 0.5 mmol.

Magnesium is excreted through the kidneys, therefore hypermagnesaemia is most commonly seen in patients with reduced glomerular filtration rate, and generally does not require specific treatment. Hypermagnesaemia associated with iatrogenic overdose has been reported (Jackson and Drobatz, 2004).

Acid–base abnormalities

Maintenance of pH within a strict range is essential for normal cellular function, as many intracellular enzymatic processes are pH-dependent. On a daily basis, the body produces large amounts of both carbon dioxide (so called volatile acid) as a by-product of the metabolism of carbohydrate and fat, and hydrogen ions (H^+) as a by-product of the metabolism of proteins and phospholipids. The carbon dioxide is excreted through the lungs and the hydrogen ions are excreted through the kidneys. Carbon dioxide is an acid in solution due to its ability to combine with water, in the presence of carbonic anhydrase, to produce carbonic acid:

$$CO_2 + H_2O \leftrightarrow H_2CO_3 \leftrightarrow H^+ + HCO_3^-$$

To facilitate handling of the daily acid load, the body has several buffer systems, the most important of which is bicarbonate. Other buffers include haemoglobin and plasma proteins. Bicarbonate is constantly regenerated and added back to the circulation by the kidneys. Many pathological processes affect the body's ability to maintain a normal pH.

Measurement of acid–base status in emergency and critically ill patients has many uses including:

- Early identification of some diagnoses, e.g. ketoacidosis in a vomiting patient with an unexplained metabolic acidosis
- Production and refinement of complete problem and differential diagnosis lists
- Monitoring response to therapy, e.g. resolution of lactic acidosis in a patient with hypovolaemic shock following appropriate fluid therapy
- Prompting specific treatment when the acid–base abnormality is severe enough to be life threatening, e.g. starting (or increasing) artificial ventilation on patients with severe hypercarbia (P_aCO_2 >60 mmHg)
- Optimizing therapy for an individual patient, e.g. choice of 0.9% NaCl as opposed to a fluid with lower chloride concentration for use in a patient with a hypochloraemic metabolic alkalosis.

Interpretation of acid–base abnormalities is often regarded as challenging and there is ongoing debate about the best way to interpret results in patients with complex acid–base disturbances. However, for the majority of patients the traditional approach to blood gas interpretation, utilizing pH, pCO_2 and bicarbonate (or base excess) provides sufficient information for effective clinical use.

Definitions

- pH: a familiar measure of acidity/alkalinity calculated as the negative log of the hydrogen ion concentration.
- Acidaemia: blood pH <7.35.
- Alkalaemia: blood pH >7.45.
- Acidosis: a process that tends to lead to acidaemia. It may not result in acidaemia if there is adequate compensation, or if there is a concurrent process tending to lead to alkalaemia.
- Alkalosis: a process that tends to lead to alkalaemia. It may not result in alkalaemia if there is adequate compensation or if there is a concurrent process tending to lead to acidaemia.

- Respiratory acidosis/alkalosis: where the process leading to the acid–base disturbance involves abnormalities of the concentration (partial pressure) of the volatile acid carbon dioxide.
- Metabolic acidosis/alkalosis: where the process leading to the acid–base disturbance involves abnormalities of acid/alkali other than carbon dioxide.
- Base excess (BE): a calculated value that is a reflection of the non-respiratory portion of acid–base balance. It takes into account all of the body's buffer systems and is closely (but not linearly) related to bicarbonate. A negative value indicates the presence of a metabolic acidosis whereas a positive value indicates the presence of a metabolic alkalosis.
- Compensation: mechanisms by which the body attempts to maintain a normal pH despite disturbances in the acid–base status. With a primary metabolic acid–base disturbance, compensation is via the respiratory system, with alterations in ventilation and the excretion of carbon dioxide. This respiratory compensation occurs very rapidly over minutes to hours. With a primary respiratory acid–base disturbance, there is compensation on the metabolic side, by alterations in the excretion of acid load through the kidneys. This metabolic compensation occurs gradually over days. Compensation can be very effective and may return the pH to within the normal range. Importantly, overcompensation never occurs.
- Primary acid–base disturbance: the initial (usually the most severe) disturbance in acid–base status. Primary acid–base disturbances may be accompanied by compensatory changes. Examples might include a cat with urethral obstruction and a primary metabolic acidosis secondary to reduced renal excretion of the daily acid load. This cat may also be tachypnoeic as acidosis leads to an increase in minute ventilation, producing a compensatory respiratory alkalosis.
- Mixed acid–base disturbances: more than one primary acid–base disturbance occurring concurrently. Examples might include:
  - A patient with pneumonia and septic shock. This patient may have a respiratory alkalosis, as it increases ventilation to try to maximize oxygenation, and a metabolic (lactic) acidosis secondary to the septic shock and inadequate tissue perfusion
  - A dog with pyloric obstruction and vomiting of gastric contents, which is also in hypovolaemic shock. This patient may have a metabolic alkalosis secondary to vomiting of hydrochloric acid-rich stomach contents, and a metabolic (lactic) acidosis secondary to hypovolaemic shock and reduced tissue perfusion. This patient may have a normal pH at presentation because the two primary processes balance each other out, but could become significantly alkalaemic as the shock is treated with intravenous fluids.

Approximate reference values for acid–base parameters in arterial blood are shown in Figure 5.8. Venous blood differs slightly because carbon dioxide produced by tissue metabolism has been added as it passes through the capillary bed, therefore venous blood tends to have a slightly lower pH and higher pCO_2. In all situations other than complete circulatory collapse venous blood is considered to be adequate for assessment of acid–base status (Ilkiw *et al.*, 1991).

Parameter	Dog	Cat
pH	7.35–7.46	7.31–7.46
pCO_2 (mmHg)	31–43	25–37
HCO_3^- (mEq/l)	18–26	14–22
Base excess (BE)	–4 to +2	–4 to +2

5.8 Approximate normal values for acid–base parameters in arterial blood (based on Haskins, 1983).

Respiratory acid–base disturbances

Respiratory acid–base disturbances occur secondary to alterations in the concentration (partial pressure) of carbon dioxide (pCO_2) in the blood. Because carbon dioxide is an acid in solution, an increase in pCO_2 leads to a respiratory acidosis and a decrease in pCO_2 leads to a respiratory alkalosis. As blood levels of carbon dioxide are determined by the state of alveolar ventilation, the causes of respiratory acidosis and alkalosis are identical to those for hypo-and hyperventilation respectively. These are summarized in Figure 5.9 and discussed in more detail in Chapter 7. In animals with chronic respiratory acid–base disturbances the kidneys can compensate by altering net acid excretion and bicarbonate resorption. Treatment for respiratory acid–base disturbances involves resolution of the underlying problem or, if severe, intubation with mechanical ventilation to normalize pCO_2. Bicarbonate should not be administered to patients

Respiratory acidosis (hypoventilation)

Upper airway obstruction
Respiratory centre depression
Central neurological disease
Spinal cord injury cranial to C4–C5
Drugs, e.g. anaesthesia
Neuromuscular disease, e.g. myasthenia gravis, botulism
Restrictive disease, e.g. pneumothorax, pleural effusion
Respiratory muscle fatigue, e.g. severe parenchymal disease
Inadequate mechanical ventilation

Respiratory alkalosis (hyperventilation)

Hypoxaemia (severe)
Pulmonary parenchymal disease
Hyperthermia
Pain
Fear/stress
Exercise
Neurological disease
Excessive mechanical ventilation

5.9 Causes of respiratory acid–base disturbances.

with severe respiratory acidosis. In this situation, bicarbonate is ineffective in improving the acidosis (and may actually worsen acidosis) as the patient is unable to excrete the carbon dioxide formed as the bicarbonate combines with hydrogen ions. Bicarbonate administration also has the theoretical potential to cause several detrimental effects, including worsening hypoxaemia, paradoxical cerebrospinal fluid (CSF) acidosis and hypotension.

Metabolic acid–base disturbances

Metabolic acid–base disturbances occur as a result of alterations in the non-volatile (i.e. non-carbon dioxide) acids in the blood. A metabolic alkalosis implies that acid has been lost from the body. A metabolic acidosis implies that an acid has been added or generated within the body, or that bicarbonate has been lost from the body. The anion gap can be used to help determine whether a metabolic acidosis was caused by addition of an acid or by loss of bicarbonate. The anion gap is calculated using the following formula:

$$\text{Anion gap} = ([Na^+] + [K^+]) - ([Cl^-] + [HCO_3^-])$$

The body must maintain electroneutrality (i.e. the number of cations in the body must equal the number of anions). The total number of cations in blood includes sodium, potassium and others, for example calcium and magnesium, which are not included in this equation and are therefore termed 'unmeasured'. Similarly, a number of 'unmeasured' anions are not included in this equation, for example sulphates and phosphates. The presence of a small anion gap in normal animals simply tells us that there are more unmeasured anions (UA) than unmeasured cations (UC). A normal anion gap is 10–27 in cats and 8–25 in dogs. An acidosis with a normal anion gap implies that no additional unmeasured anions are present in the blood, thus loss of bicarbonate is the cause of the acidosis. Conversely, an acidosis with a high anion gap implies the presence of an unmeasured anion (e.g. lactate, ketones, salicylate) and hence addition or generation of an acid within the body (Figure 5.10).

Causes of metabolic acid–base disturbances are summarized in Figure 5.11. Respiratory compensation for primary metabolic disturbances occurs rapidly and is often very effective, therefore the plasma pH may be close to normal. Treatment for metabolic acid–base disturbances involves resolution of the underlying problem (e.g. fluid therapy for lactic acidosis, insulin therapy for ketoacidosis). In animals with severe metabolic acidosis (pH <7.2) in which the primary disturbance cannot be resolved quickly, it may be necessary to administer bicarbonate. The bicarbonate deficit is calculated as below:

$$\text{Bicarbonate deficit} = \text{body weight (kg)} \times \text{base excess} \times 0.3$$

One third of the calculated deficit is administered by slow intravenous infusion over 15–30 minutes and the acid–base status is reassessed. The remainder can be added to the patient's intravenous fluids and delivered over a period of hours if necessary.

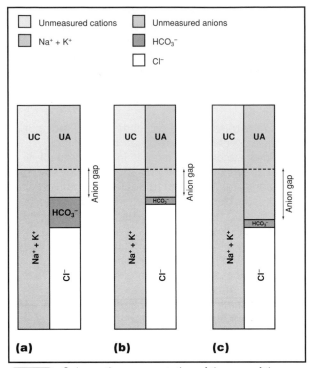

5.10 Schematic representation of the use of the anion gap for determining the cause of metabolic acidosis. Because plasma electroneutrality must be maintained, the total number of cations must equal the total number of anions. **(a)** A normal dog, in which the anion gap represents the difference between the unmeasured cations (UC) and the unmeasured anions (UA). **(b)** A patient with a metabolic acidosis secondary to loss of bicarbonate. As no other anions have been added to the body, chloride is increased so electroneutrality is maintained and the patient has a normal anion gap (or hyperchloraemic) acidosis. **(c)** A patient in which the acidosis is caused by addition of an acid (i.e. anion) to the body (e.g. lactate or phosphate). This anion is buffered by bicarbonate which decreases, but as another anion is present chloride does not change. This represents a high anion gap (or normochloraemic) acidosis.

Metabolic acidosis
High anion gap (normochloraemic)
Diabetic ketoacidosis
Lactic acidosis
Uraemic acidosis
Toxins (e.g. ethylene glycol, salicylates)
Normal anion gap (hyperchloraemic)
Diarrhoea
Renal tubular acidosis
Drugs (e.g. carbonic anhydrase inhibitors)
Dilutional acidosis

Metabolic alkalosis
Associated with hypochloraemia
Vomiting
Diuretic therapy
Following hypercapnia
Not typically associated with hypochloraemia
Primary hyperaldosteronism
Hyperadrenocorticism

5.11 Causes of metabolic acid–base disturbances. Diagnoses in italics are those encountered most frequently in clinical practice.

Interpreting acid–base results

Interpretation of acid–base results involves integrating the information provided by the pH, PCO_2 and base excess (or bicarbonate). All three parameters should be looked at every time an acid–base panel is reviewed. Electrolyte values are also essential for full interpretation, especially of metabolic acidosis. The following points should be used when interpreting acid–base results in clinical patients. Expected patterns are summarized in Figure 5.12.

1. Look at the pH:
   - Is it acidaemic (pH <7.4), alkalaemic (pH > 7.4) or normal (pH approximately 7.4)?
2. If acidaemia is present, determine whether it is respiratory or metabolic in origin:
   - If PCO_2 >45 mmHg, there is a primary respiratory acidosis
   - If BE is negative (or bicarbonate <18 mEq/l), there is a primary metabolic acidosis.
3. If alkalaemia is present, determine whether it is respiratory or metabolic in origin:
   - If PCO_2 <33 mmHg, there is a primary respiratory alkalosis
   - If BE is positive (or bicarbonate >24 mEq/l), there is a primary metabolic alkalosis.
4. Following on from point 2 or 3 above, assess whether the patient has evidence of compensation, and whether this appears to be adequate. Expected compensation for primary acid–base disturbances is shown in Figure 5.13. Inadequate compensation may be because there has been insufficient time for compensation, or because there is a second primary acid–base process that is preventing the expected compensation.
5. If pH is normal, look at PCO_2 and BE:
   - If both PCO_2 and BE are abnormal, the patient has either a fully compensated acid–base disturbance *or* two primary processes that are effectively cancelling each other out. These scenarios can be difficult to distinguish. Clinical information may be helpful. Also remember that overcompensation does not occur. In most patients with a fully compensated acid–base disturbance the pH will be only just within the normal range, and the direction of deviation from 7.4 will indicate the primary process
   - If both PCO_2 and BE are normal, then either the patient is normal *or* the patient has a primary metabolic acidosis and a concurrent primary metabolic alkalosis. Along with the clinical picture, the patient's electrolytes should help identify the latter group, as they will almost always be hypochloraemic.

Examples of acid–base disturbances, explanations of interpretation and major differential diagnoses to consider are given below.

Example 1

pH	7.48
PCO_2	27 mmHg
BE	−1
HCO_3^-	19 mEq/l

Interpretation: Acute respiratory alkalosis. The pH is increased indicating an alkalaemia and the low PCO_2 confirms that this is a primary respiratory alkalosis. There is no compensation, indicating that it is acute. Common differential diagnoses would include a dog that is stressed, in pain or hyperthermic, or an animal that is hyperventilating to improve oxygenation. If clinically indicated, pulse oximetry or arterial blood gas analysis with assessment of P_aO_2 (see Chapter 7) should be performed.

Disorder	pH	pCO₂	BE	Bicarbonate
Metabolic acidosis	↓	(↓)	Negative	↓
Metabolic alkalosis	↑	(↑)	Positive	↑
Respiratory acidosis	↓	↑	(Positive)	(↑)
Respiratory alkalosis	↑	↓	(Negative)	(↓)

5.12 Expected patterns of acid–base parameter changes in patients with primary acid–base disturbances. Trends in parentheses indicate a compensatory response (BE, base excess).

Disorder	Primary change	Expected compensatory response
Metabolic acidosis	↓[HCO₃⁻]	0.7 mmHg decrease in PCO_2 for each 1 mEq/l decrease in [HCO₃⁻]
Metabolic alkalosis	↑[HCO₃⁻]	0.7 mmHg increase in PCO_2 for each 1 mEq/l increase in [HCO₃⁻]
Acute respiratory acidosis	↑PCO_2	1.5 mmol/l increase in [HCO₃⁻] for each 10 mmHg increase in PCO_2
Chronic respiratory acidosis	↑PCO_2	3.5 mmol/l increase in [HCO₃⁻] for each 10 mmHg increase in PCO_2
Acute respiratory alkalosis	↓PCO_2	2.5 mmol/l decrease in [HCO₃⁻] for each 10 mmHg decrease in PCO_2
Chronic respiratory alkalosis	↓PCO_2	5.5 mmol/l decrease in [HCO₃⁻] for each 10 mmHg decrease in PCO_2

5.13 Expected renal and respiratory compensation for primary acid–base disturbances in dogs (modified from DiBartola, 2006a).

Example 2

pH   7.31
PCO_2 28 mmHg
BE   −8
HCO_3^- 12 mEq/l

Interpretation: Compensated metabolic acidosis. The pH is decreased indicating an acidaemia. The negative BE and low bicarbonate confirm that this is a primary metabolic acidosis. The carbon dioxide is decreased in compensation, and the magnitude of the decrease is appropriate. If the abnormal carbon dioxide was the primary process, it would tend to lead to an alkalaemia, which is not present in this patient. An underlying cause for the acidaemia should be sought. Common differential diagnoses include lactic acidosis (with poor perfusion and shock), ketoacidosis or uraemia.

Example 3

pH   7.40
PCO_2 22 mmHg
BE   −12
HCO_3^- 10 mEq/l

Interpretation: This patient has a normal pH but both the BE/bicarbonate and PCO_2 are very abnormal. The low BE/bicarbonate implies a metabolic acidosis and the low PCO_2 implies a respiratory alkalosis. Considering the pH is close to the middle of the normal range and that the BE/bicarbonate and PCO_2 are more extreme than would be expected for compensation, this is likely to represent two primary processes that are effectively cancelling each other out in terms of pH. The differential diagnosis lists for both metabolic acidosis and respiratory alkalosis should be considered when evaluating a complete problem list for this patient, and deciding upon further diagnostic tests and treatment. Treatment aimed at only one of the processes may lead to worsening of the pH as the other process can then predominate.

Conclusion

Acid–base disturbances occur frequently in critically ill patients. In many circumstances, treatment of the underlying disease leads to resolution of the acid–base problem, and improvement in pH can be a sign that treatment is succeeding. In more complex cases, an understanding of acid–base physiology and ability to interpret blood gas parameters can lead to improved patient care both in terms of completeness of the diagnostic evaluation and optimization of the treatment plan for that individual patient.

References and further reading

Bateman S (2006) Disorders of magnesium: magnesium deficit and excess. In: *Fluid, Electrolyte and Acid Base Disorders in Small Animal Practice, 3rd edn,* ed. SP DiBartola, pp. 210–226. Saunders Elsevier, Missouri

Cole SG and Drobatz KJ (2003) Influence of crystalloid type on acid–base and electrolyte status in cats with urethral obstruction. *Proceedings of the International Veterinary Emergency and Critical Care Society Meeting,* p. 162

DiBartola SP (2006) Disorders of sodium and water: hypernatremia and hyponatremia. In: *Fluid, Electrolyte and Acid Base Disorders in Small Animal Practice, 3rd edn,* ed. SP DiBartola, pp. 47–79. Saunders Elsevier, Missouri

DiBartola SP (2006a) Introduction to acid–base disorders. In: *Fluid, Electrolyte and Acid Base Disorders in Small Animal Practice, 3rd edn,* ed. SP DiBartola, pp. 229–251. Saunders Elsevier, Missouri

Haskins SC (1983) Blood gases and acid–base balance: clinical interpretation and therapeutic implications. In: *Current Veterinary Therapy VIII,* ed. RW Kirk, pp. 201. WB Saunders, Philadelphia

Ilkiw JE, Rose RJ and Martin ICA (1991) A comparison of simultaneously collected arterial, mixed venous, jugular venous and cephalic venous blood samples in the assessment of blood gas and acid base status in dogs. *Journal of Veterinary Internal Medicine* **5**, 294–298

Jackson CB and Drobatz KJ (2004) Iatrogenic magnesium overdose; 2 case reports. *Journal of Veterinary Emergency and Critical Care* **14**, 115–123

Martin L, Matteson V, Wingfield W *et al.* (1994) Abnormalities of serum magnesium in critically ill dogs; incidence and implications. *Journal of Veterinary Emergency and Critical Care* **4**, 15

Rose BD and Post TW (2001) *Clinical Physiology of Acid–base and Electrolyte Disorders, 5th edn.* McGrawHill, New York

Schenk PA and Chew DJ (2005) Prediction of serum ionised calcium concentration by use of serum total calcium concentration in dogs. *American Journal of Veterinary Research* **66**,1330–1336

Toll J, Erb H, Birnbaum N *et al.* (2001) Prevalence and incidence of serum magnesium abnormalities in hospitalised cats. *Journal of Veterinary Internal Medicine* **16**, 217–221

6

Cardiovascular emergencies

Rebecca L. Stepien and Adrian Boswood

Introduction

Emergencies involving the cardiovascular system include primary abnormalities of the heart, and extracardiac abnormalities that have a direct effect on cardiac function. Primary cardiac abnormalities include impaired function or damage to the heart muscle (e.g. cardiomyopathies or thoracic trauma), abnormal flow patterns within the heart (e.g. valvular regurgitation) or primary rhythm abnormalities (e.g. ventricular tachycardia). Extracardiac abnormalities affecting cardiac output may include pericardial effusion, systemic hypertension, thrombosis, or metabolic abnormalities, especially those involving electrolyte disorders.

Initial assessment of the cardiovascular system

Emergency presentation of patients with clinical signs of cardiovascular disease usually necessitates a quick but thorough assessment and rapid, decisive action.

Recognition of clinical signs and physical findings that are typical of various cardiovascular abnormalities should lead to appropriate ancillary cardiac testing. Many critically ill patients have abnormal findings on examination of the cardiovascular system, but differentiating whether cardiac abnormalities are a result of cardiac disease or secondary to abnormalities of other systems can be difficult. Clinical findings typical of cardiovascular disease with possible cardiac and non-cardiac causes are listed in Figure 6.1.

Physical examination

Physical examination of the critically ill cardiac patient involves rapid accumulation of numerical data as well as subjective assessment of physical examination findings. Historical findings typical of emergency cardiovascular patients include dyspnoea, collapse, syncope, cough, cyanosis or signs of peripheral thromboembolism (primarily in cats). When these historical findings are accompanied by physical examination findings supportive of cardiovascular disease (Figure 6.2), further cardiovascular testing is warranted.

Clinical finding	Possible cardiac causes	Non-cardiac causes
Dyspnoea	Pulmonary oedema Pleural effusion Pericardial effusion	Primary respiratory disease Airway obstruction Pulmonary thromboembolism Acid–base disorders Pain/anxiety Pulmonary hypertension
Cough (dogs)	Left atrial enlargement Severe pulmonary oedema	Primary respiratory disease Pyothorax
Cough (cats)	Rarely associated with CHF	Primary respiratory disease Feline asthma/bronchial disease
Cyanosis	Severe pulmonary oedema Right-to-left shunt (congenital heart disease)	Airway obstruction Severe respiratory disease Methaemoglobinaemia
Ascites	Right-sided CHF Caudal vena cava obstruction	Hypoproteinaemia Portal hypertension Abdominal distention secondary to gastric dilatation–volvulus Peritonitis Peritoneal haemorrhage
Heart murmur	Valvular disease Myocardial disease Congenital heart defects	Anaemia (PCV <25%) 'Innocent' murmurs (dogs <16 weeks old) Pyrexia

6.1 Cardiac and non-cardiac causes of abnormal cardiovascular clinical findings. Lists are not all-inclusive (CHF, congestive heart failure; PCV, packed cell volume). (continues)

Clinical finding	Possible cardiac causes	Non-cardiac causes
Syncope or collapse	Dysrhythmias Inappropriate drug therapy Pericardial effusion	Hypoglycaemia Electrolyte disorders Anaemia Neurological disorders Musculoskeletal abnormalities
Sinus tachycardia	Hypotension due to decreased cardiac output Sympathetic activation associated with CHF	Shock/blood loss Dehydration (severe) Pyrexia or hyperthermia Anaemia Pain/anxiety
Ectopic tachycardias	Primary myocardial disorder/trauma Myocardial hypoxia	Systemic hypoxia Acid–base disorders Electrolyte disorders Sepsis Drug toxicity Autonomic nervous system abnormalities
Bradycardia	Sick sinus syndrome Atrioventricular block	High vagal tone Hyperkalaemia or other electrolyte disturbances
Peripheral paresis	Systemic thromboembolism	Musculoskeletal abnormalities Neurological disorders
Peripheral oedema	Severe right-sided or biventricular CHF	Hypoproteinaemia Vasculitis Lymphatic disorder Vascular obstruction

6.1 (continued) Cardiac and non-cardiac causes of abnormal cardiovascular clinical findings. Lists are not all-inclusive (CHF, congestive heart failure; PCV, packed cell volume).

Physical parameter	Cardiovascular disease
Heart rate and rhythm	Tachycardia or bradycardia Irregular rhythm *accompanied by pulse deficits*
Respiratory rate and character	Elevated respiratory rate Dyspnoea or shallow breathing Panting (cats)
Thoracic auscultation	Gallop rhythm Heart murmur Muffled heart sounds (pericardial effusion) Pulmonary crackles Increased large airway sounds Muffled respiratory sounds (pleural effusion) Spontaneous cough (dog)
Abdominal assessment	Fluid wave or abdominal fluid distension accompanied by jugular distension Hepatomegaly
Peripheral vascular assessment	Weak or bounding pulses Pulse deficits Jugular distension Jugular pulsation Cyanosis Slow capillary refill time
Other	Peripheral paresis accompanied by pulselessness Peripheral oedema accompanied by other signs of right-sided or biventricular CHF

6.2 Physical findings associated with cardiovascular disease (CHF, congestive heart failure).

Electrocardiography

Electrocardiographic recordings are crucial in the diagnosis and therapy of cardiac dysrhythmias. All unstable emergency patients should have an electrocardiogram (ECG) recorded as a baseline assessment regardless of suspected illness. On physical examination, sinus tachycardia accompanied by weak pulses due to hypovolaemic shock may be indistinguishable from the same findings when caused by ventricular tachycardia, yet ventricular tachycardia might need to be treated directly with anti-dysrhythmic medications, whereas sinus tachycardia due to shock-related hypotension usually resolves with fluid therapy. Animals with accelerated idioventricular rhythms, second-degree heart block and junctional tachycardias due to digitalis intoxication may each have heart rates within accepted normal ranges, but ECG recognition of these abnormalities may provide critical diagnostic information.

In stable patients, a baseline ECG recording is recommended in order to provide evidence of admission status for comparison in case of dysrhythmia development later during hospitalization. For patients suspected of having cardiovascular disease, the ECG provides not only a quick assessment of rhythm status, but also provides information regarding conduction abnormalities and limited information about cardiac size.

Recording of the ECG in the critically ill patient should involve as little patient stress as possible. Lead II ECG recordings are usually adequate for rhythm diagnosis, but multiple leads may be necessary to allow scrutinization of individual recordings for the presence of P waves, or to better recognize rhythm disorders in patients in which complexes are smaller than usual. Recordings for rhythm analysis may be taken with the patient in any position; sternal recumbency is often the most comfortable for dyspnoeic patients. Electrocardiographic coupling gel, rather than alcohol (i.e. spirits), should be used to moisten the lead contact points, to avoid inadvertent ignition if emergency use of defibrillation paddles becomes necessary.

Arterial blood pressure

Arterial blood pressure (ABP) measurement is useful in the assessment of cardiovascular function and is included in the initial assessment of many emergency patients. Methods of blood pressure assessment are discussed in Chapter 3. Indirect blood pressure measurement systems (e.g. Doppler sphygmomanometric or oscillometric methods) are useful to document high blood pressure in patients with systemic hypertension, but are less useful in hypotensive patients where repeatable detection of a distal limb pulse may be difficult. Invasive methods of monitoring blood pressure involve placement of an arterial catheter (see Chapter 2) and are more accurate than non-invasive methods when blood pressure is low. The dorsal pedal artery is accessible and can be catheterized in most dogs following local anaesthetic infiltration (e.g. lidocaine); cats may require a femoral arterial surgical 'cut-down' to establish an arterial line. Once arterial access is established, baseline blood pressure is recorded, and continuous blood pressure monitoring can be used throughout initial therapy.

Dogs and cats are generally considered to be hypotensive when they have a *systolic* pressure of less than 90 mmHg, a *mean* arterial pressure less than 60 mmHg and/or a *diastolic* pressure less than 50 mmHg. In animals with heart failure it may be desirable to maintain *mean arterial pressure* (MAP) between 70 and 80 mmHg; this provides decreased afterload but preserves adequate blood pressure to perfuse end organs. In the heart failure patient, blood pressure may be increased by administration of positive inotropes (with or without addition of fluid therapy) and treatment of dysrhythmias, while blood pressure may be decreased by the use of vasodilating drugs.

Central venous pressure

Measurement of central venous pressure (CVP) is used to estimate the filling pressure of the right side of the heart (i.e. right atrial pressure). CVP is measured and monitored using a catheter placed into the cranial vena cava or right atrium via the jugular vein (see Chapters 2 and 4). Low CVP is usually a result of hypovolaemia, and high CVP may result from increased intravascular volume, decreased cardiac output in a normovolaemic patient, or right-sided congestive heart failure (CHF). CVP can also be used to monitor volume status in non-cardiogenic shock during an intravenous fluid challenge. If cardiac disease is suspected, *or* if initial CVP measurements are elevated, fluid boluses should be avoided.

Elevated central venous pressure

Elevated CVP (reflecting elevated right atrial pressure) indicates failure of the right ventricle (RV) to pump the volume of blood presented during ventricular filling adequately. This may be due to increased intravascular volume (e.g. fluid overload) or right-sided cardiac abnormalities. In cardiac patients, elevated CVP reflects RV inflow abnormalities (e.g. tricuspid valve insufficiency/stenosis, pericardial tamponade), primary myocardial disease or RV outflow obstruction (e.g. pulmonic stenosis, pulmonary hypertension, pulmonary thromboembolism). Some abnormalities are co-existent (e.g. right-sided congestive heart failure (CHF) secondary to severe tricuspid insufficiency). Notably, pulmonary arterial hypertension leading to elevations in CVP may be due to left ventricular failure and elevated left atrial pressure; CVP may therefore be serially monitored to judge the efficacy of therapy for left heart failure. CVP monitoring is not as sensitive to elevations in left atrial pressure as pulmonary arterial wedge pressure monitoring, but is easier to maintain in clinical veterinary patients. In cases of acute CHF, therapy involves controlled volume depletion of the patient, and serial CVP measurement allows the clinician to follow decreases in right atrial pressure while avoiding excessive dehydration. The target CVP to maintain optimal cardiac output without leading to fluid overload is approximately 10–15 cmH$_2$O or 7–11 mmHg in dogs, and 5–7 cmH$_2$O or 3–4 mmHg in cats.

Decreased central venous pressure

Decreased CVP usually reflects hypovolaemia. Patients with heart disease may have concurrent hypovolaemia contributing to their clinical signs. In animals with heart disease and signs of low output (exercise intolerance, collapse, slow capillary refill time), a hypovolaemic component to the poor output is suspected when there is a low CVP and no congestive signs. These patients may benefit from cautious fluid therapy with serial CVP monitoring to document increases in right atrial pressure. The aim is to restore CVP to within or slightly above normal range, to optimize ventricular filling.

Pulmonary artery wedge pressure

Pulmonary artery wedge pressure is measured using a balloon-tipped catheter in the main pulmonary artery. In veterinary patients, the catheter is usually introduced via the jugular vein and advanced through the RV to the main pulmonary artery using typical pressure tracings or fluoroscopic guidance. When the balloon is deflated, the pressure measured is the main pulmonary artery pressure, but when the balloon is inflated and carried by blood flow to 'wedge' in a smaller pulmonary artery, the 'wedge pressure' recorded is roughly equal to left atrial pressure. Pulmonary artery wedge pressure measurements are an accurate reflection of left ventricular filling pressures, and may be used serially to monitor the efficacy of CHF therapy in reducing left atrial pressure. In many clinical cases of acute CHF in veterinary patients, dyspnoea and patient anxiety are limiting factors for patient manipulation. In these cases, fast and accurate placement of a balloon-tipped catheter can be difficult. Since continuous monitoring of pulmonary artery wedge pressure is not commonly available in most veterinary clinics, other methods of monitoring will be emphasized here.

Arterial blood gases

Arterial blood gas analysis is helpful in the respiratory management of patients with dyspnoea due to CHF. Hypoxia (P_aO_2 <80 mmHg on room air), arterial desaturation as measured by pulse oximetry (arterial oxygen saturation <90% on room air) and hyperventilation (P_aCO_2 <35 mmHg) are consistent with respiratory impairment related to pulmonary oedema. In patients with fulminant pulmonary oedema, P_aO_2 is frequently 40–60 mmHg or less while the patient is breathing room air. Development of hypercarbia (P_aCO_2 >45 mmHg) is an ominous sign, reflecting profound (imminently life-threatening) pulmonary dysfunction and/or fatigue of the muscles of respiration. In these cases, assisted ventilation may be necessary.

Thoracic radiographs

Emergency radiography is covered in detail in Chapter 25. Acute pulmonary oedema is generally recognizable based on history and physical examination findings, and the stress related to positioning an animal for radiographs may worsen its clinical condition. In most cases, anaesthetized radiographs are *contraindicated*, as most anaesthetic regimens have depressant effects on the cardiovascular system. In some cases, marginal amounts of pulmonary oedema can be worsened greatly by use of negative inotropic anaesthetic regimens. Animals with severe dysrhythmias should *never* be anaesthetized until the rhythm has been stabilized. In general, while thoracic radiographs contribute greatly to diagnosis of the underlying disease and differentiation of cardiac disease from pulmonary disease, most cases of severe congestive heart failure can be diagnosed without immediate radiographs.

'Cardiac' blood tests

In human patients with cardiac disease, evaluation of B-type natriuretic peptide and troponins has been shown to assist in the discrimination of cardiac from non-cardiac causes of dyspnoea and chest pain. In order to be useful in acute management of patients these tests must be available in the emergency setting; none of the currently validated natriuretic peptide or troponin tests for dogs or cats is yet available as a 'bedside' test. In the future it might be anticipated that these will be developed and may prove very useful. Further studies will help to elucidate their value in the emergency setting but they cannot currently be considered validated for this purpose.

Acute heart failure

Algorithms for emergency patients in heart failure are presented in Figures 6.3 and 6.4. Immediate identification of key clinical signs indicative of pulmonary

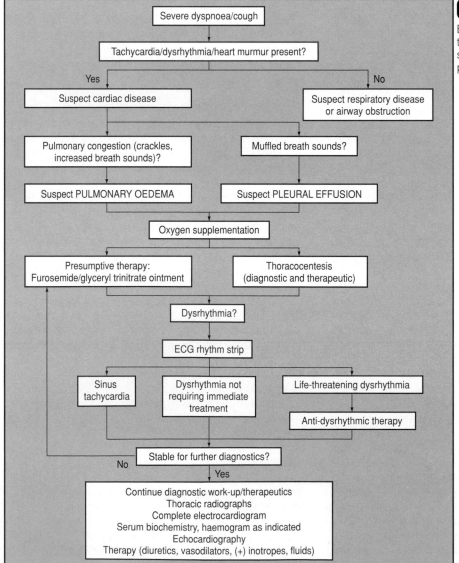

6.3 Emergency diagnostic/ therapeutic evaluation of the severely dyspnoeic cardiac patient.

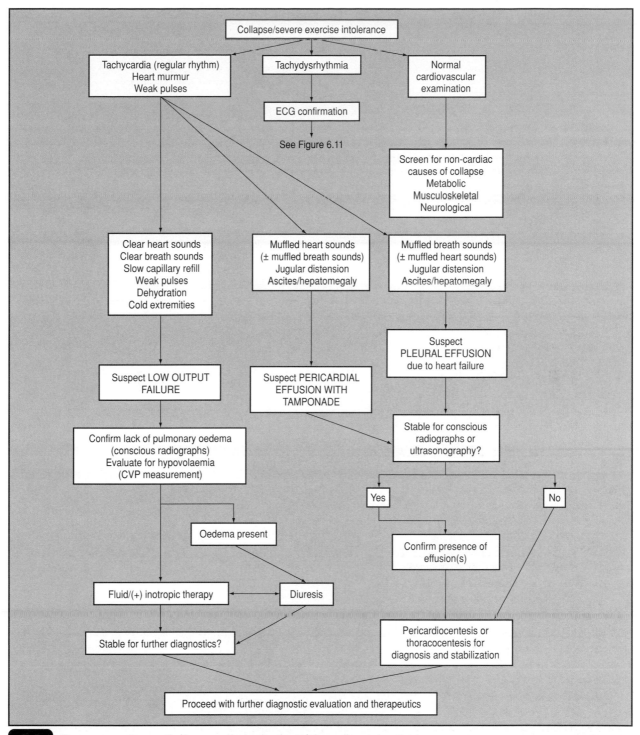

6.4 Emergency diagnostic/therapeutic evaluation of the collapsed patient.

oedema, pleural effusion, low output failure, cardiac tamponade and severe dysrhythmias may be life saving. Once the nature of the clinical presentation is recognized, emergency therapy may (and often must) proceed in the absence of an anatomical diagnosis of the underlying heart disease. Once the patient's condition is stable, further diagnostic testing may be used to establish the underlying cause of the problem and develop a definitive treatment plan. If signs of cardiogenic shock (i.e. tachycardia, cool extremities, weak pulses, prolonged capillary refill time) are present but congestive signs (e.g. pulmonary oedema or ascites)

are not, low filling pressures secondary to hypovolaemia may be complicating the underlying cardiac disease.

Most animals presented to the emergency service do not arrive with a previous diagnosis and the unstable nature of many cardiovascular emergencies makes extensive diagnostic testing dangerous. The following discussion outlines general approaches to the major presenting signs of dogs and cats with cardiovascular emergencies. Dosing regimens for commonly used drugs are outlined in Figure 6.5. Systemic hypertension (hypertensive crisis) and systemic thromboembolism are addressed separately.

Diuretics
Furosemide: (D) 2–6 mg/kg i.v., i.m., s.c. q6–12h, orally q8–24h; (C) 1–4 mg/kg i.v., i.m., s.c., orally q12–48h

Vasodilators
Acepromazine: (D,C) 0.01–0.05 mg/kg i.m., s.c. no more than q6h
Amlodipine besylate: (D) 0.05 mg/kg orally q24h; (C) 0.625 mg per cat orally q24h
Hydralazine: (D) 1–3 mg/kg orally q12h
Glyceryl trinitrate ointment (2% = 15 mg/25 mm): 1.25–2.5 mg/5 kg body wt, cutaneously q6–12h
Glyceryl trinitrate patch: (D) 2.5–10 mg/24 h as patch, 24 hours on, 24 hours off; (C) 2.5–5 mg, apply as dog
Sodium nitroprusside: (D) 1–5 µg/kg/min (start low and titrate up while monitoring blood pressure)

Inotropes
Dobutamine: (D) 2–15 µg/kg/min; (C) 1–5 µg/kg/min (start low and titrate up)
Dopamine: (D) 2–10 µg/kg/min; (C) 5–15 µg/kg/min (start low and titrate up)
Isoprenaline: (D,C) 0.04–0.08 µg/kg/min i.v.
Pimobendan (D) 0.1–0.3 mg/kg orally q12h

Anti-dysrhythmics
Atenolol (D) 1–2 mg/kg orally q12h, start low and titrate up; (C) 6.25–12.5 mg total dose orally q12h
Diltiazem: (D,C) 0.25 mg/kg i.v. (over 3 minutes), 3–6 µg/kg/min; (D) 1–2 mg/kg orally q8h; (C) 7.5 mg total dose orally q8h
Esmolol: (D,C) 0.5 mg/kg i.v. bolus, 25–200 µg/kg/min
Lidocaine: (D) 2–4 mg/kg i.v. bolus, 30–80 µg/kg/min; (C) 0.2–0.4 mg/kg i.v. slow bolus
Mexiletine: (D) 4–8 mg/kg orally q8h
Procainamide: (D) 5–15 mg/kg i.v., i.m. q6h, 10–40 µg/kg/min
Propranolol: (D) 0.1–2 mg/kg orally q8h, start low/titrate, 0.04–0.06 mg/kg i.v. slowly; (C) 2.5–5 mg total dose orally q8h, start low/titrate
Sotalol: (D) 0.5–2 mg/kg, orally q12h, start low/titrate
Amiodarone: (D) 10–15 mg/kg q12h orally for 7 days, then 5–7.5 mg/kg q12h orally for 14 days, then 7.5 mg/kg orally q24h

Sedatives
Morphine: (D) 0.05–0.1 mg/kg slow i.v. repeated every 10 minutes until effects are seen (up to 0.4 mg/kg total), dose repeated q1–4h
Butorphanol: (D,C) 0.2–0.4 mg/kg i.v., i.m. or s.c. q1–4h as needed for sedation
Buprenorphine: (D,C) 0.005–0.01 mg/kg i.v., i.m., s.c. q4–6h as needed for sedation

Other
Aspirin (for anti-thrombotic therapy): (C) 80 mg/cat q48h
Atropine: (D,C)   *atropine response test*: (D, C) 0.04 mg/kg i.m.
emergency therapy of bradycardia: 0.02–0.04 mg/kg s.c., i.m., i.v. q6–8h
Calcium gluconate (for therapy of hyperkalaemia): (D,C) 0.5–1.5 ml of a 10% solution slowly i.v.
Dextrose (for therapy of hyperkalaemia): (D,C) 5–10% dextrose-containing fluids i.v., or 1–2 ml/kg 50% dextrose i.v. (may administer with insulin, see below)
Glycopyrrolate: (D,C) 0.005–0.01 mg/kg s.c., i.m., i.v.
Insulin (for therapy of hyperkalaemia): (D,C) 0.55–1.1 IU/kg regular insulin in parenteral fluids with 2 g dextrose per unit of insulin administered
Sodium bicarbonate (for therapy of hyperkalaemia): (D,C) 1–2 mEq/kg i.v.
Unfractionated heparin (for anti-thrombotic therapy): 100–300 iu/kg s.c. q8h
Warfarin: (C) 0.25–0.5 mg/cat/day

6.5 Drugs used in therapy of cardiovascular emergency patients. Ranges are approximate; clinical evaluation of the patient dictates dosage of drug administered (D, dog; C, cat).

Severe pulmonary oedema: recognition and emergency stabilization

Key points

- Recognition:
  - Dyspnoea ± gagging cough
  - Pulmonary crackles/increased breath sounds on auscultation
  - Other physical findings typical of cardiac disease.

- Therapy:
  - Oxygen supplementation
  - Furosemide administration
  - Vasodilator administration (with some exceptions – see below)
  - Inotropic support
  - Opioid sedation
  - Low-stress environment.
- Typical underlying cardiac conditions:
  - Dilated cardiomyopathy (dog/cat)
  - Mitral insufficiency secondary to progressive

endocardiosis or acute chordae tendineae rupture (dog)
- Hypertrophic or restrictive cardiomyopathy (cat)
- Decompensated congenital heart disease (e.g. patent ductus arteriosus, ventricular septal defect, mitral dysplasia, mitral stenosis (dog/cat)).

In dogs, pulmonary oedema commonly results in respiratory difficulty and gasping, often associated with a gagging cough that may produce white or blood-tinged foam. Cats with severe pulmonary oedema often pant, but seldom cough until oedema fluid begins to fill the main airways. In both species, severe dyspnoea is accompanied by cyanosis, abdominal contraction with respiration, and signs of anxiety, including dilated pupils and resistance to restraint. Rapid appreciation of harsh or loud breath sounds, usually with pulmonary crackles, in association with other clinical findings of cardiac disease (see Figure 6.2), should lead to a tentative diagnosis of pulmonary oedema and institution of treatment (Figure 6.6).

Radiographs should not be obtained until the patient is stable enough to be manipulated. Typical radiographic findings in a dog and a cat with pulmonary oedema are shown in Figures 6.7 and 6.8.

Oxygen supplementation

The most important component of therapy for acute pulmonary oedema is *oxygen supplementation*. Supplemental oxygen should be provided immediately upon recognition of dyspnoea or cyanosis, and continued throughout stabilization. Initially, oxygen may be supplied via facemask, oxygen cage or nasal insufflation; the choice of method is dependent on availability, the patient's tolerance of administration, and manipulation requirements with regard to further diagnostic testing. If arterial blood gas analysis is available, assessment of any level of hypoxia should lead to at least temporary supplementation, but a P_aO_2 of <60 mmHg or oxygen saturation of <90% warrants aggressive oxygen therapy. Clinical status of the patient must be monitored closely. Evidence of progressive respiratory fatigue, lack of P_aO_2 response to oxygen supplementation and progressive hypercapnia are all indications for mechanical ventilation.

Medication	Action	Contraindications	Monitoring concerns	Onset of action
Butorphanol	Opioid sedative Sedative effects in depressed animals	Altered level of consciousness	Over-sedation	IV: 5–10 minutes
Buprenorphine	Opioid sedative Sedative effects in depressed animals	Altered level of consciousness	Over-sedation	IV: 5–10 minutes
Dobutamine	Catecholamine Positive inotrope	Dysrhythmias	Dysrhythmias (continuous ECG) Blood pressure	CRI: 1–2 minutes
Dopamine	Catecholamine Positive inotrope Renal vasodilator (at low doses)	Dysrhythmias Hypertension at doses >10 µg/kg/min	Dysrhythmias (continuous ECG) Blood pressure	CRI: 1–2 minutes
Furosemide	Loop diuretic Acute vasodilation (intravenous route only) Preload reduction through diuresis	Hypovolaemia	Hydration Hypokalaemia Hypomagnesaemia	IV: 5–10 minutes
Hydralazine	Arterial dilator Decrease afterload by direct arterial dilation	Hypotension Hypovolaemia Fixed or dynamic LV outflow obstruction Inability to swallow oral medication	Hypotension	Oral: 30–60 minutes
Morphine	Opioid sedative Decrease sensation of dyspnoea (CNS effect) Decrease vasoconstriction by decreasing SNS tone (decreases preload) Anti-anxiety effects	Hypercapnia (hypoventilation) Altered level of consciousness Do not use in cats	Hypoventilation Over-sedation Vomiting may be induced by acute intravenous administration	IV: 5–10 minutes
Glyceryl trinitrate ointment (2%)	Venodilator Decrease preload by systemic and pulmonary venous dilation	None	Use gloves when in contact with ointment	Peak effect: 1 hour
Sodium nitroprusside	Arterial/venous dilator Decrease preload and afterload by direct vasodilation	Hypotension Hypovolaemia Fixed or dynamic LV outflow obstruction	Acute hypotension (use invasive ABP monitoring) Thiocyanate or cyanide toxicity if administered for >48 hours	CRI: 1–2 minutes

6.6 Medications commonly used in therapy of acute congestive heart failure (ABP, arterial blood pressure; CNS, central nervous system; SNS, sympathetic nervous system; AV, atrioventricular).

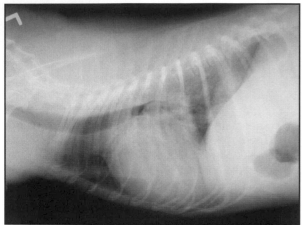

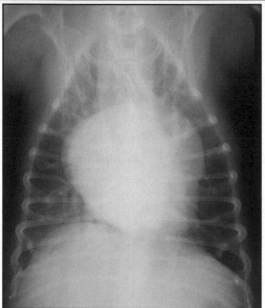

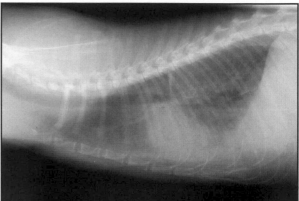

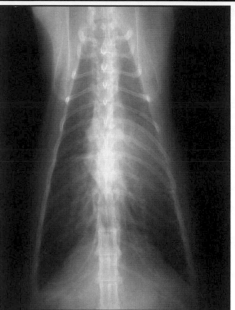

6.7 Lateral and dorsoventral radiographs of an elderly Beagle with advanced mitral and tricuspid insufficiency and congestive heart failure. Severe left ventricular and left atrial enlargement with pulmonary venous enlargement are visible on the lateral view. These findings, with the dorsal and caudal alveolar infiltrates visible in both views, are consistent with left heart failure. On the dorsoventral view, severe biatrial enlargement is visible. Note the mainstem bronchial compression caused by severe left atrial enlargement visible on the lateral view. Coughing due to bronchial compression was a prominent clinical sign in this dog.

6.8 Lateral and dorsoventral radiographs of a Domestic Short-Haired cat with restrictive myocardial disease and congestive heart failure. Moderate cardiomegaly is present in both views. Alveolar infiltrates are most visible in the left thorax on the dorsoventral view and are diffusely distributed on the lateral view. Note the engorgement of the cranial pulmonary arteries and veins visible on the lateral view.

Diuretics

After oxygen supplementation has been established, aggressive *diuretic therapy* provides the next component of stabilization. Loop diuretics are the most potent and fast-acting diuretics commonly available in veterinary practice, and immediate administration of 2–6 mg/kg of furosemide intravenously usually results in increased urine flow within approximately 30 minutes. Furosemide is also effective if given intramuscularly when intravenous access is not available. Response to furosemide administration (e.g. urination) should occur within 60–90 minutes of intravenous administration. Cats and some fastidiously trained dogs will not urinate in the cage in which they are resting; litter boxes (cats) and occasional removal from the cage to urinate (dogs) reduces additional stress

in these animals. If urination or a palpable increase in the size of the bladder does not occur in response to furosemide administration, the initial diagnosis should be reconsidered; however if CHF is still deemed to be likely, additional doses of furosemide (2–4 mg/kg i.v.) can be administered. In patients which do not produce urine after administration of furosemide, arterial blood pressure should be measured to make sure that it is high enough to maintain adequate glomerular filtration. Hypotensive animals with a combination of cardiogenic shock and congestive heart failure may be unable to respond to diuretic therapy (e.g. some cats with cardiomyopathy) until mean arterial blood pressure is above 60 mmHg. Water should be available to the patient at all times.

Vasodilators

Vasodilators, especially arterial dilators, allow rapid 'off-loading' of the ventricle and are indicated in patients with pulmonary oedema due to impaired left ventricular function, mitral insufficiency or severe systemic hypertension. By decreasing the resistance to left ventricular ejection, cardiac function is improved and, in patients with significant mitral regurgitation, the regurgitant fraction is decreased. In order to obtain this response, the left ventricle must be able to sustain an adequate stroke volume. Consequently, marked arterial vasodilation is contraindicated in animals with fixed left ventricular stroke volume (e.g. hypertrophic cardiomyopathy, mitral stenosis, aortic stenosis, many causes of RV failure) or severe hypovolaemia. Severe pulmonary oedema in animals with fixed left ventricular stroke volume must be managed primarily by preload reduction (e.g. furosemide, low-salt diet, venodilators) and judicious use of angiotensin-converting enzyme inhibitors. In hypovolaemic patients, rehydration is necessary before use of arterial vasodilators. Venodilators, such as glyceryl trinitrate ointment, are often recommended as adjunctive therapy for acute pulmonary oedema. Dermally applied glyceryl trinitrate ointment (2%) or glyceryl trinitrate-impregnated skin patches have been used to effect systemic and pulmonary venodilation and reduce preload. Although the efficacy of dermally applied glyceryl trinitrate ointment in the dog has been questioned (DeLellis and Kittleson, 1992), use of this medication remains common due to ease of application and lack of serious side effects. Angiotensin-converting enzyme inhibitors are important in the therapy of chronic CHF but are less helpful in the therapy of acute pulmonary oedema. The slower onset of action and relatively mild arterial dilation produced by this family of drugs compared with other, more potent vasodilators makes them less useful in acute emergencies.

Sodium nitroprusside (SN) and hydralazine remain the most commonly used and most effective acute arterial vasodilators in veterinary medicine. The relative advantages and disadvantages of either drug must be carefully considered in each individual patient. The potent effects of these medications make close monitoring of blood pressure during administration mandatory, and patients with acute pulmonary oedema must be continuously reassessed for moment-to-moment changes in cardiovascular status. Evidence of effective vasodilation includes bright pink mucous membranes with rapid capillary refill time, palpably warm ears and lips and gradual decreases in dyspnoea, anxiety and pulmonary oedema, as assessed by resolution of pulmonary crackles. Signs of hypotension include collapse, tachycardia and worsening renal biochemistry values.

Sodium nitroprusside: Sodium nitroprusside is a rapid-acting and potent 'mixed' vasodilator, causing both preload and afterload reduction. SN is administered intravenously, and with a half-life of minutes, can be titrated to effect. SN is used less frequently than other vasodilators in veterinary patients due to perceived monitoring problems. With careful direct blood pressure monitoring, however, SN can be used to effectively reduce arterial pressures and provide rapid relief of acute pulmonary oedema and acute hypertension. Contraindications for use of SN are listed in Figure 6.6.

Indications for use are:

- Acute pulmonary oedema due to CHF when normal to elevated systemic vascular resistance is present
- Acute pulmonary oedema secondary to mitral valve chordae tendineae rupture
- Acute hypertensive crisis.

Animals with CHF typically have low or normal arterial blood pressure, but in an animal with compromised myocardial function (e.g. dilated cardiomyopathy), normal blood pressures may represent elevated systemic vascular resistance. Therefore, known hypotension is a contraindication for SN administration, but normal to mildly elevated ABP accompanying low cardiac output and congestive signs is an indication for its use.

Direct arterial blood pressure monitoring should ideally be established prior to administration of SN. In rare cases, Doppler or oscillometric methods can be used to monitor patients receiving SN, but the tendency of these methods to be inaccurate at low ABP limits their usefulness in this setting. Once a direct ABP tracing is obtained, a continuous rate infusion (CRI) of SN can be initiated, beginning with an infusion rate of 1 µg/kg/min and titrating upwards in 0.5–1.0 µg/kg/min increments at intervals of 5–10 minutes to a target mean ABP of approximately 70–80 mmHg. A maximum rate of 10 µg/kg/min should not be exceeded. SN is light sensitive and should be prepared in relatively high concentrations allowing low fluid administration rates compatible with CHF. Any additional fluid therapy or medication infusions should be given separately to allow independent changes in administration rate. Because of the potency of SN, a fluid or syringe pump is mandatory to control infusion rate precisely. When an effective dose is ascertained, SN can be continuously administered for 48–72 hours with minimal risk of toxicity. Rapid improvement in clinical signs is usually noted in the first 3–6 hours when SN is administered concurrently with furosemide and other adjunctive therapies.

Hydralazine: Hydralazine is a potent arterial dilator. It has been used extensively in veterinary patients for both acute and chronic heart failure. The indications for use of hydralazine in the therapy of acute pulmonary oedema are the same as those for SN. Hydralazine may be chosen for acute therapy if SN is not readily available, invasive ABP monitoring or use of an infusion pump is not possible, or monetary concerns preclude the use of a CRI. If an animal is too unstable for administration of oral medications, SN should be used. Contraindications for use of hydralazine are similar to those for SN and are listed in Figure 6.6.

ABP should be obtained prior to therapy to exclude hypotension in an individual patient. Animals with fulminant pulmonary oedema are usually given a higher initial dose of hydralazine than patients with more chronic signs or animals already receiving chronic vasodilator therapy. In acute CHF, the first dose of hydralazine is approximately 1–2 mg/kg orally. Blood pressure is assessed approximately 1 hour after dosing. Target response is a mean (if measured invasively) or systolic (if measured by Doppler sphygmomanometry or oscillometry) ABP decrease of up to 20 mmHg, as long as the MAP remains higher than 60 mmHg. If such a decrease is not achieved with the initial dose, an additional 1 mg/kg is administered orally, resulting in a cumulative dose of 2 mg/kg. This may be repeated up to a cumulative dose of 3 mg/kg in most dogs. When an effective dose has been documented, that dose is repeated at 12-hour intervals.

Ancillary therapy

Opioid sedatives are used to treat acute CHF in human and veterinary patients. Morphine is the prototypical opioid for use in the setting of acute pulmonary oedema, providing both sedative and vasodilating effects. Morphine may be given intramuscularly or subcutaneously, but the intravenous route is preferred, in order to speed onset of action and assure absorption. Rapid administration of morphine intravenously may, however, cause vomiting and vagally induced bradycardia. Morphine has central respiratory depressant effects, but these effects are believed to be advantageous in CHF therapy. By blunting ventilatory reflexes, morphine lessens the sensation of dyspnoea and decreases anxiety associated with increased work of breathing. Administration also leads to vasodilation, resulting in a decrease in preload. These effects are specific to morphine; the common synthetic opioids butorphanol and buprenorphine provide variable degrees of sedation, but have no vasoactive properties. Use of intravenous oxymorphone is not recommended for patients with cardiogenic pulmonary oedema due to the increased pulmonary venous pressure associated with its administration.

Provision of a *low-stress environment* is a basic but often challenging component of therapy of acute pulmonary oedema. Most animals arriving at the veterinary surgery with pulmonary oedema have endured a car ride and multiple episodes of being coaxed, prodded, lifted and carried. The following relatively simple interventions may limit additional stress and allow for a faster and more comfortable evaluation of the patient:

- Provide oxygen immediately and supplement throughout the evaluation process, but avoid struggling with the patient who resists a facemask (consider an oxygen cage, 'flow-by', or nasal supplementation for these patients)
- Gather vital signs and perform a limited physical examination with minimal manipulation of the patient
- Attempt to position the patient in sternal recumbency whenever possible, including during thoracocentesis
- If multiple medications are to be given, organize them in advance so they can be administered with minimal manipulation
- Give as many medications as possible parenterally
- Postpone radiographs until the patient is stable
- Once medications are administered, maintain the patient with minimal handling while drug therapy takes effect
- Do not 'overwarm' the patient (no additional heat supplementation if body temperature is >38°C).

Pleural effusion: recognition and emergency stabilization

Key points

- Recognition:
  - Dyspnoea with muffled heart/breath sounds, especially ventral thorax
  - Jugular distension
  - ± Ascites
  - Other physical findings typical of cardiac disease.
- Therapy:
  - Oxygen supplementation
  - Low-stress environment
  - Thoracocentesis
  - (Opioid sedation).
- Typical underlying cardiac conditions:
  - Hypertrophic or restrictive cardiomyopathy (cat)
  - Thyrotoxic heart disease (cat)
  - Dilated cardiomyopathy (dog/cat)
  - Pericardial effusion (dog, various causes)
  - Decompensated congenital heart disease (e.g. atrial septal defect, atrioventricular canal defect, pulmonic stenosis, tricuspid stenosis)
  - Severe tricuspid insufficiency secondary to endocardiosis (dog).

Cats may develop pleural effusion when they have only severe left-sided heart disease, but in dogs pleural effusion that is not associated with pericardial effusion usually indicates biventricular heart failure. Pulmonary oedema may accompany pleural effusion in patients with biventricular failure. In some patients, the development of right-sided heart failure secondary to left-sided failure may actually result in resolution of pulmonary oedema, such that some patients with advanced left-sided heart disease may be presented with pleural effusion and ascites as their predominant clinical signs.

Once significant pleural effusion has accumulated, full expansion of the lungs is difficult, and patients eventually become overtly dyspnoeic. Cats may function quite well with significant amounts of pleural effusion but decompensate suddenly when fluid accumulation exceeds critical levels. In patients with biventricular failure, in which pulmonary oedema accompanies pleural effusion, mechanical removal of pleural fluid must be accompanied by medical therapy for pulmonary oedema.

Pleural effusion that leads to clinical signs of dyspnoea and discomfort is best treated by mechanical removal. Furosemide administration with sodium restriction may be successful in reducing effusions in chronic cases and in preventing effusions from reforming, but the effect of medical therapy on cavitary effusions is not rapid enough to be life saving in dyspnoeic patients. In severely dyspnoeic animals suspected of having significant pleural effusion, a diagnostic thoracic aspiration should be performed prior to radiographic confirmation of the presence of fluid. The presence of fluid may also be confirmed rapidly with an ultrasound examination; this is often better tolerated and less stressful for the patient than thoracic radiography. If fluid is obtained on a diagnostic aspirate, pleural effusion should be removed until the patient is comfortable. If technically adequate aspiration is performed and no pleural fluid obtained, further diagnostic investigation should be considered.

Thoracocentesis is described in more detail in Chapter 7; most animals with profound dyspnoea will tolerate the procedure with minimal restraint if supplemented with oxygen, maintained in sternal recumbency and given a local anaesthetic. Sedation may be required in anxious or fractious animals. Rapid and deft aspiration of pleural fluid leads to immediate relief of dyspnoea. In contrast to abdominocentesis, as much fluid as possible should be removed. Continuous ECG monitoring during the procedure is ideal and any necessary treatments can be continued during thoracocentesis (e.g. oxygen supplementation). Thoracic radiographs taken after thoracocentesis are more helpful than prior to the procedure, when large amounts of fluid are likely to obscure intrathoracic structures.

Low output failure and cardiogenic shock: recognition and emergency stabilization

Key points

- Recognition:
  - Collapse or weakness with tachycardia, weak pulses, slow capillary refill, cold extremities
  - Often accompanied by cardiac dysrhythmias and pulse deficits
  - Low or normal ABP
  - May be accompanied by pulmonary oedema
  - May be accompanied by significant dehydration.
- Therapy:
  - Aggressive invasive monitoring (ABP and CVP)
  - Positive inotropes administered via CRI (catecholamines) or orally (pimobendan)
  - Fluid therapy/electrolyte management
  - Cautious vasodilation
  - Furosemide, if needed.
- Typical underlying cardiac conditions:
  - Dilated cardiomyopathy (dog/cat)
  - Mitral insufficiency with dehydration (dog)
  - Hypertrophic cardiomyopathy (HCM) or restrictive cardiomyopathy (RCM) (cat).

Low output cardiac failure is one of the most problematic emergency presentations associated with cardiac disease. This clinical presentation may occur with concurrent pulmonary oedema, necessitating simultaneous CHF management, or may occur in chronic CHF patients who are experiencing complications of therapy (e.g. digoxin toxicity, or when azotaemia and electrolyte imbalances have resulted in decreased water intake, vomiting and eventual debilitating dehydration).

Recognition of cardiogenic shock leads to assessment of underlying causes. History and physical examination findings, results of quick 'bench-top' tests (e.g. packed cell volume (PCV), total protein concentration, labstick assessment of renal function) and analysis of the ECG add crucial information to divide low output failure patients into those with concurrent congestive signs, those who are markedly hypovolaemic, with or without drug toxicity, and those who are experiencing significant dysrhythmias as the basis for low output signs.

Low cardiac output with pulmonary oedema

This clinical presentation may occur in the setting of severe systolic or severe diastolic dysfunction. Poor systolic function is typical of dogs or cats with dilated cardiomyopathy, while poor diastolic function is more commonly seen in the setting of hypertrophic or restrictive myocardial diseases in cats. In the case of dilated cardiomyopathy, poor systolic function is accompanied by increased filling pressures, but cardiac output is still inadequate. This combination of physiological events is manifested clinically as a dog with clinical weakness, collapse or signs of shock accompanied by pulmonary oedema, with or without dysrhythmias. These dogs are most often normotensive or mildly hypotensive, with systolic ABP in the range of 80–90 mmHg, but are poorly perfused with cold extremities due to peripheral vasoconstriction. Cats with HCM or RCM have clinical signs due to diastolic dysfunction and are treated differently (see below).

Clinical approach to severe systolic dysfunction: Therapy of critically low cardiac output with pulmonary oedema consists of maximizing forward blood flow while limiting elevations in left atrial pressure. Dysrhythmias may be severe enough to require immediate treatment, or may be managed concurrently with other therapies (see section on 'Dysrhythmias').

Cardiac output depends on maintaining sufficient preload and heart rate (with minimal dysrhythmias) while encouraging improved systolic function with positive inotropic drugs and arterial vasodilators. The use of potent arterial dilators without inotropic and preload support frequently leads to hypotension; therefore great care must be taken and invasive monitoring is very helpful to 'balance' therapy in these patients.

After physical examination is complete and baseline data have been gathered (e.g. ECG, any blood tests), an arterial catheter and a jugular catheter should ideally be placed for measurement of ABP and CVP, respectively. Baseline measurements are recorded. Therapeutic goals consist of a mean ABP of 70–80 mmHg with CVP of less than 10–15 cmH$_2$O or 7–11 mmHg (dogs) or <5 mmHg (cats).

ABP is reduced through the cautious use of arterial dilators as described earlier. Excessive decreases in blood pressure due to vasodilation are offset by concurrently improving contractility with positive inotropic drugs. Both types of medication are simultaneously titrated, using ABP, heart rate and CVP as well as the physical condition of the patient to guide dosing. The combination of arterial dilators and positive inotropes often increases cardiac output enough to decrease left atrial pressures and relieve pulmonary oedema, making heroic doses of furosemide unnecessary. If relief of oedema does not occur rapidly enough for patient comfort, low to moderate doses of furosemide may be used to decrease preload. Rapid, aggressive diuresis should not be employed unless oedema is life threatening, because it is important to avoid dehydration which might result in worsening of low output signs.

Dobutamine is the positive inotrope recommended for most cases of CHF therapy. Dobutamine is a selective beta-1 adrenergic agonist, increasing contractility with minimal increase in heart rate. It is delivered via CRI using a syringe or fluid infusion pump, and titrated to effect. Higher doses of dobutamine may result in supraventricular or ventricular dysrhythmias, but these usually resolve when the CRI is decreased or discontinued. *Dopamine* is an alternative catecholamine often used as a positive inotrope in veterinary patients. The effects of dopamine are similar to those of dobutamine except that dopamine is an alpha adrenergic agonist at higher doses. Dopamine may be slightly more dysrhythmogenic, and higher doses may result in vasoconstriction and increased systemic vascular resistance which should be avoided in patients with heart failure (see Figure 6.6).

Pimobendan is an orally administered drug with a positive inotropic action that may be useful when a CRI is impractical, however, it should be noted that administration of an oral drug may be risky in patients with severe respiratory distress, and absorption of oral drugs may be delayed in patients with poor gastro-intestinal tract perfusion. Pimobendan is a calcium sensitizing agent with phosphodiesterase inhibiting effects. This dual mechanism of action provides pimobendan with vasodilating, positive inotropic (promoting systolic function) and positive lusitropic (promoting diastolic relaxation) effects. Acute oral administration of pimobendan has a slower onset of effect than intravenous catecholamines, but patients receiving this medication typically display noticeable clinical improvement over a period of hours. Because of the delayed onset of action, however, dobutamine infusion is preferred over pimobendan in cases where immediate increases in cardiac output are needed.

Clinical approach to severe diastolic dysfunction:
Acute low cardiac output due to diastolic dysfunction (e.g. HCM or RCM) is usually accompanied by pulmonary oedema. In diseases typified by diastolic dysfunction, systolic function is normal or increased. Relief of pulmonary oedema is achieved by administration of diuretics and venodilators as outlined above, but care must be taken to avoid over-diuresis and arterial hypotension.

Arterial vasodilation is contraindicated in acute heart failure caused by diastolic dysfunction. In some cases, diuretic and venodilating therapy may be sufficient to relieve acute pulmonary oedema associated with diastolic dysfunction, but severe cases may require dobutamine infusions to increase cardiac output and relieve oedema. Although dobutamine is usually referred to as a positive inotrope, it also has powerful lusitropic (promoting ventricular relaxation) effects. Administration of a dobutamine CRI to cats with severe pulmonary oedema, paired with judicious diuretic therapy, often results in more rapid resolution of pulmonary oedema without induction of severe dehydration. In cats that have sinus or other supraventricular tachycardias, administration of a calcium channel blocking agent, such as diltiazem, may improve diastolic function by slowing heart rate. Once pulmonary oedema has been resolved,

beta-blocking agents may be used instead of calcium channel blockers to slow the heart rate if preferred, but use of beta-blocking agents is contraindicated if CHF is present, or if calcium channel blockers or dobutamine are already being used.

Low cardiac output with hypovolaemia
The combination of low cardiac output with a hypovolaemic state in patients with cardiac disease is usually the result of complications of CHF therapy (e.g. over-diuresis or digoxin toxicity leading to dehydration). In some cases, systemic effects of non-cardiac disease (e.g. chronic renal failure) cause decreased fluid intake and eventual dehydration, leading to cardiac decompensation. The therapeutic plan includes judicious rehydration and adjustment of any electrolyte disturbances while encouraging cardiac output with positive inotropic medications.

Initial assessment of the hypovolaemic patient with heart disease that is causing low cardiac output involves serum biochemical analysis to document evidence of dehydration, organ dysfunction and any electrolyte imbalances. Serum digoxin concentrations should be measured if the patient is receiving this medication. Most animals with clinical signs of hypovolaemia and no evidence of CHF benefit from reduction or temporary discontinuation of diuretic therapy. Discontinuation of vasodilators must be approached with more caution, as rebound hypertension may occur if vasodilators are discontinued abruptly. In many cases, once diuretics are withdrawn, vasodilator doses can be decreased but usually should not be completely discontinued.

Fluid administration should precede positive inotropic therapy or, at a minimum, be administered concurrently. Traditionally, lower sodium fluids are recommended (0.45% NaCl with 2.5% dextrose), and are supplemented with potassium and magnesium based on measured blood concentrations of these electrolytes. In most cases, 'maintenance' fluid administration rates (2–3 ml/kg/h) are sufficient for initial supplementation, and the use of fluid pumps for administration is highly recommended. As rehydration is accomplished (documented through monitoring of physical examination, weight and blood tests), positive inotropic drugs are added to encourage increases in cardiac output. Continuous ABP and CVP monitoring allows rough assessment of cardiac output; rehydration at maintenance or slightly above maintenance rates continues until CVP approaches 12–15 cmH$_2$O (dogs) or 7–10 cmH$_2$O (cats); if hypotension persists when CVP is normal, an increased rate of infusion of positive inotropic drugs is warranted.

Cardiac tamponade: recognition and emergency stabilization

Key points

- Recognition:
  - Collapse or weakness with tachycardia, weak pulses, slow capillary refill, cold extremities
  - Muffled heart sounds with or without muffled breath sounds

- Jugular distension
- Ascites
- Low or normal ABP
- Small QRS complexes on ECG recording, height of R wave may vary
- Dyspnoea with normal or dull pulmonary auscultatory findings
- Pulsus paradoxus, i.e. a palpable variation in pulse quality according to the phase of respiration. The pulse becomes weaker during inspiration.
- Therapy:
  - Pericardiocentesis
  - Fluid therapy if hypovolaemia is present
  - ± Furosemide therapy to relieve ascites after pericardiocentesis.
- Typical underlying cardiac conditions:
  - Idiopathic (dog, cat)
  - Cardiac neoplasia, e.g. haemangiosarcoma (dog), lymphoma (dog/cat)
  - Extracardiac neoplasia, e.g. mesothelioma (dog)
  - Infection, e.g. feline infectious peritonitis (cat), bacterial (dog).

Pericardial effusion and tamponade may be one of the most underdiagnosed causes of collapse and ascites in dogs. Paradoxically, pericardial effusion may be one of the most over-treated abnormalities once diagnosed, when pericardiocentesis is often performed regardless of the haemodynamic need for this procedure.

Pericardial effusion may accumulate in dogs and cats due to identifiable causes (e.g. infection or neoplasia), or be idiopathic. Pericardial effusion is associated with acute development of clinical signs when tamponade occurs. Tamponade is defined as the presence of pericardial fluid at increased pressure, leading to compression of the heart and right-sided heart failure. When accumulation of the fluid is gradual, the pericardium stretches to accommodate it, and compression of the heart does not occur until large amounts of fluid are present. If effusion is acute (e.g. acute haemorrhage into the pericardium), much smaller amounts of fluid are required to raise intrapericardial pressure substantially. In most cases of pericardial effusion, underlying cardiac function is normal. Therefore, the emphasis is on immediate relief of tamponade, if present, and subsequent pursuit of underlying causes of the effusion.

If clinical signs of tamponade are not present, pericardial effusion may not need to be treated as an emergency. Clinical recognition of pericardial effusion can be difficult if tamponade is not present, and requires a high index of suspicion. In many cases, pericardial effusion is identified on echocardiographic examination when no outward clinical signs are detected. Other indicators for the presence of small-to-moderate amounts of pericardial fluid include cardiomegaly on radiographs, or attenuated QRS voltages on the ECG.

The emergency presentation of cardiac tamponade typically involves evidence of obstructive shock (i.e. weakness, tachycardia, pallor, slow capillary refill time and weak pulses) accompanied by jugular distension, hepatomegaly and variable amounts of ascites. Cardiac tamponade should top the differential diagnosis list for animals lacking a murmur that have the combination of ascites and jugular distension, especially if muffled heart sounds are noted. Pleural effusion is also commonly seen in conjunction with pericardial effusion. Documenting the presence of pericardial effusion in animals with pleural effusion helps distinguish right heart failure due to primary cardiac disease from tamponade, but may not be immediately possible (see below). Animals with cardiac tamponade are frequently tachypnoeic even though pulmonary infiltrates are not present; this tachypnoea probably reflects decreased ability to move the chest wall and diaphragm due to the presence of ascites and pleural effusion.

If the patient is stable enough for thoracic radiographs, the presence of pericardial effusion can be suspected based on the presence of an enlarged cardiac silhouette with a crisp border and the absence of indentations demarcating individual chambers ('globoid' heart) (see Figures 25.8 and 25.9). Pulmonary perfusion is usually decreased, and smaller than normal pulmonary arteries may be noted. The presence of pulmonary infiltrates with uncomplicated pericardial effusion is unusual, and should lead the clinician to look for other causes of clinical signs, or factors complicating pericardial effusion. In some cases, large amounts of pleural effusion obscure the cardiac silhouette, and radiographic analysis cannot definitively establish the diagnosis of pericardial effusion.

Emergency echocardiography is extremely useful to establish the diagnosis in cases of suspected pericardial disease. In most cases, a complete echocardiographic examination can be postponed until the animal's condition is stabilized, but a brief echocardiographic examination with the animal in sternal recumbency can confirm the presence of a large echo free space surrounding the heart, reflecting fluid accumulation within the pericardium. When tamponade is present, the right atrium and/or right ventricular wall may be seen to collapse in early diastole. Echocardiographic examination can also be used to determine the most advantageous area on the thorax from which to perform the pericardiocentesis. An area with a large amount of fluid and no interfering structures (especially lung) is the most appropriate site for centesis.

If echocardiography is not available, and the animal is not stable for conscious radiography, presumptive pericardiocentesis may be life saving. Patients with clinical signs of shock may receive intravenous fluid support as their effusion is relieved, in order to increase their cardiac output. In most cases, local anaesthetic only is used to facilitate the procedure, and a continuous ECG is recommended to monitor for centesis-related or other dysrhythmias. Samples of the fluid are saved for fluid analysis and cytology. The packed cell volume of the fluid can be compared with that of peripheral blood to establish the diagnosis of intrapericardial haemorrhage. The PCV of the effusion may be high, but is generally lower than that of peripheral blood unless the patient is actively bleeding into the pericardial sac at the time of centesis. Ensuring that this is the case helps prevent drainage of whole blood should accidental cardiac puncture have occurred.

Pericardiocentesis

The optimum site for pericardiocentesis can be selected on the basis of an echocardiographic or radiographic examination, or it can be performed blindly at the fifth or sixth rib space on the right side of the thorax. Centesis is usually carried out on the right to minimize the likelihood of damage to lung and to reduce the chances of laceration of major coronary arteries. The majority of animals will tolerate the procedure conscious, gently restrained in sternal recumbency. Animals with cardiac tamponade are unlikely to tolerate the cardiovascular effects of commonly used sedatives or general anaesthesia, and therefore in the emergency patient it is preferable to perform the procedure conscious. Local anaesthetic should be infiltrated into the skin and intercostal muscles at the site of anticipated drainage. The intercostal nerves, running down the caudal aspect of the ribs and innervating the rib spaces where drainage is to be carried out, can also be blocked dorsal to the site of introduction of the catheter.

The pericardiocentesis catheter is typically introduced about one third of the way up the thoracic wall. The hair overlying the site is clipped and the skin prepared aseptically. Several dedicated pericardiocentesis catheters are available but a large-bore (14 or 16 gauge), long (50–125 mm) intravenous catheter will often suffice. A closed system of drainage should be used with the hub of the catheter attached to a fluid administration or extension set, which is itself attached via a three-way tap to a large syringe. The catheter is introduced through the skin and directed horizontally into the thorax towards the anticipated position of the pericardial sac. Ultrasound guidance can be used but is usually not necessary. Once through the thoracic wall there is often a sensation of the pericardial sac scratching the tip of the catheter. ECG monitoring throughout the procedure allows monitoring for the presence of dysrhythmias induced by the catheter traumatizing the epicardium. A short but moderately forceful advancement of the catheter is sometimes necessary to advance the catheter into the pericardium and a 'popping' sensation may be perceived. Pericardial fluid will often appear in the hub of the catheter and is typically bloody or 'port-wine' coloured. The stylette can be removed from the catheter at this time but frequently is temporarily left in position to prevent the catheter from kinking and blocking. Fluid is drained from the pericardial space until it is no longer possible to maintain the catheter in position without sensing contact between the catheter and the epicardium. It is usually not necessary to drain all the fluid from the pericardial space for two reasons: first, draining less than half the pericardial fluid is likely to relieve the majority of the pressure that has built up in the pericardial sac and therefore relieve the signs of tamponade; and

secondly, any remaining pericardial fluid frequently drains spontaneously through the hole made in the pericardial sac into the pleural space, from which it is reabsorbed.

Management following pericardiocentesis

Moderate doses of furosemide, with concurrent cage rest, frequently lead to resolution of ascites over the first few days after pericardiocentesis. Diuretics may not always be necessary in this situation as the relief of the tamponade should result in physiological diuresis in response to the increased venous filling pressures and cardiac output. Once the tamponade has been relieved, further diagnostic testing to establish the cause of the pericardial effusion can be pursued. A complete echocardiographic examination can be used to screen for obvious right atrial masses indicative of haemangiosarcoma, but lack of an identifiable mass in the right atrium does not rule out other types of neoplasia (e.g. mesothelioma) or small masses below the size identifiable with ultrasound technology. Abdominal ultrasonography is recommended in animals that have pericardial effusion and no identifiable right atrial mass, to look for other sites of primary neoplasia. In many cases, however, diagnosis of the cause of pericardial effusion relies on excluding as many differential diagnoses as possible with diagnostic imaging, then monitoring the patient's progress. Idiopathic pericardial effusions may occur as a single event or may be recurrent until palliative pericardiectomy is performed. Survival for longer than 8 months after pericardiectomy usually indicates non-neoplastic causes for the effusion (Stepien *et al.*, 2000).

A special case of pericardial effusion occurs as a result of left atrial rupture. This situation is rare but life threatening. Left atrial rupture in the dog is usually the result of acute elevations in left atrial pressure secondary to chordae tendineae rupture, related to chronic mitral endocardiosis. Typically, the patient has a chronic history of mitral valve insufficiency, but has acutely collapsed. Signs of cardiogenic shock are common, as is jugular distension and fulminant, life-threatening pulmonary oedema. If thoracic radiographs and an echocardiogram are obtained, pericardial effusion may be documented. In these cases, pulmonary oedema is usually the life-limiting problem, and aggressive therapy of the oedema with diuretics and vasodilators is life saving. The pericardial effusion should not be removed, as decreasing the intrapericardial pressure will allow further leakage from the ruptured left atrium. If the animal survives the acute stages of CHF, many left atrial tears will heal spontaneously. Occasionally, healed but previously undiagnosed left atrial ruptures are documented as an incidental finding in dogs that have died from other causes.

Dysrhythmias

Dysrhythmias are a common finding in emergency and critically ill patients. When other overt signs of CHF are not present, it may be difficult to differentiate dysrhythmias caused by intrinsic cardiac disease from those resulting from severe traumatic or metabolic derangements. Nonetheless, rapid diagnosis and therapy of emergency dysrhythmias is of paramount importance and most dysrhythmias respond to appropriate therapy regardless of their aetiology. Once the dysrhythmia has been controlled, the underlying cause(s) can be addressed.

Underlying causes of dysrhythmias generally fall into one of several general categories (Figure 6.9). Many of these causes can be ruled out based on history, clinical examination findings, blood chemistries and other routine diagnostic tests. The presence of documented cardiac disease does not rule out other concurrent causes of dysrhythmias, especially when the patient has been receiving medications that may alter electrolyte and acid–base status. Medical therapy of CHF may alter sodium and potassium balance or affect renal function; electrolyte imbalance can directly cause or worsen pre-existing dysrhythmias and alterations in renal function may lead to decreased elimination of medications and development of toxic plasma drug concentrations.

Dysrhythmias: recognition and emergency stabilization

Key points

- Detect dysrhythmia during examination.
- Diagnose the type of dysrhythmia based on ECG recording.
- Determine haemodynamic significance of dysrhythmia.
- Begin necessary therapy while searching for underlying causes (Figure 6.9).
- In cases of probable hyperkalaemia, immediate therapy is mandatory regardless of haemodynamic status.

Suspicion of dysrhythmia in a critically ill patient is the most important step towards therapy. Detection of an inappropriately rapid or slow rhythm, especially if irregular, should prompt the clinician to examine the patient more closely for additional compatible signs of cardiac dysfunction. Although sinus arrhythmia is a commonly recognized cause of an irregular cardiac rhythm in dogs, this variation of normal rhythm is associated with resting vagal tone and is therefore not seen commonly in severely ill emergency patients. In less acute emergencies, a normal sinus arrhythmia may be clinically differentiated from a pathological dysrhythmia through a combination of auscultation and palpation of peripheral pulses, followed by confirmation with a lead II ECG recording.

Identification and characterization of a dysrhythmia based on a lead II ECG recording must be rapid and accurate. Frequently, measurement of individual wave sizes (e.g. P and R wave height and width) adds little diagnostic information in acute emergencies, but recognition of the presence or absence of individual waves and recognition of interval variations (e.g. P–Q or Q–T intervals) are an important component in rapid diagnosis. After the patient is stabilized, closer scrutiny of the ECG and exact measurements may be performed.

Intrinsic cardiovascular disease

Myocardial disease
    Cardiomyopathies
    Infiltrative (e.g. neoplasia, fibrosis)
    Myocarditis
    Myocardial trauma
Pericardial disease/neoplasia
Ischaemia
Hypotension
Hypertension
Disorders of sinoatrial function
Conduction disorders
Congenital heart disease
Acquired valvular diseases (e.g. endocardiosis, endocarditis)

Hypoxia
Systemic (pulmonary disease, anaemia, anaesthesia, etc.) Local (myocardial infarction)
Infection
Sepsis Septic shock Severe pyrexia
Metabolic disease
Acid–base disorders Electrolyte disorders Neurological (primarily intracranial) disease Organ failure Endocrine disorders
Autonomic nervous system disorders/imbalances
Vagal disorders (situational or pathological) Sympathetic nervous system stimulation (e.g. stress, drugs, pain)
Drugs/toxins

Direct effects:
    Prodysrhythmic medications
    Most anti-dysrhythmic medications
    Methylxanthines
    Anaesthetic and sedative agents
    Toxic plants
    Autonomic nervous system alteration (e.g. anticholinergics)
Indirect effects:
    Medications that alter acid–base/electrolyte status
    (e.g. diuretics, angiotensin-converting enzyme inhibitors)

6.9 Potential causes of dysrhythmias.

Stepwise emergency ECG analysis is outlined in Figures 6.10 and 6.11. Once the rhythm is identified, appropriate therapy can be instituted. Lack of response to appropriate therapy should prompt re-evaluation of the rhythm diagnosis and initiate a search for complicating issues. Hypokalaemia or hypomagnesaemia may decrease the efficacy of some anti-dysrhythmic medications and should be identified and rectified as soon as possible. Hypoxaemia and acidaemia may also limit anti-dysrhythmic drug efficacy, and are identifiable based on blood gas analysis.

Diagnosis	ECG findings	Typical clinical findings	Suggested therapy
Sinus bradycardia	Regular rhythm P waves associated with every QRS	No pulse deficits May be no clinical signs	Rule out vagal involvement with atropine response test Acute: dobutamine or isoprenaline CRI, temporary pacemaker Chronic: permanent pacemaker
Sinus arrest	Sinus bradycardia with irregular pauses >3 seconds Pauses ended by ectopic complexes (escape complexes)	Irregular Usually no pulse deficits May be associated with syncope Pulses variable in strength; pulses following pauses are typically strong	As above
Bradycardia–tachycardia (associated with sick sinus syndrome)	Very irregular rhythm Sinus bradycardia, sinus pauses interspersed with paroxysmal SVT	Often associated with syncope Pulse deficits present	Permanent pacemaker implantation precedes therapy of SVT Post-pacemaker, treat SVT as needed
Atrial asystole (atrial standstill)	No P waves Normal or wide QRS complexes T waves tall or deep, often symmetrical ('tented')	Associated with hyperkalaemia (e.g. urinary obstruction, acute renal failure, hypoadrenocorticism) Pulses usually weak Shock may be present	Check serum potassium concentration Treat presumptively if compatible disease is present and no potassium testing available EMERGENCY THERAPY FOR HYPERKALAEMIA: calcium gluconate OR dextrose OR insulin + dextrose OR sodium bicarbonate
Second degree atrioventricular block	Normal P waves Some P waves are not associated with QRS complexes, creating a pause in rhythm Pauses may be ended by escape complexes	No pulse deficits Irregular rhythm on auscultation May be associated with syncope	Atropine response test Acute: if no response to atropine, intravenous dobutamine or isoprenaline OR temporary pacemaker Chronic: permanent pacemaker implantation
Third degree atrioventricular block	Normal P waves Wide and bizarre QRS complexes at rate <P wave rate No relationship between P waves and QRS complexes	Strong pulses No pulse deficits May be associated with collapse	Immediate temporary or permanent pacemaker implantation Multiform escape QRS complexes or irregular escape rhythm are associated with increased risk of sudden death

6.10 Diagnosis and therapy of bradydysrhythmias (heart rate <60 bpm in dogs and <120 bpm in cats). In critically ill animals, the presence of a normal heart rate may be inappropriate and indicate dysfunction (CRI, continuous rate infusion; SVT, supraventricular tachycardia).

Diagnosis	ECG findings	Typical clinical findings	Suggested therapy
Sinus tachycardia	Regular rhythm P waves associated with every QRS complex	No pulse deficits Ausc: regular rhythm	Treat underlying condition
Atrial premature depolarizations	Single, tall narrow premature ectopics Ectopic depolarizations have normal or abnormal P waves	Pulse deficits Ausc: irregular rhythm	No direct treatment unless CHF present or rate of premature depolarizations >20–30/min May resolve with therapy of underlying problem Digoxin therapy if CHF present Beta blockers or calcium channel blockers if no CHF
Atrial tachycardia OR supraventricular tachycardia	Paroxysmal or sustained tachycardia, usually >250 bpm (dogs), >300 bpm (cats) Complexes tall and narrow in lead II Negative or no P waves associated with ectopic complexes	Rapid, weak pulses Pulse deficits common Ausc: irregular rhythm if paroxysmal, regular if sustained May be associated with syncope	Attempt vagal manoeuvre (e.g. ocular and carotid sinus massage) In CHF: intravenous or oral diltiazem with extreme caution No CHF: intravenous diltiazem OR propranolol OR esmolol
Atrial fibrillation	Irregularly irregular rhythm Tall, narrow complexes No P waves	Pulse deficits Ausc: irregular rhythm with variation in pitch of heart sounds	In CHF: digoxin No CHF: beta blockers OR diltiazem

6.11 Diagnosis and therapy of tachydysrhythmias (heart rate >140 bpm in dogs and >200 bpm in cats). In critically ill animals, presence of sinus tachycardia is a frequent finding, and resolves with therapy of the underlying problem. In all cases, diagnostic work-up, including measurement of electrolytes, should be performed as soon as feasible (Ausc, auscultation; CHF, congestive heart failure; VPD, ventricular premature depolarization). (continues) ▶

Diagnosis	ECG findings	Typical clinical findings	Suggested therapy
Ventricular premature depolarizations	Wide, bizarre-appearing premature QRS complexes Ectopics have no P waves Underlying rhythm usually sinus in origin	Pulse deficits Ausc: irregular rhythm 'dropped beats'	Treat if resulting in haemodynamic compromise. Typically in order to do so VPDs will need to be frequent and may be multiform in appearance Acutely: intravenous lidocaine or procainamide
Accelerated idioventricular rhythm (slow ventricular tachycardia)	Intermittent occurrence of ectopic rhythm at rate similar to sinus rate Ectopic complexes are wide and bizarre Ectopic complexes have no P waves	Ectopic depolarizations are associated with palpably weaker pulses No pulse deficits Ausc: regular or mildly irregular	No direct therapy if mean arterial pressure is normal and rate of ectopic rhythm is <160 bpm Usually resolves with resolution of underlying problems
Ventricular tachycardia	Paroxysmal or sustained tachycardia, usually >250 bpm (dogs), >300 bpm (cats) Complexes wide and bizarre in lead II No P waves associated with ectopic complexes	Weak pulses Pulse deficits Ausc: regular if sustained, irregular rhythm if paroxysmal, with variation in pitch of heart sounds	Dogs: intravenous lidocaine or procainamide Check potassium concentrations if rhythm is non-responsive to lidocaine Cats: intravenous beta blocker or procainamide. Use lidocaine with caution

6.11 (continued) Diagnosis and therapy of tachydysrhythmias (heart rate >140 bpm in dogs and >200 bpm in cats). In critically ill animals, presence of sinus tachycardia is a frequent finding, and resolves with therapy of the underlying problem. In all cases, diagnostic work-up, including measurement of electrolytes, should be performed as soon as feasible (Ausc, auscultation; CHF, congestive heart failure; VPD, ventricular premature depolarization).

The haemodynamic significance and electrical instability of the dysrhythmia should be evaluated before therapy and, if therapy is instituted, be re-evaluated throughout therapy. The haemodynamic significance of a dysrhythmia depends on the impact of the dysrhythmia on cardiac output. During tachy-dysrhythmias, premature contractions of the ventricle related to supraventricular or ventricular premature depolarizations are associated with decreased stroke volume due to incomplete diastolic ventricular filling and abnormal patterns of ventricular contraction. This decreased stroke volume is detected clinically as a 'pulse deficit', an auscultatable heartbeat that is not followed by a palpable peripheral pulse. If heart rate is within the normal range for a dog or cat and pulse deficits are not detected, it is unlikely that any dysrhythmia will require direct treatment (see 'accelerated idioventricular rhythms', below). If pulse deficits are present, the ECG should be evaluated carefully to determine whether specific anti-dysrhythmic therapy is warranted. Sinus bradycardia and sinus arrest are associated with normal to slightly augmented stroke volume, due to prolonged diastolic filling times, but patients with these dysrhythmias have decreased overall cardiac output due to their limited heart rate. Thus, even though pulses may be palpably normal and no pulse deficits may be detected, cardiac output may be compromised to a critical level in some patients with profound sinus bradydysrhythmias. Similarly, the combination of decreased stroke volume (due to abnormal ventricular contraction) and bradycardia associated with third-degree atrioventricular block (AVB) may contribute to haemodynamic compromise. As in other bradycardic patients, acceptable peripheral pulse strength does not necessarily indicate adequate cardiac output.

The choice of an anti-dysrhythmic medication or procedure is based on the clinician's knowledge of which agent or treatment modality is appropriate, effective, available, practical to administer and affordable. The clinician should always have several therapeutic options in mind when choosing an anti-dysrhythmic regimen, then tailor the regimen to fit the patient. Most dysrhythmias are treated according to the origin of the dysrhythmia (e.g. supraventricular vs. ventricular), some are treated based on the proposed mechanism of the dysrhythmia (e.g. re-entry vs. increased automaticity), and some dysrhythmias are treated by palliative methods that control the clinical signs without attempting to address the origin of the dysrhythmia directly (e.g. pacemaker implantation for third-degree AVB).

Dysrhythmias and shock

A common clinical dilemma involves the presence of a severe tachy- or bradydysrhythmia in a patient exhibiting signs of collapse or shock. The key question is whether the dysrhythmia alone could be responsible for the patient's poor perfusion or whether it is co-existing with another cause of shock, commonly hypovolaemia. In the ideal situation, co-existing abnormalities would be treated simultaneously, but in many cases, the clinician must immediately weigh the relative contributions of both abnormalities to the clinical signs, and treat accordingly. Guidelines for determining the course of therapy in dysrhythmic shock patients must be general and allow for patient variation, but some general guidelines may be followed. Specific therapeutic recommendations appear in subsequent sections.

Bradydysrhythmias and shock

Sinus bradycardia, sinus arrest, or bradycardia associated with second- or third-degree AVB is an inappropriate response to shock of any cause. The presence of an abnormally low heart rate in a patient with signs of poor cardiac output should lead the clinician to suspect primary cardiac disease (e.g. abnormal sinus node function or AVB), profound electrolyte disturbances (e.g. hyperkalaemia or hypocalcaemia), drug toxicity (e.g. digoxin) or neurological disorders, especially space-occupying lesions or cerebral oedema. When atrial standstill (also termed atrial asystole or sinoventricular rhythm) is present, hyperkalaemia should be ruled out as quickly as possible; presumptive therapy for hyperkalaemia (see Chapter 5) should be administered prior to confirmation of potassium concentrations if the patient is bradycardic with an appropriate clinical disease (e.g. urinary obstruction, acute renal failure or hypoadrenocorticism) and ECG findings suggestive of hyperkalaemia (Figure 6.12). If

third-degree block is present with an escape rhythm that is excessively slow (i.e. <30 bpm), irregular or multiform in appearance, intravenous catecholamine support should be initiated immediately and a temporary or permanent pacemaker implanted as soon as possible (Figure 6.13). Temporary transthoracic pacing can be used in patients with third-degree AVB, clinical signs and an unstable escape rhythm. This requires general anaesthesia and is usually only carried out as a prelude to permanent pacemaker implantation (DeFrancesco *et al.*, 2003).

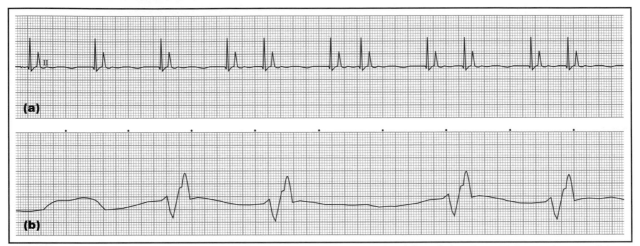

6.12 Two lead II ECG recordings (25 mm/s, dots indicate 1 sec markers) from **(a)** a dog with hypoadrenocorticism and **(b)** a cat with aortic thromboembolism. Despite similar serum concentrations of potassium (approximately 10 mmol/l in both cases), the appearance of the ECG differs. In both cases, bradycardia is present and P waves are not identifiable. Normal width QRS complexes with tall T waves are noted in strip (a), but abnormal intraventricular conduction is diagnosed based on the wide and bizarre appearance of the QRS complexes in strip (b). Immediate therapy for hyperkalaemia is indicated.

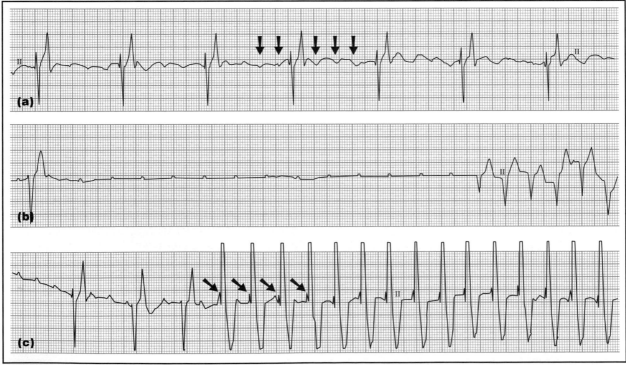

6.13 Lead II ECG recorded from a 12-year-old Chesapeake Bay Retriever with acute collapse. **(a)** Third-degree heart block is present. Unconducted P waves (arrowed) are noted with unrelated ventricular escape complexes at a ventricular rate of 40 bpm. **(b)** Failure of the escape focus leads to intermittent ventricular asystole and clinical collapse; these asystolic periods are terminated by a rapid ventricular rhythm at a rate of 100 bpm. **(c)** Successful 'capture' of the ventricular rhythm is achieved via insertion of a temporary pacing lead into the right ventricle via the jugular vein. Arrows identify pacing spikes. (continues) ▶

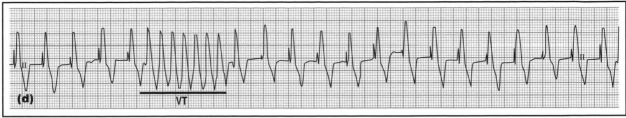

6.13 (continued) Lead II ECG recorded from a 12-year-old Chesapeake Bay Retriever with acute collapse. **(d)** Migration of the temporary pacing lead to the right ventricular outflow tract is associated with paroxysms of ventricular tachycardia (VT). The ventricular tachycardia resolved with repositioning of the lead wire. All strips are recorded at 25 mm/s.

Supraventricular tachycardias and shock

Supraventricular tachycardia (SVT) associated with signs of shock may itself be the cause of the low output signs, or may result from whatever cardiac insult led to the signs of shock. In some cases, SVT will spontaneously resolve when the patient has been stabilized. Unfortunately, it is often difficult to discern which patients will revert to sinus rhythm without direct anti-dysrhythmic therapy. In general, if the patient has no other signs of primary cardiac disease and has hypovolaemic or distributive shock, aggressive therapy for the shock usually results in slowing or conversion of the abnormal rhythm. The patient should, however, be monitored closely for development of pulmonary oedema during rapid fluid infusions. If SVT persists, direct anti-dysrhythmic therapy may be instituted. In either case, vagal manoeuvres may be attempted to convert the SVT to sinus rhythm.

Atrial fibrillation (AF) is seldom found in patients free of cardiac disease. When AF is present in a patient with cardiogenic shock, signs of CHF are treated first, especially if pulmonary oedema is present. Once CHF is stabilized, therapy of AF is pursued with the goal of limiting ventricular response rate to less than approximately 160 bpm in dogs or less than 180 bpm in cats. A special case exists when catecholamines must be administered for positive inotropic effects. In these situations, administration of drugs such as dopamine or dobutamine may increase ventricular response rate to atrial fibrillation to markedly rapid rates (>250 bpm). In these cases, simultaneous administration of diltiazem at typical clinical doses may help to limit ventricular response. In very acute and severe cases, diltiazem may be delivered as a slow intravenous bolus followed by a CRI, rather than orally.

Ventricular tachycardia and shock

Ventricular tachycardia (VT) should be treated directly with intravenous anti-dysrhythmic medications if the rate of depolarization is rapid and the patient appears haemodynamically compromised. At increasing rates of depolarization, especially those greater than 240 bpm (Figure 6.14a), VT may be electrically unstable and must be addressed immediately to support cardiac output and avoid ventricular fibrillation. Frequent ventricular premature depolarizations (VPDs), especially if multiform in appearance, or repetitive VPDs occurring in pairs or paroxysms of ventricular tachycardia, are often treated directly (Figure 6.14b), but in some cases, may resolve with therapy of underlying disease. In cases where the chances of adverse drug effects are low (e.g. use of lidocaine in dogs), presumptive administration of anti-dysrhythmic medication to patients with ventricular tachydysrhythmias may be advisable until the patient's haemodynamic situation is improved.

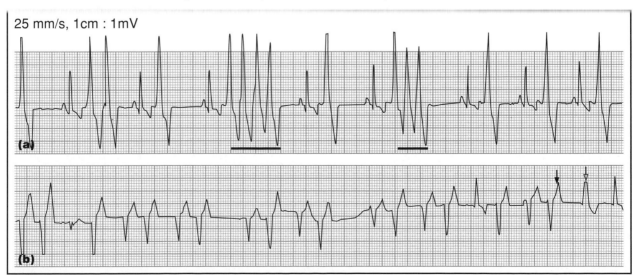

25 mm/s, 1cm : 1mV

6.14 Lead II ECG recordings (25 mm/s) from two dogs with ventricular tachycardia. In both cases, immediate therapy is recommended. **(a)** Uniform ventricular ectopics occur at an overall rate of 120 per minute, but the rate of ventricular depolarization during paroxysms of ventricular tachycardia (marked by bars) exceeds 300 bpm. **(b)** Repetitive multiform ventricular premature depolarizations occur at a rate of approximately 120 VPD/min. Closed and open arrows identify two differing ventricular complex configurations.

Therapy of bradydysrhythmias

Bradydysrhythmias may be relatively benign or may be life threatening. The primary focus of evaluation of the bradycardic emergency patient is the differentiation of vagally mediated bradydysrhythmias from pathological dysrhythmias. If the signs of low cardiac output persist after elimination of the bradydysrhythmia using vagolytic therapy, one can conclude that the slow heart rate was not the cause of the clinical signs.

Sinus bradycardia, sinus arrest, sick sinus syndrome

Sinus bradycardia with or without sinus arrest may reflect a primary problem with sinus node function or reflect systemic abnormalities, especially those which enhance vagal activity. Sinus bradycardia may be associated with the use of some sedatives, anaesthetic agents, anti-dysrhythmic medications and medications or conditions that alter electrolyte balance. These bradycardias are usually self-limiting and resolve with removal of the underlying cause. Clinical signs that may be attributed to bradycardia include exercise intolerance, weakness, lethargy and, if periods of sinus arrest occur, syncopal episodes. In some cases, sinus node disease may be suspected if 'inappropriate' bradycardia is present in a critically ill patient. Sick sinus syndrome is a clinical syndrome consisting of variable combinations of sinus bradycardia, sinus arrest and SVT (Figure 6.15). Affected animals may show no clinical signs but more often exhibit lethargy, exercise intolerance and syncope. Although death as a result of this dysrhythmia is rare, clinical signs may severely compromise quality of life in affected animals.

All animals presented for emergency examination that are found to have bradycardia on physical examination should have an ECG recorded to diagnose the dysrhythmia. Dogs with sinus rhythms at rates below 'normal range' but no other ECG abnormalities should be monitored as they are treated for their underlying disease. Dogs and cats that show clinical signs of exercise intolerance, weakness, lethargy, syncope or other 'collapse' behaviours and have sinus bradycardia should be further evaluated through the administration of atropine or glycopyrrolate. Vagally mediated (physiological) sinus bradycardia will be abolished by administration of such vagolytic drugs, and bradycardia, as an aetiology for the clinical signs, may be ruled out.

If administration of vagolytic drugs is unsuccessful in converting sinus bradydysrhythmias to a sinus rhythm at an appropriate rate and clinical signs appear to be associated with poor cardiac output, positive chronotropic drugs may be administered as temporary support until a temporary or permanent pacemaker can be implanted. Dopamine, dobutamine or isoprenaline may be used to attempt to support heart rate in affected animals. These drugs are administered via CRI and dosed 'to effect'; continuous ECG and invasive blood pressure monitoring are used to document adequate elevations in blood pressure while monitoring for dysrhythmias that may be caused by these catecholamines. If periods of sinus arrest alternate with SVT on the pre-treatment ECG, concurrent therapy for the SVT may be needed once blood pressure has been supported with the catecholamines. Temporary pacing with an intravenous pacing lead or external thoracic pacing leads, if available, may be used to support heart rate

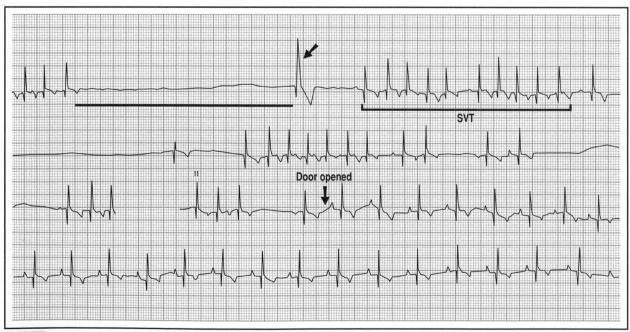

6.15 Lead II ECG recording (25 mm/s, 0.5 cm:1 mv) from a Miniature Schnauzer with sick sinus syndrome. Sinus rhythm is apparent intermittently, alternating with periods of sinus arrest (bar) terminated by a ventricular escape complex (arrow). Paroxysmal supraventricular tachycardia (SVT) is intermittently present. When the dog is stimulated ('door opened'), a normal sinus rhythm resumes. No emergency therapy for the dysrhythmia was indicated, but a permanent transvenous pacemaker was successfully implanted the following day.

until a permanent pacemaker can be implanted. Short-term catecholamine support may be necessary to maintain blood pressure during placement of the temporary pacing lead.

Atrial standstill (atrial asystole)
Atrial standstill may be a primary problem (associated with atrial myopathies) or occur as a result of systemic abnormalities such as hyperkalaemia or digitalis intoxication. When hyperkalaemia is the underlying cause, administration of anticholinergics may increase the heart rate minimally, but immediate, definitive therapy of the hyperkalaemic state is necessary to prevent ventricular asystole and death of the patient. If increased potassium concentrations are acute, serum potassium concentrations >6.5 mmol/l should be treated immediately, and the underlying cause (e.g. urethral obstruction) should be addressed. In severe cases (potassium >8 mmol/l), the hyperkalaemia should be treated prior to any other therapy; if typical ECG abnormalities are noted in a patient with compatible underlying disease, presumed hyperkalaemia must be treated even if measured serum potassium concentrations are not immediately available. Acute hyperkalaemia may be treated with intravenous calcium gluconate, intravenous glucose with or without insulin, or intravenous sodium bicarbonate (see Figure 6.5). If atrial standstill is persistent and due to pathological changes in the atrium itself, it is treated as AVB (below). Bizarre escape rhythms (see Figure 6.12) may develop in response to hyperkalaemia-associated or persistent atrial standstill; it is imperative to recognize escape rhythms as such and avoid suppressing these life-sustaining rhythms.

Atrioventricular block
High vagal tone or drug-related slowing of nodal conduction are the most common causes of first- or second-degree AVB. First-degree AVB (i.e. prolonged P–Q interval) may occur as a physiological slowing mechanism during episodes of SVT, and is not treated under this clinical circumstance. First-degree AVB seldom leads to clinical signs in itself but may reflect metabolic abnormalities (e.g. hyperkalaemia) or drug toxicities (e.g. digoxin toxicity) that may be associated with clinical signs.

Vagally mediated second-degree AVB is usually abolished by exercise, excitement or stress and therefore is rarely seen in emergency patients. Second-degree AVB resulting from AV nodal disease is permanent, non-responsive to vagolytic drugs and may lead to clinical signs of low cardiac output, especially during exercise. True syncope may occur if second-degree AVB results in long periods of ventricular asystole.

Third-degree AVB is manifest as P waves (usually occurring at a normal or increased sinus rate) with no relation to QRS complexes (see Figure 6.13). In most cases, the escape rhythm is ventricular in origin and at a slow rate (25–40 beats per minute), but escape rhythms may originate in the AV node or bundle of His, leading to a faster escape rhythm (i.e. 60–100 bpm). If clinical signs of low cardiac output are present in association with second- or third-degree AVB, temporary or permanent pacemaker implantation is warranted. Catecholamines may be administered to support heart rate but may result in serious dysrhythmias without increasing the ventricular escape rate sufficiently to support blood pressure.

In some cases, second- or third-degree AVB may be present without clinical signs. This is frequently the case when third-degree AVB is diagnosed in cats. Therapy of other diseases precedes further consideration of the bradycardia in these feline patients, but patients should be closely monitored for development of signs of fluid overload if aggressive fluid therapy is administered. In contrast, clinically silent third-degree AVB in dogs requires timely pacemaker implantation due to the significant risk of sudden death in these patients.

Therapy of tachydysrhythmias
Classification of anti-dysrhythmic agents into medications useful to treat supraventricular tachydysrhythmias, ventricular tachydysrhythmias, or both, is helpful when choosing drugs in an emergency. Division of tachydysrhythmias into supraventricular and ventricular categories allows development of a hierarchy of medications in the clinician's repertoire. In most cases, first-line or standard drug therapy is successful for dysrhythmia management. If unsuccessful, 'second-' or 'third-line' drugs may be substituted or added to first-line therapy. If a first-line medication is contraindicated in an individual patient, a second- or third-line drug may be the most appropriate therapy to be used initially.

Supraventricular tachydysrhythmias
Supraventricular tachydysrhythmias can be divided into sinus rhythms (sinus tachycardia), and non-sinus rhythms (atrial, junctional and nodal re-entry rhythms). Medications commonly used for therapy of ectopic supraventricular dysrhythmias (e.g. atrial tachycardia, atrial fibrillation) include oral digitalis glycosides (DG), oral or intravenous beta blocking agents and oral or intravenous calcium channel blocking agents (CCB) (Figures 6.16 and 6.17). Other medications that have been used when dysrhythmias are refractory or side effects limit use of first-line drugs include quinidine, sotalol, procainamide and amiodarone. These drugs may be administered to treat both supraventricular and ventricular dysrhythmias, but because of more frequent occurrence of side effects with their use, other anti-dysrhythmic medications are usually preferred as first-line agents for therapy of supraventricular dysrhythmias.

Sinus tachycardia may be associated with many systemic abnormalities and is treated by rectifying the underlying abnormality (hypovolaemia, hyperthermia, infection, etc.). Sinus tachycardia is often associated with cardiac disease, especially in the presence of CHF. Under these circumstances, control of CHF usually results in resolution of the tachycardia.

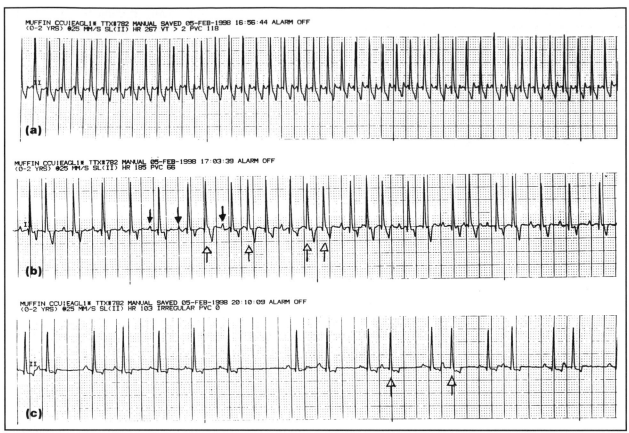

6.16 Lead II ECG recordings (25 mm/s) from a dog with severe pancreatitis but no primary cardiac disease. **(a)** Atrial tachycardia at a rate of approximately 270 bpm is present. Vagal manoeuvres were unsuccessful in converting the atrial tachycardia to sinus rhythm. **(b)** 4 minutes after intravenous administration of propranolol, sinus beats conducted with first-degree atrioventricular block are present (closed arrows). Frequent atrial premature depolarizations (open arrows) remain. **(c)** 4 hours later, a sinus rhythm is present at a heart rate of 110 bpm, but occasional atrial premature depolarizations remain (open arrows).

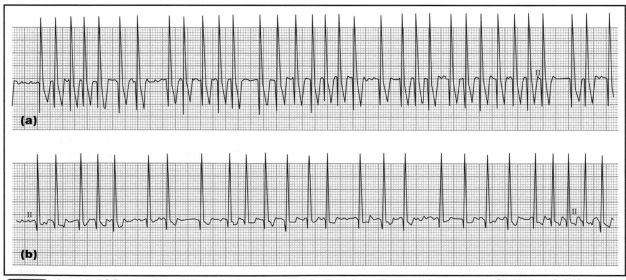

6.17 Lead II ECG recordings (25 mm/s) from a dog with dilated cardiomyopathy and atrial fibrillation. **(a)** Untreated, the ventricular response rate to atrial fibrillation exceeds 220 bpm. **(b)** 24 hours after initiation of therapy with oral diltiazem, ventricular response to atrial fibrillation is approximately 140–160 bpm.

Atrial ectopic depolarizations: Single atrial ectopic depolarizations may not require therapy if they occur at low frequency, are not related to CHF or known structural heart disease and are not associated with clinical signs. Occasionally, single atrial ectopics in an animal with a history of syncope may reflect undetected paroxysmal SVT. It is not usually necessary to treat isolated atrial ectopics on an emergency basis.

Supraventricular tachycardias: SVT (atrial tachycardia or nodal re-entry tachycardia) is not always associated with clinical signs, but if paroxysms of SVT are frequent, sustained SVT is present, or the dysrhythmia is associated with signs of overt heart failure or hypotension, emergency therapy may be required prior to definitive diagnosis. Emergency therapy for SVT includes augmentation of vagal tone via ocular pressure or carotid sinus stimulation ('vagal manoeuvre'). This procedure may abruptly abolish the tachycardia (suggesting that the dysrhythmia was SVT) or transiently slow the rate of discharge (suggesting sinus tachycardia). If these manoeuvres are unsuccessful initially, they may be successful after supraventricular anti-dysrhythmic medications have been administered (e.g. beta blocking agents). Vagal manoeuvres are frequently unsuccessful in conversion of SVT associated with primary cardiac disease. Intravenous administration of beta blocking agents (propranolol or esmolol) or CCB (diltiazem) can be used on an emergency basis to convert persistent SVT to normal sinus rhythm (see Figure 6.16). Each of these medications may have significant negative inotropic and hypotensive effects, and they are administered as a slow intravenous bolus to avoid precipitation or exacerbation of clinical signs.

Junctional tachycardia: Junctional tachycardias are usually not life threatening and if the rate of depolarization allows for adequate ventricular filling (i.e. heart rate <140 bpm with no pulse deficits), junctional tachycardia is not usually treated directly. The presence of junctional tachycardia may reflect systemic metabolic derangements (e.g. electrolyte imbalance) or drug toxicity (e.g. digoxin toxicity). Detection of this dysrhythmia should prompt investigation of the drug and metabolic status of the patient even when direct anti-dysrhythmic therapy is not needed.

Atrial fibrillation: AF is most frequently diagnosed in emergency patients as a complication of severe cardiac disease. Acute occurrence of AF in previously stable CHF patients may be associated with sudden decompensation, but conversion of AF to a normal sinus rhythm may not be feasible due to the presence of severe underlying cardiac disease. Atrial fibrillation results in a rapid and irregular ventricular response to the high rate of atrial depolarization. In cases where medical therapy is the method of choice, the therapeutic goal for most cases of atrial fibrillation is control of the ventricular response rate. In severe heart failure, the patient may be dependent on an elevated heart rate to support cardiac output, so decreasing the rate of ventricular response must be approached with caution. Anti-dysrhythmic drugs used for this purpose are often 'titrated' to the desired clinical effect. Intravenous administration of diltiazem may be used acutely to decrease the ventricular response to AF when extreme tachycardia is limiting resolution of CHF or when catecholamines must be administered for inotropic support. Close monitoring of ECG and blood pressure during administration is advisable. Acute oral administration of the CCB diltiazem is a slower method of decreasing ventricular response to AF in emergency patients but may be used if intravenous diltiazem is not available (see Figure 6.17). Side effects of slow intravenous or oral diltiazem are rare, but may include negative inotropic effects (worsening of CHF signs) or acute hypotension. Acute administration of beta blockers will slow the ventricular response rate in AF, but negative inotropic effects make the use of these drugs contraindicated in CHF patients. Atrial flutter is a rare dysrhythmia that involves very high rates of atrial depolarization and very rapid ventricular response. It is treated similarly to atrial fibrillation.

Ventricular dysrhythmias

Ventricular anti-dysrhythmics may be divided into medications used intravenously (e.g. lidocaine, procainamide) and those used chronically (usually orally) to treat various types of ventricular ectopy (quinidine, sotalol, atenolol, propranolol, mexiletine) (see Figure 6.5).

Ventricular premature depolarizations: VPDs may or may not require direct intervention. In veterinary emergency cases, VPDs should be treated directly under the following circumstances:

* If the patient is symptomatic for the dysrhythmia (e.g. syncope, weakness, hypotension)
* If paroxysmal or sustained fast ventricular tachycardia (VT) (three or more ventricular depolarizations in a row) is present.

In addition, therapy of VPDs may be considered if multiform VPDs are present or single VPDs occur frequently and the patient is considered to be at high risk of the development of a worse dysrhythmia. Hypotension in the presence of ventricular dysrhythmias warrants anti-dysrhythmic therapy in addition to therapy for blood pressure support.

Ventricular tachycardia: In dogs, VT is treated with parenteral ventricular anti-dysrhythmic medications. Lidocaine is the first-line drug of choice for dogs with VT, and administration of one to three boluses of lidocaine intravenously will lead to the conversion of the majority of VT to sinus rhythm. Lidocaine has a short half-life and usually needs to be given as a CRI after bolus loading has achieved therapeutic blood levels. Additional boluses of lidocaine may be necessary to control tachycardia until stable therapeutic levels are reached and maintained. Lidocaine toxicity is enhanced when there is hepatic compromise and when lidocaine is administered in the presence of several medications, including beta blockers and cimetidine. The dose of lidocaine should be halved and titrated to effect when these medications are used, or intravenous procainamide may be substituted as emergency therapy. Common signs of lidocaine toxicity are depression, nystagmus, head-bobbing, salivation, vomiting or seizures. If any signs of toxicity occur after bolus administration, further administration should be avoided and intravenous diazepam may be used to control seizures temporarily. Ultimately, neurological side effects related to lidocaine administration cease with discontinuation of the drug. Lidocaine is less effective in the presence of hypokalaemia; normal potassium balance should be restored to allow maximal beneficial effect of lidocaine administration.

If lidocaine administration fails to control ventricular tachycardia, intravenous procainamide is recommended as a second-line drug. Other possibilities include quinidine, beta blockers or other anti-dysrhythmic agents, or combinations of these medications. Procainamide, sotalol or quinidine may also be administered parenterally. Procainamide appears to be associated with fewer side effects than quinidine and is recommended acutely if lidocaine is ineffective. Intravenous quinidine has significant myocardial depressant and hypotensive effects and this route of administration is usually not recommended unless other, less hypotensive, drugs have failed to control the dysrhythmia and acute therapy is required. If CHF is not present and the patient is no longer hypotensive after acute resolution of VT, oral sotalol or mexiletine (with or without atenolol) may be initiated as administration of intravenous therapy is gradually decreased. Refractory ventricular tachycardia may respond to synchronized direct current (DC) cardioversion if this is available (see below).

Cats with ventricular dysrhythmias are treated differently to dogs. When VT is present in hypoxic patients, resolution of hypoxia may lead to resolution of the dysrhythmia. If VT must be treated directly, beta blocking agents are the ventricular anti-dysrhythmic agents of choice. Intravenous propranolol (non-selective beta blocker) or esmolol (cardioselective beta blocker) is given as a slow bolus and continued as a CRI as required. Oral beta blockers (e.g. propranolol, atenolol) may be administered as needed to control dysrhythmias if intravenous access is not available, but onset and effects may be less predictable. Procainamide may also be used as a ventricular anti-dysrhythmic in cats, but quinidine may not be tolerated due to frequent gastrointestinal side effects. Lidocaine is tolerated by cats *if given slowly at doses much lower than those recommended for dogs*; toxicity usually results in neurological signs.

Accelerated idioventricular rhythms (idioventricular tachycardias): Accelerated idioventricular rhythms are ventricular rhythms with a slower rate of depolarization than ventricular tachycardia. Most accelerated idioventricular rhythms depolarize at a rate close to the sinus rate. In some cases, the accelerated idioventricular rhythm will become manifest intermittently when sinus rate slows slightly due to respiratory sinus arrhythmia (Figure 6.18). These rhythms are usually diagnosed in patients with significant systemic disease or trauma, and are thought to be related to changes in autonomic tone or myocardial perfusion (Abbott, 1995). ECG characteristics of idioventricular tachycardia include a rate of depolarization of <160 bpm (usually <140 bpm) with a regular and uniform appearance. Initial ventricular ectopics in a 'run' usually occur late in diastole and fusion beats may be present. The rhythm disappears when sinus rate increases (e.g. excitement or administration of vagolytic drugs), but does not typically respond to lidocaine administration. Patients with idioventricular rhythms do not typically display overt signs of hypotension. Although qualitative decreases in pulse pressure may be detectable, pulse deficits are usually not significant. Direct therapy of an accelerated idioventricular rhythm in an animal without signs of primary cardiac disease is often unnecessary; the rhythm will resolve with resolution of the underlying systemic abnormalities. Direct anti-dysrhythmic therapy may become necessary if idioventricular tachycardia is complicated by other ventricular ectopics and detection of pulse deficits should lead to reconsideration of a previous decision not to treat. If the ventricular rate exceeds 160 bpm, in conjunction with clinical signs suggestive of compromised perfusion, anti-dysrhythmic therapy should be considered.

Synchronous DC cardioversion

Synchronous DC cardioversion is an electrical treatment method that can be used in an attempt to manage both supraventricular and ventricular tachydysrhythmias. The technique relies on the fact that certain types of dysrhythmia, particularly those dependent on macro or micro re-entry (which usually cannot be determined from the surface ECG) need to be conducted into areas of non-refractory myocardium in order to be sustained. In theory therefore, if all of the myocardium can be simultaneously rendered refractory, i.e. if all the myocardium can be depolarized simultaneously, the rhythm disturbance will no longer be sustainable. Delivery to the heart of an electrical shock of sufficient magnitude may allow this to happen. In order to avoid the induction of worse dysrhythmias, particularly ventricular fibrillation, it is important

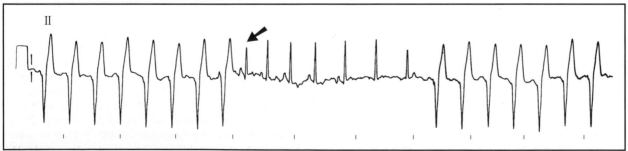

6.18 Lead II ECG (25 mm/s, dots along the bottom are 1 second markers) recorded from a systemically ill dog with no evidence of primary cardiac disease. An accelerated idioventricular rhythm is noted at the beginning of the recording, with a ventricular rate of approximately 140 bpm. When the sinus rate exceeds the ventricular depolarization rate (instantaneous heart rate approximately 160 bpm at arrow), the sinus node resumes control of the heart rate. When the sinus node slows, the ventricular rhythm is again apparent. Mean arterial pressure remained normal throughout the recording. No direct anti-dysrhythmic medications were indicated; this rhythm abnormality resolved within 24 hours.

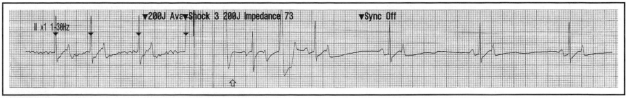

6.19 DC cardioversion of atrial fibrillation to sinus rhythm. The first four QRS complexes on the ECG are indicated by solid arrows, demonstrating that the defibrillator is adequately sensing the QRS complexes. The ECG baseline prior to the delivery of the shock shows coarse undulation and no evidence of P waves, consistent with atrial fibrillation. Immediately after the fourth QRS complex a 200 Joule shock is delivered. This shock is delivered very shortly after the peak of the R wave to ensure that it does not occur during the vulnerable period of ventricular repolarization. The shock is followed by a supraventricular depolarization with a biphasic P wave, a ventricular premature depolarization and then resumption of sinus rhythm with normal P wave configuration. This represents successful cardioversion.

that this shock should not be delivered during the vulnerable phase of repolarization. This can be avoided by delivering the shock almost immediately after a detected QRS complex (hence the word synchronous). This method can be used to attempt to treat medically refractory ventricular tachycardia, atrial tachydysrhythmias and atrial fibrillation. It is currently most widely used in dogs for treatment of atrial fibrillation (Bright *et al.*, 2005). Figure 6.19 shows a successful conversion from atrial fibrillation to sinus rhythm following the administration of a shock. Any patient with a sustained haemodynamically significant, medically refractory tachydysrhythmia could be considered to be a candidate for cardioversion. However, patients must be anaesthetized prior to delivery of the shock, which may limit the usefulness of the technique in haemodynamically unstable patients.

Vascular emergencies

Hypertension: recognition and emergency stabilization

Key points

- Systemic hypertension in veterinary patients is usually secondary to metabolic disease.
- Acute blindness due to retinal detachment may be the only presenting sign of systemic hypertension.
- Hypertensive crisis may result in neurological signs.
- Aggressive vasodilating therapy is indicated to prevent permanent debilitation.

Recognition and chronic management of systemic hypertension is a relatively recent development in clinical veterinary medicine, and little clinical literature is available addressing the therapy of acute, naturally occurring hypertension in dogs and cats. Management of hypertension is complicated by lack of agreement regarding methods of measurement and 'cut-off' values for diagnosis. The term 'hypertensive crisis' is used in human medicine to refer to clinical circumstances requiring rapid reduction of blood pressure. Clinical abnormalities may include acute damage to retinal vessels (haemorrhage, exudates, oedema or detachment), encephalopathic signs, cerebral infarction, acute aortic dissection and acute CHF. In dogs and cats, acute ocular signs are the most frequent

indicator of malignant hypertension, but neurological signs (e.g. seizures, ataxia) may be seen. Congestive heart failure is a rare presentation of systemic hypertension in veterinary medicine, but cardiac murmurs are common in hypertensive animals. Diagnosis of acute retinal detachment, especially with hyphaema, or the coincidence of compatible ocular signs with neurological signs should lead the clinician to suspect hypertensive crisis and act quickly to diagnose and treat the abnormality.

Diagnosis

Systemic hypertension must be suspected before it can be diagnosed. Animals presented for acute blindness, intraocular haemorrhage or epistaxis should have their blood pressure assessed at initial presentation. In addition, animals noted to have signs associated with hypertensive retinopathy (e.g. tortuous retinal vessels, retinal haemorrhage, papilloedema) on routine fundic examination, especially if concurrent neurological abnormalities are present, should have their blood pressure assessed immediately. Any patient presented with intracranial neurological signs, such as stupor, mentation changes or photophobia, should be screened for hypertension. Lastly, because several systemic diseases are known to be associated with hypertension in dogs (e.g. hyperadrenocorticism, protein-losing nephropathy) and cats (e.g. chronic renal disease, thyrotoxicosis), routine blood pressure assessment should be part of the routine diagnostic testing and monitoring of these diseases.

Several methods of blood pressure measurement have been used clinically in veterinary patients. The usefulness and repeatability of any method is user-dependent; the goal of any method is to produce repeatable results with minimal stress to the patient. In some cases, more invasive methods are less stressful. If an arterial catheter is placed, once the catheter is in place in the artery, repeated manipulation of the animal is unnecessary. Direct or Doppler-measured values are recommended in cases of suspected hypertension; oscillometric methods, while useful for monitoring trends, may be time-consuming and unreliable as single-assessment measurements, and may underestimate values at higher pressures.

Non-invasively measured blood pressure values diagnostic of hypertension are >160 mmHg (systolic) and >100 mmHg (diastolic) for both dogs and cats, regardless of the method of blood pressure measurement. Even though a large range of normal values exist, depending on the technique used and operator-dependent effects, the presence of clinical signs of hypertension is usually associated with values well above normal ranges. Abnormal elevation in either systolic pressure, diastolic pressure or both should be considered consistent with hypertension, and further clarification of the patient's clinical signs and any co-morbid conditions should be sought. Arterial catheterization can be used to diagnose or to confirm hypertension in dogs but is typically used only for monitoring during anaesthesia or intensive care in cats.

The rapidity with which a patient's blood pressure has increased is more important in the generation of clinical signs than the absolute value of the blood pressure. Animals with rapidly developing increases in blood pressure will show clinical signs at values slightly higher than normal range, while some animals with chronically extremely high pressures show no outward clinical signs. When associated with any measured elevation in blood pressure, any combination of the following signs is indicative of a hypertensive crisis and warrants aggressive interventional therapy:

- Acute blindness, hyphaema or visible retinal detachment
- Acute onset of intracranial neurological abnormalities (e.g. seizures, nystagmus, head pressing, circling, mentation changes, focal cranial nerve abnormalities)
- Epistaxis.

Therapy (hypertensive crisis)

Acute therapy of hypertension is based on aggressive use of vasodilating drugs. Blood pressure should be monitored frequently throughout initial therapy. Furosemide may be a useful adjunct to vasodilating therapies for hypertensive crisis, especially when hypertensive encephalopathy is present. Care is taken not to cause dehydration with overzealous use of diuretics. The target blood pressure range for treatment of the hypertensive crisis is a reduction of blood pressure by 25%, rather than immediate reduction to normal levels. In patients with hypertension associated with renal failure, urine output should be closely observed during therapy, as reduction of blood pressure may cause decreases in glomerular filtration and anuria.

Drugs which may be used to treat a hypertensive crisis include:

- Sodium nitroprusside: intravenous SN is the drug of choice for rapid reduction of critical hypertension. CRI of SN allows rapid titration of blood pressure to desired levels. Continuous invasive blood pressure monitoring is required when using SN for this purpose. SN should only be used for the first 48–72 hours of therapy to avoid toxicity; chronic oral anti-hypertensive therapy should be initiated as soon as possible
- Hydralazine: as a direct acting arterial dilator, hydralazine causes reliable decreases in blood pressure within 1–2 hours after oral administration. Patients must be monitored for side effects such as tachycardia or inappetence. Concern regarding neurohumoral activation after hydralazine

administration has led to concurrent administration of spironolactone or angiotensin-converting enzyme inhibitors in some cases
- Angiotensin-converting enzyme inhibitors: in animals that are in a hypertensive crisis, angiotensin-converting enzyme inhibitors may be administered as a single therapy or as adjunctive therapy with other vasodilators. The unreliable and sometimes delayed response to these medications makes them less effective than other vasodilators in an acute crisis
- Calcium channel blockers: amlodipine besylate, a long-acting CCB, has been advocated for chronic therapy of systemic hypertension (Henik and Snyder, 1997). The slow onset of action of this drug makes it less useful for acute therapy of hypertension, but it may be administered simultaneously with faster-acting agents, then continued chronically once blood pressure is controlled.

A typical therapeutic protocol for hypertensive crisis includes documentation of elevated blood pressure, placement of an intra-arterial catheter for continuous blood pressure monitoring if needed (arterial catheters may be difficult to place in cats and small dogs, and Doppler monitoring is typically used instead in small patients) and administration of intravenous or oral vasodilators. Clinical signs of hypertensive encephalopathy should subside rapidly when blood pressure decreases, but ocular signs may take days to weeks to resolve. In many cases, retinal detachment is permanent, but some animals regain some visual ability. Once blood pressure is decreased acutely and clinical improvement is noted, oral anti-hypertensive agents may be initiated. Rapid and consistent control of blood pressure is necessary to prevent permanent neurological, ocular and renal damage; underlying causes of systemic hypertension should be addressed as soon as feasible. In cases of endocrine-related hypertension (e.g. hyperadrenocorticism or thyrotoxicosis), adequate control of the underlying disease may allow reduction or discontinuation of anti-hypertensive medications.

Thromboembolism: recognition and emergency stabilization

Key points

- Thromboembolism in cats is usually associated with primary cardiac disease.
- Thromboembolism in dogs is usually secondary to systemic disease.
- Aortic thromboembolism (ATE) should be suspected in any case of sudden lameness in cats.
- Diagnosis is based on physical findings.
- Analgesia is a mainstay of emergency management.
- Careful fluid therapy is recommended to support perfusion.

ATE is a common and serious complication of the feline cardiomyopathies. Thromboembolic events may occur in dogs, but are usually associated with systemic illness (e.g. hyperadrenocorticism, neoplasia) rather than primary cardiac disease. In cats, acute decompensation of cardiac disease may occur due to the pain and stress of ATE.

Many ATE patients are euthanased due to the severity of the signs, severity of concurrent heart disease or overall guarded prognosis for return to function, but some animals can survive to live comfortably for many additional months. Patients who are systemically stable or can be rapidly stabilized often exhibit slow, steady progress toward improved function of the affected limbs. Improvement in motor function of affected limbs may be seen as early as 3 days after ATE, and supportive care at home can result in gradual return to function over a period of weeks. If absolutely no improvement is seen in the first week, or if the limb itself deteriorates (cutaneous oedema formation, gas gangrene), full recovery of limb function is unlikely, but amputation of the affected limb is a viable possibility in stable patients.

Diagnosis
Physical findings in cases of peripheral thromboembolism are specific. Affected limbs are paretic or paralysed; there is pallor of the affected footpads or nailbeds and a lack of arterial pulse to the affected leg(s). The leg(s) are cool to the touch and may be stiff if contracture of major muscle groups is present. Complete paralysis may not be present; peripheral pulses should be carefully evaluated in any case of acute lameness in cats. Affected animals are usually painful and may vocalize. Cats with ATE related to cardiomyopathy are frequently in CHF at the time of presentation and may be markedly dyspnoeic. Dysrhythmias may be detected on auscultation, and confirmed with an ECG recording. Life-threatening CHF and dysrhythmias are treated acutely, before management of ATE begins.

Diagnosis of ATE or thromboembolism of other sites is usually based on physical examination, compatible history and physical evidence of cardiac disease. Although angiography or echocardiography may confirm the diagnosis and document underlying disease, these tests are not usually necessary for initial management. Extensive testing may add unacceptable stress to hospitalization and pose a significant risk to the patient. If biochemical evaluation is performed, abnormalities may include evidence of severe muscle injury and organ damage including metabolic acidosis and elevations in lactate dehydrogenase, creatine kinase, creatinine, aspartate aminotransferase and alanine aminotransferase. Evidence of disseminated intravascular coagulation (DIC) may be present on a haemostasis screen. Hyperkalaemia and hypermagnesaemia are occasionally noted, reflecting acidosis, muscle damage, acute renal failure or reperfusion phenomena.

Therapy of aortic thromboembolism
Therapy of CHF, if present, is the highest priority in the management of ATE patients. Some therapies (e.g. acepromazine maleate) may be of benefit for therapy of CHF and ATE simultaneously. Acute CHF therapy consisting of diuretics, vasodilators and anti-dysrhythmic therapy, if needed, is administered. Specific therapy for ATE may consist of surgical removal of the thrombus, administration of thrombolytic drugs (e.g. tissue plasminogen activator (t-PA), streptokinase), or supportive medical therapy. Surgical removal of the thrombus, while a possibility in stable patients, in contraindicated in patients with unstable CHF or metabolic status. Supportive therapy often includes the use of anticoagulants to prevent further thrombosis.

Thrombolytic therapy: Despite initial hopes for thrombolytic drugs as acute therapy for ATE in cats, consistent success with this mode of therapy has been elusive. While t-PA or streptokinase therapy has been used in cats with acute ATE, the unfavourable side-effect profile and high mortality associated with the use of these drugs is discouraging. Acute reperfusion of ischaemic tissue may lead to hyperkalaemia, hypermagnesaemia and acidosis (i.e. reperfusion syndrome). Successful treatment of peripheral thrombosis in dogs has been described (Ramsey et al., 1996; Clare and Kraje, 1998), but at this time, acute administration of thrombolytic drugs should be considered experimental and, in general, is not recommended for cats with ATE.

Medical therapy: Before treatment neurological, muscular and vascular function is assessed and metabolic status is established via biochemical analysis and blood gas measurements. Stabilization of CHF status is an important first step, but care must be taken to avoid dehydration, which may make recovery from metabolic and thromboembolic problems more difficult. The goals of emergency medical therapy for ATE include alleviation of pain, support of collateral circulation to affected muscles and, ultimately, prevention of further embolization.

Alleviation of pain associated with acute muscle ischaemia is a major goal of therapy of ATE patients. Analgesics recommended for use in cardiac patients include morphine, butorphanol, buprenorphine, fentanyl or oxymorphone. Each of these opioids has advantages and disadvantages; clinicians should use an available opioid with which they are comfortable. The importance of aggressive analgesic therapy cannot be over-emphasized as pain itself and the stress related to pain are severely debilitating. Analgesic drugs should be administered on a strict schedule rather than 'as needed': there is little doubt that even quiet-appearing animals are in pain if major muscle groups have become acutely ischaemic or are reperfusing. Epidural analgesia, where available, is an effective means of controlling the patient's pain while allowing the patient to remain alert, allowing their condition to be monitored effectively.

Support of collateral circulation may be achieved through the use of vasodilators. Acepromazine maleate is the drug most often recommended because of its vasodilating and sedating effects. The effect of angiotensin-converting enzyme inhibitors on perfusion in cases of ATE is unknown, but if they are used to treat concurrent CHF, hydration and renal function must be closely monitored. Hydration is maintained with controlled delivery of intravenous fluids.

Prevention of further embolization is unreliable at best. Current recommendations consist of administration of sodium heparin to decrease the probability of additional clot formation. Although the success of heparin therapy in this regard is unproven, its use is typically associated with minimal side effects. Some clinicians advocate simultaneous use of warfarin in cats with acute ATE; extensive clinical data regarding this use have not been published. Aspirin administration, while sometimes recommended for prevention of ATE, is not recommended in the acute therapy of an existing thrombus.

References and further reading

Abbott JA (1995) Traumatic myocarditis. In: *Kirk's Current Veterinary Therapy XII: Small Animal Practice*, ed. RW Kirk and JD Bonagura, pp. 846–850. WB Saunders, Philadelphia

Bright JM, Martin JM and Mama K (2005) A retrospective evaluation of transthoracic biphasic electrical cardioversion for atrial fibrillation in dogs. *Journal of Veterinary Cardiology* **7**, 85–96

Clare AC and Kraje BJ (1998) Use of recombinant tissue-plasminogen activator for aortic thrombolysis in a hypoproteinemic dog. *Journal of the American Veterinary Medical Association* **212**, 539–543

DeFrancesco TC, Hansen BD, Atkins CE, Sidley JA and Keene BW (2003) Noninvasive transthoracic temporary cardiac pacing in dogs. *Journal of Veterinary Internal Medicine* **17**, 663–667

DeLellis LA and Kittleson MD (1992) Current uses and hazards of vasodilator therapy in heart failure. In: *Kirk's Current Veterinary Therapy XI: Small Animal Practice*, ed. RW Kirk and JD Bonagura, pp. 700–708. WB Saunders, Philadelphia

Henik RA and Snyder PS (1997) Treatment of systemic hypertension in cats with amlodipine besylate. *Journal of the American Animal Hospital Association* **33**, 226–234

Ramsey CC, Burney DP, Macintire DK and Finn-Bodner S (1996) Use of streptokinase in four dogs with thrombosis. *Journal of the American Veterinary Medical Association* **209**, 780–785

Stepien RL, Whitley NT and Dubielzig RR (2000) Idiopathic or mesothelioma-related pericardial effusion: clinical findings and survival in 17 dogs studied retrospectively. *Journal of Small Animal Practice* **41**, 342–347

7

General approach to dyspnoea

Lori S. Waddell and Lesley G. King

Definition and diagnosis

Dyspnoea may be defined as the sensation of difficulty in breathing that is experienced by patients with compromised respiratory function. This sensation of respiratory distress is caused by a low arterial partial pressure of oxygen (P_aO_2) (hypoxaemia), a high arterial partial pressure of carbon dioxide (P_aCO_2) (hypercapnia), or a significant increase in the work of breathing. Normally, ventilation is stimulated by increases in arterial carbon dioxide concentration, and decreased by hypocapnia. Hypoxia only acts as a respiratory stimulus if P_aO_2 falls below 50 mmHg, when hypoxic drive overrides the effects of hypocapnia that may be present due to hyperventilation.

It is essential that patients in respiratory distress are recognized immediately. In the emergency room, observation of the patient and a detailed physical examination of the respiratory system are the most important tools for diagnosis and treatment, often providing clues about the causes of dyspnoea when more stressful diagnostic procedures are not possible. The clinician attempts to localize the disease process to the airways, lungs or pleural space, facilitating immediate steps to stabilize the patient.

Observation of respiratory patterns in the dyspnoeic patient

Dogs and cats with dyspnoea may be recognized by an increase in respiratory rate and effort. Increased respiratory effort is a manifestation of recruitment of the secondary muscles of respiration. This includes the scalene and sternomastoid muscles of the neck and chest, the alae nasae which dilate the nostrils, and the muscles of the abdominal wall, which contract when expiration becomes an active rather than a passive process. Recruitment of the secondary muscles of respiration is a non-specific response to increased respiratory drive and does not necessarily confirm the presence of dyspnoea or hypoxia. Normal respiration is characterized by concurrent outward movement of both the chest and abdomen during inspiration. 'Paradoxical respiration' is recognized by a lack of synchronous movement of the chest and abdominal walls – the diaphragm and caudal intercostal and abdominal muscles tending to collapse inwards and forwards during inspiration. Unlike increased respiratory effort alone, paradoxical respiration is a specific indication of dyspnoea, increased work of breathing and the presence of respiratory

muscle fatigue. It may also be seen less commonly in patients with abnormal diaphragmatic movement secondary to paralysis or rupture.

Postural adaptations are common in patients with respiratory distress, minimizing resistance to air flow. Many patients in severe respiratory distress breathe through an open mouth to remove the resistance to airflow produced by the nasal turbinates. Similarly, the neck is often extended and the head lifted to straighten the trachea. Most dyspnoeic patients demonstrate some degree of orthopnoea, preferring to stand or lie in sternal recumbency and abducting their elbows to minimize compression of the chest wall (Figure 7.1). Any restraint that limits postural adaptations may lead to further hypoxaemia and decompensation, a fact that must be borne in mind when restraining these animals for diagnostic procedures such as radiography.

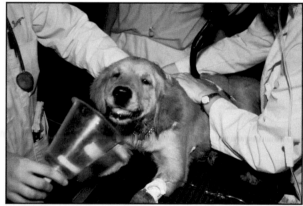

7.1 Severe respiratory distress due to neurogenic pulmonary oedema after a choking incident in a 6-month-old Golden Retriever. Notice the pale mucous membranes, extended neck, abducted elbows and reluctance to have an oxygen mask placed over the face. (Courtesy of Dr Ken Drobatz, University of Pennsylvania)

Physical examination of the dyspnoeic patient

Mucous membrane colour can yield important information about the functional status of the respiratory system. Owing to the shape of the oxyhaemoglobin dissociation curve (Figure 7.2), cyanosis only occurs with severe hypoxaemia (less than 80% saturation of arterial blood). When moderate hypoxaemia is present, the mucous membranes may still be pink. Clinicians should therefore not be lulled into a false sense of security by pink mucous membranes. At least

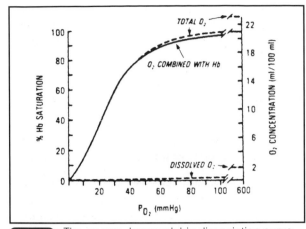

7.2 The oxygen–haemoglobin dissociation curve demonstrates the relationship between partial pressure of oxygen dissolved in the blood and the saturation of haemoglobin with oxygen. The sigmoid shape of the curve occurs as a result of a conformational change in the haemoglobin molecule following binding of the first molecule, allowing binding of the remaining three molecules to occur more rapidly. This facilitates both oxygen uptake in the lungs and oxygen release to the tissues. The plateau of >90% haemoglobin saturation also provides a wide margin of safety – lung disease may result in significant decreases in P_aO_2 without a concurrent decrease in saturation. Desaturation can occur rapidly, however, once the P_aO_2 decreases to a value of <60 mmHg. (Reproduced from West JB (1985) *Respiratory Physiology – The Essentials, 5th edn*, p.69, with permission of Williams & Wilkins, Baltimore)

50 g/l of desaturated haemoglobin must be present for the blue colour of cyanosis to be detectable. Thus, anaemia or peripheral vasoconstriction may lead to pale mucous membranes and inability to detect cyanosis. Cherry red or muddy chocolate mucous membranes can indicate the presence of toxins such as cyanide and paracetamol (acetaminophen), respectively. Carbon monoxide can also cause bright red mucous membranes (carboxyhaemoglobin). These toxicities all cause respiratory distress, despite a normal P_aO_2, by interfering with haemoglobin binding and release of oxygen.

A limited physical examination of the respiratory and cardiovascular systems can be performed rapidly and can be very rewarding. Auscultation of the chest and cervical trachea may detect wheezes, crackles, harshness or increased bronchovesicular sounds, as well as areas of dullness (dorsal, ventral, unilateral). Wheezes are musical or squeaky sounds associated with narrowing of the airways secondary to inflammation, mucosal oedema, mucus or masses. If wheezes occur during inspiration, upper airway pathology should be suspected, whereas disease of the small bronchi or lower airways, such as feline asthma, generally produces expiratory wheezes. Crackles are discontinuous popping sounds that usually indicate the presence of fluid in the alveoli and airways. They are caused by air bubbling through fluid, but can also be caused by the opening and closing of small bronchi and alveoli. Soft end-inspiratory crackles occur with parenchymal disease and often indicate pulmonary oedema, haemorrhage or purulent exudate in the alveoli. Loud snapping airway crackles can be heard in dogs with pulmonary

fibrosis or chronic bronchitis. If the lung or heart sounds are dull, muffled or difficult to hear, pleural space disease should be considered. The most common pleural abnormalities include pneumothorax, pleural effusion, diaphragmatic hernia and neoplastic masses. In cats, diminished chest compressibility can suggest an effusion or mediastinal mass.

Auscultation of the heart and simultaneous palpation of the pulses help to determine whether cardiovascular disease is contributing to respiratory dysfunction. In dogs with congestive heart failure, a mitral murmur or supraventricular dysrhythmia (often atrial fibrillation) is usually heard. In the absence of these findings, heart failure as a cause of dyspnoea is extremely unusual. Use of auscultation to rule out cardiovascular disease may be more difficult in cats, as murmurs and dysrhythmias may be absent or intermittent in cats with heart disease, even those with congestive heart failure.

Emergency stabilization

Initial stabilization of patients with severe respiratory distress should include increasing the inspired oxygen concentration (oxygen therapy), while a rapid but thorough physical examination is performed. Ideally, the patient should be allowed to rest briefly in an oxygen-enriched environment before further diagnostic investigation and manipulation. This is particularly important for cats, as it allows calming and recovery from transport. A more complete examination and further investigations are performed only when tolerated and shown not to exacerbate signs of distress. An exception is made when lung sounds are auscultated to be dull either dorsally or ventrally, suggesting the presence of pleural space disease. In this situation, thoracocentesis should be attempted promptly, to remove pleural air or fluid (see below), even before radiographs are obtained. Dyspnoeic patients may not be stable enough for radiography or other diagnostic procedures, and thoracocentesis may not only be diagnostic but therapeutic.

Oxygen supplementation
Emergency oxygen therapy can be supplied in several ways. Mask oxygen can be used on any patient that is lying still and tolerates the mask. It may be poorly tolerated in distressed patients and persistent attempts to place the mask over the muzzle of the animal can increase stress (see Figure 7.1). With a tight-fitting mask at high oxygen flow rates (5–6 l/min), a fractional inspired oxygen concentration (F_iO_2; room air $F_iO_2 = 0.21$) of 0.7–0.8 can be achieved. Care must be taken that the mask is not so tight as to cause rebreathing of carbon dioxide and consequent hypercarbia.

Flow-by oxygen is achieved by holding the oxygen supply tubing near the nostrils or mouth of the animal and provides a similar effect to a mask, with much less stress.

An oxygen pipe from an anaesthetic machine can supply oxygen (5–8 l/min) to an Elizabethan collar covered with clingfilm, leaving 2.5–5 cm open at the top of the Elizabethan collar to allow for carbon dioxide and water vapour to be eliminated. This technique allows the animal to be visible and minimizes stress, but is not tolerated by all patients. The humidity and temperature within the enclosed space of the Elizabethan collar may increase fairly rapidly, which can limit the duration for which this technique can be employed.

Oxygen cages are one of the easiest methods of oxygen administration, but they isolate the patient, making it difficult to examine, monitor and treat these dynamic cases (Figure 7.3). This may be an advantage in some stressed and dyspnoeic cats, however, that may benefit from enforced isolation from strange people in a strange environment. Initial crisis management of dyspnoeic animals may require high oxygen concentrations (F_iO_2 up to 0.9) until the patient has been stabilized. The oxygen percentage in the cage is determined by the extent of filling with 100% oxygen. Although it should be possible to reach an F_iO_2 of up to 1.0, some oxygen cages cannot raise the F_iO_2 above approximately 0.5, which may be too low for severely dyspnoeic animals. Opening the cage door drops the F_iO_2 to that of room air almost immediately. Oxygen cages may also be associated with inappropriate patient warming and consequent hyperthermia. Large dogs may not fit into standard oxygen cages. Despite these limitations, oxygen cages may represent a useful investment for the emergency practice. At present, no commercially available oxygen supplementation cages are available in the UK, although they may be purchased from the USA. Paediatric incubators, into which oxygen is piped, provide a suitable alternative for cats, small dogs and neonates, attaining oxygen concentrations of 80–90%. These allow good observation of the patient and, although expensive when purchased new, are often available second-hand from human hospitals.

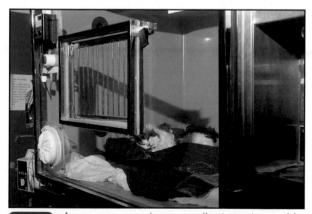

7.3 An oxygen cage is an excellent way to provide oxygen supplementation in extremely stressed or fractious animals. Temperature, inspired oxygen concentration and humidity can be controlled in these units.

For more prolonged oxygen supplementation, nasal oxygen can be provided with nasal oxygen prongs that are manufactured for human patients (Figure 7.4), or by placing a catheter in one or both nostrils and suturing or glueing it in place (Figure 7.5). Nasal prongs penetrate approximately 1 cm into both nostrils and usually work well in large-breed dogs that are relatively immobile. Nasal catheters can be used in dogs or cats of almost any size. Any type of catheter can be used for this purpose; most commonly 5–8 French red rubber urinary catheters or soft feeding tubes are used (Figure 7.6). Brachycephalic breeds are poor candidates for nasal oxygen supplementation: catheter prongs cannot be adjusted to fit comfortably on their faces; nasal catheters may not fit due to stenotic nares or do not stay in place because their noses are short; and they may have increased vagal tone, which may be aggravated by the nasal catheter. Animals that are mouth breathing because of dyspnoea or excitement are also poor candidates for this technique, as increased air mixing in the pharynx leads to a reduced effective F_iO_2. Generally, nasal oxygen is thought to give an F_iO_2 of approximately 0.4 depending on the flow rate of oxygen, the size of the animal and its minute ventilation. The F_iO_2 can be increased by placement of a second nasal catheter in the other nostril. Alternatively, a long intravenous catheter can be placed percutaneously into the trachea following the instillation of surface local anaesthetic. Humidified oxygen is supplied at similar flow rates to those used with the nasal catheter. This system may be especially useful in individuals with laryngeal or upper tracheal obstruction.

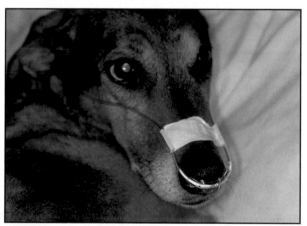

7.4 Nasal oxygen prongs that are manufactured for human patients can be used in many canine patients to provide oxygen supplementation.

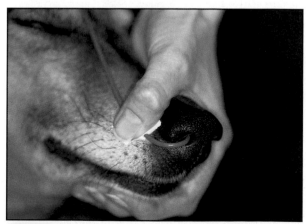

7.5 Nasal oxygen can also be provided by suturing a red rubber catheter into one nostril and inserting it a premeasured length equal to the distance from the nostril to the medial canthus of the eye.

Used to provide supplemental oxygen in patients that are not tolerating nasal prongs and are too large to fit into oxygen cage or oxygen cage is not available

Red rubber catheter/soft feeding tube, usually 8 French (or 5 French in small dogs) is used

1. The distance from the nose to the medial canthus of the eye is measured and marked on the catheter.
2. The nostril is numbed with topical anaesthetic such as lidocaine gel or one to two drops of 2% lidocaine dripped into the nostril.
3. The catheter is inserted through the nostril into the ventral meatus to the premeasured distance.
4. Catheter is sutured in place using 2 metric nylon and tape butterflies, just beside the nostril and again on the side of the face or on top of the head.

Single or bilateral nasal catheters can be used depending on the percentage of oxygen supplementation that is required

An Elizabethan collar may be necessary to prevent the patient from removing the catheter. Complications may include excessive sneezing, dislodgement, epistaxis or increased dyspnoea if upper airway disease is present

7.6 Nasal oxygen catheter.

Oxygen for long-term therapy should be humidified (saturated with water vapour) to prevent desiccation of the airways, especially if the turbinates are bypassed, as occurs with nasal or tracheal oxygen catheters. Specially designed units that heat and humidify the inspired air are available for placement in anaesthetic and ventilator circuits, but nasal or cage oxygen humidification can be simply accomplished by bubbling the oxygen through a chamber of distilled water (Figure 7.7).

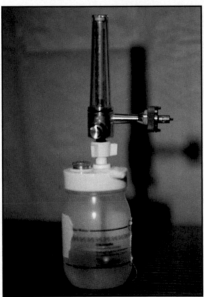

7.7

Oxygen can be humidified by bubbling it through a chamber filled with distilled water. This reduces airway irritation by preventing desiccation.

Long-term therapy with high concentrations of oxygen (F_iO_2 >0.6 for more than 12 hours) is associated with damage to the lung called oxygen toxicity. Inflammatory injury is caused by toxic metabolites of oxygen, including oxygen free radicals and superoxide molecules. Clinically, oxygen toxicity is difficult to diagnose, but changes in the lungs are similar to those seen in the acute respiratory distress syndrome

(ARDS). Every effort should be made to minimize the F_iO_2 used to maintain critical patients. In the presence of severe dyspnoea, however, it may not be possible to decrease the F_iO_2 without provoking severe distress, and the clinician may have to accept the risk of oxygen toxicity in the interests of survival of the patient.

Intravenous access

Intravenous access with an indwelling peripheral catheter placed in the cephalic or saphenous vein should be obtained early during the hospitalization of all dyspnoeic patients. The catheter should be placed with minimal restraint and stress. Establishment of intravenous access allows administration of drugs and, if the animal decompensates, provides a means to administer intravenous anaesthesia to facilitate rapid control over the airway.

Thoracic radiography in dyspnoeic patients

Thoracic radiographs represent one of the most useful diagnostic tools for the clinician faced with a patient in respiratory distress. Detailed information about thoracic radiography is available in Chapter 25. Although valuable information is provided, radiography is a stressful procedure that can cause significant respiratory decompensation and may not be advisable in patients with severe dyspnoea. To minimize stress, dorsoventral radiographs are obtained with the patient restrained in sternal recumbency. Although this view provides less useful diagnostic information, it is also less likely to compromise remaining ventilatory function. Alternatively, horizontal beam lateral views may be obtained where suitable radiographic protection protocols are available. The animal should be measured and radiograph settings calculated in advance of moving and positioning for radiography. Supplementation of inspired oxygen should be continued during the procedure. If the animal can tolerate the manipulation, it is ideal to obtain at least two and ideally three views of the thorax.

Thoracic ultrasonography

Thoracic ultrasonography can be very useful in confirming the presence of pleural effusion in dyspnoeic patients. It is a rapid, relatively non-stressful diagnostic tool that can be used to diagnose pleural effusion and aid in performing thoracocentesis by identifying areas with the greatest amount of fluid accumulation and structures that need to be avoided. In many patients, it is a much quicker and less stressful procedure than thoracic radiography, especially since the patient can remain in sternal recumbency.

Approach to undiagnosed respiratory distress

When the initial history does not provide specific useful information, the approach to the patient in respiratory distress is to treat according to the apparent site of respiratory pathology. The history, signalment and physical examination are often sufficient to determine which areas of the respiratory system are involved.

For this purpose, the respiratory tract is divided into the airways (upper and lower), the pulmonary parenchyma and the pleural space. After determining which of these are affected, a list of differential diagnoses, diagnostic procedures and therapeutic strategies is then formed for the individual patient.

Upper airway disease

Clinical signs of upper airway disease

The clinical signs of disease of the upper airway are listed in Figure 7.8. Because they commonly involve the larynx, upper airway disorders often cause loud stridor that is audible without a stethoscope. On auscultation, upper airway noise is loudest over the trachea. Referred sounds may also be heard on auscultation of the lungs. Most dogs with dynamic upper airway obstruction (such as brachycephalic airway syndrome or laryngeal paralysis) have stridor or stertor primarily on inspiration. Negative inspiratory pressure tends to close the upper airway, whereas during expiration the airway opens. Animals with fixed upper airway obstructions (such as masses or abscesses) tend to have difficulty during both inspiration and expiration.

Differential diagnosis of upper airway obstruction

Brachycephalic syndrome
Laryngeal paralysis
Tracheal collapse
Nasopharyngeal polyps (cats)
Aspirated foreign bodies
Upper airway neoplasia
Retropharyngeal masses, abscesses or haematomas

Clinical and historical signs associated with upper airway obstruction

Dyspnoea
Audible stridor or stertor
Increased respiratory effort with prolonged inspiratory time (gasping respiration)
Change in vocalization (bark or meow)
Exercise intolerance – clinical signs most severe when stressed or exercising
Excessive panting
Hyperthermia

7.8 Common differential diagnoses and clinical and historical signs associated with upper airway or laryngeal obstruction in dogs and cats.

Dyspnoea in animals with upper airway obstruction is made worse by exercise or excitement and is improved or almost absent at rest. Increased respiratory drive results in enhanced negative inspiratory pressures during exercise, leading to more severe narrowing of the airway. Tests of pulmonary function during dyspnoeic episodes often reveal significant hypoxia and hypercarbia, whereas these parameters may become almost normal at rest. This return of pulmonary function to normal at rest is one of the hallmark signs of upper airway obstruction; blood gases usually remain abnormal at rest in animals with parenchymal or pleural disease.

Many dogs with upper airway obstruction suffer from concurrent hyperthermia. They are unable to thermoregulate effectively because an insufficient volume of air passes over the tongue during panting. Hyperthermia starts a vicious cycle, as it stimulates an increased respiration rate and panting, which further narrows the airway.

General approach to management of patients with upper airway obstruction

Management of animals with upper airway obstruction is summarized in Figure 7.9. The most important priority is to encourage the animal to rest quietly in an oxygen-enriched environment. Many benefit considerably from sedation; acepromazine is the drug of choice provided that the animal is not hypovolaemic (phenothiazines may be associated with vasodilation, which exacerbates signs of hypovolaemia) or brachycephalic (brachycephalic breeds may have increased sensitivity to phenothiazines). The dose of acepromazine should be kept at a minimum and may be more effective if combined with an opioid analgesic (neuroleptanalgesia). Opioids may also be used in isolation where there is hypovolaemia, as these agents produce minimal cardiovascular effects. Occasionally, opioids may lead to the detrimental effect of narcotic-induced panting. Suggested agents include morphine, methadone (UK), pethidine (UK), oxymorphone (USA) or butorphanol, any of which may be combined with a sedative such as diazepam if they trigger excessive panting.

Oxygen supplementation: oxygen cage best

Rest, sedation if necessary

Acepromazine 0.01–0.05 mg/kg i.v. or i.m. if cardiovascularly stable

If collapsed or sedated, extend head and neck and pull tongue out of the mouth

Vascular access

Minimal stress

Anti-inflammatory to immunosuppressive doses of corticosteroids unless contraindicated (dexamethasone 0.25–0.5 mg/kg i.v. or i.m.)

Monitor temperature, vigorous efforts to cool if needed

Fluid therapy if dehydrated or hypovolaemic

Emergency tracheostomy or intubation if no response to medical management

---

7.9 Management of patients with upper airway obstruction.

Manipulation and stress should be kept to a minimum, but if the animal is collapsed or sedated, the head and neck should be extended and the mouth opened with the tongue pulled forward to minimize airway resistance. Corticosteroids at anti-inflammatory doses are often very helpful if significant airway oedema or inflammation is present. They should be avoided initially if neoplasia such as lymphoma is one of the differential diagnoses. Corticosteroids may cause lysis of malignant lymphocytes, thereby making it difficult to confirm the diagnosis. Core body temperature should be monitored carefully and vigorous attempts made to cool the patient with fans, ice, alcohol or cool intravenous fluids if the temperature is greater than 40°C.

Animals that do not respond to this approach should be anaesthetized and intubated, or a tracheostomy performed if necessary (Figures 7.10 and 7.11). Ideally, these animals should not remain intubated through the larynx for more than a few hours, as the tube triggers swelling that may exacerbate the problem following extubation.

1. Patient placed in dorsal recumbency, with the neck extended. A sand bag placed beneath the neck will help with positioning. The ventral cervical region should be clipped and aseptically prepared if time permits.
2. A ventral cervical midline incision is made from the caudal aspect of the cricoid cartilage to the sixth tracheal ring.
3. The sternohyoid muscles are separated on the midline and retracted laterally.
4. The trachea should be isolated and a full thickness stab incision should be made through the annular ligament between the third and fourth tracheal rings.
5. The incision in the trachea is extended laterally so that approximately 50–60% of the tracheal circumference is incised.
6. A tracheostomy tube approximately 50% of the tracheal diameter is placed into the lumen.
7. Two stay sutures are placed in the rings adjacent to the tracheostomy site to facilitate exposure for placement of the tracheostomy tube.
8. The subcutaneous tissues and skin are apposed cranial and caudal to the tracheostomy site allowing a large enough opening for re-intubation if necessary.
9. The tube is then secured with umbilical tape tied around the neck.

Patients with a temporary tracheostomy require careful 24-hour monitoring due to the risk of tube occlusion or dislodgement. Sterile technique should be used when handling the site, tracheostomy tubes, and suction catheters

Postoperative treatment includes nebulization of the tube site to humidify the airways, frequent removal and cleaning of the inner cannula (if present) to prevent obstruction with mucus, airway suctioning and observation for swelling and irritation. Short-term complications can include haemorrhage, obstruction of the tube, dislodgement, infection and damage to the peritracheal structures

7.10 Emergency tracheostomy.

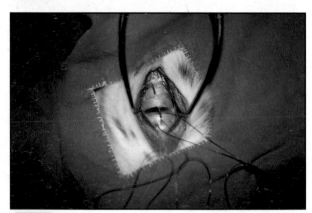

7.11 Tracheostomy. A 50% circumferential incision has been made into the trachea, and stay sutures are being placed around tracheal rings on both sides of the incision. (Courtesy of Dr Robert White)

In many syndromes of upper airway obstruction, pharyngoscopy and laryngoscopy under general anaesthesia are required to confirm the diagnosis. Following this, steps should be taken to relieve the airway obstruction prior to anaesthetic recovery. Attempts to recover patients with severe upper airway obstruction from anaesthesia without supporting the airway are hazardous and often fail. If the underlying disease cannot be corrected, a tracheostomy should be considered prior to extubation. In less severe cases, particularly those with a dynamic airway obstruction, a slow, non-stressful recovery may be successful, allowing definitive surgical correction of the airway problem to be planned in the near future.

Syndromes of upper airway obstruction

Brachycephalic obstructive airway syndrome: This is a common cause of respiratory distress in affected breeds such as English Bulldogs, Boston Terriers, Boxers, Pekingese and Pugs. The components of this syndrome are stenotic nares, redundant pharyngeal soft tissue, excessively long soft palate and hypoplastic trachea. Chronic obstruction of the upper airway causes increased negative inspiratory pressure leading to further airway occlusion, inflammation and oedema of the redundant tissue, eversion of the laryngeal saccules and eventually, in end-stage cases, complete laryngeal collapse. In patients with brachycephalic obstructive airway syndrome (BOAS), mouth breathing often improves the clinical signs because some of the airway resistance caused by the stenotic nares is eliminated. These animals often present with hyperthermia and acute respiratory distress during hot humid weather, after exercise or when extremely excited. Careful questioning of the owners often reveals a history of chronic airway obstruction (snoring and airway noise), which the owners may interpret as 'normal for the breed'.

Treatment is as described above, including oxygen supplementation, sedation, cooling and corticosteroids. Most patients can be managed medically through the presenting crisis, but surgical intervention to prevent future episodes is strongly recommended. Surgical correction of the stenotic nares and the overlong soft palate can greatly improve these patients, especially if performed in young dogs (less than 2 years of age).

Laryngeal paralysis: Laryngeal paralysis occurs in dogs and cats due to disruption of innervation of the muscles of the larynx and is classified as either congenital or acquired (idiopathic, traumatic, polyneuropathic or iatrogenic). Idiopathic acquired laryngeal paralysis is the most common form, most often seen in large-breed dogs such as Labrador Retrievers, Golden Retrievers and St Bernards. Affected dogs can present in severe respiratory distress with cyanosis and collapse. They often have loud inspiratory stridor and may be hyperthermic. The history may include voice change, gagging while eating and drinking, progressive exercise intolerance and noisy breathing.

Immediate therapy is as described above, with severely affected animals requiring intubation or a temporary tracheostomy. Thoracic radiography should be performed, as aspiration pneumonia and non-cardiogenic pulmonary oedema are common. Definitive diagnosis is made by laryngeal examination on induction of anaesthesia, to determine whether the vocal folds abduct effectively and symmetrically during inspiration. Since anaesthesia affects movement of the larynx, anaesthesia must be light enough that the patient is almost coughing during the laryngeal examination. Paradoxical laryngeal motion is another source of error of interpretation during laryngoscopy. If the larynx is paralysed, inspiration may be accompanied by closure of the larynx because of negative inspiratory pressures, and exhalation may tend to 'blow the larynx open'. This creates a paradoxical motion of the larynx, which on casual inspection may simulate normal function. Therefore, while performing a laryngeal examination, any observed movement of the larynx must be carefully correlated with the phase of respiration.

Surgical intervention may be delayed until the respiratory crisis has passed, allowing resolution of laryngeal inflammation and oedema. The surgical method of choice is a laryngeal tie-back (arytenoid cartilage lateralization). Postoperative concerns include aspiration pneumonia, laryngeal inflammation and oedema, haemorrhage, or breakdown of the surgical repair. Postoperative complications can be minimized by keeping the animal as calm as possible and reducing vocalization or coughing in the first 24 hours after surgery.

Tracheal collapse: This is a common problem in middle-aged to older small-breed dogs with a progressive history of cough and exercise intolerance. A cough is usually easy to induce on tracheal palpation. Excitement often triggers a paroxysmal 'honking' cough and dyspnoea. The tracheal rings in these animals are often abnormally C-shaped and fibrodysplastic, and the dorsal tracheal membrane is stretched, floppy and weak. Obstruction of the tracheal lumen occurs in the cervical and/or thoracic trachea. Compression, elevation and collapse of the left main-stem bronchus may mimic the clinical signs of collapsing trachea in dogs with mitral regurgitation and enlargement of the left atrium, before congestive heart failure occurs. Coughing due to mainstem bronchus compression is medically managed in a similar way to tracheal collapse, in addition to concurrent management of the primary cardiac disease.

Animals with tracheal collapse can present with varying degrees of dyspnoea. In the most severe cases, complete collapse of sections of the trachea can cause upper airway obstruction. Other animals can become hypoxic because of spasms of paroxysmal coughing. The diagnosis can be suggested using plain thoracic radiography. Severe collapse can appear radiographically similar to a tracheal soft tissue mass. One method of confirming the clinical diagnosis is observation of the trachea while coughing under fluoroscopy. The gold standard for diagnosis is bronchoscopy, but this requires anaesthesia, recovery from which is associated with a high degree of risk in severely affected patients if surgical correction is not performed at the time of diagnosis.

Management is as described above, with the addition of cough suppressants. Opioids, especially butorphanol and with the possible exception of pethidine (meperidine), are antitussive at low doses and are often beneficial. If medical management is ineffective, surgical placement of extraluminal rings or non-surgical placement of intraluminal stents may produce good results even in patients with end-stage disease. Tracheostomy is usually not of benefit in these patients because the collapse typically occurs throughout the cervical region and intrathoracic trachea or mainstem bronchi. Surgical options currently used in the UK include extraluminal ring prostheses with or without concurrent laryngeal surgery.

Inflammatory nasopharyngeal polyps: These occasionally cause respiratory stridor and dyspnoea in young, otherwise healthy cats. Polyps are often associated with inflammatory disease of the tympanic bullae or auditory canals. These cats may have an inspiratory stridor, a nasal discharge and otitis externa. The polyp is occasionally visible on oral examination in the awake patient, but sedation is usually required for adequate visualization. The soft palate should be palpated and retracted to detect polyps in the nasopharynx, and a thorough otoscopic examination should be performed. Radiographs of the skull, bullae and nasal cavity should be obtained (Figure 7.12). Polyps may arise from the bullae, ear canals or nasopharyngeal mucosa and must be removed surgically. If there is evidence of otitis, bulla osteotomy may be considered to resolve the underlying cause of the polyp. If the entire polyp is removed, surgery is generally curative.

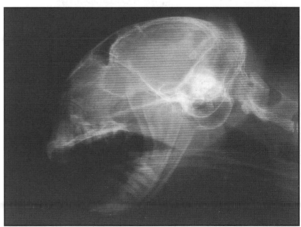

7.12 A lateral radiograph of a cat's skull showing an extremely large pharyngeal polyp occluding the pharynx. This cat presented with very loud upper airway stridor. (Reproduced with permission of Veterinary Learning Systems, Trenton, NJ)

Aspirated foreign bodies: These can cause sudden onset of respiratory distress if the foreign body obstructs the airway. Large upper airway obstructions require immediate action, since they may completely block all air flow. The animals often panic and are difficult to restrain, and sedation or anaesthesia may be necessary. If possible, vascular access should be established to allow intravenous administration of anaesthetic drugs. Because it may be impossible to remove the foreign body fast enough, preparation for an emergency tracheostomy is prudent. After expeditious removal of the object, supplemental oxygen should be administered. If the animal is unconscious after foreign body removal, it should be intubated and ventilation assisted until spontaneous breathing and consciousness return.

Upper airway masses: Upper airway neoplasia also occasionally causes upper airway obstruction. Neoplasia usually causes a slow onset of respiratory distress unless the tumour is very rapidly growing or associated with an abscess. Lymphoma is the most commonly observed neoplasm, especially in cats, but any oral neoplasm may be involved. Oxygen supplementation and sedation may be sufficient to improve clinical signs if the animal is not too severely affected. If necessary, when the neoplasm is in the proximal trachea or above, emergency tracheostomy can provide an adequate airway until more definitive surgery is performed. If the neoplasm is in the thoracic trachea and the patient cannot be stabilized medically, intubation (if possible), thoracotomy or palliative placement of an intraluminal stent are the only options.

Retropharyngeal masses, abscesses and haematomas are an occasional cause of respiratory distress. The most common retropharyngeal neoplasm is lymphoma, while abscesses can result from haematogenous spread or foreign body penetration. Rapid diagnosis by pharyngoscopy, ultrasonography, needle aspiration or even exploratory surgery is essential. These animals can easily progress to complete obstruction of their airway and require emergency tracheostomy. Haematomas can occur secondary to anticoagulant rodenticide ingestion, *Angiostrongylus vasorum* infection or trauma. In animals with coagulopathies, needle aspiration and surgery are contraindicated. Haemostasis can be difficult to achieve, but plasma transfusions and specific antidotes such as vitamin K1 should eventually lead to cessation of haemorrhage.

Lower airway disease

Clinical signs of lower airway disease

Clinical signs of animals with lower airway disease are summarized in Figure 7.13. Disease of the lower airways usually refers to abnormalities of the small bronchi and is commonly inflammatory in origin. Coughing is the most common historical finding. Typically, the cough is harsh or honking and non-productive, and is not beneficial to the patient as it tends to exacerbate inflammation, thereby promoting more coughing. In contrast, animals with productive coughing (usually a soft moist sound that is followed by swallowing when the animal expectorates material into the pharynx) should be evaluated for other disorders such as pneumonia. In pneumonia, the cough is a necessary part of the clearance mechanism of the lung, rather than being due to bronchial disease alone. On auscultation, most dogs with lower airway disease have increased bronchovesicular sounds and/or wheezes. Patients with

end-stage disease may have significantly increased respiratory rate and effort associated with hypoxia. Thoracic radiographs usually reveal minimal evidence of alveolar disease.

Hypoxia in animals with chronic bronchitis is thought to be attributable to inequality of ventilation and pulmonary perfusion (V–Q mismatch), mainly caused by bronchial obstruction. Bronchial obstruction follows increased mucus production, mucosal hyperaemia and oedema, as well as early collapse of abnormal and weakened small airways. Obesity often contributes to the severity of clinical signs, causing diminished ability to expand the lungs and pressure on the thorax from the chest wall and abdomen. Bronchopneumonia is a common complication because of diminished lung defences. Although some degree of bronchoconstriction can occur, dogs do not suffer from smooth muscle spasm as seen in cats with feline allergic airway disease (asthma). Acute severe bronchoconstriction in cats with hyper-responsive airways contributes significantly to dyspnoea in affected animals. Animals with severe lower airway disease therefore present with dyspnoea caused by end-stage chronic obstructive pulmonary disease, superimposed bronchopneumonia and, in cats, bronchospasm.

General approach to management of patients with lower airway disease

Priorities for management of lower airway disease are summarized in Figure 7.14. Animals brought to the emergency room because of lower airway disease are usually presented during exacerbations and crises, or when the disease has become end stage. Dyspnoea is a common presentation, especially in cats with asthma. As usual, oxygen supplementation is the first priority. Animals that are extremely distressed may benefit from sedation. Early diagnostic investigation should include thoracic radiography. Most patients with bronchial disease have little or no alveolar disease visible on thoracic radiographs. A peribronchial pattern may be present, with 'doughnuts' and 'tramlines', but alveolar disease should be absent unless pneumonia or another secondary process is present.

Cough

Exercise intolerance

Dyspnoea (severe cases, expiratory dyspnoea in cats with feline asthma)

Increased bronchovesicular sounds

Wheezes

7.13 Clinical and historical signs associated with lower airway (bronchial) disease in dogs and cats.

Oxygen supplementation

Rest, sedation not usually required

Minimal stress

Vascular access

Anti-inflammatory to immunosuppressive doses of corticosteroids
  Dexamethasone 0.25–0.5 mg/kg i.v. or i.m.
  or prednisolone 0.5–1 mg/kg i.v., i.m. or orally

Bronchodilators
  Terbutaline 0.01 mg/kg i.v. or i.m.
  or aminophylline 5.5 mg/kg i.v.

Cough suppressants
  Butorphanol 0.2–0.4 mg/kg i.v. or i.m. or 0.5–1.0 mg/kg orally
  or hydrocodone 1.25–5 mg/kg orally

Antibiotics

Thoracic radiographs to rule out pulmonary alveolar disease

Consider tracheal wash for culture and cytological examination

---

7.14 General approach to emergency management of dogs and cats with lower airway disease.

If bronchial disease is suspected, corticosteroids can be extremely helpful because of the role of inflammation in the disease process. Initially, high doses are indicated, reducing to the minimal effective dose as soon as possible. Bronchodilators are also considered first-line drugs in these patients. Beta agonists such as terbutaline have superseded aminophylline in clinical use. Administration of bronchodilators and corticosteroids by aerosolization can be helpful, but may not be tolerated by extremely dyspnoeic animals, and should supplement, rather than replace, parenteral drug administration in an emergency situation. Refractory coughing may respond to antitussive drugs such as butorphanol. Since exacerbation of signs may occur due to secondary bacterial infection and even pneumonia, antibiotics may be of value in some cases to diminish exudate production. Ideally, cytology and cultures from the airway (usually obtained by tracheal wash, Figures 7.15 and 7.16) should be obtained prior to starting

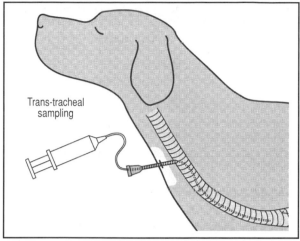

Trans-tracheal sampling

7.16 Method for trans-tracheal wash. (Modified from the *BSAVA Manual of Small Animal Cardiorespiratory Medicine and Surgery*, with the permission of Vicki Martin Design)

Trans-tracheal wash (TTW)

Used in medium to large-sized dogs

TTW can usually be performed without sedation unless the dog is fractious. Ideally, the animal should be alert enough to cough to aid in sample collection. An 18 gauge 'through-the-needle' catheter is used to collect the sample: 20 cm length in smaller dogs; 30 cm length in larger dogs

1. The skin of the ventral neck from the larynx to the mid-trachea should be clipped and sterilely prepared.

2. A local anaesthetic such as lidocaine is infiltrated to the level of the trachea at the site of planned catheter placement. The site of insertion is typically between two and five tracheal rings distal to the larynx; precise counting of tracheal rings is not necessary.

3. The catheter is pushed through the skin. The trachea is isolated and stabilized between the thumb and forefinger, and the tip of the catheter is placed against the trachea between two rings. The tip of the catheter is held perpendicular to the trachea with the bevel of the needle facing down, and is 'popped' into the lumen of the trachea.

4. The needle is then angled downward and the catheter's entire length is fed down the trachea.

5. If the catheter does not feed easily, the needle is backed out of the trachea about 0.25 cm as the tip of the needle may be pressed up against the back wall of the trachea, and the catheter is again fed into the trachea.

6. Once the full length of the catheter is in the trachea, the needle is withdrawn from the neck, the needle guard is placed around the needle, and the stylet is removed from the catheter.

7. Approximately 5–10 ml of sterile saline is injected into the catheter.

8. Coupage is performed on the dog's chest to encourage coughing and productive sampling.

9. This injection procedure can be repeated up to three times if necessary to obtain an adequate sample. Only a small proportion of the instilled fluid will be recovered.

10. The sample is submitted in a sterile container for culture and cytology.

11. The catheter is removed from the dog's neck and a gauze square is placed over the entry point to stop any minor bleeding.

Alternatively, if a long 'through the needle' catheter is not available, a standard 'over the needle' catheter may be used. The catheter is placed in the trachea as described above and the stylet removed. A long male dog urinary catheter is then threaded through the intravenous catheter to approximately the level of the carina. This can be estimated by premeasuring the catheter to the fourth intercostal space. The saline is instilled though the urinary catheter. Typically a 4–6 French urinary catheter is used with a 12–14 gauge intravenous catheter, depending on patient size

Complications can include subcutaneous emphysema, pneumomediastinum, pneumothorax, bleeding, catheter breakage and aspiration of the catheter into the airway, and worsening respiratory status due to the stress of the procedure

Endotracheal wash (ETW)

Endotracheal washes can be used in small dogs, large dogs that are anaesthetized for another procedure and cats. The patient should be stable enough to be lightly anaesthetized

1. A sterile endotracheal tube is inserted into the trachea, avoiding oral contamination.

2. A sterile dog urinary catheter or red rubber catheter is used to inject sterile saline beyond the lumen of the endotracheal tube.

3. The catheter is then aspirated while an assistant performs coupage on the patient.

An alternative method uses a suction catheter and sterile suction trap to collect the samples. This requires mechanical suction; the sample is automatically collected into the sterile suction trap

Patients that have an ETW performed should be closely monitored during recovery to ensure that they have adequate ventilatory function and oxygenation

7.15 Tracheal washes.

antibiotic therapy. Most respiratory crises caused by bronchial disease respond well to medical management, minimal stress and an oxygen-enriched environment.

Syndromes of lower airway disease

Feline asthma: Feline asthma, also referred to as allergic bronchitis, is the most common cause of lower airway disease in cats (Figure 7.17). The clinical signs result from bronchial inflammation with peribronchial infiltrates, mucosal oedema, increased mucus production, bronchiolar smooth muscle hypertrophy and reversible airway obstruction caused by excessive bronchoconstriction. Airway obstruction is most severe during expiration and may lead to air trapping and alveolar hyperinflation. Cats may present with disease at any age, but signs often first appear in young adults. Clinical signs can range from severe dyspnoea to intermittent cough. In severe cases, the cats open-mouth breathe, have pale to cyanotic mucous membranes and may have an abdominal component to respiration, especially during expiration. On auscultation, expiratory wheezes are often heard. In the most severe cases, respiratory sounds may be almost absent, as air movement is almost cut off by the severity of bronchial obstruction.

Feline asthma
Chronic bronchitis
Neoplasia
Aspirated foreign body

7.17 Common differential diagnoses for lower airway disease in dogs and cats.

If the cat is in severe distress, obtaining a definitive diagnosis should be delayed until the cat is more stable. The cat should be placed in an oxygen cage, thereby minimizing stress and allowing it to relax after transport. Since bronchoconstriction occurs as a result of inflammation, corticosteroids should be given intravenously if possible (otherwise, intramuscularly). Bronchodilators such as terbutaline have proven to be useful in acute management, and can be given by inhalation as well as parenterally. In agonal cases, adrenaline should be administered intramuscularly (0.5–0.75 ml of 1:10,000 solution i.m.), for its profound vasoconstrictive, inotropic and bronchodilator effects. If there is no response to medical management and the cat remains in severe distress, anaesthesia (halothane is particularly useful for its bronchodilatory effects) and intubation may be required. Occasionally, cats may have pneumothorax secondary to rupture of the hyperinflated alveoli.

Radiographic findings include a bronchiolar pattern, collapse of the right middle lung lobe and pulmonary hyperinflation (Figure 7.18). Findings may, however, be normal, especially if radiography is delayed in unstable animals. Definitive diagnosis requires the demonstration of inflammation on tracheal wash cytology.

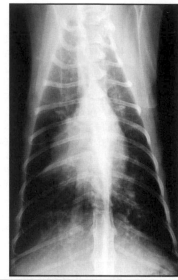

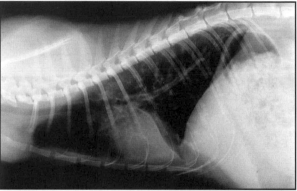

7.18 Lateral and ventrodorsal thoracic radiographs of a 3-year-old Domestic Longhair cat that presented with a 3-month history of coughing and acute respiratory distress. The radiographs show the typical bronchial pattern of feline asthma, often described as 'doughnuts and tramlines', collapse of the right middle lung lobe and pulmonary hyperinflation.

Canine chronic bronchitis: This is recognized as a persistent cough occurring for at least two consecutive months in the absence of another specific pulmonary disease. Hyperplasia and hypertrophy of bronchial glands, increased goblet cells, increased airway secretion and increased infiltrates of inflammatory cells are seen. This produces thickened, hyperaemic bronchial walls, obstruction of small airways with mucus and proliferation of epithelial surfaces. Patients with exacerbated or end-stage disease can present with severe distress and cyanosis.

Physical examination findings may include increased airway sounds with wheezes and coarse crackles on chest auscultation caused by opening and closing of small bronchi. Thoracic radiographs usually show a bronchial pattern and the extent of the changes does not always correlate with the severity of clinical signs. Immediate management is as described above. In addition, saline nebulization may assist with mobilization of secretions.

Lower airway masses and foreign bodies: Foreign bodies and tumours can also occur in the lower airways. Radiographs may assist in confirming the diagnosis. Chronic bronchial obstruction causes gradual collapse and absorption atelectasis of the affected lung lobe. Even if a foreign body or neoplasm is not visible on radiographs, the presence of one completely collapsed lung lobe should prompt suspicion of complete bronchial obstruction and absorption atelectasis. Sudden onset of respiratory distress can be seen after aspiration of a foreign body into the bronchi (Figure 7.19). Foreign bodies may be retrieved with the aid of bronchoscopy or fluoroscopy or removed at the time of thoracotomy. Neoplasia of the lower airways is usually characterized by a slower, more gradual onset of respiratory distress. Thoracic radiographs and bronchoscopy can aid in the diagnosis, and biopsy assists in its confirmation. Debulking or removal of the mass (often including lung lobectomy) may be necessary, unless the biopsy reveals lymphoma, which may respond to chemotherapy.

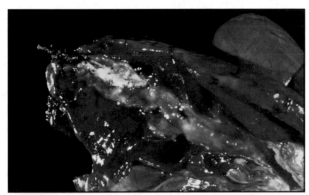

7.19 A postmortem examination of this 4-year-old cat revealed aspirated plant material in a bronchus. (Reproduced with permission of Veterinary Learning Systems, Trenton, NJ)

Pulmonary parenchymal disease

Clinical signs of pulmonary parenchymal disease
Clinical signs of pulmonary parenchymal disease are summarized in Figure 7.20. Pulmonary parenchymal disease is commonly associated with varying degrees of hypoxia and dyspnoea. Typically, the lungs have decreased compliance. A restrictive pattern of respiration (rapid shallow breathing) is observed and severe hypoxia may be manifested by paradoxical respiration. Hypoxia in patients with pulmonary parenchymal disease is usually caused by ventilation/perfusion mismatch due to filling and collapse of alveoli. Some patients may also have an increased diffusion barrier caused by thickening or infiltration of the alveolar membrane.

Pale or cyanotic mucous membranes

Increased respiratory rate or dyspnoea

Restrictive respiratory pattern

Harsh bronchovesicular sounds

Crackles

Nasal discharge

Cough (often productive)

7.20 Clinical and historical signs associated with pulmonary parenchymal disease in dogs and cats.

On auscultation, harsh bronchovesicular sounds and/or crackles are common. Careful auscultation of the heart should be performed to detect the presence of a murmur which might indicate congestive heart failure. Nasal discharge can occur in patients with bronchopneumonia or profound pulmonary oedema. Coughing may be a feature of pulmonary parenchymal disease if there is bronchial irritation or inflammation. Typically, coughing is productive: a soft moist cough is an important part of clearance of secretions from the pulmonary parenchyma.

Animals with pulmonary parenchymal disease usually have an alveolar pattern on thoracic radiographs. The distribution of the alveolar pattern can give important information about the aetiology of respiratory failure. Occasionally animals may have minor or absent radiographic changes; for example those with pulmonary thromboembolism or interstitial fibrosis.

General approach to management of patients with pulmonary parenchymal disease
The approach to management of animals with pulmonary parenchymal disease is summarized in Figure 7.21. Patients that are dyspnoeic due to suspected pulmonary parenchymal disease should receive oxygen supplementation immediately. Physical examination and historical findings often give an indication of

Oxygen supplementation

Rest and minimal stress

Vascular access

Thoracic radiographs (if possible)

Medical management according to most likely differential diagnoses:

Bacterial bronchopneumonia:
Tracheal wash for culture and cytological examination
Stable:
- Enrofloxacin 5–15 mg/kg orally q24h *or*
- Amoxicillin/clavulanate 14–22 mg/kg orally q12h
Unstable:
- Enrofloxacin 5–15 mg/kg i.v. q24h and ampicillin 22 mg/kg i.v. q8h *or*
- Amikacin 15 mg/kg i.v. q24h and ampicillin 22 mg/kg i.v. q8h *or*
- Cefotaxime 20–50 mg/kg i.v. q6h *or*
- Ticarcillin/clavulanate 50 mg/kg i.v. q6h
Nebulization and coupage

Pulmonary oedema:
- Furosemide 0.5–2 mg/kg i.v. or i.m. q4–12h
- Glyceryl trinitrate paste 6–25 mm cutaneously *or*
- Nitroprusside 2–10 µg/kg/min
- Dobutamine 5–10 µg/kg/min

Haemorrhage
Fresh whole blood, fresh frozen plasma, or packed red blood cell transfusions
- Vitamin K1 2 mg/kg s.c. or orally q12h

Pulmonary thromboembolism
Fresh frozen plasma
- Unfractionated heparin 100–300 IU/kg q6h s.c. or 10–50 IU/kg/h i.v. CRI

Pulmonary inflammatory disorders
- Dexamethasone 0.25–0.5 mg/kg i.v. or i.m. q12–24h *or*
- Prednisolone 0.5–1 mg/kg i.v., i.m. or orally q12–24h

7.21 General approach to emergency management of dogs and cats with pulmonary parenchymal disease.

the cause of the dyspnoea. Thoracic radiographs are a valuable diagnostic tool at this stage. If respiratory distress is so severe that thoracic radiographs cannot be obtained safely, empirical treatment for the most common causes of pulmonary parenchymal disease should be initiated. Often, empirical medical management, combined with oxygen supplementation, can improve the condition of the patient to the point that radiographs can be obtained. If the patient does not improve, or even deteriorates in spite of medical management, an aggressive approach may be required, including general anaesthesia and intubation of the patient to facilitate diagnostic testing and therapy. The most common medical problems and their management are described below.

Syndromes of pulmonary parenchymal disease

Pneumonia: Pneumonia is one of the most common causes of pulmonary parenchymal disease (Figure 7.22). It is categorized as aspiration, bacterial, parasitic, viral or fungal, occurring alone or in combination. Pneumonia is more common in dogs than in cats. Physical examination usually reveals increased respiratory rate and effort, pale to cyanotic mucous membranes and harsh lung sounds or crackles. If the animal is stable, the diagnosis is confirmed by radiographic findings of alveolar disease (Figure 7.23), cytology showing acute neutrophilic inflammation, and culture and sensitivity testing of airway aspirates obtained by tracheal wash or bronchoalveolar lavage. Serology may be used to assist diagnosis of viral or fungal pneumonia.

Pneumonia
Pulmonary oedema (cardiogenic and non-cardiogenic)
Haemorrhage
Pulmonary thromboembolism
Neoplasia: primary or metastatic
Pulmonary inflammatory disease (PIE and LG)
Acute lung injury and acute respiratory distress syndrome (ARDS)

7.22 Differential diagnoses for pulmonary parenchymal disease in dogs and cats. (PIE, pulmonary infiltrate with eosinophils, LG, lymphomatoid granulomatosis.)

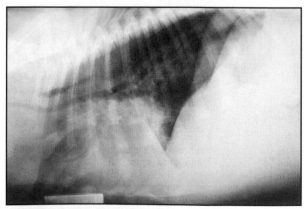

7.23 Severe aspiration pneumonia in the cranioventral and right middle lung lobes. An alveolar pattern with air bronchograms is present.

Aspiration pneumonia is caused by inhalation of foreign material. This typically comprises oral secretions or gastrointestinal tract contents subsequent to vomiting or regurgitation. Animals with underlying conditions such as pharyngeal/laryngeal dysfunction, megaoesophagus, cleft palate, abnormal mentation, recumbency or debilitation have an increased risk of aspiration. The acidic pH of gastric reflux material determines the extent of bronchoconstriction and injury to the pulmonary parenchyma. Liquids reach the alveoli within minutes, making attempts to perform suction of the airways futile in most cases. The resultant inflammation impairs lung defences and allows bacteria in the aspirated material to colonize the lungs. By the time most aspiration pneumonia cases are recognized, bacterial infection has occurred. These patients are therefore treated in the same way as those with primary bacterial pneumonia.

Bacterial bronchopneumonia usually occurs as a consequence of bronchogenous invasion (inhalation) of pathogenic bacteria, or occasionally by haematogenous spread. Animals with bronchogenous pneumonia typically have a cranioventral pattern of alveolar disease on radiographs, whereas those with haematogenous pneumonia often have a patchy or nodular distribution. Bacterial pneumonia can be caused by primary respiratory tract pathogens such as *Bordetella bronchiseptica*, or by opportunistic pathogens that proliferate because of suppression of respiratory tract defences. With the exception of animals suspected of *Bordetella* infection, dogs and cats that present with bacterial pneumonia should be carefully evaluated for underlying disorders.

Other causes of pneumonia include parasitic pneumonia (*Angiostrongylus vasorum*), viral agents (canine distemper), protozoal organisms (toxoplasmosis) and fungal invasion (histoplasmosis, blastomycosis and coccidioidomycosis). In addition to general pneumonia management, specific therapy should be directed against individual organisms.

Bacterial cultures should be obtained before starting antibiotic therapy whenever possible. Gram-negative pathogens and polymicrobial infections are common. Broad-spectrum antibiotic treatment should be started while waiting for the culture results. Oral drugs such as amoxicillin/clavulanate or fluoroquinolones can be used if the animal is not systemically ill. If the patient is hypoxic, dyspnoeic or febrile, intravenous antibiotics must be used until the animal is stable. Combinations of antibiotics that provide broad-spectrum coverage include ampicillin/aminoglycosides, ampicillin/fluoroquinolones or second- or third-generation cephalosporins. Another potentially valuable therapy is that of nebulization with sterile saline followed by coupage to loosen and mobilize airway secretions, promote coughing and improve airway clearance. Nebulized mucolytic agents are not typically used as they can cause bronchospasm. Oxygen supplementation should be administered as required, and severely affected cases may require positive pressure ventilation.

Pulmonary oedema: This is the accumulation of fluid in the alveoli and pulmonary interstitium and is divided by initiating cause into cardiogenic and non-cardiogenic forms. Cardiogenic oedema is more common, and is seen in animals with left-sided heart failure and elevated pulmonary venous pressure. On auscultation, crackles are often evident and may be accompanied by a mitral murmur in dogs or a gallop rhythm in cats. Thoracic radiographs usually reveal cardiomegaly and a perihilar alveolar pattern in the dog. In cats, distribution of oedema is less specific. Details of diagnosis and management of cardiogenic pulmonary oedema are given in Chapter 6.

Neurogenic pulmonary oedema is a form of non-cardiogenic pulmonary oedema that can be caused by seizures or head trauma, choking or airway obstruction and electric shock. Although the pathophysiology is not well understood, it is thought that massive sympathetic discharge results in increased peripheral resistance, which raises systemic blood pressure. Blood therefore moves transiently from the systemic circulation into the low-pressure pulmonary vasculature which has relatively few catecholamine receptors. This volume shift dramatically and transiently elevates pulmonary venous pressures. The end result is increased capillary permeability and fluid redistribution to the interstitium and alveoli. The pressures rapidly return to normal, but the changes in permeability remain for several hours.

Affected animals may develop respiratory distress immediately or over several hours after the inciting incident. Varying degrees of respiratory distress occur; some animals have minimal signs, and others can rapidly become agonal because of fulminant pulmonary oedema. Crackles are often heard on auscultation. The diagnosis can be confirmed by thoracic radiography, which reveals an interstitial or alveolar pattern in the dorsocaudal lung fields (Figure 7.24). The extent of lung involvement is determined by arterial blood gas analysis. Typical findings include hypoxia and a P_aCO_2 that is low, normal or high, depending on the severity of the oedema.

Treatment consists of supportive care, with oxygen supplementation as needed. Diuretics may be administered, but are less effective than in cardiogenic oedema because the oedema is caused by a vascular permeability change, rather than by a sustained increase in pulmonary venous pressure. The use of corticosteroids in these patients remains controversial and is not currently recommended. Mildly affected animals improve dramatically in 24–48 hours, while the most severely affected animals with fulminant pulmonary oedema may require positive pressure ventilation and often do not recover.

Pulmonary haemorrhage: Pulmonary haemorrhage can occur secondary to trauma (pulmonary contusions), coagulopathies (rodenticide ingestion, *Angiostrongylus vasorum* infection) and neoplasia. Haemorrhage into the parenchyma is commonly seen following anticoagulant rodenticide ingestion. These animals are presented with coughing (which may include a productive cough with blood-tinged sputum), lethargy or dyspnoea. Varying degrees of anaemia and pale mucous membranes are seen due to blood loss. Radiographs usually reveal a patchy alveolar pattern or pleural effusion. Treatment consists of oxygen support, fresh frozen plasma or fresh whole blood in addition to vitamin K1 therapy (see Chapters 14 and 19).

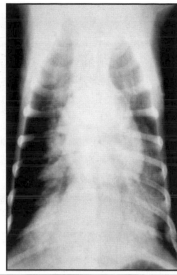

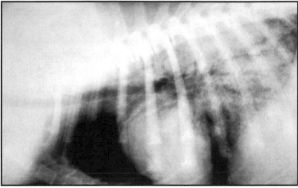

7.24 Lateral and ventrodorsal thoracic radiographs of a dog with neurogenic pulmonary oedema following airway obstruction. The typical caudodorsal patchy alveolar pattern is present.

Pulmonary thromboembolic disease: This is caused by pulmonary arterial obstruction by thrombi and results in respiratory distress by producing severe ventilation/perfusion mismatch. Thrombi form because of systemic hypercoagulability, stasis of blood within vessels or direct endothelial damage. Thrombi can form in disease states such as protein-losing nephropathy, hyperadrenocorticism, immune-mediated haemolytic anaemia, bacterial endocarditis and dirofilariasis, as well as post surgery. Affected patients often have a sudden onset of respiratory distress, increased respiratory rate and effort, generalized harsh lung sounds and pale to cyanotic mucous membranes. When thrombus accumulation in the lungs is extensive, an occlusive reduction in pulmonary venous return to the heart may occur, which will be detected as reduced pulse quality and hypotension. Thoracic radiographs are often normal, but may reveal varying interstitial or alveolar patterns, pleural effusion and dilated or truncated pulmonary arteries (Figure 7.25). The most common clinicopathological findings are elevation of serum D-dimers and thrombocytopenia. A definitive diagnosis can sometimes be made using non-selective computed tomography (CT) angiography, but unstable patients may not tolerate this procedure. Ventilation/perfusion scanning with radioisotopes is a non-invasive procedure that can provide useful diagnostic information, but the equipment is not widely available.

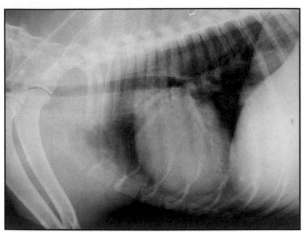

7.25 A lateral thoracic radiograph of a mixed breed dog with severe, autoagglutinating haemolytic anaemia that developed acute respiratory distress. A presumptive diagnosis of pulmonary thromboembolism was made based on the severity of the hypoxia and lack of radiographic abnormalities.

The prognosis for thromboembolic disease is fair to guarded, depending on the extent of lung involvement and the nature of any underlying disease condition. Oxygen supplementation should be provided, but may not lead to dramatic improvement because of pulmonary shunting. Therapy consists of supportive care, treatment of the underlying disease and prevention of further thrombosis using anticoagulants. Heparin can be administered subcutaneously or as an intravenous constant rate infusion (see Figure 7.21). If the predisposing disease is established and considered ongoing, warfarin therapy can also be instituted for long-term maintenance. In such cases, treatment with heparin is tapered and discontinued. Thrombolytic agents, such as streptokinase and tissue plasminogen activator, have been used with mixed success in a limited number of patients.

Neoplasia: Primary pulmonary neoplasia or metastatic disease can also cause severe respiratory distress. Patient history varies from acute signs to a gradual onset of exercise intolerance and laboured breathing, with or without coughing. Thoracic radiographs and identification of a distant primary neoplasm are often diagnostic. A definitive diagnosis can often be made following cytological examination of pleural fluid or fine needle aspiration of the mass. If cytological evaluation and other diagnostics provide equivocal results, exploratory thoracotomy may be required. Supportive care should be provided as needed, but treatment options may be limited. Unless the neoplasm is either responsive to chemotherapy or can be removed in its entirety at the time of surgery, euthanasia is often indicated.

Pulmonary inflammatory disease: This is an uncommon cause of respiratory distress in small animals. Reported pulmonary inflammatory diseases include pulmonary infiltrate with eosinophils and lymphomatoid granulomatosis. Pulmonary tissue is infiltrated by a non-neoplastic proliferation of eosinophils or lymphocytes, respectively. Clinical findings vary from sudden to gradual onset of respiratory distress or coughing. Radiographic findings include mass lesions or infiltration. The diagnosis may be confirmed by a cytological finding of inflammatory cells on samples obtained by tracheal wash or fine needle aspiration. Other underlying causes, such as pulmonary parasites, must also be ruled out. Apart from routine respiratory supportive care, therapy includes immunosuppressive doses of corticosteroids. More aggressive cytotoxic drugs may be required in refractory cases. Many animals respond well to this therapy.

Acute lung injury and acute respiratory distress syndrome: Acute lung injury (ALI) and ARDS are terms that refer to a syndrome of generalized inflammatory lung injury. Inflammation can be triggered by systemic inflammatory disorders, such as septic shock or pancreatitis, or by a severe pulmonary insult, such as aspiration pneumonia, pulmonary contusions or smoke inhalation. In ALI, pulmonary inflammation manifests as vasculitis, interstitial and alveolar permeability oedema, and infiltration of inflammatory cells such as neutrophils and macrophages. ARDS is a more severe form, manifested by inflammation as in ALI, accompanied by proliferation of type II pneumocytes, hyaline membranes and eventually interstitial fibrosis. Animals with ALI-like syndrome have mild to moderate degrees of dyspnoea and hypoxia and often respond to fluid restriction, colloid support, low doses of diuretics and treatment of the underlying disease. Despite the fact that this is an inflammatory disease, corticosteroids have been shown to have no effect on mortality rates in human patients with these syndromes, and may be contraindicated because of their immunosuppressive effects. Animals with ARDS have severe pulmonary dysfunction and very poor lung compliance. They usually require positive pressure ventilation and the prognosis is grave.

Pleural space disease

Clinical signs of pleural space disease
The clinical signs of pleural space disease are summarized in Figure 7.26. Pulmonary dysfunction can be caused by accumulation of fluid, air or soft tissue within the pleural cavity. Pleural space disease is suggested by physical examination findings that include increased respiratory rate or effort, dyspnoea and auscultation of diminished or dull lung and heart

Increased respiratory rate and effort, short shallow respiratory pattern
Dyspnoea
Cough
Dull or diminished lung and heart sounds on auscultation
Fever
Weight loss and lethargy

7.26 Clinical and historical signs associated with pleural space disease in dogs and cats.

sounds. Depending on the cause, other signs such as fever may also be present. Because the pleural pathology prevents lung expansion, hypoxia is caused by atelectasis and ventilation/perfusion mismatch. Radiographic changes are compatible with either the presence of free air or increases in fluid or soft tissue density in the pleural space. Increased soft tissue density may occur secondary to neoplasia or diaphragmatic herniation into the pleural space.

General approach to management of patients with pleural space disease

The approach to management of patients with pleural space disease is summarized in Figure 7.27. If pneumothorax or pleural effusion is suspected and the animal is in severe respiratory distress, routine oxygen supplementation should be provided and thoracocentesis should be performed immediately and before radiographs have confirmed the diagnosis. Thoracocentesis is both a therapeutic and diagnostic procedure and can be life saving in severely compromised patients (Figures 7.28 and 7.29). Thoracic radiographs obtained after thoracocentesis are more valuable than those obtained prior to removal of the fluid or air. Once the fluid has been removed, radiographs may reveal the cause of the effusion, and allow evaluation of the cardiac silhouette and demonstration of masses.

Oxygen supplementation

Rest and minimal stress

Vascular access

Thoracocentesis

Thoracic ultrasonography

Thoracic radiography (if possible) after thoracocentesis

Fluid analysis:
    Cell counts
    Cytology
    Aerobic and anaerobic culture
    Biochemical analysis if indicated (triglycerides)

7.27 General approach to emergency management of dogs and cats with pleural space disease.

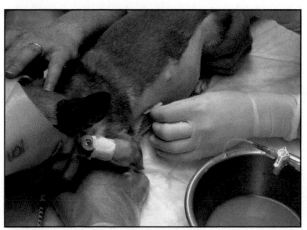

7.28 Thoracocentesis is performed in this small dog using a butterfly catheter and a three-way stopcock.

Indications

- Patients with respiratory distress and dull lung sounds on auscultation.
- Patients that present after trauma (RTA, bite wounds, falling from height).
- Patients that are undergoing positive pressure ventilation with sudden deterioration.

Contraindications

- Severe coagulopathy.

Procedure

Position patient, preferably in sternal recumbency or standing. Lateral recumbency is also acceptable for pneumothorax. An assistant should be available to restrain patient or give sedation as needed. In many cats a minimal restraint technique is preferred and is generally better tolerated

1. Clip and aseptically prepare appropriate rib space:
   - If expecting fluid, the 7th or 8th intercostal space, at approximately the level of the costo-chondral junction
   - If expecting air, the 8th or 9th intercostal space approximately one third of the way down the chest.
2. Use sterile gloves for the insertion of the appropriate size needle or butterfly catheter:
   - Large dogs – 40 mm needle or even longer catheter
   - Medium dogs and large cats – 25 mm needle or catheter
   - Cats and small dogs – 18–22 mm butterfly needle.
3. Insert the needle slowly just cranial to the rib to avoid intercostal blood vessels.
4. Observe the hub of needle for any signs of fluid:
   - If a small amount of frank blood is aspirated or if the lungs can be felt rubbing against the needle, the needle should be withdrawn and moved to a different location
   - If a large amount of blood is obtained, place 1–2 ml in an empty blood collection tube to see if it clots. Blood from haemothorax should not clot, while blood from the heart or a blood vessel should clot normally, if patient does not have a significant coagulopathy
   - For any other fluid, aspiration should continue until no more can be removed.
5. Directing the needle ventrally, rolling the patient slightly to the side on which thoracocentesis is being performed, and re-aspirating from a more ventral location can facilitate removal of as much fluid as possible.
6. Fluid is saved for fluid analysis, cytology, and possibly culture.
7. Aspiration of air will turn the tubing a slightly foggy, white colour as the warm air from the thoracic cavity encounters the room temperature tubing.
8. Aspirate until negative pressure is reached. If negative pressure is never obtained, a tension pneumothorax may be present, and chest tubes with continuous suction are needed (see Figure 7.32).

7.29 Thoracocentesis.

Pleural effusions are classified according to the type of fluid obtained (Figure 7.30). Gross examination can identify whether the fluid is haemorrhagic, purulent, chylous or a transudate. All fluid should be analysed further including determination of protein content, cytology and cell counts. In addition, specific chemical analysis, such as triglyceride concentration, or microbiological culture may be indicated. The character of the pleural effusion determines the course of further diagnostic evaluation and the likelihood of recurrence. Specific management will depend on the findings of fluid analysis and presence of underlying disease.

Pleural effusion:
    Pyothorax
    Non-bacterial exudates (FIP or neoplasia)
    Chylothorax
    Transudates (pure or modified)
    Haemothorax
    Sanguineous effusions (lung lobe torsion)
Pneumothorax
Diaphragmatic hernia
Pleural neoplasia or masses

7.30 Common differential diagnoses for pleural space disease in dogs and cats (FIP, feline infectious peritonitis).

Syndromes of pleural space disease

Pyothorax: This is the accumulation of a purulent exudate in one or both sides of the pleural space and is more common in cats than in dogs. The aetiology includes idiopathic causes, penetrating chest wounds, haematogenous spread, extension from adjacent structures or fascial planes, aspirated foreign bodies, ruptured pulmonary abscesses and ruptured oesophagus. Presenting complaints include lethargy, anorexia, respiratory distress, fever and/or weight loss. The diagnosis is confirmed by high nucleated cell counts in the pleural fluid, with a large number of degenerate neutrophils. Bacteria may be visible, but are not always evident. Both aerobic and anaerobic cultures should be submitted because of the high incidence of anaerobic bacteria in pleural infections. Polymicrobial infections are common.

Treatment in cats should consist of thoracic drainage and administration of broad-spectrum intravenous antibiotics until the rate of effusion diminishes, followed by oral antibiotics once culture results become available. Since this is a deep tissue infection, prone to recurrence in individual animals, antibiotic therapy is typically continued for 2–3 months. Thoracic drainage can be accomplished by repeated needle thoracocentesis, however it is a painful procedure that may not be well tolerated, and may not effectively drain the exudate if it is viscous or loculated. Placement of one or more chest drains allows continuous drainage of the fluid as it forms (Figures 7.31 and 7.32). Frequency of drainage will depend on the rate of fluid production but gentle aspiration of the chest tube is usually performed several times daily. Alternatively, the drain may be attached to a pleural suction device which provides gentle continuous negative pressure to the drain and is ideal if large volumes of fluid are produced. Lavage of the thoracic cavity with 5–20 ml/kg of warmed sterile saline once or twice daily has been recommended but should be reserved for patients that have very viscous effusions. Thoracic drainage should continue until the fluid character has changed to a serosanguineous effusion containing non-degenerate neutrophils, and the volume has diminished to 5 ml/kg/day or less. On average, thoracic drainage is required for about 1 week, but the range varies from 2 days to 3 weeks. If patients fail to respond, careful evaluation for underlying causes of pyothorax, such as lung abscesses, should be considered and exploratory thoracotomy may be required.

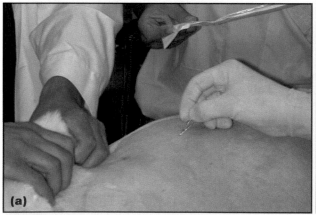 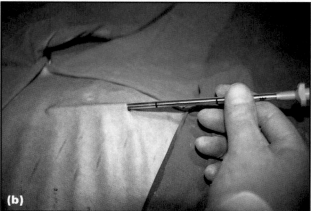

7.31 Chest tube placement. **(a)** Prior to placement of the chest tube, the thoracic skin is pulled cranially by an assistant; release of the skin will create a subcutaneous tunnel for the tube. (Courtesy of Dr David Holt, School of Veterinary Medicine, University of Pennsylvania) **(b)** The trochar thoracostomy tube has been inserted through a skin incision (10th intercostal space), and is being directed subcutaneously in a cranial direction. (Courtesy of Dr Robert White)

Indications
• Pyothorax
• Rapidly-forming pleural effusion
• Recurring pneumothorax requiring repeated thoracocentesis
• Tension pneumothorax
• Postoperative management of thoracotomy patients

Contraindications
• Severe coagulopathy

7.32 Chest tube placement. (continues) ▶

Procedure
1. General anaesthesia (preferable), can be done with sedation only in emergency.
2. Place patient in lateral recumbency.
3. Clip lateral thorax from just caudal to the front legs to the last rib and from dorsal spine to ventral midline.
4. Aseptically prepare and drape area.
5. Loosen stylet from chest tube. Extra holes can be carefully made in the chest tube to aid drainage if fluid is present in the pleural space. The holes are made with a scalpel blade and should not exceed 50% of the diameter of tube to prevent tube breakage within the thoracic cavity.
6. A small stab incision should be made in the skin over the highest point of the thorax at intercostal space 9–10.
7. Skin is then pulled forward (by assistant) to create tunnel and allow the chest tube to be placed in intercostal space 7–8 (Figure 7.31a).
8. Lidocaine (maximum total dose of 7 mg/kg) is injected into intercostal muscles at tube insertion site or intercostal block can be performed, injecting lidocaine just ventral and caudal to transverse processes of the thoracic vertebrae/head of ribs one space cranial and caudal, and at the site of insertion. Before injecting, aspirate to determine that the needle is not in the intercostal artery or vein.
9. Haemostats are used to dissect bluntly into the pleural space, then spread wide enough to allow the tube to be passed through the hole created. The tube and stylet are inserted into the pleural space and advanced very slightly as a unit in a cranioventral direction. At this time, the tube/stylet unit should be being held parallel to the thoracic wall. The tube should then be fed off the stylet again in a cranioventral direction. Tubes without trochars can also be placed using this technique.
10. Stop manual ventilation while inserting the tube, to allow lungs to deflate and decrease risk of trauma to lungs.
11. Assess placement of the tube by using the stylet to measure the distance the tube has been advanced within the thorax.
12. Connect the tube to a three-way stopcock and injection caps or a pleural drainage system.
13. As soon as the drain is in place, aspirate as much of the air/fluid as possible. Record the amount and keep samples for further analysis if required.
14. Secure to the skin with a purse-string suture around the tube at the entry site and a 'Chinese finger trap' suture pattern to reduce sliding of the tube.
15. Place sterile dressing and light bandage.
16. Tube connection sites can be secured with orthopaedic wire in figure-of-eight patterns.

Alternative method – trochar technique
1. Sedation or anaesthesia should be provided if possible.
2. Steps 2–6 as above.
3. The tube is tunnelled subcutaneously two to three rib spaces (Figure 7.31b), then positioned perpendicular to the chest wall and grasped tightly 2.5–5.0 cm from its distal tip to prevent the tube from penetrating too deeply into the chest cavity.
4. The top of the tube is hit bluntly with the palm of other hand, popping the tube through into the pleural space.
5. The tube is then slid off the stylet, directing it cranially and ventrally, then connected and secured as described above.
This is a very rapid placement technique, but is not recommended unless in an emergency situation with no other options, due to increased risk of iatrogenic trauma. It is never recommended in cats due to their small size and very compliant chest walls

Following placement (either method)
• Thoracic radiographs (lateral and ventrodorsal or dorsoventral) to check tube(s) placement should be performed
• The tube(s) should be securely bandaged to prevent patient interference. An Elizabethan collar may also be used
• Pain management with injectable opioids or intrapleural bupivicaine should be used. Non-steroidal anti-inflammatory drugs (NSAIDs) may be administered if patient has a stable cardiovascular system
• Bupivicaine can be given at a dose of 1.5 mg/kg through the tube every 6–8 hours
• 24-hour monitoring is required due to the risk of disconnection and the development of a pneumothorax

7.32 (continued) Chest tube placement.

In dogs, surgical treatment with thoracotomy has been shown to be beneficial in pyothorax, improving outcome and reducing recurrence rate when compared to medical therapy alone. Recently, the use of thoracoscopy for treatment of pyothorax in both dogs and cats has been discussed. This treatment modality allows thorough lavage of the pleural space while guaranteeing removal of the fluid. It also provides an opportunity to examine the lungs and mediastinum for obvious abscessation, masses or foreign material. Thoracoscopy is frequently used in human patients with pyothorax, and has the potential to become the treatment of choice in veterinary patients as well.

Non-bacterial exudates: Feline infectious peritonitis virus can cause pleural effusion in affected cats, recognized by a sticky yellow effusion that has a high protein and low cellularity. The prognosis is very poor for affected cats.

Chylothorax: This is the accumulation of a milky effusion within the pleural space, which has a triglyceride concentration higher than that of a concurrently obtained plasma sample. A true chylous effusion contains chylomicrons, but a pseudochylous effusion, although the same on gross inspection, contains only cholesterol. Chylothorax can occur whenever there is obstruction or leakage of chyle due to disruption of the thoracic duct (Figure 7.33). Common causes include idiopathic disease, trauma, neoplasia and feline cardiomyopathy.

Treatment of chylous effusion aims to remove the underlying cause and decrease the rate of formation. With the exception of chylous effusions caused by heart failure or lymphoma where specific medical therapy is indicated, empirical medical management with Rutin (a flavonoid compound) and low-fat diets is often disappointing. Surgical management is associated with a poor prognosis for complete correction. Thoracic duct

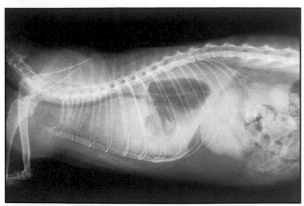

7.33 A 5-year-old Domestic Longhair cat that presented for progressive respiratory distress. Thoracic radiographs were taken and show a marked pleural effusion. Thoracocentesis was performed and 150 ml of a chylous effusion was removed.

ligation accompanied by pericardectomy and omentalization of the thoracic cavity is generally regarded to be the best option, but is associated with a relatively high rate of recurrence. An alternative option is placement of a pleuroperitoneal shunt device.

Transudates: Transudates (pure and modified) are recognized as clear to yellow fluid which has low cellularity and low protein content. The most common cause is right-sided congestive heart failure, management of which is discussed in Chapter 6. A complete cardiac evaluation should be performed, and cardiac disease should be treated appropriately to prevent or reduce recurrence of pleural effusion. Transudates can also develop or be exacerbated by factors such as hypoproteinaemia and low oncotic pressure, or vasculitis. For these reasons, modified transudates in the pleural cavity are common in patients with sepsis or pancreatitis and in patients with pulmonary thromboembolism. Neoplasia may also cause a modified transudate, which may contain exfoliated neoplastic cells. This emphasizes the need for cytological evaluation of all effusions. Thoracic radiographs should be obtained following thoracocentesis to evaluate the cardiac silhouette and to look for evidence of neoplasia. Occasionally, in the absence of cardiac disease, a definitive diagnosis cannot initially be made. As the disease progresses and the effusion returns, the underlying cause can usually be identified.

Haemothorax and sanguineous effusions: Haemothorax may be produced following trauma, as a result of a coagulopathy, or may be caused by neoplasia. Anticoagulant rodenticides are considered the most common non-traumatic cause of haemothorax. Animals with rodenticide poisoning may present in acute respiratory distress with no other obvious signs of bleeding. Treatment requires a source of coagulation factors via fresh whole blood or plasma transfusions as well as vitamin K1 therapy. Thoracocentesis should only be performed if the animal's respiratory status is severely compromised by the pleural effusion. Congenital coagulopathies such as haemophilia A can also lead to haemothorax, but are less common. Neoplasms such as haemangiosarcoma can also result

in a rapidly forming haemothorax, which should also be managed by transfusions and thoracocentesis (with cytological evaluation of the fluid). Patients that do not respond to conservative therapy may require exploratory thoracotomy to establish a diagnosis and to resect bleeding masses, although long-term prognosis is poor.

A sanguineous effusion can be defined as an accumulation of grossly bloody pleural fluid that does not have a high enough packed cell volume to be classified as haemorrhage. The most common causes of sanguineous effusions are lung lobe torsions and neoplasia. Lung lobe torsions are most commonly diagnosed in deep-chested dogs, with a predilection in Afghan Hounds and Borzois, although they have also been reported in pugs. Affected animals present with an acute or chronic history of progressive dyspnoea and weight loss. On physical examination typical findings include dull lung sounds in the ventral portion of the lung fields. Pleural fluid accumulates because of obstruction of venous outflow from the twisted lung lobe, and the fluid is typically bloody with numerous neutrophils and macrophages on cytology. Chylous effusions are also seen. Thoracic radiographs should be obtained after the fluid has been removed from the pleural cavity. The most common finding is complete collapse of a single lung lobe, which can appear consolidated or with an unusual 'honeycomb' pattern (Figure 7.34). The bronchus of the affected lobe may appear distorted or extend in the wrong direction. Ultrasonography with colour-flow Doppler can help confirm the diagnosis by showing lack of blood flow in the twisted lung lobe. Once lung lobe torsion is suspected, an emergency thoracotomy is indicated to resect the affected lobe before tissue necrosis triggers the systemic inflammatory response syndrome (SIRS). If the lobe is resected early in the course of the disease process the prognosis is good, but occasionally effusions recur in the days and weeks following surgery. In these cases the character of the effusion may change from sanguineous to chylous. The risk of chylous effusion appears to be particularly high in Afghan Hounds and Borzois, and in these breeds the prognosis for long-term survival is guarded.

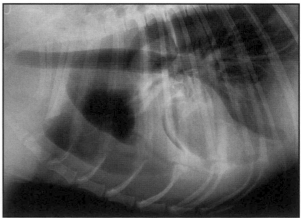

7.34 A 3-year-old intact male Afghan Hound presented with acute respiratory distress. Thoracic radiographs revealed a pleural effusion and possible lung lobe torsion. Ultrasonography confirmed this diagnosis and the dog underwent a thoracotomy to remove the right cranial lung lobe.

Neoplastic effusions may also be sanguineous. Exfoliated neoplastic cells may be evident on cytological evaluation of the fluid, but the absence of neoplastic cells does not rule out neoplasia. The most common neoplasm that is easily diagnosed on cytology is lymphoma in cats, which is usually associated with a mediastinal mass that can reduce chest compressibility (Figure 7.35). Other neoplasms that can cause a pleural effusion include carcinomas, chemodectomas, thymomas, sarcomas and mesotheliomas.

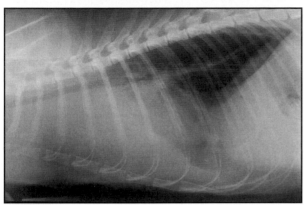

7.35 A 9-year-old Siamese cat that presented for increased respiratory rate and effort. Decreased chest compressibility and dull ventral lung sounds were noted on physical examination. This lateral thoracic radiograph shows a marked pleural effusion and elevation of the carina and narrowing of the trachea caused by a large cranial mediastinal mass.

Pulmonary function testing in the dyspnoeic patient

Apart from clinical examination, useful methods for pulmonary function testing in the dyspnoeic patient include arterial blood gas analysis, pulse oximetry and end-tidal capnography.

Arterial blood gas analysis

The most definitive method of assessment of lung function is measurement of partial pressures of oxygen (PO_2) and carbon dioxide (PCO_2) in arterial blood. Commonly used analysers directly measure pH, PO_2 and PCO_2. A variety of instruments is available to measure blood gases in veterinary practice, including relatively inexpensive hand-held instruments.

Samples of arterial blood can be obtained by direct puncture of any artery. Most commonly, the dorsal pedal artery is used, but other sites include the femoral, brachial and auricular arteries. Samples can also be obtained from catheters placed in the dorsal pedal, femoral or auricular artery (see Chapter 2). Blood gas syringes should be preheparinized, either by using heparin sodium solution to flush the syringe, or by use of specially made blood gas syringes which contain lyophilized lithium heparin.

To obtain a sample by direct puncture, one or two assistants will be required to restrain the animal. The artery is palpated such that the operator can feel the pulsations with one hand and use the other to direct the needle at about a 60 degree angle towards the palpated artery. When the artery has been penetrated, a flash of blood will be seen in the hub of the needle, and the syringe is aspirated to obtain the sample. Proprietary pre-set syringes contain a filter through which air is displaced, and the syringe fills by direct arterial pressure, without the need for aspiration on the plunger. On removal of the needle, direct pressure should be applied to the artery for a few minutes to prevent haematoma formation. All air bubbles should be removed immediately, and the sample capped with an airtight seal to prevent exposure to room air. The sample should be analysed as soon as possible, and kept on ice until analysis. Ideally, analysis should occur within 2 hours of sample collection.

A considerable degree of error can be introduced into blood gas analysis by operator technique and sample maintenance. If exposed to room air or if there are air bubbles in the sample, PCO_2 will decrease and PO_2 will increase as the sample equilibrates with room air gas tensions. Dilution of the sample with heparin also introduces error. Excessive heparinization of the syringe leads to reduction in measured PCO_2, but little change in pH. This error can be minimized by expelling all of the heparin from the syringe after flushing, leaving only the heparin that fills the dead space of the hub of the needle, or by using lyophilized heparin.

Storage of the sample leads to changes in measured gas tensions as a result of ongoing metabolism by the cells. Anaerobic glycolysis by red blood cells leads to production of carbon dioxide. Oxygen utilization for aerobic metabolism by leucocytes and reticulocytes leads to a decrease in PO_2. The longer the sample is stored, and the higher the white cell count, the more pronounced these changes become. Maintenance of the sample on ice between collection and analysis minimizes this effect by reducing metabolism by the cells. Small samples of blood quickly cool to 0°C when placed in ice water, and therefore do not maintain cell metabolism for more than a few minutes.

P_aO_2 and hypoxaemia

PO_2 represents the oxygen dissolved in plasma. The P_aO_2 then determines the oxygen saturation of haemoglobin in a sigmoid relationship according to the oxygen dissociation curve (see Figure 7.2). Haemoglobin is expected to be fully saturated at a P_aO_2 between 60 and 70 mmHg. Animals with normal lung function, breathing room air, should have P_aO_2 values greater than 85 mmHg. Increases in inspired oxygen concentration lead to further increases in P_aO_2. A useful clinical rule of thumb is that the P_aO_2 should roughly equal five times the inspired oxygen concentration: an animal on 100% oxygen (anaesthetized and intubated) should have a P_aO_2 of about 500 mmHg, and an animal on 40% oxygen (nasal oxygen or oxygen cage) should have a P_aO_2 of 200 mmHg. The great majority of oxygen is carried in blood as oxyhaemoglobin, and relatively small amounts are carried as dissolved oxygen. Thus, once the haemoglobin is fully saturated, little overall increase in oxygen delivery to the tissues will occur by dissolving more oxygen in the plasma. If the inspired oxygen concentration has been changed, equilibration to the new P_aO_2 occurs within 2–3 minutes.

P_aO_2 values less than 75 mmHg are usually treated by oxygen supplementation and addressing the underlying cause of the hypoxaemia. Values less than 55 mmHg are imminently life threatening and require immediate action. Decreases in P_aO_2 result from one of the following:

- Decreased oxygen in inspired air (e.g. decreased barometric pressure at high altitudes)
- Hypoventilation (decreased movement of air into the lungs) leading to less availability of oxygen in the alveoli for gas transfer (see below)
- Venous admixture, resulting from:
    - Shunting
    - Ventilation–perfusion mismatch
    - Diffusion impairment.

Shunting implies that blood completely bypasses functional alveoli. This can occur either by venous–arterial shunts that deliver venous blood directly to the arterial circulation (e.g. reverse patent ductus arteriosus (PDA), bronchial anastomoses), or by blood flow to completely non-functional areas of lung, such as severely atelectatic areas or neoplastic masses. In either case, blood with the same oxygen content as systemic venous blood returns to the systemic circulation and mixes with arterial blood, resulting in an overall decrease in P_aO_2. If shunting is the cause of hypoxaemia, the hypoxaemia will not be correctable, no matter how much the inspired oxygen concentration is increased.

The second cause of venous admixture is ventilation–perfusion mismatch. In normal animals, ventilation (the delivery of air to alveoli) and perfusion of the alveoli with blood are fairly closely matched in order to maximize gas transfer. Disease processes such as airway or alveolar disease can change the pattern of ventilation. Similarly, vascular disorders such as thromboembolic disease can change the pattern of perfusion. Significant mismatch of ventilation and perfusion can result, causing hypoxaemia. In such cases, providing an increased inspired oxygen concentration may result in increases in P_aO_2. Ventilation–perfusion mismatch is the most common cause of hypoxaemia in veterinary patients with parenchymal disease.

Diffusion of oxygen across the alveolar capillary membrane may be impaired by any process that leads to thickening of that membrane. Since there is a great reserve for diffusion of oxygen, it is unusual for diffusion to be the limiting factor for oxygen transfer, except in very severe disease processes. Since carbon dioxide is about 20 times more soluble than oxygen, diffusion almost never limits carbon dioxide transfer in the lungs.

P_aCO_2 and hypercarbia

The rate of elimination of carbon dioxide from the body directly influences the **arterial** partial pressure of carbon dioxide (P_aCO_2), whereas the production of carbon dioxide by tissue metabolism is most closely related to **venous** partial pressure of carbon dioxide (P_vCO_2). Since carbon dioxide is very soluble and has an almost linear dissociation curve, it easily diffuses out of blood into the alveoli, and there is a huge reserve for carbon dioxide elimination from the lung. Thus, P_aCO_2 primarily depends on the extent of ventilation. Minute ventilation is a measure of the total amount of gas moved in and out of the lung per minute, and is a function of respiratory rate and tidal volume. Hyperventilation, such as might occur with fear, pain or pulmonary parenchymal disease, results in low P_aCO_2. Hypoventilation leads to increases in P_aCO_2, and is commonly seen with disorders that affect the mechanical ability to move air into the lungs, and occasionally in animals with severe pulmonary parenchymal disease.

P_aCO_2 values above 50 mmHg are significant and require treatment, and values above 70 mmHg are imminently life-threatening. P_aCO_2 values below 20 mmHg may result in excessive cerebral vasoconstriction, and should be treated aggressively.

Increased P_aCO_2 in hypoventilation is accompanied by decreased P_aO_2. In a hypoventilating patient, oxygen supplementation will increase the P_aO_2, but will result in no change in P_aCO_2 values because it does not change the total volume of air moved into and out of the lungs per minute. Examples of the most common causes of hypoventilation include:

- Neurological disease or anaesthesia affecting central medullary respiratory drive
- Spinal cord dysfunction cranial to C4–C5
- Phrenic nerve dysfunction or neuromuscular junction disease
- Chest wall injury
- Respiratory muscle dysfunction
- Airway obstruction.

If P_aCO_2 is high, the animal experiences dyspnoea. Profound respiratory acidosis may result from the hypercarbia, which can become life threatening by causing decreased cardiac output, hypotension and neurological depression due to carbon dioxide narcosis. Thus, if hypoventilation is found in clinical patients, measures must be taken to improve ventilatory status by addressing the cause of hypoventilation. If correction of the underlying cause is impossible or will take time, positive pressure ventilatory support should be considered.

Indices based on oxygen tension

The measured value for P_aO_2 depends on the extent of ventilation and the inspired oxygen concentration, as well as the presence of lung disease. A number of calculations can be performed to allow meaningful comparison between abnormal P_aO_2 values at different ventilation rates and while the patient is receiving oxygen supplementation.

Calculation of the alveolar–arterial oxygen gradient ($P_{A-a}O_2$) gives an estimate of the effectiveness of gas transfer, while removing the variable contribution of the extent of ventilation. As lung dysfunction worsens, the oxygen gradient between the alveoli and the arteries increases. To calculate the $P_{A-a}O_2$, the partial pressure of oxygen in the alveoli (P_AO_2) must first be estimated, using the alveolar gas equation:

$$P_AO_2 = F_iO_2 (P_b - P_{H2O}) - P_aCO_2/RQ$$

where F_iO_2 is the fractional inspired oxygen concentration, P_b is barometric pressure, P_{H2O} is saturated water vapour pressure at body temperature and RQ is the respiratory quotient. At sea level, in room air and assuming RQ for the dog to be about 0.9 on typical diets, the alveolar gas equation can be simplified as:

$$P_AO_2 = 150 - (P_aCO_2)1.1$$

This equation provides a very useful clinical estimate of alveolar PO_2. Measured arterial PO_2 is subtracted from P_AO_2 to give the alveolar–arterial gradient:

$$P_{A-a}O_2 = P_AO_2 - P_aO_2$$

The reference range for $P_{A-a}O_2$ in patients breathing room air is less than 15 mmHg. Increased gradients are seen in patients with pulmonary parenchymal disease, and the gradient would be expected to be normal in patients with hypoxaemia secondary to pure hypoventilation with no parenchymal lung disease. Calculation of $P_{A-a}O_2$ allows clinical comparison of serial blood gases in patients with variable ventilatory status.

A second clinically useful index based on oxygen tension is the ratio of $P_aO_2:F_iO_2$. Many arterial blood gases are obtained in critically ill patients that are receiving oxygen supplementation. In such patients, removal of oxygen support in order to obtain arterial samples on room air may be unsafe or inhumane. Calculation of $P_aO_2:F_iO_2$ ratios allows comparison of serial samples that are obtained at varying concentrations of inspired oxygen. Normal animals usually have a $P_aO_2:F_iO_2$ >400. Values less than 200 imply serious lung disease.

Pulse oximetry

Pulse oximetry is used to determine indirectly the arterial haemoglobin saturation with oxygen. Oxygen is carried to the tissues attached to haemoglobin in the red blood cells. Each haemoglobin molecule is capable of binding four molecules of oxygen; thus haemoglobin carries the majority of the oxygen in the blood, with only a relatively small proportion carried as dissolved oxygen in the plasma. The relationship between the P_aO_2 and the amount of oxygen attached to haemoglobin (expressed as percent saturation, S_aO_2), is not linear. When one molecule of oxygen binds to haemoglobin, the haemoglobin molecule undergoes a conformational change that allows three more oxygen molecules to bind much more easily. Thus, the oxygen dissolved in the plasma and that carried on the haemoglobin are in fact related by means of a sigmoid curve.

In normal arterial blood, the haemoglobin should be >95% saturated with oxygen. Observation of the curve (see Figure 7.2) demonstrates that the normal animal operates with quite a large safety margin with regard to haemoglobin saturation. Haemoglobin becomes close to fully saturated (>90%) at a P_aO_2 of about 70 mmHg; at this point the curve plateaus and despite higher P_aO_2, haemoglobin saturation, and therefore oxygen transport, cannot be increased much more. In animals with lung disease, decreases in oxygenation may occur. Once the P_aO_2 becomes as low as 70–75 mmHg (corresponding to an S_aO_2 of 90–92%), the animal comes perilously close to the 'shoulder' of the curve.

The pulse oximeter is a dual wavelength spectrophotometer that measures haemoglobin saturation by transmitting light through a pulsating arterial vascular bed. Transmission of light through tissue is not constant, but varies with each cardiac pulse. The variation in transmitted light is entirely due to arterial blood, with the contribution of venous blood and tissue remaining constant. By using the appropriate transmitted light wavelengths for oxyhaemoglobin and deoxyhaemoglobin, the microprocessor can continuously calculate oxygen saturation. Pulse oximetry readings of 93% or higher are acceptable in non-anaemic critically ill patients breathing room air. Oxygen supplementation should be considered in patients with haemoglobin saturation of less than 93%. Saturation values of 90% correlate with a P_aO_2 of approximately 60–70 mmHg and indicate severe hypoxaemia. Values below 90% should be addressed immediately by providing supplemental oxygen or positive pressure ventilation.

The pulse oximeter has been validated to be accurate in dogs. In cats and dogs, the small pulse oximeter probe can be placed on a shaved area of the pinna of the ear, the lip, or a fold of skin at the axilla or the inguinal area. In anaesthetized patients, the tongue is the most useful site. The pulse oximeter is non-invasive and very well tolerated by the majority of animals. It provides a continuous read-out of haemoglobin oxygen saturation and pulse rate, thus it is a useful tool for continuous monitoring of the hypoxaemic patient. When arterial blood gas analysis is unavailable, or when arterial blood cannot be obtained, the pulse oximeter can provide a useful indication of arterial saturation and a means of assessing disease progression.

In humans, the accuracy of the pulse oximeter reading has not been noted to change significantly with skin colour, serum quality, or mild to moderate anaemia. In dogs, it seems that extremely dark skin pigmentation, as in Newfoundlands or black Labrador Retrievers, impedes effective pulse oximetry readings. The major limiting factor in the use of pulse oximetry is tissue perfusion. Any condition that diminishes tissue blood flow, such as hypotension or shock, will prevent the pulse oximeter from accurately reading and measuring haemoglobin saturation. Motion of the probe also can decrease the ability to obtain a signal. Despite these limitations, the pulse oximeter provides us with a clinically useful and simple measure of haemoglobin saturation. Newer technology in pulse oximetry, which is now beginning to be clinically available, may help to address some of the limitations relating to poor perfusion and motion artefact.

End-tidal capnography

End-tidal capnography is another indirect technique for respiratory monitoring. This instrument measures the amount of carbon dioxide in exhaled air, and thus can give an indirect estimate of ventilation status. End-tidal carbon dioxide is most frequently measured in anaesthetized and intubated patients. A T-piece is inserted into the system at the end of the endotracheal tube. Some instruments have side-stream ports that aspirate air into the machine where it is analysed, others with main-stream ports measure carbon dioxide at the airway. Alternative approaches include placement of the sampling tube at the nares, or its attachment to the end of a tracheostomy tube. The end-tidal capnograph continuously measures the carbon dioxide content of inhaled and exhaled air.

Because it is so easily diffusible, the carbon dioxide in pulmonary capillaries equilibrates almost immediately with alveolar air. If carbon dioxide in alveolar air could be measured, it would almost exactly represent that of pulmonary capillary blood (Figure 7.36). In a single breath, air sampled during inspiration should represent room air and therefore contain virtually no carbon dioxide. As exhalation begins, the air passing the instrument initially represents dead space which has not been in contact with alveolar air. It therefore contains virtually no carbon dioxide. As exhalation continues, alveolar air begins to mix with air from dead space, with a resultant gradual increase in the amount of carbon dioxide measured by the instrument. Eventually, all the air passing the sampling port is alveolar air, and the partial pressure of carbon dioxide reaches a plateau, which is reported by the instrument as the end-tidal carbon dioxide.

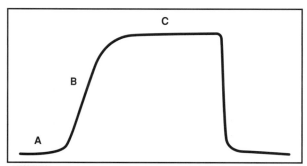

7.36 The capnograph tracing. (A) Phase I: represents airway deadspace, the portion of the breath being exhaled from the conducting airways, which does not contain any measurable amount of carbon dioxide. (B) Phase II: represents the mix of airway deadspace gases with alveolar gas, and typically shows a significant rise in carbon dioxide. (C) Phase III: represents effective alveolar ventilation. The plateau value is the value that is reported as end-tidal carbon dioxide.

Errors in end-tidal carbon dioxide monitoring are primarily related to respiratory rate, especially in panting animals or extremely tachypnoeic patients. Further errors might occur if lung disease results in uneven emptying of alveoli, thus preventing the end-tidal carbon dioxide concentration from reaching a measurable plateau. Another factor to bear in mind when using this type of instrumentation is the volume of air aspirated from the anaesthetic circuit during side-stream monitoring. Instruments in veterinary use aspirate air at a rate of 50–150 ml/min, and gas flow rates should be adjusted accordingly. If this type of instrument is being used with inhalant gas in an anaesthetic circuit, the sampled air should be returned to the circuit or vented to the exterior, rather than allowing release of inhalant gas into the room.

End-tidal carbon dioxide should approximate the venous partial pressure of carbon dioxide, providing an estimate of ventilation status. There is usually a variable gradient, however, between the end-tidal result and the venous partial pressure of carbon dioxide. This instrument should therefore be used

primarily to follow trends. Normal values should be in the 35–45 mmHg range. If the end-tidal carbon dioxide concentration is >50 mmHg, this result is highly specific for clinically significant hypoventilation, which should be treated immediately.

Intubation and positive pressure ventilation

Extremely dyspnoeic animals that cannot adequately ventilate or oxygenate may require anaesthesia and intubation to establish control over the airway and to provide short-term positive pressure ventilation (PPV) (Figure 7.37). This aggressive approach is reserved for the most severe cases of respiratory distress. Clinical parameters indicating that the animal should be intubated include severe distress that is non-responsive to therapy, persistent cyanosis that is not responsive to oxygen supplementation and a fractious patient that cannot be restrained for diagnostics or therapy. In any of these situations, anaesthesia eliminates distress and facilitates handling for diagnostic investigation. On blood gas analysis general indicators for PPV are a P_aO_2 of 60 mmHg or less on oxygen supplementation, or a P_aCO_2 >50 mmHg.

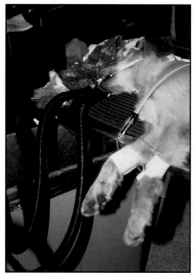

7.37 The Golden Retriever puppy pictured in Figure 7.1 after failing to respond to oxygen therapy. He required anaesthesia, intubation and positive pressure ventilation. A large amount of sanguineous fluid has flowed out of his airways and pooled on the table in front of him. (Courtesy of Dr Ken Drobatz, University of Pennsylvania)

Induction of anaesthesia for intubation
Care must be taken when choosing an anaesthetic agent for induction. Often there is concurrent cardiovascular system instability and myocardial irritability due to hypoxaemia. Since the clinician will be establishing control over the airway and taking over respiratory function, concerns about ventilatory depression by anaesthetic agents are reduced. Intravenous anaesthetic agents are ideal because they allow rapid induction, intubation and therefore airway management. Mask induction or the use of intramuscular agents are associated with a high risk of cardiopulmonary arrest when severe respiratory distress is present. If upper airway obstruction is suspected, before inducing anaesthesia the clinician should organize all of the materials required to perform an emergency tracheostomy in the event that endotracheal intubation is not possible (see Figure 7.10).

Where there is no evidence of hypovolaemia, propofol may be administered by intravenous injection to effect, although this drug may be associated with vasodilation and production of intrapulmonary arteriovenous shunting. Shunting may severely aggravate pre-existing hypoxia and, although temporary, is not responsive to increased inspired oxygen concentration or assisted ventilation. Thiopental is not associated with intrapulmonary shunting, but may produce ventricular premature contractions if there is myocardial hypoxia and hypotension when there is hypovolaemia. Alternatively, low doses of intravenous opioid analgesics, such as fentanyl or morphine, combined with a benzodiazepine sedative agent, such as diazepam or midazolam, may produce adequate sedation and muscle relaxation to allow endotracheal intubation in critically ill patients (see Chapter 21). Respiratory arrest may be temporarily produced with this technique and it is important immediately to intubate and ventilate the patient.

Anaesthesia must then be maintained to allow continued intubation using either volatile agent inhalation or repeated administration of injectable drugs. Once the animal has been intubated, it should be immediately placed on 100% oxygen and positive pressure ventilation should be initiated by manually bagging the animal until more information is available about respiratory function. The haemodynamic status of the patient should be carefully monitored, body temperature measured and supported if necessary and the administration of anaesthetic drugs kept at the minimum required to maintain unconsciousness and lack of response to gentle movement of the endotracheal tube.

Positive pressure ventilation

Because it is labour intensive, invasive and associated with numerous complications, positive pressure ventilation in dogs and cats is reserved for severely affected patients when all other treatment possibilities have failed. Hypoxaemia can usually be managed by increasing the concentration of oxygen in inspired air using an oxygen cage, nasal oxygen or mask. If these measures fail, positive pressure ventilation becomes the only option for continued treatment. Similarly, hypoventilation can sometimes be treated by effective management of the underlying problem, but if that fails to result in satisfactory improvement, positive pressure ventilation is required. Positive pressure ventilation requires 24-hour nursing and veterinary care and, ideally, a specialized intensive care unit (ICU) ventilator, especially if this type of respiratory support needs to be continued beyond 12–24 hours.

Ventilators

Volume-cycled ventilators are programmed to deliver a given volume of oxygen–air mix. Once a given volume is chosen, this volume will be delivered irrespective of the airway pressure that is reached. Problems such as mucous plugs in the endotracheal tube or airways are easily detected, as narrowing of the functional airway causes an increase in the peak airway pressure for a given tidal volume.

Pressure-cycled ventilators are programmed to deliver oxygen–air up to a given airway pressure, irrespective of the volume delivered. In this mode, unless tidal volume is measured frequently, it can slowly decrease over time as mucus accumulates, and the animal may be ventilated with smaller and smaller volumes to reach a given pressure. This can lead to problems with hypoventilation that may be difficult to detect, especially if they occur acutely. Peak pressures vary depending on the requirements of individual patients: patients with very stiff (poorly compliant) lungs may require higher pressures in order to achieve adequate ventilation.

Modes of ventilation

There are two basic ventilator modes (Figure 7.38): assist/control (AC), or synchronous intermittent mandatory ventilation (SIMV). The choice of mode depends on the degree of ventilatory support that is

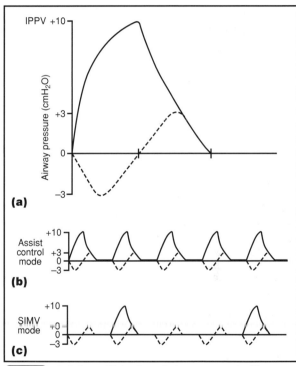

7.38 **(a)** A ventilator breath is compared with a spontaneous patient breath. The spontaneous breath (dotted line) begins as a negative inspiratory effort, followed by a slightly positive airway pressure during exhalation. In contrast, the ventilator breath (solid line) generates exclusively positive airway pressure. **(b)** In *assist/control ventilation*, the ventilator delivers a set number of breaths, to a set pressure or tidal volume. The machine delivers these breaths when the patient creates a negative pressure in the airway; if the patient is not breathing, the machine will automatically deliver the set respiration rate. If the patient breathes faster than the set rate, the machine is also triggered, and it will deliver the desired tidal volume for each patient-initiated breath. **(c)** In *synchronous intermittent mandatory ventilation*, the ventilator is set to deliver a desired number of breaths, just as in AC. The breaths are delivered when the machine senses a negative pressure effort by the patient ('synchronous'). Between each breath, if the patient breathes spontaneously, the machine does not 'kick in' with a breath of its own, and these patient-induced breaths only reach the negative pressure and tidal volume determined by the patient.

desired: AC controls ventilation completely with very little effort from the patient; SIMV assists ventilation, but requires varying amounts of patient effort. In the majority of cases AC is used initially, and then the patient is switched to SIMV when it is ready to be weaned from the ventilator.

In AC ventilation, the ventilator delivers a set number of breaths, to a set pressure or tidal volume. The machine delivers these breaths when the patient creates a negative pressure in the airway; if the patient is not breathing, the machine will automatically deliver the set respiration rate. If the patient breathes faster than the set rate, the machine is also triggered, and it will deliver the desired tidal volume or pressure for each patient-initiated breath. Therefore, if the patient is breathing spontaneously, the machine will deliver a full breath for every patient-initiated breath. This results in the ventilator performing almost all of the work of breathing in this mode. This mode can become problematical in patients with a rapid and shallow respiratory rate; hyperventilation can result as each breath taken by the patient will result in delivery of a full tidal volume.

In SIMV the ventilator is set to deliver a desired number of breaths, just as in AC. The breaths are delivered when the machine senses a negative pressure effort by the patient ('synchronous'). Between each breath, if the patient breathes spontaneously, the machine does not 'kick in' with a breath of its own, and these patient-induced breaths only reach the negative pressure and tidal volume determined by the patient. This causes the animal to perform a varying proportion of the work of respiration on its own. The amount of spontaneous ventilation, and therefore the work of respiration, can be increased or decreased depending on the rate that is set on the ventilator. Thus this mode of ventilation is very useful for weaning from the ventilator, since the amount of ventilatory support can be slowly reduced, requiring more and more patient work. It is also useful in patients with rapid, shallow respiratory patterns, as it prevents the hyperventilation that was mentioned above with AC mode.

Positive end expiratory pressure

Positive end expiratory pressure (PEEP) can be used to improve oxygenation in the hypoxaemic patient. It should be used for hypoxaemic animals that are being adequately ventilated based on P_aCO_2 levels, but remain hypoxaemic in spite of oxygen supplementation. By applying small amounts of positive pressure to the airway, complete expiration is prevented, resulting in:

- Increased functional residual capacity
- Increased alveolar size and recruitment
- Prevention of early closure of small airways.

This can sometimes lead to marked improvement of oxygenation, particularly in animals with pulmonary oedema or haemorrhage. It usually does not significantly affect carbon dioxide. However it is not without its drawbacks; high levels of PEEP will decrease venous return to the heart, increase central venous pressure (CVP) and increase the mechanical work of breathing. The use of PEEP to improve oxygenation

sometimes allows decreases in the concentration of inspired oxygen. This can be particularly useful in animals that are being ventilated with very high oxygen concentrations, and thus are at risk of oxygen toxicity. PEEP should be started at 5 cmH$_2$O, and slowly increased until the desired endpoint is reached. It is important to watch haemodynamic variables closely as PEEP is increased, since it may lead to increased incidence of cardiovascular instability.

Goals of ventilation

The aim should be to maintain the P_aO_2 at 80–100 mmHg or higher; and to keep the P_aCO_2 between 30 and 40 mmHg, depending on the condition of the animal, its acid–base status and whether or not efforts are being made to wean the animal from the ventilator. P_aCO_2 should be at the lower end of the range in animals with cerebral oedema or head trauma or in animals that have severe metabolic acidosis. The P_aCO_2 is adjusted to the desired level by manipulation of the respiratory rate and tidal volume. P_aO_2 achieved in the ventilated animal depends on:

- Extent of lung disease
- The concentration of oxygen
- Ventilation rate
- The use of PEEP.

General recommendations suggest that during positive pressure ventilation, peak airway pressures of 10–20 cmH$_2$O should be the goal. In animals with normal lungs, the low end of this airway pressure range will usually be achieved if the patient is ventilated with tidal volumes of 8–12 ml/kg. Numerous studies confirm adverse effects in the lungs if airway pressures exceed 30 cmH$_2$O, including alveolar inflammation, rupture of alveolar septae, emphysema and pneumothorax. In contrast to normal lungs, the diseased lung can be very heterogeneous. Lung units with normal alveoli may be side-by-side with lung units with severely abnormal alveoli. If the lung contains many abnormal alveoli, positive pressure ventilation with normal tidal volumes can result in very high peak airway pressures and over-distension of normal alveoli, which are relatively compliant. Over-distension of the normal alveoli results in alveolar inflammation. In addition, some alveoli and terminal bronchioles may be 'recruitable': collapsed at end expiration but expanded during inspiration. In these recruitable alveoli and the alveoli immediately adjacent to them, further lung injury and inflammation may occur due to shear stress as they are opened and closed with each breath. Pneumothorax is the most dramatic and easily recognised complication of barotrauma and volutrauma in the ventilated patient.

Multiple recent studies suggest that lung protective ventilation strategies may result in decreased lung inflammation and improved survival. High levels of PEEP are used to recruit alveoli and increase functional residual capacity, thereby preventing the cycle of alveolar re-opening and stretching with each breath. Current recommendations suggest that tidal volumes and peak airway pressures should be kept as low as possible (ideally 6–8 ml/kg and <30 cmH$_2$O) in order to prevent over-distension of relatively normal alveoli and shear stress. Increased physiological and anatomical dead space and low tidal volumes can result in problems with carbon dioxide elimination during PPV, particularly at low tidal volumes. The term 'permissive hypercapnia' refers to acceptance of a higher than normal P_aCO_2 (as long as respiratory acidosis is not severe), in order to minimize tidal volumes and airway pressures.

Animals being managed with positive pressure ventilation are at a high risk of developing pneumonia because airway intubation bypasses upper airway defences, atelectasis predisposes to impaired bacterial clearance from the alveoli and there are often increased populations of resistant Gram-negative bacteria in the oropharynx, especially if the animal is receiving antibiotics or H_2 blockers. In addition, most critically ill ventilator patients can be expected to be immunocompromised because of their illness and often decreased nutrition. Pneumonia is a potentially serious complication in the ventilated patient because it predisposes to sepsis and worsening of SIRS and multiple organ failure. In addition it can lead to progressive worsening of hypoxia and delay of weaning, and therefore can potentially contribute to mortality. Ideally, surveillance bacterial cultures should be submitted daily from the airway. The use of prophylactic antibiotics is not generally considered ideal; the optimal approach is to diagnose infection at as early a stage as possible, and to initiate targeted therapy at that time. If there is clinical evidence of pneumonia, broad-spectrum antibiotic therapy should be immediately administered, pending the result of bacterial cultures.

Monitoring the ventilated patient
Blood gases should be measured at least every 6 hours, in order to assess progress and monitor for deterioration in pulmonary function or changes in acid–base status. The ventilator settings should be adjusted based on these results. Packed cell volume, total solids/protein and serum electrolytes are measured at least every 6 hours, and abnormalities are corrected. Continuous monitoring of oxygen saturation using the pulse oximeter will give warning if the animal suddenly desaturates. End-tidal carbon dioxide can be monitored, providing an estimation of the P_aCO_2, and can therefore be used to adjust the ventilation volumes and pressures.

The endotracheal tube should be aspirated daily and cytology and cultures performed on the aspirates. The ventilated animal should have chest radiographs frequently to monitor for deterioration or to note improvement. Ideally chest radiographs should be obtained once daily, but they are indicated if there is any deterioration of the clinical condition of the animal.

Continuous electrocardiograph (ECG) monitoring is necessary to monitor heart rate and the presence of dysrhythmias. Arterial pressure should be monitored frequently, ideally using continuous direct arterial monitoring via an arterial catheter, which is also useful for obtaining regular blood gases. Hypotension should be treated as required. Urine output should be monitored, and should be at least 1–2 ml/kg/h. Body temperature should be monitored and heat support provided as needed.

Selected respiratory distress syndromes

Patient history often provides a significant insight into possible causes of respiratory distress. Trauma, exposure to smoke and certain infectious diseases are examples of situations in which historical information can be extremely important. Other common presentations, including congestive heart failure or toxicoses, such as anticoagulant rodenticide toxicity, are addressed in the relevant chapters of this manual.

Trauma
Trauma is a common cause of respiratory distress, most commonly following a road traffic accident (RTA). When a patient is presented with dyspnoea and a history of trauma, the clinician has a limited list of possible differential diagnoses. Specifically, dyspnoea in trauma patients is usually associated with pneumothorax, pulmonary contusions, haemothorax, rib fractures or diaphragmatic hernia, occurring alone or in any combination.

Pneumothorax
Pneumothorax is the most common result of blunt trauma to the chest. It is caused by leakage of air from the parenchyma or airways into the pleural space, resulting in atelectasis or collapse of the lung lobes (Figure 7.39). Many trauma patients have a small air leak that quickly seals over and may not lead to clinical signs. Where clinical signs of dyspnoea are absent and pneumothorax is an incidental finding on a screening radiograph, it is not necessary to remove the air which will be gradually absorbed by the body. At the other end of the spectrum, tension pneumothorax is a serious condition in which a large pulmonary leak acts as a ball-valve, allowing air to enter the pleural cavity with each inspiration, but preventing air from leaving during expiration. This results in progressively increasing interpleural pressure, resulting in further compression of the lungs and a mediastinal shift away from the pneumothorax.

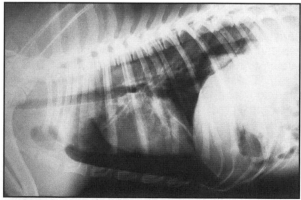

7.39 A Pit Bull Terrier after sustaining blunt vehicular trauma to the chest. A pneumothorax can be diagnosed on this lateral thoracic radiograph by elevation of the cardiac silhouette off the sternum and collapse and retraction of the lung lobes. Thoracocentesis resulted in removal of 1500 ml of air.

Animals with pneumothorax present with varying degrees of dyspnoea depending on the amount of air that has leaked into the pleural cavity. Physical examination findings include a rapid shallow respiratory rate, orthopnoea, pale, pink or cyanotic mucous membranes and diminished dorsal lung sounds. Concurrent signs of hypovolaemic shock (tachycardia, poor pulse quality or bounding pulses and delayed or rapid capillary refill time) are common. These may be caused by haemorrhage or by obstruction of venous return to the heart due to the increased interpleural pressure exerted by a tension pneumothorax.

Because pneumothorax is a common finding following an RTA, the first priority for stabilization of any dyspnoeic trauma patient with dull lung sounds is to perform thoracocentesis, even before radiographs are obtained. Most traumatic pneumothorax patients require thoracocentesis once or twice at presentation, and because the leak seals spontaneously, do not require further treatment for this problem. Some animals have a significant leak of air that continues after the initial thoracocentesis and, although they may show a good initial clinical response, they can become dyspnoeic again within minutes or hours of the procedure, necessitating repeated thoracocenteses. If needle thoracocentesis is required on more than two occasions; if the volumes obtained each time are large; or if the clinician fails to reach a negative pressure end-point of thoracocentesis (probable tension pneumothorax), placement of chest tubes is indicated. If considerable volumes of air are leaking into the pleural cavity, management may be facilitated by attachment of the chest tubes to a water-sealed continuous evacuation device. These devices apply a negative pressure of 10–15 cmH$_2$O to the pleural cavity, simulating normal interpleural pressure, and continuously aspirate air from the chest as it leaks from the lungs. In most cases, the leak seals within 48 hours, and no further treatment is necessary. On rare occasions, if the leak fails to seal, exploratory thoracotomy may be required to resolve the problem. Ongoing leaks that have failed to seal spontaneously may represent tears of major airways and are often also accompanied by pneumomediastinum or subcutaneous emphysema.

Pulmonary contusions

Pulmonary contusions are the second most common cause of dyspnoea following blunt thoracic trauma, representing haemorrhage into the pulmonary interstitium and alveoli from ruptured capillaries (Figure 7.40). These animals are often in hypovolaemic (haemorrhagic) shock, combined with respiratory distress and increased bronchovesicular sounds or even crackles. Even though these patients are usually in shock, caution should be exercised when giving intravenous fluids, since fluid loading can worsen the severity of pulmonary haemorrhage and can cause accumulation of oedema in addition to blood. Although crackles may sometimes be heard on chest auscultation, diuretics are contraindicated in the presence of shock. Diuretics do not prevent further haemorrhage into the pulmonary parenchyma nor promote reabsorption of erythrocytes from the lung. Rather, by causing diuresis, they may exacerbate hypovolaemia.

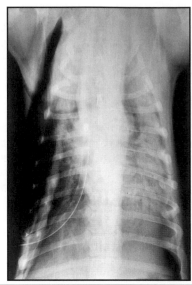

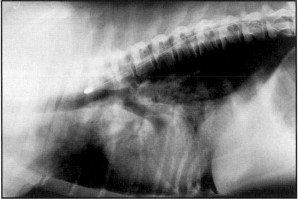

7.40 Lateral and ventrodorsal thoracic radiographs of an 11-month-old Basset Hound after sustaining blunt trauma to the chest. A chest tube has been placed in the right side of the chest. Pulmonary contusions are evident in the left lung lobes and several ribs are fractured on that side. A small amount of air remains in the right side of the chest and subcutaneous emphysema is also present on that side.

Pulmonary contusions should be treated by cautious fluid therapy and supportive care (oxygen supplementation) until the lungs have a chance to reabsorb the blood. In severe cases, PPV and/or PEEP may be required to support oxygenation. If pulmonary function deteriorates following fluid therapy, but the cardiovascular system has stabilized, it is likely that pulmonary oedema is present, superimposed on the haemorrhage. In this event, judicious use of furosemide can be helpful to resolve the oedema.

Bacterial pneumonia is an uncommon complication of pulmonary contusions, and prophylactic antibiotic therapy is not recommended. Prophylactic antibiotics result in selection for resistant bacterial populations and may not change the incidence of pneumonia. Instead, the patient should be monitored for signs that pneumonia has developed: a productive cough, fever or failure of dyspnoea to resolve within 48–72 hours. If pneumonia occurs, a tracheal wash with culture and sensitivity testing, followed by appropriate antibiotic therapy, nebulization and coupage are recommended.

Haemothorax

Serious haemothorax (haemorrhage into the pleural cavity) is an uncommon complication of thoracic trauma. Dull ventral lung sounds may be evident, as well as decreased heart sounds. Patients with significant haemothorax have usually sustained massive trauma to the chest cavity, and other problems, including fractured ribs and pulmonary contusions, should be suspected. If the amount of pleural haemorrhage is small and respiratory distress is believed to be due to other causes such as pulmonary contusions, the pleural blood should not be removed. Minimal invasion of the chest prevents disruption of any clots that have formed and also allows reabsorption of erythrocytes and gradual 'autotransfusion'. If the animal has significant respiratory compromise because of blood in the pleural space, then thoracocentesis should be performed. In the most severe cases of haemothorax, an emergency thoracotomy may be required to identify and ligate a bleeding vessel.

Rib fractures and flail chest

Rib fractures are another common sequela of blunt thoracic trauma and are commonly accompanied by pulmonary contusions. Fracture of one or several ribs (see Figure 7.40) does not usually require any specific treatment other than rest, pain management and oxygen supplementation. If several ribs are each fractured in more than one place, a flail chest segment can occur. The flail segment is not stabilized by attachment to the spine or sternum and can be observed moving paradoxically relative to the rest of the chest wall during respiration. During inspiration, when the rest of the chest is moving outward, the flail segment is pulled inward by the negative intrapleural pressure.

Small to moderate-sized sections of flail chest should be managed medically, with oxygen supplementation and analgesia as needed. Dyspnoea in these patients is thought to be primarily caused by concurrent pulmonary contusions. Large flail chest segments can contribute to dyspnoea by preventing effective movement of the chest wall, resulting in hypoventilation. Placing the animal with the affected side down can help stabilize the segment and promote better ventilation. Large flail segments may require surgical stabilization, and some of these animals require postoperative mechanical ventilation if severe pulmonary contusions are also present.

Diaphragmatic hernia

Animals that have sustained trauma may also develop a diaphragmatic hernia: rupture of the diaphragm with penetration of abdominal contents into the thoracic cavity. A variety of organs may be involved in the hernia, including liver, spleen, stomach, omentum and intestines (Figure 7.41). Dyspnoea is caused by the physical presence of these organs, as well as the accumulation of pleural fluid due to inflammation and occlusion of venous return from the viscera. Vascular compromise associated with strangulation may cause tissue necrosis, further compromising organ and pulmonary function. Acute onset of respiratory distress may occur if the stomach herniates and becomes bloated with gas due to occlusion of the cardia. The

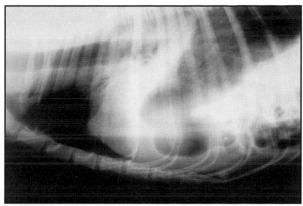

7.41 A dog that presented in acute respiratory distress several months after sustaining blunt vehicular trauma to the chest. On this lateral thoracic radiograph, the diaphragm cannot be visualized and abdominal organs, including liver, stomach and loops of bowel, can be seen in the thoracic cavity, indicating that there is a diaphragmatic hernia. This dog underwent an emergency thoracotomy to repair his diaphragmatic hernia.

size of the stomach can increase rapidly due to gas distension. This represents an immediate surgical emergency and the gas distension of the stomach should be relieved by trocharization while the animal is being prepared for surgery.

Diagnosis of diaphragmatic hernia is suggested by clinical findings including diminished lung sounds or auscultation of bowel sounds in the thorax. Some patients may also have signs of dysfunction of the displaced organs such as vomiting or icterus. The diagnosis should be confirmed by plain radiography or by administration of contrast media. If the stomach or intestines are in the chest, they can be easily outlined by a small amount of oral barium. Other techniques, including positional lateral beam radiography or ultrasonography, can also provide valuable information.

Diaphragmatic hernias should be repaired surgically as soon as possible. Some patients with diaphragmatic hernia do not have clinical evidence of respiratory distress at the time of trauma and may present years later with their first signs of respiratory compromise. Animals with chronic diaphragmatic hernias may be extremely difficult to treat surgically because of the presence of adhesions and the high likelihood of postoperative re-expansion pulmonary oedema. Thus, early diagnosis and surgical treatment is essential for animals with this problem, even if clinical signs are not initially evident. Thoracic radiography is therefore recommended in all cases of trauma to rule out the presence of an occult diaphragmatic hernia.

Smoke inhalation

Animals that present after exposure to smoke from house fires can have varying degrees of respiratory difficulty. Damage is caused by direct thermal injury and by inhalation of noxious substances produced by combustion. The gases produced in the largest amounts during combustion are carbon monoxide, hydrogen cyanide and carbon dioxide. All three of these gases, combined with low concentrations of oxygen, can cause narcosis. They combine very rapidly with haemoglobin, diminishing its availability and effectiveness for oxygen transfer. Animals that have been exposed to smoke in fires should be immediately treated with a high inspired concentration of oxygen to attempt to displace these gases from haemoglobin. Oxygen therapy should be continued for at least an hour. Other gases produced by combustion vary depending on the materials that have burned and some can be extremely toxic.

The upper airway can become so inflamed and oedematous from thermal burns that obstruction can occur. Patients should be monitored for signs of laryngeal or upper airway obstruction, and tracheostomy or intubation performed if necessary. Airway damage often includes severe necrotizing tracheobronchitis, which is accompanied by exudate and cough. Bacterial pneumonia is a common sequela due to damaged lung defences and proliferation of bacterial pathogens. In worst-case scenarios, diffuse inflammatory damage to the lung may be recognized, manifesting as generalized acute lung injury that can progress to ARDS.

Treatment of smoke inhalation should consist of oxygen supplementation, saline nebulization and coupage to promote clearance of material from the airways, bronchodilators and supportive care. Corticosteroids are not recommended in these patients because they are already immunosuppressed. Prophylactic antibiotics should be avoided, as their use prior to the development of pneumonia will only select for resistant bacteria. As with all patients at risk for pneumonia, careful monitoring for signs of pneumonia should be followed by a tracheal wash for cytology, culture and sensitivity testing before starting antibiotic therapy.

Animals that are caught in fires may suffer skin burns as well as lung injury. Particular attention should be given to the corneas and oronasal mucosa. The corneas should be stained with fluorescein, and ulceration treated if present. Patients with skin burns suffer from profound fluid and protein loss and are among the most critically ill animals, with potential for rapid development of multiple organ dysfunction or failure.

Selected infectious and parasitic disease syndromes

Infectious tracheobronchitis ('kennel cough')
Kennel cough is a syndrome of acute infectious tracheobronchitis in dogs, caused by infection with a number of different organisms, of which the most clinically important is *Bordetella bronchiseptica*. Other bacteria, such as *Streptococcus*, *Staphylococcus* and *Klebsiella*, have also been implicated. The most common viruses include canine parainfluenza virus, canine adenovirus-1 and -2, canine distemper virus, canine herpesvirus and reoviruses-1, -2 and -3. The typical history involves exposure to a coughing dog. After an incubation period of 2–7 days, affected dogs develop an acute hacking cough. Although the cough can be distressing to the owner, typically these dogs are otherwise systemically healthy, active, eating normally and afebrile. In dogs with an acute onset of cough associated with concurrent dyspnoea, systemic illness

or depression, alternative diagnoses (including pneumonia secondary to *Bordetella bronchiseptica*) should be considered.

Bordetella bronchiseptica is specially adapted to infect the ciliated epithelium of the upper respiratory tract, attaching via fimbriae to the cilia of the mucociliary escalator. It secretes exotoxins that cause paralysis of the cilia, thereby eliminating one of the most important lung defence mechanisms, allowing the organism to persist in the airway for a prolonged period of time. Infectious tracheobronchitis is associated with acute inflammation of the upper airways, and increased production of thick, viscous mucus.

Antibiotics used to treat infectious tracheobronchitis should be effective against *Bordetella*, and should achieve adequate penetration through the blood–bronchus barrier into the mucus lining the bronchi. In adult dogs, good choices include doxycycline or fluoroquinolones. In puppies, azithromycin or doxycycline should be considered. Antitussive, expectorant and anti-inflammatory drugs may also contribute to the comfort of the patient and the client. Care should be taken not to over-use corticosteroids, however, because of the infectious nature of the disease.

Parenteral and nasal vaccines are available for prevention of infection, but are typically not used in animals already showing clinical signs. Vaccines may not completely prevent clinical illness; however the severity of disease is likely to be considerably less in vaccinated dogs. Importantly, the duration of protection following vaccination is relatively short, and for continued protection dogs should be vaccinated every 3–4 months. Typically, vaccines are administered prior to anticipated exposure, for example prior to boarding.

Feline viral upper respiratory tract disease
Viral upper respiratory disease is a common cause of nasal and ocular discharge, sneezing, fever and debilitation in cats. Feline calicivirus and feline herpesvirus (feline rhinotracheitis) are the most common viruses involved. Following exposure, there is an incubation period of 2–5 days. Calicivirus infection usually manifests by acute onset of lethargy and fever, typically followed by mild hypersalivation, sneezing, conjunctivitis and oculonasal discharge. Ulcers are often evident on the tongue and soft palate. The cat usually recovers in 7–10 days. In contrast, feline herpesvirus often causes more severe illness with fever, profound serous to mucopurulent oculonasal discharge and excessive salivation. Severely affected cats may also have coughing and dyspnoea because of viral pneumonia. Clinical signs usually resolve in 2–3 weeks, although in some cases nasal turbinate damage can be so severe that the cat is prone to bacterial upper respiratory tract infections over a prolonged period of time. Following recovery from acute infection with herpesvirus, clinically normal cats may remain persistently infected and act as carriers that continuously or intermittently shed virus.

Most cats that are experiencing an acute viral upper respiratory infection respond well to supportive care and antibiotic therapy to treat secondary bacterial infections. In cats with severe oral ulceration or difficulty swallowing, broad-spectrum antibiotic therapy may need to be administered parenterally rather than orally. Nutritional support is important; food may need to be heated in order to increase its palatability, and some severely affected cats may require tube feeding (see Chapter 23). Nursing care should include careful cleaning of discharges from the face. Antiviral drugs are usually unnecessary. Minimal data are available regarding the use of non-specific immune stimulants such as feline interferon. Numerous vaccines are available and are routinely used as part of the feline annual vaccination strategy, but are generally not used in cats that are already showing clinical signs. Although most vaccines confer good protection against clinical signs of disease, they do not prevent infection and the subsequent development of a carrier state.

Lungworms

A variety of parasitic nematodes can cause clinical signs of respiratory disease including coughing and dyspnoea. *Angiostrongylus vasorum* (French heartworm) is a metastrongylid nematode; the adult worm lives in the pulmonary arterioles. It can cause both respiratory signs, which may be severe, and a coagulopathy, and occurs most commonly in young dogs throughout the south of England. *Oslerus osleri* is found in small nodules on the mucosa of the tracheal bifurcation and bronchi of dogs, and usually causes chronic coughing, but occasionally can cause dyspnoea due to airway obstruction. *Aelurostrongylus abstrusus* primarily infects cats, is found in the terminal bronchioles and alveoli, and causes bronchiolitis and pneumonia. *Filaroides hirthi* and *Crenosoma vulpis* are found in the lower airways of dogs, and cause bronchitis and eosinophilic or granulomatous pneumonia. Both dogs and cats can be infected with *Capillaria aerophila*, which lives in coiled masses embedded in the tracheal and bronchial mucosa and causes chronic coughing or pneumonia. Occasionally, dogs and cats heavily infested with ascarids may have respiratory signs associated with lung migration.

Clinical signs in dogs and cats with lungworms typically include chronic coughing, but may include dyspnoea and fever in severe cases. Radiographic signs are generally non-specific although a peripheral alveolar–interstitial pattern has been reported with *Angiostrongylus vasorum* infection and mucosal nodules are occasionally visible radiographically in dogs with *Oslerus osleri*. As the life cycle of most of the parasites involves production of first-stage larvae in the lung that are expectorated into the mouth and swallowed, diagnosis is achieved by identifying the larvae in faeces (Baermann technique or direct smear). Larvae may also be identified in lung wash samples along with neutrophilic or eosinophilic inflammation. With *Oslerus osleri* the nodules and adult parasites may be directly visualized at the time of bronchoscopy. Although some parasites, such as *Oslerus osleri* and *Filaroides hirthi*, are directly transmitted, most other lungworms require a paratenic host such as a slug, snail or earthworm. Treatment of lungworms typically involves the use of fenbendazole, milbemycin or ivermectin. Fenbendazole should be administered for a minimum of 14 days, and as long as 20 days in cats with *Aelurostrongylus abstrusus*.

Further reading

Berry CR, Moore PF, Thomas WP *et al.* (1990) Pulmonary lymphomatoid granulomatosis in seven dogs (1976–1987). *Journal of Veterinary Internal Medicine* **4**, 157–166

Buback JL, Boothe HW and Hobson HP (1996) Surgical treatment of tracheal collapse in dogs: 90 cases (1983–1993). *Journal of the American Veterinary Medical Association* **208**, 380–384

Cooper E, Syring R and King LG (2003) Pneumothorax in cats with a clinical diagnosis of feline asthma: 5 cases (1990–2000). *Journal of Veterinary Emergency and Critical Care* **13**, 95–101

Costello MF, Keith D, Hendrick M and King LG (2001) Acute upper airway obstruction due to inflammatory laryngeal disease in 5 cats. *Journal of Veterinary Emergency and Critical Care* **11**, 205–210

Drobatz KJ and Concannon K (1994) Noncardiogenic pulmonary edema. *Compendium on Continuing Education for the Practicing Veterinarian* **16**, 333–346

Dye JA, McKiernan BC and Rozanski EA (1996) Bronchopulmonary disease in the cat: historical, physical, radiographic, clinicopathologic and pulmonary functional evaluation of 24 affected and 15 healthy cats. *Journal of Veterinary Internal Medicine* **10**, 385–400

Fossum TW (1993) Feline chylothorax. *Compendium on Continuing Education for the Practicing Veterinarian* **15**, 549–567

Hackner SG (1995) Emergency management of traumatic pulmonary contusions. *Compendium on Continuing Education for the Practicing Veterinarian* **17**, 677–686

Kapatkin AS, Matthiesen DT, Noone KE *et al.* (1990) Results of surgery and long-term follow-up in 31 cats with nasopharyngeal polyps. *Journal of the American Animal Hospital Association* **26**, 387–392

Keyes ML, Rush JE and Knowles KE (1993) Pulmonary thromboembolism in dogs. *Journal of Veterinary Emergency and Critical Care* **3**, 23–32

King LG and Boothe DM (1997) *Bacterial Infections of the Respiratory Tract in Dogs and Cats.* Bayer, Shawnee Mission, Kansas

Lotti U and Niebauer GW (1992) Tracheobronchial foreign bodies of plant origin in 153 hunting dogs. *Compendium on Continuing Education for the Practicing Veterinarian* **14**, 900–904

Moritz A, Schneider M and Bauer N (2004) Management of advanced tracheal collapse in dogs using intraluminal self-expanding biliary wallstents. *Journal of Veterinary Internal Medicine* **18**, 31–42

Neath PJ, Brockman DJ and King LG (2000) Lung lobe torsion in the dog: A retrospective study of 22 cases (1981–1999). *Journal of the American Veterinary Medical Association* **217**, 1041–1044

Ogilvie GK, Haschek WM, Withrow SJ *et al.* (1989) Classification of primary lung tumours in dogs: 210 cases (1975–1985). *Journal of the American Veterinary Medical Association* **195**, 106–108

Ogilvie GK, Weigel RM, Haschek WM *et al.* (1989) Prognostic factors for tumour remission and survival in dogs after surgery for primary lung tumour: 76 cases (1975–1985). *Journal of the American Veterinary Medical Association* **195**, 109–112

Padrid PA, Hornof WJ, Kurpershoek CG *et al.* (1990) Canine chronic bronchitis: a pathophysiologic evaluation of 18 cases. *Journal of Veterinary Internal Medicine* **4**, 172–180

Parent C, King LG, van Winkle TJ *et al.* (1996) Respiratory function and treatment in dogs with acute respiratory distress syndrome: 19 cases (1985–1993). *Journal of the American Veterinary Medical Association* **208**, 1428–1433

Parent C, King LG, Walker LM *et al.* (1996) Clinical and clinicopathologic findings in dogs with acute respiratory distress syndrome: 19 cases (1985–1993). *Journal of the American Veterinary Medical Association* **208**, 1419–1427

Puerto DA, Brockman DJ, Lindquist C and Drobatz K (2002) Surgical and nonsurgical management of and selected risk factors for spontaneous pneumothorax in dogs: 64 cases (1986–1999). *Journal of the American Veterinary Medical Association* **220**, 1670–1674

Rooney MB and Monnet E (2002) Medical and surgical treatment of pyothorax in dogs: 26 cases (1991–2001). *Journal of the American Veterinary Medical Association* **221**, 86–92

Sauve V, Drobatz KJ, Shokek AB, McKnight AL, King LG (2005) Clinical course, diagnostic findings and necropsy diagnosis in dyspneic cats with primary pulmonary parenchymal disease: 15 cats (1996–2002). *Journal of Veterinary Emergency and Critical Care* **15**, 38–47

Waddell LS, Brady CA, Drobatz KJ (2002) Risk factors, prognostic indicators, and outcome of pyothorax in cats: 80 cases (1986–1999). *Journal of the American Veterinary Medical Association* **221**, 819–824

8

Renal and urinary tract emergencies

Karol A. Mathews

Introduction

Renal emergencies may primarily involve the kidneys (Figure 8.1), or be secondary to prerenal (Figure 8.2) or postrenal (Figure 8.3) disease. Similarly, lower urinary tract pathology may be primary, or secondary to other initiating factors. A thorough history, physical examination and laboratory information are required to diagnose renal dysfunction or disease, and in many

Ischaemia
Severe persistent prerenal causes
Renal vascular thrombosis
Renal parenchymal injury/trauma

Infectious
Bacterial pyelonephritis
Leptospirosis
Lyme nephropathy
Feline infectious peritonitis

Structural
Nephroliths
Polycystic

Immune-mediated
Glomerulonephritis
Amyloidosis
Interstitial nephritis
Systemic lupus glomerulonephritis

Neoplastic
Lymphoma
Haemangiosarcoma

Toxins
Aminoglycosides
Other antibiotics, including polymyxin B, sulphonamides, cephaloridine and tetracyclines
Amphotericin B
Thiacetarsamine
Non-steroidal anti-inflammatory drugs
Methoxyflurane
Carbon tetrachloride
Ethylene glycol
Heavy metals
Myoglobin
Haemoglobin and red cell stroma
Unknown substances associated with compost ingestion
Easter Lily (cats)
Grapes/raisins (dogs)

8.1 Examples of renal emergencies caused by primary renal disease.

Inadequate intravascular volume due to fluid translocation or loss
Vomiting
Diarrhoea
Third space losses
Thermal burns
Heatstroke
Blood loss
Hypoadrenocorticism
Hypoalbuminaemia
Vasculitis
Pancreatitis
Shock
Diabetes inspidus (central or renal, e.g. endotoxin)
Diabetes mellitus
Overzealous diuretic use

Increased renal and systemic vascular resistance
Increased circulating catecholamines
Renal sympathetic nervous stimulation (e.g. unilateral nephrectomy affecting contralateral renal function)
Angiotensin II
Hypothermia

Inadequate intravascular volume due to vasodilation
Anaphylaxis
Inhalational anaesthetics
Sepsis
Heatstroke
Vasodilator therapy

Inadequate cardiac output
Congestive heart failure
Cardiac tamponade
Restrictive pericardial or cardiac disease
Dysrhythmias
Positive pressure ventilation
Following cardiac arrest
Selective anaesthetic protocols

Hyperviscosity
Polycythaemia
Hyperproteinaemia/hyperglobulinaemia

Miscellaneous (reduced urine volume but not necessarily azotaemia)
Antidiuretic hormone (ADH) secretion due to hypotension or hypovolaemia
Opioids (ADH-like effect)
Lung pathology (ADH activity)
Ventilator patients

8.2 Examples of renal emergencies due to prerenal disease.

Trauma
Ruptured bladder
Herniated bladder
Ruptured/avulsed ureters
Ruptured/avulsed urethra
Post-traumatic scarring of ureters or urethra
Bladder or urethral haematoma
Iatrogenic ligation of ureters or urethra

Obstruction
Uroliths
Granulomatous urethritis
Neoplasia (extra- or intraluminal or intramural)
Prostatic disease
Stump pyometra
Functional spasm – reflex dyssynergia
Urethral inflammation
Herniated, retroflexed bladder
Urethral haematoma
Technical problems associated with an indwelling urinary catheter

Neurological
Spinal injury/disease

8.3 Examples of renal emergencies due to postrenal disease.

instances diagnostic imaging is necessary to diagnose lower urinary tract injuries or disease accurately. Renal biopsy is required for definitive diagnosis of most renal diseases, although it is rarely performed. Attention to these diagnostic details should help prevent misdiagnosis and inappropriate prognostication, which may lead to incorrect therapy or euthanasia.

Questions to the owner should include those pertaining to prerenal, renal and postrenal causes of azotaemia:

- Voiding behaviour and frequency
- Urine volume and colour
- Water consumption
- Overall activity
- Appetite
- Vomiting and diarrhoea
- Trauma (within past 7 days)
- Medications, including over-the-counter non-steroidal anti-inflammatory drugs (NSAIDs)
- Access to toxins and owner medication
- Acuity of onset of signs
- Previous history of renal or urinary tract disease, cardiac or other system disease
- Recent anaesthesia (surgical, dental or diagnostic procedures)
- Travel history.

The physical examination should include evaluation of:

- Hydration status
- Mucous membrane colour and capillary refill time
- Heart and respiratory rates
- Pulse pressure
- Jugular vein distension
- Presence of pleural or abdominal effusions
- Abdominal palpation to assess kidney, uterus, prostate size, abdominal masses, fluid (intraperitoneal or subcutaneous) or pain

- Body temperature
- Penis (crepitus, lacerations), prepuce (haemorrhage), scrotum or vulva
- Perineum (cellulitis, bruising) and anus
- Rectal examination, especially in males and where pelvic injury is present
- Hind limbs for swelling, cellulitis
- Overall examination to rule out trauma, especially abdominal and pelvic, and to check for enlargement of peripheral lymph nodes.

Based on the history and physical findings, immediate and appropriate testing should be performed to evaluate and treat imminently life-threatening problems (trauma and haemorrhage, hyperkalaemia, severe metabolic acidosis or dehydration).

Azotaemia

Definition of terms and concepts related to azotaemia

Azotaemia is defined as an abnormal concentration of urea, creatinine and other nitrogenous substances in blood, and is a laboratory diagnosis. Both urea and creatinine may be increased due to diminished elimination by the kidneys and/or the lower urinary tract. A high urea may also occur due to increased production of urea by the liver secondary to gastrointestinal haemorrhage or a high-protein meal, starvation, fever or dehydration. A low urea may be seen with liver insufficiency/failure and following administration of anabolic steroids. Creatinine may be elevated by increased muscle mass or decreased due to muscle wasting. Azotaemia may be transient and therefore does not always imply renal disease, renal failure or insufficiency. Commonly used formulae related to renal function are shown in Figure 8.4.

Fractional excretion of sodium
= (Urine [Na$^+$]/Plasma [Na$^+$]) x (Plasma [Cr]/Urine [Cr]) x 100 Normal tubular function or prerenal disease: <1% Acute tubular necrosis: >2% Invalid in such conditions as congestive heart failure, hepatic failure or nephrotic syndrome, as excretion of sodium is impaired and retention of sodium may persist despite renal dysfunction

Anion gap
= ([Na$^+$] + [K$^+$]) – ([HCO$_3^-$] + [Cl$^-$]) Normal value = 15–25 Total CO_2 can be used instead of HCO_3^- where venous blood gases cannot be measured

Urine protein:creatinine ratio
Urine protein (mg/dl)/Urine creatinine (mg/dl) or Urine protein (g/l)/Urine creatinine (µmol/l) x 8.84 Normal value = <0.5

Average daily maintenance fluid requirements for ill animals (ml)
= 1.2 (70 x $BW^{0.75}$) for all animals or = (30 x BW) + 70 for animals between 2 and 40 kg, where BW = body weight in kg

8.4 Commonly used formulae.

115

The term *uraemia* is used when azotaemia is associated with metabolic and physiological alterations, including depression, anorexia, nausea, vomiting, diarrhoea, melaena, dehydration, stupor, coma or seizures. These occur due to the polysystemic toxic syndrome that results from abnormal renal function. For uraemia to develop, the function of both kidneys must be reduced by at least 75%. Uraemia may occur in animals with primary renal failure/insufficiency or pre- or postrenal disorders, and may be reversible or irreversible.

Renal disease is not always associated with renal failure, insufficiency or azotaemia and may regress, persist or increase in severity. Renal disease has many aetiologies and may involve the glomeruli, tubules, interstitial tissue, blood vessels, or a combination of these.

The terms *renal failure* and *renal insufficiency* describe failure of the kidney to concentrate or dilute urine, or to eliminate the products of metabolism appropriately, resulting in azotaemia. Inability to concentrate or dilute the urine usually occurs when there has been approximately a 66% reduction in renal function, whereas recognizable failure to eliminate products of metabolism occurs following 66–75% reduction in renal function. As an early indicator, when the creatinine value of a well hydrated animal lies in the upper end of the normal range, this may be consistent with a 50% or greater reduction in renal function.

Whenever possible, a urine sample should be obtained prior to fluid therapy in order to assess the concentrating ability of the kidneys. The urine specific gravity is helpful in localizing the cause of azotaemia (Figure 8.5). Dehydrated azotaemic patients with urine specific gravity >1.030 (in dogs) and >1.045 (in cats) are most likely to have prerenal azotaemia. Some cats can effectively concentrate their urine despite significant reduction in renal function; therefore concentrated urine in cats may not exclude intrinsic renal failure. Azotaemic dehydrated animals that cannot concentrate urine may be receiving medication (e.g. furosemide, corticosteroids) or have an illness (e.g. hypoadrenocorticism, diabetes mellitus, hypercalcaemia, bacterial cystitis) that interferes with urine-concentrating ability, and therefore they also may not have intrinsic renal dysfunction. Cystitis caused by *Escherichia coli* (and possibly other bacteria) can cause a profound polyuria resulting in dehydration, without other typical signs of cystitis.

The packed cell volume and plasma total protein in prerenal azotaemia tend to be increased above normal, unless blood loss or anaemia is present. Response to intravenous fluid therapy usually distinguishes between prerenal and renal azotaemia. Postrenal azotaemia, due to partial or total urinary tract obstruction, is diagnosed based on history and physical examination (discussed later) and may be associated with pollakiuria, dysuria or stranguria. With pre- and postrenal disease or injury excluded, a presumptive diagnosis of renal failure can be made when azotaemia is associated with isosthenuria (urine specific gravity <1.025 or more commonly 1.008–1.015). Primary renal failure is confirmed once diseases or drugs that can affect the kidney's ability to concentrate urine have been ruled out.

Patient assessment

The diagnostic tests and treatment for renal or urinary tract emergencies are based on the underlying

Laboratory test	Prerenal azotaemia	Parenchymal acute renal failure	Postrenal azotaemia
Urine specific gravity	>1.035 dogs >1.045 cats	1.008–1.029 dogs 1.008–1.034 cats	Variable
Urine to plasma osmolality Urinary sodium concentration Fractional excretion of sodium Urine creatinine:plasma creatinine Urine protein:urine creatinine Urine glucose	>5:1 <20 mmol/l <1% >20:1 <0.5 Absent	 >40 mmol/l >1% <10:1 1 to >13 Variably present	 <0.5
Urine sediment			
Proteinuria Granular casts Renal epithelial cells Red blood cells >5/hpf	Absent/trace Absent Absent Cardiac/emboli Exercise Coagulopathy	Present Present Present Glomerular injury	 Absent to many
Red blood cell ghosts White blood cells >5/hpf Cellular debris Neoplastic cells	Cardiac/emboli Absent Absent Absent	Renal tubular injury Present Present Renal neoplasia	Absent to many Absent/present Absent/present Bladder/urethral neoplasia
Urine colour			
Dark red/brown		Myoglobin Haemoglobin	
Red	Blood		Blood

8.5 Differentiation of prerenal and postrenal azotaemia and parenchymal acute renal failure based on urine analysis. All or individual components of the urine sediment may be present depending on severity, the time from onset of renal injury to presentation and aetiology.

problem as discussed below. Patient monitoring is similar in most instances and is outlined at the end of this chapter.

Emergency minimum database
See Figure 8.6.

- Serum creatinine and urea, plasma glucose, phosphorus, calcium, electrolytes, packed cell volume (PCV) and total protein (TP), total carbon dioxide or venous blood gases. Note that urea (or blood urea nitrogen (BUN)) is not a reliable definitive test for renal assessment as outlined above; however it is a good screening test.
- Measured serum osmolality if ethylene glycol or salicylate intoxication is suspected.
- Urine specific gravity, sediment, protein, glucose, urine culture and sensitivity.
- Cytology, urea, creatinine, PCV and TP of abdominal fluid if present.
- Abdominal and pelvic radiographs ± abdominal ultrasonography ± contrast studies.
- Arterial and central venous blood pressure monitoring.

Additional diagnostic testing

- Complete biochemical profile and complete blood count.
- Urine protein:creatinine ratio if indicated.
- Urine electrolytes and creatinine if indicated for lesion localization.
- Serology if indicated (e.g. *Leptospira*, *Borrelia*).
- Renal biopsy if indicated.

Urine output
Assessment of urine production is one of the most important tools for immediate monitoring of renal function in critical patients. Normal urine production is 1–2 ml/kg/h but may be reduced in dehydrated animals, and should be expected to be higher in animals receiving large volumes of intravenous fluids. In all emergency situations, the volume of urine within the bladder should be assessed immediately by abdominal palpation, abdominal radiography or ultrasonography, urinary bladder catheterization or voiding. Wherever possible, a urine sample should be obtained for laboratory analysis prior to institution of therapy, via urinary bladder catheterization (Figure 8.7), cystocentesis (Figures 8.8 and 8.9) or a voided sample. If culture and sensitivity testing are warranted, a sample obtained via cystocentesis is recommended. Injury to the urinary system may interfere with urine output. As various problems unrelated to renal function may impair spontaneous voiding, the urinary bladder may require catheterization, palpation or imaging to assess whether urine is being produced over time.

Laboratory test	Prerenal azotaemia	Parenchymal acute renal failure	Postrenal azotaemia
Packed cell volume Total protein	>Normal >Normal	Normal [a] Normal [a]	>Normal [a] >Normal [a]
Serum potassium	Normal High (hypoadrenocorticism) Low (loop diuretic)	Normal or high	Normal or high
Serum sodium	Normal High Low [b]	Normal	Normal
Metabolic acidosis Anion gap	Present Increased	Present Increased	Present Increased

8.6 Database, electrolyte and blood gas findings in prerenal, renal and postrenal azotaemia. [a] Assuming blood loss or anaemia of systemic illness, including chronic renal failure, is not present. [b] ADH release due to ineffective circulating volume.

The technique of urethral catheterization varies between the sexes and between dogs and cats. Most male dogs can be catheterized without chemical restraint but bitches and cats, especially males, usually require sedation or anaesthesia. Urethral catheterization techniques have been well reviewed by Holt (1994).

Many catheters are commercially available for the urethral catheterization of small animals. The majority of catheters are manufactured from polyurethane, red rubber or silicone. Metal catheters cannot be recommended because of the increased likelihood of trauma to the urethra and/or bladder. Silicone has certain advantages for the patient, including softness, flexibility and biological inertness. These allow for atraumatic placement, minimal epithelial irritation and long-term patient comfort.

Urethral catheters for use in cats are generally sized between 3 and 4 French (Fr). Catheters for use in small dogs are usually sized between 3 and 5 Fr and catheters for use in medium to large/giant-sized dogs are usually between 8 (male and female) and 10–12 Fr (female). A number of urethral catheters are specifically designed to be used as indwelling catheters. Catheters manufactured from silicone or other soft materials may require a wire guide stylet to assist their introduction. Narrow gauge paediatric feeding tubes may be used as indwelling catheters in cats, do not require a stylet and are easily placed. In bitches, Foley catheters can be utilized as indwelling catheters. Their placement typically uses a nylon stylet which is contained within the catheter, and is removed following insertion. Longer Foley catheters for male dogs are now available. Some urethral catheters have a detachable Luer lock fitting, allowing them to be trimmed to any length. This is of considerable use when these catheters are used as indwelling systems.

8.7 Catheterization of the urethra and urinary bladder. (continues) ▶

Indwelling catheters should ideally be connected to a sterile closed urine collecting system, which can be constructed in an aseptic manner from an intravenous fluid administration set and bag. Commercially available systems are also available. One-way valves in the urinary bag have the advantage of preventing retrograde flow of urine and consequently reducing urinary bladder infection. If these valves are not present in the collection system, unless the line is clamped, the urine collection bag should not be raised above the animal, which would allow retrograde flow of urine.

Urethral catheterization in the male dog

1. Clean the prepuce of all debris and discharge with chlorhexidine soap and rinse with warm water.
2. As an estimate of the length of catheter to be inserted into the urinary bladder, premeasure the catheter from the prepuce along the course of the urethra, around the ischial arch and to the approximate level of the mid-urinary bladder, while avoiding contamination of the catheter. If a paediatric feeding tube is used, coil this length of the catheter into the palm of the sterile-gloved hand. This will give the operator an idea of the length of catheter to be inserted and avoid the potential of extra length being inserted and potential 'looping' within the lumen of the bladder.
3. Grasp the caudal os penis with one hand and retract the prepuce caudally with the other hand, exposing the glans penis. Aseptic handling and placement of the catheter is facilitated if an assistant is available who can perform this part of the procedure.
4. One of the fingers of the hand grasping the os penis is used to keep the prepuce retracted and the glans exposed.
5. The catheter to be inserted should be lubricated with sterile water-soluble jelly.
6. The catheter is then inserted into the urethra under aseptic conditions (either by wearing a sterile glove or by handling the catheter through its sterile polythene bag).
7. Once the catheter is inserted to the level of the caudal os penis, the grip of the hand holding the penis is relaxed allowing further unobstructed passage of the catheter.
8. As soon as the catheter tip enters the bladder and urine appears in the catheter hub, pass an additional 2 cm to ensure adequate length beyond the trigone.
9. The catheter may be sutured to the cranial preputial skin using butterfly tapes or the Chinese finger trap technique, and maintained as an indwelling catheter.
10. An Elizabethan collar should be fitted initially to prevent self-removal of the catheter, however this can often be removed based on the individual's tolerance of the catheter.

Urethral catheterization in the bitch

1. The dog is positioned in sternal recumbency with hind limbs draped over the edge of the table or in lateral recumbency (right lateral recumbency if right handed, left lateral recumbency if left handed), and the vulva is cleaned with chlorhexidine soap and rinsed with warm water.
2. Sterile lidocaine jelly contained within a 'syringe-like cartridge' can be introduced into the vulva and 2 mg/kg deposited into the vaginal vault to confer local anaesthesia. The vulva is held closed for 5 minutes prior to catheter placement.
3. A vaginal speculum is inserted into the vestibule/vagina taking care not to enter the ventrally placed clitoral fossa.
4. The slit of the speculum is positioned ventrally allowing the raised external urethral orifice to be identified on the floor of the cranial vestibule. Visualization of the external urethral orifice is often made easier if an assistant pulls the ventral vulva caudally.
5. If a vaginal speculum is not available, the catheter can be inserted blindly using digital palpation of the urethral papilla. While sterile gloves are recommended, they are not necessary if the hands have been washed three times with chlorhexidine soap, with the final soap suds remaining on the hands. Sterile water lubricant is placed on the catheter and the index finger of the non-dominant hand. The non-dominant index (or smaller) finger, depending on the size of the animal, is placed into the vestibule and while gently applying pressure to its floor, is moved cranially. The urethral papilla is palpated as a slight 'bulge' of mucosa. While applying gentle pressure over the papilla, the catheter is fed under the finger and guided into the urethra. The catheter is then sensed to 'disappear' into the urethra. Should the catheter be palpated high within the vagina, then urethral catheterization was unsuccessful. Residue of soap is rinsed off with warm water.
6. The catheter is inserted into the urethra in an aseptic manner (when using soft rubber or silicone catheters it may be advantageous to stiffen the catheter with a stylet) until urine is seen. If a Foley catheter is used, the full length of the catheter is placed into the bladder, then the balloon is inflated with the recommended volume of sterile saline, and the catheter is gently pulled back out until resistance is felt. Complete insertion is required to avoid inflating the balloon within the urethra.
7. The non-Foley catheter may be sutured to the perivulval skin using butterfly tapes, and maintained as an indwelling catheter.
8. An Elizabethan collar should be fitted to prevent self-removal of the catheter if necessary.

Urethral catheterization in the male cat

1. A Jackson tom cat catheter or a 3.5 Fr paediatric feeding tube may be used as a urinary catheter.
2. The cat is positioned in lateral recumbency and the prepuce is cleaned with chlorhexidine soap and rinsed with warm water.
3. For right-handed operators, the thumb and index finger of the left hand are used to push the prepuce cranially and expose the glans penis.
4. The tip of the catheter is inserted into the penile urethra (lubrication of the catheter tip with a water-soluble lubricant may prove advantageous).
5. To allow the safe advancement of the catheter, the prepuce is grasped with the left hand and pulled in a caudal direction (this aligns the penile and membranous urethrae, making further catheter passage possible).
6. As soon as the catheter tip enters the bladder and urine appears in the catheter hub, insert the catheter 1 cm further.
7. When the Jackson's catheter is used, it may be sutured to the preputial skin using the holes in the catheter flange, and maintained as an indwelling catheter for short periods. Softer catheters are recommended for long-term catheterization.
8. An Elizabethan collar should be fitted to prevent self-removal of the catheter.

8.7 (continued) Catheterization of the urethra and urinary bladder. (continues) ▶

Urethral catheterization in the queen

The anatomy of the queen is such that the external urethral orifice is found as a depression on the vaginal floor. This anatomical situation allows 'blind' urethral catheterization. A 3.5 Fr paediatric feeding tube is preferred. If 'blind' catheterization fails, an otoscope may be used as a vaginoscope to identify the external urethral orifice, allowing urethral catheterization.

1. For the right-handed operator, the cat is positioned in right lateral recumbency.

2. The left hand is used to grasp the vulval lips, allowing the right hand to pass the catheter along the vestibular floor in the midline.

3. This passage of the catheter will commonly result in entrance to the urethra.

4. As soon as the catheter tip enters the bladder and urine appears in the catheter hub, continue to advance the catheter another 1 cm.

5. When a Jackson's catheter is used, it may be sutured to the vulval skin using the holes in the catheter flange, and maintained as an indwelling catheter for short periods. Softer catheters are recommended for long-term catheterization.

6. An Elizabethan collar should be fitted to prevent self-removal of the catheter.

8.7 (continued) Catheterization of the urethra and urinary bladder.

Cystocentesis allows a urine sample to be obtained without contamination from the urethra, the genital tract or the skin. It reduces the risk of producing an iatrogenic urinary tract infection that may occur with urinary catheterization. Cystocentesis may also be required to decompress a severely over-distended bladder in patients with urethral obstruction when urethral catheterization is not possible. For cystocentesis, the bladder must contain a reasonable volume of urine such that it can be safely identified and immobilized. If a small volume of urine is present, the bladder is difficult to palpate or the animal is obese, ultrasonography may be used to help guide the needle into the bladder.

1. The skin of the caudoventral abdomen is clipped if required and prepared aseptically.

2. In the cat and small dog, the technique is most readily performed with the animal in either lateral or dorsal recumbency.

3. In larger dogs, the procedure may be performed with the animal in either lateral recumbency or standing.

4. In all instances, an assistant is required to restrain the subject.

5. The operator's free hand is used to palpate and stabilize the bladder by pushing it in a caudal direction against the pelvic brim.

6. The needle (22 or 23 gauge, 25–50 mm (1–2 inches) in length) is attached to a 5 or 10 ml syringe and inserted through the abdominal wall, on the midline, just in front of the pelvic brim.

7. The ideal site of bladder penetration is a short distance cranial to the junction of the bladder with the urethra (this will permit removal of urine and decompression of the bladder without the need for re-insertion of the needle into the bladder lumen).

8. The needle is inserted in a caudal direction at a 45-degree angle. Once the needle has penetrated the abdominal wall slight negative pressure should be applied to the syringe.

9. Alternatively, in standing dogs, the operator can obtain the sample from the right side (to avoid penetrating the descending colon), while gently stabilizing and pushing the bladder from the left side towards the right side of the caudal abdomen (Figure 8.9a).

10. Once the bladder lumen is penetrated, urine will be seen filling the syringe.

11. When only a small volume of urine is present, the animal is placed in dorsal recumbency and a 22 gauge 25–50 mm (1–2 inch) needle on a syringe is placed into the midline of the caudal abdomen between the two caudal mammary glands in bitches and cats, and at the same level slightly lateral to the penis in male dogs (Figure 8.9b).

8.8 Cystocentesis.

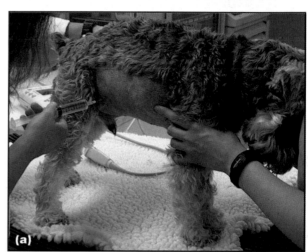

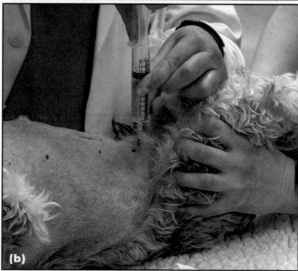

8.9 **(a)** In standing dogs, the operator can obtain a urine sample by cystocentesis from the right side (to avoid penetrating the descending colon), while gently stabilizing and pushing the bladder from the left towards the right side of the caudal abdomen. **(b)** Alternatively, the animal is placed in dorsal recumbency and a 22 gauge, 25–50 mm (1–2 inch) needle on a syringe is placed into the midline of the caudal abdomen between the two caudal mammary glands in bitches rend queens, and at the same level slightly lateral to the penis in male dogs. (Note: the extensive hair clipping in this dog was required for ultrasonographic examination of the abdomen, and not for cystocentesis.)

Approach to oliguria and anuria

The definition of oliguria is urine production <0.27 ml/ kg/h, but if the animal is receiving intravenous fluid therapy, <1–2 ml/kg/h may represent oliguria. The cause of decreased urine output should be defined, as specific therapy depends on aetiology. The history may reveal a period of polyuria and polydipsia, or an abrupt reduction in urine production (frequently associated with postrenal obstruction, see below). Bradycardia, hypothermia, pale mucous membranes with prolonged capillary refill time, hyperpnoea and halitosis are evident in animals with prolonged anuria, and indicate severe metabolic and electrolyte derangements that can occur with prerenal, postrenal or primary renal disease.

Initial treatment

An intravenous catheter is placed and enough blood obtained for an emergency minimum database. Immediate concerns include: the adequacy of circulating blood volume; hypotension; electrolyte imbalance, especially hyperkalaemia; metabolic acidosis; and the severity of underlying disease. A urine sample should be obtained as soon as possible, and ideally prior to fluid therapy. Where indicated, a urinary catheter is passed to assess urethral patency, facilitate voiding and measure urine production. Electrocardiographic monitoring is advised to detect cardiac dysrhythmias associated with hyperkalaemia, primary cardiac disease or caused by other metabolic or traumatic disorders. Therapeutic suggestions are outlined below under the specific problems. Guidelines for fluid therapy are described in the section on acute intrinsic renal failure.

Approach to urine leakage due to renal, ureteral, bladder or urethral injury

Renal parenchymal injury may be due to blunt or penetrating trauma, which may involve one or both kidneys. Renal injury may cause retroperitoneal haemorrhage, haemorrhage into the abdomen or haemorrhage into the parenchyma and pelvis of the kidney, with haematuria and obstruction to urine flow by haematoma formation. Nephroliths may obstruct urine flow from the pelvis of the kidney, causing hydronephrosis with possible traumatic injury and rupture. If the nephrolith is associated with bacterial infection, abscessation and rupture may occur, resulting in peritonitis. Ureteral obstruction may also occur with similar consequences. If one kidney or ureter is involved, the other unit may function adequately, resulting in normal serum urea and creatinine levels. However, if there is urine leakage into the peritoneal cavity, serum urea and creatinine levels will increase. Bladder or urethral rupture may be caused by blunt trauma, erosion of a tumour, cystic calculi obstructing urine flow, aggressive palpation, cystocentesis, especially in patients with a compromised bladder wall, or attempts at unblocking an obstructed urethra. Injuries or obstruction to any part of the urinary tract may also result from calculi, abscesses, neoplasia, perineal, inguinal or abdominal hernias and iatrogenic injuries.

Urinary tract injury should be suspected in all trauma patients, with a high level of suspicion in patients sustaining abdominal or pelvic injuries. The incidence of urinary tract injury associated with pelvic trauma was 39% in one study (Selcer, 1982). Gentle and thorough palpation of the abdomen and sublumbar area should be performed whilst noting areas of tenderness, bladder size, abdominal girth, evidence of free abdominal fluid and injuries to the abdominal wall. Preputial or vulval bleeding, haematuria, dysuria and anuria may also be associated with urinary tract injuries. The inguinal region and perineum should be monitored carefully for swelling or discoloration associated with urine leakage from a ruptured urethra. Repeated physical examination should be performed to detect early signs of intra-abdominal injury. In a study of hospitalized animals only 40% of the diagnoses of ruptured bladder were made within 12 hours after trauma and 22.7% were not diagnosed until necropsy (Burrows, 1974).

Diagnosis

Diagnosis and localization of urinary tract injury is based on history, physical findings and the emergency minimum database, repeated physical examination and diagnostic imaging. Metabolic changes associated with urine leakage include increased serum urea and creatinine, increased serum potassium with reduced serum sodium and chloride and a gradually increasing PCV and white blood cell count. Blood bicarbonate and PCO_2 levels gradually decrease as acidosis worsens. Should vomiting be significant, a mixed metabolic alkalosis and acidosis may be present.

Urinalysis may be abnormal (see Figure 8.5). When haematuria is present, reproductive disease should be ruled out in both males and females, and oestrus and whelping history in bitches and queens should be ascertained. When abdominal distension is noted, or urinary leakage or haemorrhage is suspected, abdominocentesis should be performed. If the fluid is negative for urea nitrogen on a reagent strip, it is not urine. A positive finding, however, may or may not indicate urine, as false-positive results may occur. For definitive diagnosis, the urea, creatinine and potassium in the fluid should be measured. If these values are greater than those in a concurrently obtained peripheral blood sample, this indicates that the fluid is urine. Blood easily obtained on abdominocentesis indicates severe haemorrhage, which may be associated with renal parenchymal, blood vessel, hepatic or splenic injuries. Injuries associated with urine or haemorrhage that is contained within the retroperitoneal space will not be detected on abdominocentesis.

Diagnostic imaging should be performed in all highly suspect cases of urinary tract trauma. Abdominal radiographs may reveal a loss of detail within the abdomen, indicating free fluid, or retroperitoneal changes associated with fluid accumulation (mass effect with ventral displacement of the colon or streaky increased density in the retroperitoneal space). Non-visualization, displacement or asymmetry of one or both kidneys suggests renal injury. Reduced size or absence of the urinary bladder may indicate rupture or avulsion from the urethra, although a normal radiographic appearance of the bladder does not rule out rupture. Uroliths (excluding ammonium urate and cystine) may also be visualized within the urinary tract. Pelvic radiographs should be performed to identify fractures. Urethral tears may result from laceration by the sharp bone segments of pelvic fractures; it is therefore important to evaluate the pelvis in any patient with a history of trauma and uroabdomen or perineal cellulitis. Ultrasonographic examination of the urinary system may be useful in identifying renal pathology, hydroureter, uroliths, bladder pathology and urethral dilation and obstruction. Excretory urography is required to identify injury, obstruction and perfusion of the kidneys and ureters definitively. This should be performed prior to cystourethrogram if both are being considered. If a rupture of the lower urinary tract (urinary bladder or urethra) is suspected, a contrast cystourethrogram should be performed using iodine-based contrast material. Even when a urethral catheter can be passed easily into the bladder, urethral injury may still be present and a urethrogram is recommended if there is extensive injury to the pelvic region. Contrast urethrography and cystography are extremely useful for identifying rupture, with leakage of the contrast agent being evident (see Chapter 25). Depending on the location of the urethral tear, urine may leak into the peritoneal cavity, the perineal area (perineal urethral tear or rarely, urethral avulsion), or the dorsal lumbar subcutaneous tissue (dorsal tear in the proximal urethra). If urethral rupture is not identified promptly and urine leakage has been present for some time (days), urine and contrast material may dissect through the subcutaneous tissue down the hind limbs or along the dorsum as far cranial as the scapulae.

Treatment

Renal parenchymal injuries
Renal parenchymal injuries may require surgical treatment if they are associated with significant haemorrhage or urine leakage. Leakage of contrast during excretory urography, or obstruction of urine flow due to haematomas or other masses, are both indications for laparotomy. Contusions and intracapsular fractures do not require treatment. Severe renal injuries may require partial nephrectomy, and repair of capsular haemorrhage by deep sutures or omental wrap. If more than 50% of the kidney is destroyed or the pedicle is avulsed, nephrectomy is indicated. A complete examination of both kidneys should be performed prior to surgical intervention unless severe ongoing haemorrhage is occurring.

Ureteral trauma
Ureteral trauma may result in crush injury, laceration or contusions, usually in the proximal or distal regions. Incomplete tears are debrided and sutured with 1 metric (5-0 USP) absorbable suture in a simple interrupted pattern. If the ureter is transected, the ends are debrided, spatulated and anastomosed using 1 metric (5-0 USP) absorbable suture in a simple interrupted pattern. The use of a soft catheter

stent, which is placed into the ureter to bridge the anastomotic site, passed into the bladder and exteriorized through the urethra, may facilitate ureteral repair. The catheter is removed after 5–7 days. Ureters avulsed from the bladder can be reimplanted (see Further reading). If the ureter is significantly damaged and repair or reimplantation is not an option, renal autograft into the iliac fossa should be considered (Mathews *et al.*, 1994) or nephrectomy performed.

Urinary bladder injuries
Urinary bladder contusions result in haemorrhage, which frequently resolves spontaneously. Rupture due to blunt trauma occurs most frequently at the apex. The bladder neck and trigone, urethra or prostate may be lacerated or punctured by pelvic fracture fragments. Since bladder filling and voiding may still be present, frequent examination of the abdomen is necessary to detect uroperitoneum. A urinary catheter may pass easily into the bladder, and urethral injury may not initially be suspected. In some animals with bladder injury, urinary catheters can be difficult to pass into the bladder and may continue into the peritoneal cavity. Where pelvic injury is severe, it is advisable to perform a contrast urethrogram and cystogram to rule out large defects such as complete or partial avulsion of the bladder from the proximal urethra (see Chapter 25).

When the bladder is ruptured, debridement is carried out and repair is performed using 1 metric (5-0 USP) absorbable suture in a simple interrupted pattern. Placement of a urinary catheter postoperatively may facilitate healing. Where urinary leakage is occurring and surgical correction cannot be performed immediately, a urinary catheter can be passed into the bladder and connected to a closed urinary collection system (Figure 8.10). If a ureteral tear is present, or uroperitoneum persists, it is necessary to place a catheter into the peritoneal cavity to remove urine and reduce peritonitis, uraemia and hyperkalaemia (Figure 8.11).

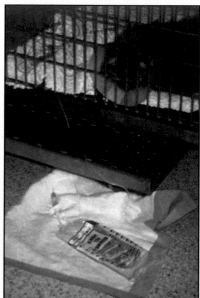

8.10

A sterile intravenous delivery set and fluid bag are attached to the urinary catheter. The bag may be hooked to a lower cage, or as in this case, placed on a clean barrier on the floor.

1. Strict aseptic technique is imperative.
2. Place a urinary catheter to remove urine or ensure that the bladder is empty.
3. Clip and surgically prepare and drape the mid-caudal abdomen.
4. Place 1 ml 1% lidocaine into the skin, subcutaneous tissues and abdominal wall on the midline, 1–2 cm caudal to the umbilicus.
5. Make a small incision through skin and subcutaneous tissues. The incision should just go to the depth of the linea alba if a manufactured peritoneal catheter (Abbot Laboratories) is used, as the stylet may facilitate passage through the linea alba. The incision should go through the linea alba if a sterile feeding tube is used. When using a sterile feeding tube, multiple holes must be made in this tube. Insert a 16 gauge over-the-needle catheter through the incision and infuse 10 ml/kg warm dialysate into the abdomen to elevate the abdominal wall prior to catheter placement. Place two stay sutures, one at each end of the proposed incision site, elevate the abdominal wall, and remove the 16 gauge catheter.
6. Direct the peritoneal dialysis catheter through the incision towards the pelvic inlet. Retract the stylet slightly prior to advancing the catheter. Be sure all holes in the catheter are in the abdomen otherwise urine or dialysate will leak into the subcutaneous tissue. The catheter is secured to the abdominal wall as instructed or with a purse-string and Chinese finger-trap technique.
7. A Jackson-Pratt suction drainage tubing system (without the vacuum bulb) is an excellent alternative to a commercial dialysis catheter. Alternatively, commercial over-the-wire peritoneal dialysis catheters (Mila, Arrow) can be placed using the Seldinger technique. Sterile feeding tubes, or 12 or 16 Fr Argyle trocar thoracic catheters can also be used for dialysis.
8. The peritoneal catheter is attached to a three-way stopcock. A sterile intravenous delivery set with an in-line roller clamp is attached to the stopcock and the other end attached to a sterile fluid bag for collection of urine or dialysate. The third port of the stopcock may be attached to a sterile intravenous line and used for delivery of dialysate if required.
9. A sterile dressing and bandage are applied. All connections should be covered with gauze sponges soaked in chlorhexidine or povidone–iodine.

8.11 Peritoneal dialysis: catheter placement.

Urethral injury

For small tears in the urinary bladder or proximal urethra, an indwelling urinary catheter or cystostomy tube may be used to divert urine while the injury heals. If urine leakage originates from the pelvic or distal urethra, or if a catheter cannot be passed, a tube cystostomy (Figure 8.12) should be placed into the bladder to divert the urine. Placement of a catheter or cystostomy is preferable to performing multiple cystocenteses while stabilizing the patient for definitive surgical correction.

Although small urethral tears can heal over a urinary catheter in 5–7 days without surgical intervention, larger ones require repair. The surgical approach to the intrapelvic urethra requires osteotomy of the pubis. The torn edges of the urethra are debrided and closed with 1 metric (5-0 USP) absorbable suture in a simple interrupted pattern. If the prostate is injured or opened during the surgical procedure, the capsule is closed. For complete instruction on surgical correction of urological injuries, a specialist surgical text should be consulted (Stone and Barsanti, 1992).

1. An appropriate analgesic or anaesthetic regimen is selected, and the skin and abdominal wall are infiltrated with 1–2 ml of 1% lidocaine.
2. A small incision, the size of an 8 Fr Foley catheter, is made lateral to the midline, midway between the umbilicus and pubis.
3. An 8 Fr Foley urinary catheter is placed through the incision and tunnelled through the subcutaneous tissue, to the midline.
4. On the midline, a 2–3 cm incision is made through the skin and abdominal wall, midway between the umbilicus and pubis.
5. The bladder is exteriorized through the midline incision and stabilized using two retention (stay) sutures with the needles left attached.
6. A purse-string suture is placed through the serosa and muscular layers of the ventral apical region of the bladder. A stab incision is made within the purse-string suture and the Foley catheter is introduced.
7. The balloon is inflated with sterile saline and the purse-string suture is carefully tightened snugly. Tying too tightly should be avoided or suture line necrosis may occur. Each retention suture is passed through the linea alba and tied as a simple interrupted suture.
8. The midline incision is closed routinely.
9. The catheter is connected to a closed collection system.

Note: While the lateral incision and tunnelling of the catheter are ideal, due to potential discomfort if local anaesthesia at the site is inadequate, direct entry into the abdomen may be considered.

8.12 Tube cystostomy.

If a urinary catheter is used in these patients, it should be placed very carefully to prevent iatrogenic damage to the urethra or urinary bladder. The patient should be monitored for adequate urine flow. If urine flow decreases, it may be due to improper positioning of the catheter or tube, blockage or kinking of the catheter, or poor urine production. Catheters should remain in place for up to 7 days while the tear heals.

Approach to acute intrinsic renal failure

Renal failure is described as acute or chronic. Acute renal failure (ARF) is an abrupt, severe reduction in renal function, commonly caused by ischaemic or toxic insults or infectious agents. Animals may be polyuric, oliguric or anuric, depending on the stage of the disease and the aetiology of the renal insult. The kidneys are either normal in size or large and painful. ARF can occur as a complication in hospitalized animals, especially if high-risk patients are not identified and are therefore managed inappropriately. Risk factors are additive: a geriatric patient may be more susceptible to ischaemic or toxic drug injuries than a younger animal. Animals with chronic renal failure usually have a history of polyuria and polydipsia and may have weight loss, reduced exercise tolerance, non-regenerative anaemia and small, irregularly shaped kidneys. Acute-on-chronic renal failure can occur both in and out of the hospital.

Diagnosis of renal failure is based on history, physical examination and laboratory data. ARF occurs in three phases:

- Initial phase, where the insult occurs and oliguria or polyuria and azotaemia are present
- Maintenance phase, where loss of renal function is established and progression to irreversible failure is possible
- Recovery phase, where resolution of azotaemia, nephron repair and functional compensation occur. The prognosis for recovery is difficult to define until appropriate therapy has proved unsuccessful.

Diagnostics for acute intrinsic renal failure

The history may reveal exposure to environmental toxins (e.g. ethylene glycol) or medications (e.g. aminoglycosides, NSAIDs), lack of vaccination for *Leptospira* spp., urinary tract infection or systemic illness. Physical examination should include: temperature; abdominal/bladder palpation; search for systemic illness; body condition and hydration status; weight; and neurological, respiratory and cardiovascular assessment. Hypotension is frequently associated with volume loss and systemic sepsis, however, hypertension is frequently associated with primary renal disease or infection. Prior to commencing fluid therapy, blood should be obtained for emergency and routine minimum databases (see Figure 8.6), and a urine sample should be obtained and tested if possible (see Figures 8.7 and 8.8). Diagnosis is based on serum biochemistry, urinalysis, urine culture, complete blood count, ultrasonography and serology. The underlying cause of the ARF should be aggressively investigated as specific therapy (e.g. antibiosis) may be indicated.

Abnormalities on haematological and biochemical testing may suggest the underlying cause. Infectious causes of ARF are frequently associated with leucocytosis or leucopenia, and occasionally non-regenerative anaemia. Thrombocytopenia may also be associated with rickettsial disease, vasculitis, disseminated intravascular coagulation, advanced renal disease or ethylene glycol intoxication. Hyperglycaemia has been reported in dogs with ethylene glycol intoxication. Hypocalcaemia is a frequent finding in ethylene glycol intoxication and pancreatitis. Hypercalcaemia may be associated with advanced renal disease, cholecalciferol (vitamin D3) rodenticide intoxication and neoplastic disease. Where possible, it should be ascertained whether the hypercalcaemia represents an increase in ionized or total calcium as this may have diagnostic implications (see Chapter 5).

Electrolyte and acid–base information is vital to aid immediate therapy, especially of hyperkalaemia. Hyperkalaemia should be suspected in any patient with a low (or normal) heart rate when in ARF. Occasionally, tachycardia may be present during the early stage of hyperkalaemia. If potassium measurement is not immediately available, an ECG can be used to evaluate the effects of the hyperkalaemia on the conduction system of the heart and to guide therapy.

Of infectious causes, leptospirosis in dogs has increased markedly in incidence in the United States and Canada over the past 6 years (Prescott *et al.*, 2002). Typically, acute leptospire infections occur during the autumn months, which tend to have higher rainfall. The major clinical presentation is acute onset of depression, anorexia, vomiting and fever accompanied by haematological and biochemical changes associated with inflammation and multi-organ dysfunction. Increased serum creatinine and urea may also be associated with increased serum alkaline phosphatase, alanine aminotransferase and bilirubin due to associated liver infection. Increased serum creatine kinase is frequently present. A leucocytosis with a marked neutrophilia occurs, and is associated with thrombocytopenia in approximately one third of affected dogs (Prescott *et al.*, 2002). Leptospirosis may be diagnosed by demonstrating a four-fold rise in agglutination titre over a 1–2-week period. A single high titre associated with clinical signs is suggestive of active leptospirosis. The major serovars involved are *Leptospira bratislava, L. grippotyphosa, L. pomona* and *L. autumnalis.* In one study, *Leptospira autumnalis* was the most common serovar isolated, however, this was felt to be an erroneous representation or 'paradoxical' reaction of early leptospiral serology (Prescott *et al.*, 2002). Similarly, other infectious causes of ARF (e.g. ehrlichiosis) may be diagnosed based on clinical signs and serological testing.

Treatment

The goals of treatment are to correct fluid, electrolyte and acid–base disorders, establish or maintain urine flow, and treat the underlying cause of renal failure. Potentially nephrotoxic drugs must be discontinued. An intravenous catheter is placed using strict aseptic technique, either peripherally for rapid fluid resuscitation, or into the jugular vein for fluid therapy and measurement of central venous pressure (CVP). If oliguria or anuria is suspected, an indwelling urinary catheter is placed to monitor urine output.

Intravenous fluid therapy is the most important treatment for ARF. An isotonic, alkalinizing, replacement electrolyte solution (e.g. Hartmann's) is preferred to improve acidaemia, thus facilitating potassium translocation into cells. If renal failure is associated with hypercalcaemia, 0.9% sodium chloride is preferred to enhance calciuresis. Fluids correct dehydration and expand the intravascular space, with subsequent improvement in systemic perfusion. In addition, fluid therapy may overcome some forms of intrarenal vasoconstriction, improve renal perfusion, initiate diuresis, hasten removal of nephrotoxic substances and prevent or correct renal tubular obstruction with cellular debris.

As a guide to the volume of fluid required to rehydrate an animal, the hydration deficit is calculated by estimating percentage dehydration and multiplying by body weight in kilograms. A 10 kg dog that is 10% dehydrated will require 10 x 10/100 litres = 1.0 litre of fluid to correct the deficit (see Chapter 4). Ongoing and maintenance losses are estimated (see Figure 8.4) and added to the volume deficit. The rate of administration depends on the acuity of the loss and the volume of urine being produced. In chronic dehydration, when urine is being produced and the patient is not azotaemic, the deficit should be replaced over 24–48 hours. In anuric or acutely oliguric animals, regardless of their hydration status, a fluid bolus of 20 ml/kg (dogs) and 10 ml/kg (cats) should be administered over 10 minutes, while monitoring the animal's ability to tolerate this volume. If urine flow is not established and the animal is showing no signs of fluid overload, the remaining deficit should be administered over the next 1–2 hours. If the animal is judged not to be clinically dehydrated at presentation, it is best to assume 3–5% dehydration and administer this volume over 1–2 hours, or rapidly as previously described, to ensure volume expansion (e.g. 10 kg x 3–5/100 = 0.3–0.5 litres). If the patient is considered to be at high risk of fluid overload (e.g. concurrent cardiac disease), the deficit should be administered over 4 hours and the animal monitored carefully. The goal is to ensure optimal expansion of the intravascular volume, to replace fluid deficits and to initiate urine production at 1–2 ml/kg/h. Close monitoring is vital to avoid overhydration and to ensure that urine production is maintained.

If an adequate volume of crystalloid has been administered based on physical examination and appropriate calculation of the deficit, and urine production remains less than 1 ml/kg/h, or the patient is hypotensive, hypoproteinaemic (TP <50 g/l) or anaemic (PCV <25%), further measures are required. As appropriate, hydroxyethyl starch, plasma or whole blood should be administered to increase or maintain oncotic and systemic arterial pressures and to improve renal blood flow and oxygen delivery. If systemic arterial pressures are still unacceptably low, dopamine (5–10 µg/kg/min to effect) should be added to improve cardiac output. At this point, hypoadrenocorticism should also be ruled out and treated if necessary. Adrenal insufficiency may be primary or secondary, permanent or transient, and may develop following trauma or surgery and during sepsis and other critical illness. If poor cardiac contractility is thought to be contributing to hypotension, dobutamine can be used, starting at 5 µg/kg/min in dogs. In cats, dobutamine should be started at an initial rate of 1 µg/kg/min and slowly increased to effect, with a maximum dose of 4 µg/kg/min. Dobutamine and dopamine can be administered simultaneously in dogs. Should hypotension persist, dobutamine should be discontinued and noradrenaline can be used (constant rate infusion (CRI) 0.01–0.1 µg/kg/min, rarely higher dosages may be required). Dopamine can be discontinued or maintained during noradrenaline therapy.

The overall goals are to expand intravascular volume, replace fluid deficits and normalize oncotic and blood pressures, thereby initiating urine production at 1–2 ml/kg/h, without overhydration. Once volume expansion and normotension have been established, if urine production remains less than 1 ml/kg/h, diuretics should be administered. Their use should not be postponed, as renal failure may be difficult to reverse at a later time. Furosemide and/or mannitol are preferred. If acute tubular necrosis is suspected and there are no contraindications, mannitol may be the better choice. Contraindications to the use of mannitol include evidence of overhydration including pulmonary or interstitial oedema, hyperosmolarity (e.g. hypernatraemia, ethylene glycol or salicylate toxicosis, hyperglycaemia), the presence of ongoing haemorrhage, or if there is evidence or concern for capillary leak. Mannitol produces an osmotic diuresis and reduces cellular oedema and reperfusion injury by scavenging oxygen free radicals. It is given at 0.25

g/kg i.v. over 5–10 minutes and repeated after 30–40 minutes to maintain diuresis. Mannitol should not be repeated if urine flow is <1 ml/kg/h within 60 minutes of the initial bolus.

If there is no response to mannitol, or furosemide is preferred or indicated (see contraindications for mannitol above), furosemide should be administered intravenously at 2–4 mg/kg (dog), or 2 mg/kg (cat). Furosemide enhances aminoglycoside nephrotoxicity, therefore the use of these drugs concurrently should be avoided. If no beneficial effect on urine output is seen in 30 minutes, the dose should be repeated once in the cat, or once or twice, at 6 mg/kg, in the dog at 1-hour intervals. If mannitol or furosemide are not available, hypertonic dextrose in water (20% solution), at 2–10 ml/kg over 1–5 minutes, may establish diuresis. Glucosuria does not necessarily indicate success of diuresis unless urine output approaches 1–4 ml/kg/h.

If urine flow is established but the patient remains oliguric, a CRI of furosemide at 0.1–1 mg/kg/h may facilitate diuresis. Although it is currently controversial, dopamine at 1–3 µg/kg/min can be administered in combination with furosemide to maintain adequate renal perfusion. If tachycardia or other dysrhythmia develops during dopamine administration, the drug should be discontinued and restarted at a lower dose.

This author has found diltiazem useful in establishing and maintaining urine flow in dogs with leptospirosis, and enhancing renal recovery when compared to standard therapy (Mathews and Monteith, in press). Diltiazem (0.3–0.5 mg/kg) is administered slowly intravenously while assessing systemic blood pressure and heart rate, followed by a CRI at 2–5 µg/kg/min (0.9–2.3 µg/lb/min) if systemic blood pressure and heart rate are not adversely affected. The CRI is maintained until serum creatinine falls to within normal range, and is then discontinued by reducing the dose over a few hours. Furosemide administration (as described above) may be combined with diltiazem but should be withdrawn when urine output is more than adequate.

Peritoneal dialysis (Figures 8.11 and 8.13) or haemodialysis should be considered in the anuric animal when attempts at establishing urine flow have failed.

If urinalysis indicates the presence of infection, pyelonephritis may be the cause of renal failure. Antibiotic therapy should be based on culture and antibiogram. Commonly isolated bacteria include the Gram-negative rods *Escherichia coli*, *Klebsiella pneumoniae*, *Pseudomonas aeruginosa* or *Proteus mirabilis*, and the Gram-positive cocci *Staphylococcus aureus* or *Streptococcus* spp. While waiting for culture and sensitivity results, depending on whether cocci or rods were identified on urinalysis, antibiotic choices can include amoxicillin/clavulanic acid 10 mg/kg q12h orally, ampicillin–sulbactam 20 mg/kg (ampicillin component) q8h i.v. or i.m., cefazolin 20 mg/kg q6h i.v. or trimethoprim–sulfamethoxazole/sulfadiazine 30 mg/kg q12h orally or i.v. (check formulation). If the animal is vomiting or systemically ill, oral drugs should be avoided. Considering its capability to induce antibiotic resistance, enrofloxacin (10 mg/kg q24h i.v. or orally in dogs, or 5 mg/kg q24h i.v. or orally in cats) should only be used if indicated. Indications include the suspicion of *Pseudomonas*, the absence of

1. Commercial dialysate (Dianeal, Baxter) with dextrose 0, 1.5, 2.5 or 4.5%, or homemade dialysate using lactated Ringer's solution or 0.45% or 0.9% saline with the appropriate volume of dextrose added, should be used. Do not use acetate or gluconate-containing solutions as they are painful when infused. Select 1.5% dextrose if normally hydrated and 4.5% if oedematous, overhydrated or hyperosmolar. The concentration can be reduced as the hydration status and osmolarity improves. The dialysate should be warmed and maintained at body temperature.

2. In a small patient where multiple infusions can be obtained from a single dialysate bag, attach the intravenous delivery tubing to one arm of the three-way stopcock and the collection bag to the second arm.

3. Initially infuse 20 ml/kg of the dialysate into the peritoneal space slowly by gravity, while watching the patient's response. Record the volume infused. Overload is detected by an increase in respiratory rate, anxiety, leakage through the insertion site or overly distended abdomen. Close the stopcock. Allow a 45-minute dwell time.

4. If all the dialysate is used, close the roller clamp and place the bag below the patient (on sterile paper or towel). Open the roller clamp to allow slow drainage (over 15 minutes) by gravity. Drain as much as possible. Record the volume and discard.

5. If only a portion of the dialysate is used, close the roller clamp and the stopcock to the dialysate, and allow slow drainage by gravity into the collection bag.

6. The dialysate remaining in the bag must be kept warm.

7. Repeat every hour initially. As the patient improves or stabilizes, the procedure can be extended to every 4–6 hours.

8. Initially, volumes of dialysate recovered may be less than infused. Once dehydration is corrected, volumes should equalize or the volume recovered may increase due to ultrafiltration in the oedematous patient.

9. Monitor for fluid overload and assess the patient daily.

10. White blood cell count and Gram stain should be performed on the dialysate daily.

8.13 Peritoneal dialysis technique. For peritoneal dialysis catheter placement, see Figure 8.11.

Gram-positive cocci on Gram stain and ineffectiveness of other antibiotic therapy. If leptospirosis is suspected, ampicillin is used at 20 mg/kg q8h i.v. While many antibiotics concentrate in urine and will therefore be effective in treating cystitis, this concentration effect does not apply to the renal parenchyma, which should be considered similar to any other organ with respect to penetration and appropriate antibiotic levels.

Metoclopramide (1 mg/kg/24h CRI, or 0.2 mg/kg q8h s.c.) can be used to control vomiting, and H_2 blockers at half the recommended dose, with sucralfate, should be considered for ulcer treatment and prophylaxis. Hyperphosphataemia may be treated with phosphate binders or sucralfate. Nutritional support should be considered. Treatment for specific causes of renal failure should also be pursued.

Approach to proteinuria

Patients with uncomplicated proteinuria rarely present as emergencies but increased urinary protein levels may be identified on urine dipstick evaluation during assessment of the critically ill animal. Proteinuria may or may not be associated with azotaemia and is often secondary to underlying disease. The urine protein:creatinine ratio (UP/UC) is a sensitive, rapid and convenient test for the detection and quantification of protein in randomly collected urine samples (see Figures 8.4 and 8.5). Lower urinary tract sources of increased urinary protein should be ruled out to allow valid interpretation of the UP/UC as a marker of glomerular disease. UP/UC values <0.5 are normal; values between 0.5 and 1.0 are questionable and values >1.0 are abnormal. There are many causes of increased urine protein, but UP/UC values of 1–5 are usually associated with pre- and postrenal causes or glomerulosclerosis/atrophy; values of 5–13 are associated with non-amyloid glomerulopathy; and values >13 usually indicate severe glomerulopathy or amyloidosis (Lulich and Osborne, 1990). As severe proteinuria is associated with a hypercoaguable state, proteinuric patients may occasionally present as emergencies with signs of thromboembolic disease, such as dyspnoea (see Chapter 13).

Approach to lower urinary tract obstruction

Most commonly, either the bladder or urethra is obstructed. The history includes stranguria (owners may mistakenly report constipation), dysuria, pollakiuria or anuria, and males are more frequently affected. The clinical condition of a dog or cat with urethral obstruction depends on the duration and severity (partial, total or functional) of the obstruction. Although the animal may be straining to urinate, systemic signs are usually not present in the first 24 hours following obstruction. Postrenal azotaemia develops within 48 hours with signs of uraemia occurring shortly afterwards. With total urethral obstruction no urine is voided, but an occasional drop of urine may drip from the penis or vulva. The abdomen must be palpated gently to avoid exacerbating pain or rupturing a large tense urinary bladder. If a bladder cannot be palpated in an animal in which urethral obstruction is highly likely, a ruptured bladder should be suspected. Rarely, ureteroliths may result in bilateral ureteral obstruction and anuria. In this situation the bladder is empty.

Idiopathic, non-obstructive feline lower urinary tract disease

Diagnosis

Idiopathic, non-obstructive feline lower urinary tract disease, also called 'idiopathic cystitis' (interstitial cystitis in humans), is a diagnosis of exclusion. Suggested pathophysiology and clinical experience is reported elsewhere (Buffington and Chew, 1995). The behaviour of cats with this disease is similar to that of cats with obstructive disease, but physical obstruction is usually not a feature. Voiding appears painful, and haematuria and pollakiuria may be associated with dysuria. The cat may void in inappropriate places, groom the caudal abdomen and genitals frequently and resent abdominal palpation. These cats are usually presented as an emergency due to dysuria, inappropriate urination or haematuria. Occasionally the cat develops a functional obstruction and has a hard, moderately enlarged bladder associated with azotaemia or uraemia. A urinary catheter is passed easily into the urethra and bladder. Crystals and 'mucus-like' material may be present. The urinalysis is usually normal except for the presence of microscopic or grossly visible blood. The pH of the urine is frequently <6.5 and no bacteria are seen. Ultrasonography and contrast cystography reveal thickening of the bladder wall and contrast material may dissect under the urothelium.

Treatment

If an enlarged bladder is palpated, a urinary catheter should be passed to rule out obstruction and obtain urine for sediment and crystal identification. Urine culture is usually unnecessary, as this disease is not associated with bacteria. If frequent urethral catheterization has been performed, infection may be present and culture is warranted. When cats have been unable to void, presumably due to reflex dyssynergia secondary to cystitis, the urinary catheter must usually remain in place for at least 2 days until medical management has taken effect. Cats that have experienced functional urethral obstruction may be azotaemic, requiring fluid therapy (see acute renal failure) to reverse the azotaemia/uraemia. Phenoxybenzamine (0.5 mg/kg q24h orally or 0.25 mg/kg q12h orally) is administered to reduce urethral spasm but may require 24–48 hours for full effect. Hypotension is a possible but rare side effect related to α-adrenergic blockade, and this drug should not be used in cats with cardiovascular disease. If detrusor dysfunction is identified, bethanechol (1.25–5.0 mg q8h orally) may be administered to enhance bladder emptying, after urethral patency and function have been established. Bethanechol may cause bladder rupture if there is resistance to urine flow. Amitriptyline (2.5–12.5 mg (5 mg/cat typical dose) q24h orally at bedtime for 5–7 days) may be used and dosed to produce a barely perceptible calming effect. The analgesic, anti-inflammatory, anticholinergic and reduced adrenergic effects of amitriptyline may also contribute to relief of symptoms in these cats. Possible side effects include urine retention and increased liver enzymes. In addition, increasing water intake, including feeding canned food, reducing stressors in the environment and identifying associated crystalluria, are all necessary to treat the cystitis.

Urethral obstruction

Diagnosis

Urethral obstruction due to uroliths (dogs and cats) or urethral plugs (cats) is a common cause of anuria in dogs and cats, but other causes must also be considered. Transitional cell carcinoma and granulomatous urethritis may produce similar clinical signs of obstruction. The animal may appear physiologically normal or may be depressed, vomiting, in shock or unconscious. A large hard painful bladder may be palpable in the abdomen. Bradycardia, hypothermia, pale mucous membranes with prolonged capillary refill time, hyperpnoea and halitosis may be present. In cats with urethral obstruction, the tip of the penis is often dark red/

purple and swollen. In dogs, a urolith may be palpated anywhere from the ischial arch to the os penis and the penis may be discoloured. If uroliths are ruled out, a rectal examination of the prostate and bladder trigone should be performed in the male dog and a vaginal examination for vaginal/urethral masses in the bitch. Ultrasonography and/or contrast urography and cystography, in addition to urine cytology and urethral or bladder biopsy, are required for diagnosis of granulomatous and neoplastic lesions. Inability to void may also be associated with spinal disease or injuries, especially those that involve the sacrum (Kuntz et al., 1995). These patients require a full neurological evaluation.

Emergency stabilization

If the animal is extremely depressed, oxygen should be administered by mask, an intravenous catheter placed, and blood should be obtained for an emergency minimum database. Fluid therapy should be instituted immediately with the rate based on the degree of hypoperfusion and/or dehydration present. The degree of dehydration is estimated and an isotonic replacement electrolyte solution is administered over 12 hours if the animal is minimally dehydrated, over 4 hours if it is moderately dehydrated, and over 1–2 hours if shock is present. These rates of administration may be modified according to response to therapy, which should be reassessed every 5–10 minutes. If a bradydysrhythmia is detected, an electrocardiogram (ECG) should be obtained. Hyperkalaemia, if associated with bradycardia, should be treated aggressively (see Chapter 5) prior to relieving the obstruction. If acidosis is present and hyperkalaemia is not associated with life-threatening signs, fluid resuscitation alone will often be sufficient to correct the values. A balanced electrolyte solution, which contains potassium, does not have a negative effect on outcome.

Relieving the obstruction

If the patient is severely depressed, sedation may not be required. If in pain or alert, the dog or cat should be sedated or anaesthetized using one of the following:

* Morphine (0.1–0.3 mg/kg i.m.)
* Butorphanol (0.2–0.4 mg/kg i.v. or i.m.)
* Propofol (2–4 mg/kg i.v.)
* Short-acting thiobarbiturate (5 mg/kg i.v.)
* Mask isoflurane anaesthesia
* Ketamine (2.5–5.0 mg/kg i.v.) mixed with diazepam (0.125–0.25 mg/kg i.v.) or midazolam (0.125–0.25 mg/kg i.v. or i.m.).

Caution should be exercised with ketamine combinations if renal compromise is suspected in cats (ketamine is metabolized by the liver in dogs), and vomiting may occur following morphine administration. With any medication, the lowest dose possible should be used. Prior to anaesthesia, plasma potassium should be estimated where possible and an ECG trace obtained. Severe hyperkalaemia should be addressed (see Chapter 5).

If the bladder requires immediate decompression, cystocentesis (see Figure 8.8) can be performed prior to relieving the obstruction. A 22 gauge over-the-needle catheter can be used, the needle removed and an extension with three-way stopcock attached. Care must be taken not to move the catheter and to aspirate carefully, as the bladder might tear. As much urine as possible should be removed to reduce the risk of urine leakage into the abdomen at the cystocentesis site. Urethral catheterization should be performed as soon as possible after the cystocentesis. Only one cystocentesis should be performed, to avoid urine leakage into the abdomen. As urethral catheterization can often be achieved rapidly, the risks of cystocentesis in a patient with a compromised bladder wall should be carefully considered.

In male cats, the penis is gently massaged between the thumb and forefinger and extremely gentle pressure is applied to the bladder. If the obstruction is not immediately relieved, hydropulsion should be attempted using a lubricated (water-soluble lubricant) polypropylene tom cat catheter, an ophthalmic lacrimal duct flush cannula, or a 22 gauge over-the-needle catheter without its stylet. The prepuce is cleaned with chlorhexidine soap and rinsed with warm water. A 10–20 ml syringe is filled with sterile saline, the penis is extended caudally (making the urethra as straight as possible), the catheter is engaged in the tip of the penis and the urethra is flushed while advancing the catheter. Gently twisting the catheter can sometimes aid its passage. If the bladder is turgid, a single cystocentesis may relieve pressure within the bladder to facilitate hydropulsion. Once the catheter has been passed into the bladder, the bladder is pressed gently to empty it, then flushed multiple times slowly with warm sterile saline until clear, emptying the bladder each time. In large cats, the tom cat catheter may not reach the bladder and a 3.5 Fr rubber urinary catheter or paediatric feeding tube is recommended for longer-term catheterization. The bladder should remain catheterized if:

- Relief of the obstruction was difficult
- The urine stream is small
- The bladder was overly distended and detrusor function may be questionable
- The animal is uraemic or markedly azotaemic and diuresis is necessary
- If post-obstructive diuresis is likely and measurement of urine output is necessary in the immediate post-obstructive phase.

For indwelling catheters, the catheter is advanced into the bladder until urine appears, then advanced 1 cm further; it is secured to the patient by placing an adhesive tape butterfly around the proximal end of the catheter and suturing it to the prepuce in a horizontal pattern. A sterile intravenous administration set and empty fluid bag are attached to the urinary catheter and then maintained as a closed collection system (see Figure 8.10).

Urethral catheterization of queens is performed blindly with the cat in lateral or sternal recumbency; however, if preferred, dorsal recumbency may also be appropriate. The vulva is cleaned with chlorhexidine soap and rinsed with warm water. A lubricated (water-soluble lubricant) 3.5 Fr paediatric feeding tube is passed into the vagina along the ventral aspect of the vestibular floor. The catheter commonly passes into the entrance of the urethra. The remaining technique is similar to that for the male above but with suturing to the vulva. An otoscope may be useful to identify the external urethral orifice should the blind technique fail.

In dogs with urethral obstruction, cystocentesis may be performed if necessary. Attempts are made to pass a small-gauge catheter beyond the obstruction into the bladder to remove the urine. In males, if the obstruction is due to a urolith (frequently in or just caudal to the os penis), the urolith should be hydropulsed into the bladder using as short a catheter as possible, or a round-ended teat cannula. Two people are required for this procedure; one occludes the proximal urethra via rectal palpation and compression against the pubic symphysis and the other retracts the penis, cleans the urethral orifice and passes the catheter a short distance into the urethra. The external urethral orifice is then manually occluded. A 35–60 ml syringe is filled with equal volumes of well mixed sterile saline and sterile aqueous lubricating jelly and the mixture is injected into the urethra. Once the urethra is distended, the proximal per rectum occlusion is released while fluid injection is continued, and the urolith is flushed into the bladder. Lubricating jelly should not be used in the flush if a tear or deep abrasion of the urethra or bladder is suspected.

In bitches with urethral obstruction, a Foley catheter is placed into the urethral orifice and the balloon inflated. The urethra is flushed without proximal occlusion of the urethra. If hydropulsion is not successful in relieving the obstruction, caution must be used to avoid injuring the urethra, and surgical removal is advisable.

A cystotomy is required to remove uroliths retropulsed into the bladder, while urethrostomy is required to remove uroliths that continue to obstruct the urethra. In some dogs voiding urohydropropulsion, a non-surgical technique for removal of urocystoliths (Lulich and Osborne, 1995a), may be attempted. If attempts to relieve the obstruction fail, emergency decompression of the bladder via catheter cystostomy may be necessary while the patient is stabilized.

If hydropulsion is successful, a urinary catheter is passed into the bladder to remove the urine (see Figure 8.7). The bladder should be gently flushed to remove the lubricating jelly, blood clots or crystals. If the catheter remains in place, it should be attached to a closed urinary collection system. The duration of urinary catheter placement depends on the severity of the problem, but is usually a minimum of 24 hours.

Treatment

The cause of granulomatous urethritis in bitches is unknown, but it is frequently associated with primary or secondary bacterial cystitis. Catheterization of the urinary bladder is necessary to permit emptying. Immunosuppressive doses of prednisolone (2–3 mg/kg daily) have been suggested, with antibiotic therapy based on culture and sensitivity results.

Urethral obstruction due to neoplasia and associated inflammation may be successfully managed with a temporary indwelling urinary catheter, empirical or specific antibiotic therapy based on culture and sensitivity and piroxicam (0.3 mg/kg q24h for 3 days, then every 48 hours or to effect). If reflex dyssynergia is likely, this therapy in addition to phenoxybenzamine (5–15 mg/dog q24h orally for 5–7 days), may be effective.

Haematomas of the bladder or urethra may require hydropulsion and bladder flushing, while maintaining urine flow with an indwelling urinary catheter. If a coagulopathy is present, it should be identified and treated (see Chapter 13) to prevent further bleeding. If the haematoma is due to trauma, the injury should be identified via contrast urography. Inadvertent obstruction of urine flow due to iatrogenic ligation of the urethra may occur after any surgical procedure associated with the urethra (e.g. perineal hernia, castration, urethral surgery) or bladder (e.g. hysterectomy, prostatic surgery).

Perineal hernia with prolapsed urinary bladder may result in anuria and obstructed passage of a urinary catheter. Cystocentesis is required while planning emergency surgical correction. Similarly, prostatomegaly may cause urethral obstruction (see Chapter 15).

A tube cystostomy (see Figure 8.12) should be placed if urine leakage originates from the pelvic and distal urethra, or if a urinary catheter cannot be passed into the bladder in any animal. Due to the risk of complications, emergency urethrostomy should only be performed if absolutely essential. For emergency decompression of the bladder, a catheter or tube cystostomy is preferred to multiple cystocenteses, while stabilizing the patient for definitive surgical correction. After relief of any obstruction, if urine production is <0.5 ml/kg/h and non-responsive to estimated fluid requirements, consider treatment for oliguric/anuric renal failure as above.

Monitoring

Monitoring fluid administration

After urine flow has been established, regardless of the underlying problem, ongoing fluid requirements may be calculated as follows:

1. Divide the day into six 4-hour intervals, four 6-hour intervals or three 8-hour intervals, depending on severity of illness and availability of staff.
2. Determine urine produced during each time interval and add the estimated insensible loss for that period.
3. Determine ongoing losses in vomitus, diarrhoea and saliva over this same interval.
4. Determine insensible loss, 20 ml/kg/day, and for each degree Celsius above 38.5, add 10% of normal daily maintenance fluid requirement (for example if normal daily requirement is 1 litre and temperature is 40.5°C then 200 ml should be added). Divide this amount by 6, 4 or 3 depending on intervals selected above.
5. This total volume of fluid is to be delivered over the next time period.

Any fluid challenge must be monitored closely but if cardiac or pulmonary disease is present, CVP monitoring is advised. An increase in CVP >4 cmH$_2$O, with a slow decrease to baseline, indicates hypervolaemia or right-sided cardiac disease. Fluid therapy should be discontinued temporarily if the CVP reaches 13 cmH$_2$O (dogs) or increases by 2 cmH$_2$O or more in any 10-minute period. In addition to CVP (or if CVP is not available) the following signs can also indicate overhydration:

- Shivering
- Restlessness
- Serous nasal discharge
- Tachypnoea
- Nausea
- Vomiting
- Tachycardia (followed by bradycardia when severely overloaded)
- Subcutaneous oedema (especially the hock joint and intermandibular space)
- Pulmonary crackles and oedema
- Exophthalmos
- Chemosis
- Cough
- Dyspnoea
- Polyuria
- Diarrhoea
- Depressed mentation
- Ascites.

Monitoring ongoing therapy

The following parameters must be monitored during ongoing patient management, to assess efficacy of therapy and to prevent, identify and treat abnormalities that arise:

- Creatinine or urea or both (daily). Urea (or BUN) is not a reliable test for renal assessment as it will increase when blood is present in the gastrointestinal tract, following a high-protein meal and during starvation, fever and infection, and will decrease in hepatic insufficiency/failure and following administration of anabolic steroids. However, for monitoring trends, and whilst keeping these shortcomings in mind, it is still useful and inexpensive (BUN stick)
- Urine specific gravity (with urine volume measurement every 1–8 hours)
- Urine sediment (every 48 hours if acute tubular necrosis)
- Weight gain or loss (every 8–24 hours to assess fluid loss/gain)
- Serum electrolytes, specifically potassium (every 4–24 hours with hypo- or hyperkalaemia) and phosphorus
- Venous blood gases, or total carbon dioxide (every 6–24 hours to assess metabolic status)
- Anion gap (with electrolyte and blood gas or total carbon dioxide measurements) (see Figure 8.4)
- Urine sodium and creatinine (where indicated to assess prerenal versus renal problem) (see Figure 8.4)
- Urine protein:creatinine ratio (every 72 hours) to assess therapy and prognosis (see Figure 8.4)
- Urine production (hourly to every 8 hours depending on situation).

Monitoring urine output

The volume of urine output depends on the underlying problem. The goal is to maintain at least 1–2 ml/kg/h. However, in the presence of renal tubular injury or loss of concentrating ability for other reasons, urine output can be extremely high (25–40 ml/kg/h). In this situation it is important to measure urine output and use this to guide adequate fluid replacement. Urine volume can be measured by collection when the animal voids, use of a metabolism cage, by intermittent or continuous urinary bladder catheterization or by placing preweighed towels under the vulva or penis and weighing them after voiding. Any increase in towel weight over baseline, unless otherwise soiled, is assumed to be due to urine. Assuming 1000 ml equals 1000 g, the volume of urine voided can be estimated. This technique usually underestimates urine produced, as some urine may remain in the cage. Weighing the animal several times daily assists in estimating urine output. Should the animal's weight decline despite fluid therapy, it is assumed that ongoing losses such as high urine output, vomiting, diarrhoea, salivation, fever or hyperthermia are in excess of fluid administration. A weight loss of 0.1–0.3 kg body weight/1000 kcal energy requirement should be assumed in an anorexic animal.

When the animal is recumbent and monitoring urine output is especially important, most critical care clinicians prefer to use an indwelling urinary catheter attached to a sterile intravenous fluid delivery line and urine collection bag (see Figure 8.10). The exterior of the catheter is cleaned several times a day with chlorhexidine. Should the prepuce or vulva become soiled, it is cleaned with chlorhexidine soap and rinsed with warm water. Antibiotics are avoided unless required to treat an existing infection. The urine is cultured after 72 hours or sooner if indicated. The catheter is removed as soon as possible and the urine cultured following removal. The tip of the urinary catheter should not be cultured, as a positive result does not necessarily reflect infection in the urinary bladder.

References and further reading

Binns SH (1994) Pathogenesis and pathophysiology of ischemic injury in cases of acute renal failure. *Compendium on Continuing Education for the Practicing Veterinarian* **16**, 31–40

Bjorling DE (1993) The urinary system. In: *Textbook of Small Animal Surgery, 2nd edn*, ed. D Slatter, pp. 1368–1495. WB Saunders, Philadelphia

Buffington CAT and Chew DJ (1995) Does interstitial cystitis occur in cats? In: *Kirk's Current Veterinary Therapy Small Animal Practice XII*, ed. J Bonagura, pp. 1009–1011. WB Saunders, Philadelphia

Buffington CAT and Chew DJ (1997) Lower urinary tract diseases in cats: the Ohio experience. Proceedings of the 15th American College of Veterinary Internal Medicine Forum, Buena Vista, Florida, pp. 343–346

Burrows CF (1974) Metabolic changes due to experimentally induced rupture of the canine urinary bladder. *American Journal of Veterinary Research* **35**, 1083–1088

Forrester SD (1996) Acute renal failure due to systemic diseases. Proceedings of the 14th American College of Veterinary Internal Medicine Forum, San Antonio, Texas, pp. 362–364

Forrester SD and Brandt KS (1994) The diagnostic approach to the patient with acute renal failure. Symposium on acute renal failure. *Veterinary Medicine* **89**, 212–218

Forrester SD, Jacobson JD and Fallin EA (1994) Taking measures to prevent acute renal failure. Symposium on acute renal failure. *Veterinary Medicine* **89**, 231–236

Hitt ME (1986) Hematuria of renal origin. *Compendium on Continuing Education for the Practicing Veterinarian* **8**, 14–19

Holt PE (1994) Other diagnostic aids. In: *Colour Atlas of Small Animal Urology*, pp. 33–54. Mosby-Wolfe, London

Kuntz CA, Waldron D, Martin RA *et al.* (1995) Sacral fractures in dogs: a review of 32 cases. *Journal of the American Animal Hospital Association* **31**, 142–150

Lane IF and Grauer GF (1994) Management of acute renal failure. Symposium on acute renal failure. *Veterinary Medicine* **89**, 319–230

Lane IF, Grauer GF and Fettman MJ (1994a) Acute renal failure. Part I. Risk factors, prevention, and strategies for protection. *Compendium on Continuing Education for the Practicing Veterinarian* **16**, 15–28

Lane IF, Grauer GF and Fettman MJ (1994b) Acute renal failure. Part II. Diagnosis, management, and prognosis. *Compendium on Continuing Education for the Practicing Veterinarian* **16**, 625–642

Lee JA and Drobatz KJ (2003) Characterization of the clinical characteristics, electrolytes, acid-base, and renal parameters in male cats with urethral obstruction. *Journal of Veterinary Emergency and Critical Care* **13(4)**, 227–233

Ling GV (1995) Nephrolithiasis: prevalence of mineral type. In: *Kirk's Current Veterinary Therapy Small Animal Practice XII*, ed. J Bonagura, p. 980. WB Saunders, Philadelphia

Ling GV and Sorenson JL (1995) CVT Update: management and prevention of urate lithiasis. In: *Kirk's Current Veterinary Therapy Small Animal Practice XII*, ed. J Bonagura, pp. 985–989. WB Saunders, Philadelphia

Lulich JP and Osborne CA (1990) Interpretation of urine protein-creatinine ratios in dogs with glomerular and nonglomerular disorders. *Compendium on Continuing Education for the Practicing Veterinarian* **12**, 59–72

Lulich JP and Osborne CA (1995a) Voiding urohydropulsion: a non-surgical technique for removal of urocystoliths. In: *Kirk's Current Veterinary Therapy Small Animal Practice XII*, ed. J Bonagura, pp. 1003–1007. WB Saunders, Philadelphia

Lulich JP and Osborne CA (1995b) Canine calcium oxalate uroliths. In: *Kirk's Current Veterinary Therapy Small Animal Practice XII*, ed. J Bonagura, pp. 992–996. WB Saunders, Philadelphia

Mathews KA, Holmberg DL, Johnston K *et al.* (1994) Renal allograft survival in outbred mongrel dogs using anti-dog thymocyte serum in combination with immunosuppressive drug therapy with or without donor bone marrow. *Journal of Veterinary Surgery* **23**, 347–357

Mathews KA and Monteith G (in press) A pilot study evaluating the safety and efficacy of diltiazem therapy for acute renal failure in 18 dogs with leptospirosis. *Journal of Veterinary Emergency and Critical Care*

Morgan RV (1982) Urogenital emergencies. Part 1. *Compendium on Continuing Education for the Practicing Veterinarian* **4**, 908–915

Osborne CA (1983) Azotemia: a review of what's old and what's new. Part 1. Definition of terms and concepts. *Compendium on Continuing Education for the Practicing Veterinarian* **5**, 497–510

Osborne CA, Klausner JS and Lulich JP (1995) Canine and feline calcium phosphate urolithiasis. In: *Kirk's Current Veterinary Therapy Small Animal Practice XII*, ed. J Bonagura, pp. 996–1001. WB Saunders, Philadelphia

Osborne CA, Lulich JP and Thumchai R (1995) Feline calcium oxalate uroliths. In: *Kirk's Current Veterinary Therapy Small Animal Practice XII*, ed. J Bonagura, pp. 989–992. WB Saunders, Philadelphia

Pechman RD (1982) Urinary trauma in dogs and cats: a review. *Journal of the American Animal Hospital Association* **18**, 33–40

Prescott JF, McEwen B, Taylor J *et al.* (2002) Resurgence of leptospirosis in dogs in Ontario: recent findings. *Canadian Veterinary Journal* **43**, 955–961

Selcer BA (1982) Urinary tract trauma with pelvic trauma. *Journal of the American Animal Hospital Association* **18**, 785–793

Stone EA and Barsanti JA (1992) *Urologic Surgery of the Dog and Cat.* Lea and Febiger, Philadelphia

9

Neurological emergencies

Charles H. Vite and Sam N. Long

Introduction

Relatively few diseases that affect the nervous system endanger the life of the patient sufficiently to constitute a true emergency. However, those that do must be recognized as such and dealt with appropriately. Perhaps more importantly, several conditions affect the nervous system in a delayed manner, and if these are not identified and treated at an early stage, they can lead to a chain of events that cause a self-propagating deterioration in the patient's condition. These conditions may arise quietly, with little fanfare, and if the clinician does not pay close attention to the hallmarks of their development, they can be relentless in their progression.

Performing an emergency neurological examination

Whenever possible it is best to perform a full neurological examination early in the patient's evaluation. However, if time is of the essence, an abbreviated neurological examination can be performed that will give enough information to draw up a problem list, localize the lesion(s) and prioritize care.

Broadly speaking, the emergency neurological examination involves evaluation of three components:

- **A**mbulation
- **M**ental status
- **C**ranial nerve function.

Ambulation

- Is the animal walking? If yes, is the animal walking normally or abnormally? If abnormally, is the animal ataxic? How many limbs are affected: pelvic limbs, all four, or one side of the body? Is there circling, or is the animal walking compulsively or head pressing?
- If the animal is not walking, is there evidence of voluntary motor function in the affected limbs? Is there involuntary motor function (i.e. seizure activity)?
- A brief proprioceptive function test should be performed in each limb: ability to replace a knuckled-over paw and hopping are sufficient.
- Withdrawal reflexes should be assessed in all four limbs. While this is being performed, look for conscious recognition of stimulation (head turning, vocalizing etc.) in addition to palpating the limb for muscle tone and evidence of muscle atrophy.

Mental status

- Assess the level of consciousness of the animal. Alert? Depressed? Sleepy but rousable by voice/touch? Unrousable?
- Look for response to a single clap of the hands. Does the animal sit up/turn around? Do the ears twitch? Is there no response?
- Look for response to touching around the face, especially nasal planum, medial canthus of the eye and ears.
- If there is no response to either sound or touch, look for a response to noxious stimulus (e.g. pinch the nasal planum or lips with haemostats, look for conscious recognition when performing the withdrawal response).

Cranial nerves

In an emergency, testing of the following cranial nerves is often sufficient to localize the lesion and provide an indication of the severity of clinical signs at the same time. The cranial nerves that should be tested include:

- Pupil size (cranial nerve (CN) III): look for symmetry and note size (small, medium, large)
- Menace response (CN II/forebrain): is there a blink and/or retraction of the globe when the eye is menaced?
- Pupillary light reflex (CN II/III): look for response to light (direct and consensual)
- Examine the oculovestibular reflex (CN III/IV/VI/VIII): look for normal physiological nystagmus with horizontal and vertical movements of the head. Also look for abnormal nystagmus when the head is at rest and positional nystagmus when the patient's position is altered (e.g. turned on their back)
- Look for a gag reflex (CN IX/X/XII)
- The ocular fundus should also be examined for the presence of chorioretinitis or papilloedema.

Triaging the neurological patient

When dealing with any emergency, it is important to prioritize the problems of the patient and deal with these in an appropriate and systematic order. This applies as much to the neurological emergency as it does to emergencies affecting other body systems. Following the neurological examination, it should be possible to localize the patient's lesion into one or more of the following categories (Figure 9.1):

- Intracranial:
  - Abnormal mental status
  - Seizure activity
  - Abnormal cranial nerve examination
  - Compulsive pacing/head pressing (if walking)
- Spinal. Normal mentation with:
  - C1–C6: proprioceptive deficits in all four limbs, normal or exaggerated withdrawal reflexes in all four limbs
  - C6–T2: proprioceptive deficits in all four limbs (usually worse in pelvic limbs), normal or exaggerated withdrawal reflexes in pelvic limbs but abnormal/reduced withdrawal reflexes in the forelimbs
  - T3–L3: proprioceptive deficits in pelvic limbs only, normal or exaggerated withdrawal reflexes in the pelvic limbs
  - L4–S3: proprioceptive deficits in the pelvic limbs, reduced or absent withdrawal reflexes in the pelvic limbs, possible urinary/faecal incontinence and reduced anal sphincter tone
- Peripheral nerve:
  - Proprioceptive deficits in one or more limbs with decreased withdrawal reflexes
  - Normal mentation
  - Hypoventilation possible
- Multifocal: neurological dysfunction indicating involvement of more than one region.

	Cerebral hemispheres/ diencephalon	Midbrain	Pons/medulla
Mental status	Depression, disorientation, stupor, coma; other abnormalities such as aggression and hyperexcitability	Depression, stupor or coma	Depression, stupor or coma
Gait	Circling (frequently toward the side of the lesion), pacing, or head pressing. Otherwise gait is normal	Ataxia and spastic tetraparesis/ paralysis. Contralateral spastic hemiparesis/paralysis and ataxia if the lesion is lateralized	Ataxia and spastic tetraparesis/ paralysis. Ipsilateral spastic hemiparesis/paralysis and ataxia if the lesion is lateralized
Postural ability	Postural reaction deficits contralateral to the lesion	Postural reaction deficits contralateral (common) or ipsilateral (less common) to the lesion. Increased extensor tone of the limbs contralateral to the lesion. Decerebrate posture, characterized by opisthotonus with rigid extension of all limbs	Postural reaction deficits and increased extensor tone of the limbs ipsilateral to the lesion, or of all four limbs if lesion involves both sides of the pons/medulla
Segmental reflexes	Normal	Hyper-reflexia of the limb reflexes contralateral to the lesion	Hyper-reflexia of the limb reflexes ipsilateral to the lesion; or of all four limbs if lesion involves both sides of the pons/medulla
Sensation	Depressed over the face and limbs contralateral to the lesion	Depressed below the level of the lesion	Decreased over the side of the face ipsilateral to the lesion
Cranial nerve function	Blindness contralateral to the lesion with normal pupillary responses. Bilateral miosis with responsive pupils with diffuse cerebrocortical disease. Dilated pupils, non-responsive to light (fixed) when disease involves the optic chiasm	A dilated and fixed pupil and ventrolateral strabismus ipsilateral to the lesion due to CN III involvement. Bilateral miosis due to CN III stimulation. Dorsolateral rotation of the globe (CN IV)	Decreased sensation of the face, decreased jaw tone, masticatory muscle atrophy (CN V); decreased palpebral reflex (CN V and VII); medial strabismus, decreased globe retraction (CN VI); drooping lips, inability to blink the eyelids or move the ears (CN VII); nystagmus, head tilt and positional ventral strabismus (CN VIII); dysphagia, dysphonia, decreased gag reflex (CN IX and X); regurgitation, megaoesophagus (CN X); and decreased tongue motion and tongue muscle atrophy (CN XII) ipsilateral to the lesion
Other	Seizures. Abnormalities associated with hypothalamic involvement. Cheyne–Stokes respiration	Hyperventilation	Rapid, shallow breathing; irregular, ataxic breathing; or apnoea

9.1 Clinical signs of neurological diseases. (continues) ▶

	Cerebellum	Cervical spinal cord segments 1–5 (C1–C5)	Cervical spinal cord segment 6 to thoracic cord segment 2 (C6–T2)
Mental status	Normal	Normal	Normal
Gait	Dysmetria ipsilateral to the lesion. (An over-stepping or goose-stepping gait with a delayed onset of voluntary motion which, when initiated, is exaggerated.) Spasticity ipsilateral to the lesion without paresis/paralysis	Ataxia and spastic hemi- or tetraparesis/paralysis	Hindlimbs: ipsilateral or bilateral ataxia and spastic paresis/paralysis Forelimbs: ipsilateral or bilateral flaccid paresis/paralysis Movement is characterized by scuffing the paws; a stiff, short-strided gait; or inability to support weight
Postural ability	A broad-based stance, swaying of body from side to side and a tremor of the head and neck most noticeable when fine movements are required. Dysmetric, spastic postural reactions ipsilateral to the lesion	Ipsilateral or bilateral postural reaction deficits and increased extensor tone of the limbs	Hindlimbs: ipsilateral or bilateral postural reaction deficits and increased extensor tone of the limbs Forelimbs: ipsilateral or bilateral postural reaction deficits and decreased extensor tone of the limbs
Segmental reflexes	Normal	Ipsilateral or bilateral hyper-reflexia of limb reflexes	Hindlimbs: ipsilateral or bilateral hyper-reflexia of the limb reflexes Forelimbs: ipsilateral or bilateral hyporeflexia of the limb reflexes
Sensation	Normal	Decreased at and below the level of the lesion	Decreased at and below the level of the lesion
Cranial nerve function	An absent menace response, although the eye appears able to see, ipsilateral to the lesion. Off-balance, head tilt, nystagmus and strabismus	No abnormalities	No abnormalities
Other	Intention tremor. Truncal ataxia	Cervical muscle spasms. Horner's syndrome (uncommon). Respiratory muscle paresis/paralysis. Urinary incontinence and decreased ability to express the bladder	Horner's syndrome ipsilateral to the lesion. Diaphragmatic breathing. Ipsilateral or bilateral depressed cutaneous trunci reflex. Urinary incontinence and decreased ability to express the bladder

	Thoracic spinal cord segment 3 to lumbar cord segment 3 (T3–L3)	Lumbar cord segment 4 through sacral spinal cord segment 1 (L4–S1)	Sacral spinal cord
Mental status	Normal	Normal	Normal
Gait	Hindlimbs: ipsilateral or bilateral ataxia and spastic paresis/paralysis Forelimbs: normal	Hindlimbs: ipsilateral or bilateral flaccid paresis/paralysis Movement characterized by scuffing the paws; a stiff, short-strided gait; or inability to support weight Forelimbs: normal	Hindlimbs: normal gait or ipsilateral or bilateral scuffing of the paws Forelimbs: normal
Postural ability	Hindlimbs: ipsilateral or bilateral postural reaction deficits and increased extensor tone of the limbs Forelimbs: normal	Hindlimbs: ipsilateral or bilateral postural reaction deficits and decreased extensor tone of the limbs Forelimbs: normal	Hindlimbs: normal or ipsilateral or bilateral plantigrade posture Forelimbs: normal
Segmental reflexes	Hindlimbs: ipsilateral or bilateral hyper-reflexia of the limb reflexes Forelimbs: normal	Ipsilateral or bilateral hyporeflexia of the hindlimbs	Normal or hyporeflexive sciatic nerve reflexes. Decreased anal sphincter tone. Depressed bulbocavernosus reflex
Sensation	Decreased at and below the level of the lesion	Decreased at and below the level of the lesion	Decreased sensation of the perineal area, tail and skin over the limb innervated by the sciatic nerve
Cranial nerve function	No abnormalities	No abnormalities	No abnormalities
Other	Schiff–Sherrington posture. Urinary incontinence and decreased ability to express the bladder	Schiff–Sherrington posture. Urinary incontinence and decreased ability to express the bladder	Urinary incontinence with an easily expressible bladder

9.1 (continued) Clinical signs of neurological diseases. (continues) ▶

	Peripheral nerves	Skeletal muscle
Mental status	Normal	Normal
Gait	Monoparesis, hemiparesis or tetraparesis. Movement is characterized by scuffing the paws; a short-strided gait; or inability to support weight	Monoparesis, hemiparesis or tetraparesis. Movement is characterized by scuffing the paws; a short-strided gait; or inability to support weight
Postural ability	Postural reaction deficits and decreased extensor tone of the affected limbs	Postural reaction testing may be normal if the animal is supported; however, postural reaction deficits may occur in affected limbs
Segmental reflexes	Hyporeflexia in affected limbs. Decreased anal tone	Normoreflexia or hyporeflexia in affected limbs. Decreased anal tone
Sensation	Normal or decreased sensation of affected regions	Normal, or muscle may be painful on palpation
Cranial nerve function	Decreased sensation of the face, decreased jaw tone, masticatory muscle atrophy (CN V); decreased palpebral reflex (CN V and VII); medial strabismus, decreased globe retraction (CN VI); drooping lips, inability to blink the eyelids or move the ears (CN VII); nystagmus, head tilt and positional ventral strabismus (CN VIII); dysphagia, dysphonia, decreased gag reflex (CN IX and X); regurgitation, megaoesophagus (CN X); and decreased tongue motion and tongue muscle atrophy (CN XII) ipsilateral to the lesion	Decreased jaw tone; ipsilateral or bilateral masticatory muscle atrophy; drooping lips; decreased ability to blink or to move the ears; dysphagia; dysphonia; decreased gag reflex; regurgitation; megaoesophagus; and decreased tongue motion with atrophy of the tongue muscle
Other	Urinary incontinence with an easily expressible bladder. Faecal incontinence. Quickly progressing and severe muscle atrophy. Exercise intolerance	Quickly progressing and severe muscle atrophy. Exercise intolerance. Limited joint motion

9.1 (continued) Clinical signs of neurological diseases.

Spinal cord disorder results in no abnormalities of mental status or cranial nerve function. Deficits in gait, postural ability, reflexes and sensation occur at or caudal to the level of the lesion and ipsilateral to the lesion. Bilateral deficits may occur if the lesion crosses the midline of the spinal cord.

Ataxia: incoordination; may be characterized by crossing over of the the limbs, increased stride length, abduction or circumduction of a limb or limbs, walking on the dorsum of the paw, or the failure of an observer to be able to predict where a paw will land.

Paresis: partial loss of voluntary motor ability; may be characterized by an inability to support weight fully while walking or standing, scuffing of the paws when walking and tremoring when trying to stand.

Paralysis: complete loss of voluntary motor ability.

Spasticity: increased extensor tone of the limbs.

Abnormalities associated with hypothalamic involvement: diabetes insipidus, diabetes mellitus, hyperadrenocorticism and acromegaly; abnormalities in appetite, thirst, sleep, sexual behaviour, temperature regulation and electrolyte regulation.

Cheyne–Stoke's pattern of respiration: a repeating pattern of deep and shallow respiration followed by periods of apnoea.

Dysmetria: a form of ataxia, characterized by abnormal rate or range of a movement.

Horner's syndrome: miosis, ptosis, prolapsed third eyelid and enophthalmosis.

Schiff–Sherrington posture: characterized by increased extensor tone and normal postural ability of the forelimbs.

Bulbocavernosus reflex: squeezing the bulb of the penis or the vulva causes contraction of the anal sphincter in normal animals.

Prioritizing care

The results of the neurological examination help to identify which parts of the nervous system show evidence of malfunction. The next step is to determine what disease process is likely to be causing the neural dysfunction. This may not always be possible in the emergency room environment. Therefore, the clinician should attempt to identify problems that can immediately endanger the life of the patient, which include loss of consciousness and coma, head trauma and seizures or status epilepticus. These will be addressed first in this chapter.

Vascular disease and its associated complications, whilst common in human patients, rarely result in critical disease in veterinary patients. Metabolic encephalopathies, vestibular and cerebellar disorders, diseases causing paraparesis or tetraparesis and diseases causing episodic weakness are unlikely to result in the sudden death of the patient. However, failure to identify these disorders and institute appropriate therapy promptly may result in deterioration of the patient with possible life-long consequences. For example, it is common for a client to discontinue further therapy once a dog with neuromuscular disease deteriorates to the point of developing aspiration pneumonia. It is also common for a client to elect to euthanase a dog that is paraplegic but otherwise normal. Spinal cord and neuromuscular disorders will be presented at the end of this chapter.

Loss of consciousness and coma

Stupor is a state of depressed consciousness in which the animal is responsive only to strong, often noxious stimuli. Coma is a state of unconsciousness in which the animal is not aroused even by noxious stimuli. Both may result from: severe, bilateral and diffuse dysfunction of the cerebral hemispheres; destructive lesions of the brainstem; compression of the brainstem due to a mass or occipital lobe herniation; severe metabolic encephalopathies or severe vascular disease.

Evaluation of the stuporous or comatose patient

The neurological examination should be used to localize the likely site of the pathology leading to the stupor/coma. Regardless of neurolocalization, gait and postural ability are non-existent in stuporous or comatose animals. Segmental reflexes are normal or hyper-reflexive.

Cerebral hemispheres/diencephalon

Cranial nerves: Diffuse bilateral disease of the cerebral hemispheres and diencephalon may cause blindness and bilaterally miotic pupils that are responsive to light. No abnormalities of physiological nystagmus are found.

Other: Cheyne–Stokes respiratory pattern may occur (periods of tachypnoea interspersed with prolonged apnoea). Rhythmic walking movements may be elicited if the animal is supported.

Brainstem

Cranial nerves: The animal may or may not respond to visual testing. Unilateral or bilateral fixed mid-position or dilated pupils, ipsilateral or bilateral ventrolateral strabismus and abnormal or absent physiological nystagmus may occur. Absent physiological nystagmus may be a poor prognostic sign in animals with brainstem disease. Physiological nystagmus occurs as a result of vestibular centre projections to the nuclei of cranial nerves III, IV and VI along the medial longitudinal fasciculus (MLF). The MLF runs deep within the brainstem, and as a result lesions that are severe enough to disrupt the MLF indicate severe brainstem damage. However, depressed or absent oculovestibular movements have also been seen in some animals with severe metabolic disease, and have resolved following therapy of the underlying metabolic defect. Signs of cranial nerve V–XII dysfunction may occur.

Other: Apnoea or hyperventilation may occur. A decerebrate posture may be seen with extension of all four limbs and opisthotonus.

Causes and treatment of stupor or coma

Diffuse dysfunction of the cerebral hemispheres

Inflammatory diseases, lysosomal storage diseases, metabolic diseases, neoplasia with associated oedema, and hydrocephalus can cause signs of diffuse, cerebral hemisphere/diencephalic dysfunction. Treatment is directed at the inciting cause and at decreasing intracranial pressure (ICP) (see Head trauma).

Brainstem disease

Destructive brainstem disease: Neoplasia and encephalitis of the brainstem may result in an acute or progressive onset of brainstem dysfunction. Chemotherapy, antimicrobials/antifungals or anti-inflammatories may be required. Trauma and haemorrhage in the brainstem may also result in acute onset of dysfunction. Traumatic brainstem haemorrhage is treated by support of the patient with careful monitoring. When haemorrhage is due to an underlying clotting disorder this should be treated specifically if possible (see Chapter 13).

Herniation: Neoplasia, inflammation (e.g. canine distemper virus, granulomatous meningoencephalitis, necrotizing encephalitis, feline infectious peritonitis, toxoplasmosis/neosporosis, mycotic diseases) or trauma of the cerebral hemispheres may result in increased ICP, unilateral or bilateral occipital lobe herniation and brainstem compression. Herniation is often preceded by hours to days of progressive cerebral hemisphere/diencephalon dysfunction, including progressive depression of consciousness. Occipital lobe herniation is suspected from the development (over hours to days) of unilateral or bilateral non-responsive dilated or mid-position pupils; progressive loss of physiological nystagmus; and alterations in respiratory patterns. Interestingly, significant occipital lobe herniation can occur even in the absence of clinical signs (Walmsley *et al.*, 2005). Herniation of the cerebellum through the foramen magnum may result in apnoea. Increases in ICP causing herniation should be treated without delay by the methods discussed in the section on head trauma.

Metabolic causes

Metabolic disease and toxins rarely result in deficits related to discrete lesions of the nervous system. Rather, bilaterally symmetrical deficits that suggest diffuse cerebrocortical dysfunction or diffuse brain disease are usual. Signs are often progressive. Evidence of vision is present until stupor is profound or coma occurs. Pupils are responsive and usually of normal diameter but may be bilaterally miotic. Physiological nystagmus is generally present unless profound stupor or coma occurs. Metabolic causes for stupor or coma include: diabetic coma, heat stroke, hepatic encephalopathy, hypo- and hypernatraemia, hypoglycaemia, hypothyroid coma, hypoxia, renal encephalopathy and thiamine deficiency (see later). Toxic causes include heavy metals, ethylene glycol, barbiturates, narcotics, ivermectin and tranquillizers. Intoxication is treated by gastric lavage, activated charcoal, specific antidotes and chelating agents and by support of the patient (see Chapter 19).

Vascular causes

Stupor or coma may result from infarction/haemorrhage of the midbrain, or from infarction/haemorrhage in the cerebral hemispheres and diencephalon, resulting in increased ICP and occipital lobe herniation. Causes of cerebrovascular accidents in animals include trauma, metastatic neoplasia, coagulation disorders, cardiac disease, hypertension, parasitic emboli and feline ischaemic encephalopathy, although it is most common that an underlying cause is not identified. Predisposing vascular disease, so common in humans, is rare in animals. If vascular disease is suspected, coagulation screens and blood pressure should be assessed. Infarction is treated by supporting the patient, treating any underlying disease and decreasing ICP.

Head trauma

A global assessment of the patient must be performed, paying specific attention to ensuring a patent airway, providing respiratory support if necessary and maintaining cardiovascular function. Ideally, the initial assessment should be performed on a board or firm table where the neck and back can be immobilized and assessed for fractures or luxations. Manipulation for radiography of any suspicious areas should be done with care. The nasal cavity, ear canals and nasopharyngeal region should be examined for haemorrhage, which may imply a skull fracture with the possibility of entry of bacteria into the brain. The jugular vein should not be used to collect blood since even temporary occlusion may increase ICP.

Neurological assessment

In general, trauma to the cerebral hemispheres causes less severe neurological dysfunction and a better prognosis than trauma to the brainstem. Trauma to the cerebellum alone is uncommon. The progression of clinical signs over time plays a large role in determining prognosis. Deterioration of mental status may indicate increasing ICP and the possibility of impending brain herniation, therefore immediate therapeutic intervention is necessary. Prolonged (greater than 48–72 hours) stupor or coma suggests severe brainstem disease and indicates a poor prognosis. In general, pupillary abnormalities which become normal over time are a good prognostic sign; pupils which change to mydriasis or to mid-position and are unresponsive to light, and loss of normal physiological nystagmus are poor prognostic signs indicating oedema, herniation and compression of the brainstem, warranting more aggressive intervention. Progressive alterations in breathing patterns, or increases in mean arterial blood pressure accompanied by bradycardia, may indicate increases in ICP requiring immediate therapy.

Intracranial pressure

The objective of management of head trauma is to prevent the brain from undergoing any further insult due to ischaemia, inflammatory mediators or the effects of increased ICP. Findings indicative of raised ICP include: papilloedema; abnormal pulsing of retinal vessels; depression, stupor or coma; and elevated blood pressure with a low heart rate. ICP is rarely measured directly in small animal patients, therefore, increased ICP is frequently suspected but rarely confirmed.

ICP is the pressure exerted by tissues and fluids within the cranial vault. In normal animals, ICP ranges between 5 and 12 mmHg. Three 'compartments' exist within the skull: brain parenchyma (80%), blood (10%), and cerebrospinal fluid (CSF) (10%). If ICP is to remain constant, an increase in the volume of one of these components must be accompanied by a decrease in the volume of one (or both) of the others. In most diseases affecting the brain, a volume increase occurs in one or more compartments. Most commonly this is in the form of cerebral oedema which adds to the volume of brain parenchyma, although haemorrhage and hydrocephalus can also add to the volumes of blood and CSF respectively. In the initial stages of an increase in intracranial volume, mechanisms exist to minimize the consequent rise in ICP, first by displacing CSF out of ventricles into the subarachnoid space outside the skull, and then by reducing the blood volume contained within intracerebral vessels. However, once this initial compliance has been exhausted, small increases in volume of any compartment result in large increases in ICP in an exponential fashion.

A separate, but related, concept is that of cerebral perfusion pressure (CPP). CPP determines the cerebral blood flow (CBF) and therefore the delivery of oxygen and nutrients to brain tissue. CPP is defined by the following equation:

$$CPP = MAP - ICP$$

where MAP is mean arterial pressure. In patients with mean arterial blood pressure in the normal range (50–150 mmHg), ICP is maintained within normal limits by the phenomenon of *pressure autoregulation*: as blood pressure rises, vasoconstriction occurs to minimize the volume of blood within the cerebral vasculature and thus prevent increases in ICP. Conversely, if ICP rises, autoregulation of cerebral perfusion should result in an elevation of MAP in an attempt to maintain CPP. This increased MAP may then provoke a baroreceptor-mediated bradycardia, the so-called Cushing reflex. However, if ICP rises excessively, autoregulatory mechanisms may not be sufficient to compensate. This is especially true if there is a concurrent drop in MAP, leading to a drop in CPP and insufficient blood delivery to the brain, resulting in tissue hypoxia and ultimately necrosis of brain tissue. Importantly, in regions of the brain that have suffered significant trauma, these mechanisms do not function normally, and may fail even before ICP rises above the normal range.

Tissue hypoxia and necrosis result in a complex chain of biochemical events that culminate in progressive cerebral oedema, setting up a self-propagating spiral of rising ICP. In this situation, systemic blood pressure may rise and heart rate may fall, in a last-resort attempt to maintain cerebral perfusion. For this reason, it is vital to monitor the patient's blood pressure if there is concern about elevated ICP.

Treatment

The following treatment recommendations are made by the authors for the care of the closed head trauma patient (Bagley, 1996).

Elevate the head and neck at a 30-degree angle above heart level

The patient may be placed on a solid board and the board elevated at a 30-degree angle, thereby facilitating venous drainage from the cranial vault. It is important to avoid bending the neck by elevating the head only. Make sure no blankets compress the jugular veins, which would decrease venous drainage.

Control of ventilation

Hyperventilation can rapidly decrease ICP because hypocapnia causes cerebral vasoconstriction, thereby decreasing CBF. Studies have revealed, however, that its clinical use may be contraindicated (Obrist *et al.*,

1984; Muizelaar *et al.*, 1991; Fortune *et al.*, 1995; Skippen *et al.*, 1997). After cranial trauma, oxygen extraction is maximal and blood flow is the limiting factor for cerebral oxygen utilization. Cerebral vasoconstriction induced by hypocapnia should therefore be avoided because oligaemia might result in inadequate cerebral oxygen delivery. Assisted ventilation is recommended if P_aCO_2 (as determined by blood gas analysis, or inferred from capnography) is elevated, but the goal should be to maintain it within normal limits (35–45 mmHg). For the same reasons, hypoxaemia must be avoided and positive pressure ventilation should be considered to maintain oxygenation if the patient is stuporous or comatose. If the patient is not stuporous and is stable, supplemental oxygen, in the form of nasal oxygenation or via an oxygen cage, may be provided.

Maintainence of perfusion

Hypotension, hypoxia and hypertension must be avoided. In order to maintain CPP, fluid therapy should be used to maintain mean arterial pressure between 70 and 110 mmHg (see Chapters 3 and 4). Hypotension that is non-responsive to fluid therapy should be treated with inotropes or pressors as indicated. Hypertension due to excitement and pain may be addressed with sedation or analgesics. Occasionally, a comatose animal may present with hypertension and bradycardia (Cushing reflex) due to increased ICP; treatment should be aimed at decreasing ICP.

Furosemide and mannitol

Mannitol can rapidly decrease ICP by drawing water out of oedematous cells into the intravascular space by osmosis, and then inducing an osmotic diuresis. Its effect is greatest 30–60 minutes after administration, and lasts 2–4 hours. A dose of 0.5–1 g/kg of a 25% solution administered over 20 minutes can be repeated every 3–8 hours, with a maximum of three doses over a 24-hour period. Mannitol causes an initial expansion followed by a significant contraction of the intravascular volume and is therefore contraindicated in patients with shock, hypotension, dehydration, congestive heart failure, anuric renal failure or pulmonary oedema. Serum electrolytes and osmolality should be monitored because of the potential for free water loss in the diuresis. Furosemide (1–4 mg/kg i.v.) may be given as a bolus prior to administration of mannitol. The aim is to prevent an initial rise in ICP associated with the expanded intravascular volume that occurs immediately following mannitol administration. Furosemide should be avoided in hypovolaemic patients.

Corticosteroids

Although steroids are frequently used to treat head trauma, there is little evidence to support their efficacy, and they are currently not part of the standard of care for patients with head trauma in our hospital.

Craniotomy

Craniotomy produces a rapid decrease in ICP and may be performed when managing skull fractures with depressed displacement of bone more than the thickness of the calvarium in the fractured area, to remove projectiles, or to treat progressive increases in ICP

that are refractory to medical management. In the future, the routine availability of ICP monitoring and computerized tomography (CT) may aid in determining when craniotomy is necessary.

Anaesthetic concerns

In patients with head trauma, drugs that do not increase ICP or cause large changes in blood pressure should be used. Premedication may be limited to use of an intravenous benzodiazepine immediately prior to induction. This minimizes the required dose of induction agents and their cardiovascular effects. Opioids do not increase ICP unless there is associated respiratory depression. Lidocaine (2 mg/kg i.v.) may be given for its antitussive effect immediately before intubation. Isoflurane is the maintenance agent of choice, because cerebral autoregulation is preserved if the inspired concentration is <1.5 x MAC (minimum alveolar concentration). When inhalants are contraindicated or insufficient, supplemental agents such as fentanyl or propofol may be used. During anaesthesia, end-tidal carbon dioxide monitoring (or blood gas analysis) coupled with intermittent positive pressure ventilation (IPPV) is important to maintain arterial carbon dioxide levels within normal limits of 35–45 mmHg. Hyper- or hypoventilation must be avoided.

Sedation

Frequently, trauma-related pain or agitation may result in the patient flailing or constantly vocalizing. Both behaviours may increase ICP. Diazepam (0.2–0.5 mg/kg) or phenobarbital (5 mg/kg) may be used to sedate the patient, potentially combined with butorphanol (0.2–0.4 mg/kg) or other narcotics, especially if the patient is thought also to be in pain. Cardiorespiratory function must be carefully monitored. In the rare instance when these drugs do not result in a calm patient, small doses of acepromazine (0.01–0.02 mg/kg i.v.) may be given. Although acepromazine has been implicated in increasing the possibility of seizure induction, the authors have not found this to be common.

Seizures and status epilepticus

Seizures result from a sudden uncontrolled discharge of neurons in the cerebral cortex or diencephalon. The manifestation of a seizure depends on the area and extent of the brain affected by the abnormal electrical activity. Primary generalized seizures occur when both cerebral hemispheres are affected. The patient may show symmetrical abnormalities of movement of the head and limbs (tonus, clonus, atony, myoclonus) with a loss of consciousness. Partial seizures occur when a group of neurons in a region of the cerebral cortex is affected. The patient shows signs indicative of stimulation of the cortical region: asymmetrical signs such as tonus or clonus of one or more limbs, turning the head and neck to one side, and twitching of one side of the face, or sudden changes in behaviour may occur. Consciousness may or may not be affected and focal seizures may or may not progress to generalized seizures.

The term 'epilepsy' means recurrent seizures. Epilepsy may be classified according to its cause into three categories: idiopathic, symptomatic and cryptogenic (Berendt and Gram, 1999). Idiopathic epilepsy is the consequence of intrinsic chemical abnormalities that are not associated with structural cerebral pathology or extracranial disease. It is characterized by predominantly generalized seizures that typically begin between 6 months and 5 years of age. The animal is neurologically normal during the inter-ictal period. A hereditary cause may or may not be found. Symptomatic (secondary) epilepsy occurs when structural disease of the brain (brain tumours, encephalitis, malformations, sclerosis or trauma) provokes seizures. It is characterized by partial or generalized seizures that may begin at any age. The animal frequently, but not always, has neurological deficits that are recognized during the inter-ictal period. Cryptogenic epilepsy is used to designate recurrent seizures for which a symptomatic cause is suspected but has not been found. It is suspected when an animal has partial seizures, but brain imaging does not reveal a structural cause for the seizures.

Single or recurrent seizures can also occur due to extracranial disease, in which the normal brain is stressed by metabolic or toxic abnormalities (e.g. hepatic encephalopathy, uraemic encephalopathy, hypoglycaemia, hypocalcaemia, polycythaemia and toxins) (Podell *et al.*, 1995). These have been referred to as reactive seizures.

Obtaining a good history

When presented with a patient who is having seizures the goals are:

- To confirm that the event is/was a seizure
- To stop the seizure and treat secondary metabolic derangements
- To determine the cause of the seizure.

Confirmation that a seizure occurred is based on the owner's description of the event or observation of the event by the veterinarian (either directly or by observing videotape). Non-convulsive seizures and sudden changes in behaviour present the most difficulty in determining whether or not a seizure has occurred. Differential diagnoses must include syncope, cataplexy, narcolepsy and behavioural disorders. While electroencephalography could be used to confirm epileptiform activity in the brain, it is not routinely performed due to the need for sedation.

The following questions may be asked of the client while assessing the patient.

- What did the seizure look like? What did the animal look like immediately before and immediately following the seizure? The presence of pre- or post-ictal signs may help confirm that a seizure has occurred and may suggest a structural cause if a partial seizure is described.
- Is the animal vaccinated?
- Has there been any exposure to toxins? Strychnine, lead, mercury, metaldehyde, moulds, organophosphates, chlorinated hydrocarbons, ethylene glycol, amphetamines, caffeine, theobromine, cocaine, 5-fluorouracil, ivermectin and others may cause seizures.
- Has the animal had seizures in the past? Is the animal currently taking anticonvulsants? How many seizures have occurred within the past year, 6 months or month? Generalized seizures occurring infrequently over years suggest idiopathic epilepsy or a static, structural lesion.
- How old is the animal? The onset of seizures in dogs due to idiopathic epilepsy is principally between 6 months and 5 years of age. Idiopathic epilepsy is uncommon in cats.
- What time of day did the seizure occur? Seizures following feeding may be associated with hepatic encephalopathy. Seizures occurring when a meal has been missed, soon before a meal or associated with exercise may indicate hypoglycaemia.
- Is the animal neurologically normal between seizures? Animals with idiopathic epilepsy appear normal between seizures. Animals with symptomatic epilepsy may be normal between seizures or may be behaviourally abnormal, dull, circle, or show other signs of nervous system disease. These animals may also show signs of systemic disease.

Clinicopathological testing

Ideally blood should be drawn for analysis prior to initiating therapy. It is recommended that a complete blood count, blood smear evaluation for inclusion bodies (seen with canine distemper virus infection) and nucleated red cells (seen with lead toxicity), urinalysis and blood gas measurements be performed. Levels of serum electrolytes, blood glucose, alanine aminotransferase, blood urea nitrogen, serum ammonia, serum creatinine, albumin and cholesterol should be determined. Additional serum may be refrigerated for future determination of anticonvulsant, insulin, thyroid hormone or bile acid concentrations, or for antibody titres for infectious diseases.

Seizures due to metabolic causes require specific therapy in addition to anticonvulsant medications (see Abnormal mental status and metabolic encephalopathies for the treatment of hypoglycaemia, hypocalcaemia and thiamine deficiency).

Status epilepticus and cluster seizures may result in hypoxia, acidosis and/or hyperthermia, which require specific treatment. Seizures commonly result in hyperglycaemia. Rarely, however, prolonged status epilepticus may result in hypoglycaemia and the patient may require supplementation with dextrose.

Treatment

If the seizure lasts less than 2 minutes and is not repeated, no medication is required.

Seizures over 2 minutes, seizure clusters or status epilepticus

Cluster seizures are two or more seizures occurring over a 24-hour period. Status epilepticus is defined as a seizure which lasts longer than 5 minutes, or recurrent seizures without recovery of full consciousness between seizures. Initial treatment recommendations include:

- Diazepam: 0.2–0.5 mg/kg i.v. or 0.5–1.0 mg/kg rectally, may be repeated two to three times over 5–10 minutes
- Phenobarbital: a loading dose of 16 mg/kg i.v. is given divided into three or four doses over several hours. It may take up to 30 minutes before an effect is noted. If the animal is currently on an adequate dose of phenobarbital, there is little evidence that increasing the dose by another 16 mg/kg has any beneficial effect
- Diazepam and phenobarbital may be given concurrently.

If status epilepticus or cluster seizures continue, one of the following regimens may be used:

- Continuous rate intravenous infusion of diazepam administered at a rate of 0.1–0.5 mg/kg/h in a 5% dextrose solution
- Intravenous administration of 10–20 mg/kg thiopental (given as 2–4 mg/kg boluses to effect), endotracheal intubation with or without isoflurane anaesthesia
- Intravenous administration of 6 mg/kg propofol (given as 1–2 mg/kg boluses to effect), followed by a continuous rate intravenous infusion of propofol at 0.1–0.2 mg/kg/min. If hepatic disease is suspected, propofol may be more appropriate than administration of barbiturates
- Intravenous administration of 2–6 mg/kg pentobarbital. This drug may lead to prolonged anaesthesia. Although a total dose of up to 15 mg/kg can be used, this should be administered as small boluses of 2–3 mg/kg. There should be at least 15 minutes between these boluses due to the prolonged nature of the drug's effects.

When intermittent dosing of diazepam or phenobarbital does not control seizures and any of the above protocols are used, profound sedation may result. Endotracheal intubation and careful monitoring of respiratory and cardiovascular status may be required. The patient should be anaesthetized for 15–30 minutes with propofol or thiopental. If seizures continue after recovery from anaesthesia, repeated anaesthesia for longer periods of time may be attempted. If seizures continue after a more prolonged period of anaesthesia, patients should receive a loading dose of potassium bromide (400 mg/kg) either rectally or via stomach tube before recovery from anaesthesia is once again attempted.

Maintenance medication

- Phenobarbital (3–5 mg/kg orally every 12 hours). Serum concentration attains a steady state within 2 weeks.
  or
- Potassium bromide (30–40 mg/kg orally every 24 hours). Serum concentration attains a steady state in 2–4 months.

Prognosis
Idiopathic epilepsy is rarely life threatening unless status epilepticus develops. However, blindness, weakness or changes in behaviour may continue for days to weeks following a seizure and may be made temporarily worse by anticonvulsant medications. If status epilepticus does occur, it is important to treat secondary problems such as hyperthermia, metabolic disturbances, aspiration pneumonia, acid–base imbalance and myoglobinuria.

Animals with symptomatic epilepsy require further diagnostic testing including CSF analysis and brain imaging. If symptomatic epilepsy is suspected, medication in addition to anticonvulsants may be required (e.g. mannitol, steroids, antifungals, antibacterials). Animals with reactive epilepsy require treatment of the underlying metabolic disease.

Abnormal mental status

Abnormal mental status may result from disease of the cerebral hemispheres or brainstem, with the most common emergency presentations being due to encephalitis, neoplasia or metabolic encephalopathy.

Encephalitis
Common causes of encephalitis in dogs include steroid-responsive meningitis/arteritis, protozoal diseases (*Toxoplasma*, *Neospora*), canine distemper virus, inflammatory diseases in which no aetiological agent can be identified (granulomatous meningoencephalitis (GME), necrotizing encephalitis) and, in some locations, rickettsial diseases (Rocky Mountain spotted fever, *Ehrlichia*) and fungal diseases (*Cryptococcus*, *Blastomyces*, *Aspergillus*). In cats, feline infectious peritonitis, feline immunodeficiency virus, *Toxoplasma* and fungal disease are the most common causes of encephalitis.

Animals with encephalitis are commonly depressed or disorientated, and a recent onset of seizures is common. Evidence of systemic disease is useful in making a tentative diagnosis of some causes of encephalitis but two of the more common causes, GME and necrotizing encephalitis, are typically not associated with extracranial disease. Examination of the ocular fundus is strongly recommended, since ocular disease occurs commonly with some encephalitides (canine distemper virus, *Toxoplasma*, *Cryptococcus*, feline infectious peritonitis) and since the presence of papilloedema is supportive evidence for increased intracranial pressure.

It is useful to submit titres for infectious diseases, but the results of these tests may not be available for several days. CSF analysis may reveal fungal organisms (occasionally) or inclusion bodies (rarely) but more commonly shows inflammation without evidence of aetiology. CSF is readily collected under general anaesthesia at the cerebellomedullary cistern using a spinal needle (Figures 9.2 and 9.3). Normal CSF protein is <0.25 g/l and normal cellularity is <4 white blood cells per microlitre. Some CSF analysis findings support specific diagnoses. For example, a mononuclear pleocytosis with mild to moderate increases in protein is consistent with GME, necrotizing encephalitis and lymphoma. Moderate increases in neutrophils in addition to mononuclear cells may be seen with GME, toxoplasmosis,

1. Place the animal in lateral recumbency under general anaesthesia.

2. Clip the skin and prepare for an aseptic procedure.

3. Flex the head to 90 degrees and have an assistant hold it in place.

4. The occipital protruberance and the spinous process of C2 are palpated; an imaginary line is drawn through these two points; this line should be parallel to the table surface (if not, the nose is either raised or lowered).

5. The most rostral extents of the wings of the atlas are palpated and an imaginary vertical line is drawn between the two wings.

6. The 20 or 22 gauge CSF needle is inserted parallel to the table surface and parallel to the nose, on the midline of the patient, halfway between the occipital protuberance and an imaginary line between the wings of the atlas (see Figure 9.3).

7. The needle should be held securely and slowly advanced. The stylet is removed every 5 mm or so to look for fluid. Once fluid is seen in the hub of the needle, it is held in place while the sample is collected.

8. The needle should not be redirected once it has entered the muscle as side-to-side motion of the needle can damage the spinal cord.

9.2 Method for cerebrospinal fluid tap.

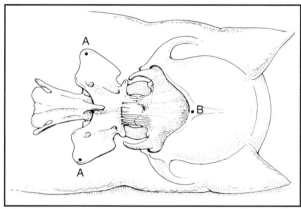

9.3 Anatomical landmarks for atlanto-occipital CSF collection. A = wings of the atlas vertebra. B = occipital protruberance. Reproduced from the *BSAVA Manual of Canine and Feline Neurology, 3rd edition.*

neosporosis and fungal disease. Marked increases in neutrophils are common with feline infectious peritonitis and steroid-responsive meningitis/arteritis. Moderate to marked increases in eosinophils can be seen with parasitic diseases, protozoal diseases and eosinophilic meningitis.

When encephalitis is suspected, the clinician must frequently institute therapy prior to obtaining a definitive diagnosis through titres or biopsy. Emergency therapy should therefore be directed at the most common causes of encephalitis found in the geographic region. For example, in the Philadelphia region, treating dogs with doxycycline and prednisolone is common, due to the prevalence of Rocky Mountain spotted fever, GME and necrotizing encephalitis in our patient population. Mannitol may also be required to treat increases in intracranial pressure. When a definitive diagnosis is made, therapy is altered to treat the specific cause.

Neoplasia
Primary intracranial neoplasia is one of the most common causes of altered mental status and seizures in older patients (Troxel *et al.*, 2003; Snyder *et al.*, 2006). Definitive diagnosis in an emergency setting may be hindered by the absence of advanced imaging capabilities. A CSF analysis showing a significant increase in protein without a significant increase in cellularity (albuminocytological dissociation) is supportive but not definitive for intracranial neoplasia. When neoplasia is suspected, the animal may be treated with steroids to decrease vasogenic oedema and mannitol to decrease ICP, until the brain can be imaged with CT or MRI.

Metabolic encephalopathies
Metabolic encephalopathies result in seizures, bilaterally symmetrical signs of cerebrocortical dysfunction, or signs of diffuse brain disease. Abnormalities of mental status may progress to stupor and coma (see Loss of consciousness and coma). History and blood work are essential in determining that the signs are due to metabolic disease. However, CSF analysis, titres for infectious disease and brain imaging are frequently necessary to rule out other causes of encephalopathy.

Calcium
Hypocalcaemia (serum calcium <1.6 mmol/l; ionized calcium <0.6 mmol/l) may cause muscle twitching and spasms, disorientation, restlessness and seizures. Intravenous administration of 10% calcium gluconate (50–150 mg/kg) over 15 minutes, followed by calcium gluconate diluted in saline and given subcutaneously (50–150 mg/kg q6–8h; Feldman, 2005) or 10 mg/kg/h i.v. by continuous rate infusion (CRI) often resolves clinical signs until the specific cause is identified. Hypoglycaemia and hypomagnesaemia may occur concurrently and supplementation may be necessary. Diazepam may be necessary to control seizures.

Hypercalcaemia (>3.0 mmol/l) may cause muscle weakness, seizures, depression, stupor or coma. Diuresis with 0.9% sodium chloride i.v. and furosemide may be performed until the cause is determined.

Sodium
Severe hyponatraemia (Na⁺<120 mmol/l) may cause disorientation, seizures, stupor or coma. Ideally, plasma sodium concentration is corrected at the rate at which it was lost, i.e. acute decreases in plasma sodium may be corrected quickly, while chronically low sodium concentrations should be gradually increased. Excessively rapid correction of chronic hyponatraemia (>10 mmol/l/day) may cause weakness, hypermetria, ataxia and myoclonic jerking of the limbs 3–5 days after treatment (O'Brien *et al.*, 1994).

If hypernatraemia (Na⁺ >170 mmol/l) occurs acutely, restlessness, irritability, seizures, stupor and coma may occur. If hypernatraemia is chronic, only depression and disorientation may be noted. Chronic hypernatraemia must be treated slowly, at a correction rate no greater than 0.5 mmol/l/h (over 2–3 days) to avoid cerebral oedema. Further details can be found in Chapter 5.

Glucose

Hypoglycaemia (blood glucose <2.5 mmol/l) may cause weakness, muscle tremors, blindness, seizures, stupor or coma. Intravenous administration of 0.5 g/kg of 10–25% dextrose solution may be given until signs resolve. Anticonvulsants may be necessary to control seizures. When an insulin-secreting tumour is present, dextrose (by CRI), diazoxide (10 mg/kg q12h) and prednisolone (0.5 mg/kg/day) are often necessary to maintain serum glucose concentrations.

Hyperglycaemia and hyperosmolality (>340 mOsm/l) may cause stupor and coma. Sodium chloride 0.45–0.9% i.v. and insulin may be given to gradually correct hyperglycaemia over 24–36 hours and reduce the risk of cerebral oedema. Potassium supplementation should be provided (see Chapter 16).

Heat stroke

A body temperature of >41°C may result in blindness, ataxia, disorientation, stupor or coma. Cooling and hydrating the patient and correcting any acidosis, hypernatraemia, hypokalaemia, hypophosphataemia and hypocalcaemia are recommended. If neurological dysfunction progresses, increased ICP may be present (see Head trauma for treatment).

Hepatic encephalopathy

Disorientation, pacing, blindness and circling often develop with hepatic encephalopathy; seizures, stupor and coma occur less often. Treatment is directed at decreasing the intake and absorption of protein-derived toxins from the large intestine (Bunch, 1995). Warm-water cleansing enemas and lactulose enemas retained for 20 minutes (20 ml/kg of 3 parts lactulose to 7 parts water) may be given every 4–6 hours. Neomycin sulphate (22 mg/kg orally q8h) and metronidazole (7.5 mg/kg orally q8h) may be administered to decrease the bacterial load. Serum glucose and potassium concentrations should be monitored and deficits corrected. Hydration should be maintained and gastrointestinal bleeding must be controlled. Hepatic encephalopathy is associated with the presence of increased numbers of GABA receptors, and administration of GABA receptor antagonists such as flumazenil (20 µg/kg i.v.) may result in improved mental status in these patients.

Seizures occasionally occur after surgery for portosystemic shunt ligation. These seizures are notoriously difficult to control with phenobarbital or diazepam. The use of potassium bromide or propofol has been more effective, however, the prognosis for many of these animals remains poor, and postmortem examination has revealed severe cerebrocortical necrosis.

Hypoadrenocorticism

Depression, lethargy, weakness and shock may occur. Depending on the severity of signs, intravenous 0.9% saline, dexamethasone sodium phosphate (0.5–2.0 mg/kg), dextrose and/or sodium bicarbonate may be necessary (see Chapter 16).

Hypoxia and ischaemia

Changes in mental status, blindness and ataxia may occur with P_aO_2 values <55 mmHg, especially if hypoxia is also associated with decreased cerebral blood flow, for example following successful resuscitation from cardiopulmonary arrest. Treatment includes providing supplemental oxygen, treating the underlying cause of the hypoxia and if necessary providing mannitol to decrease cerebral oedema. Blindness and changes in mental status will often resolve over weeks but may be permanent.

Lead poisoning

Whole blood lead concentrations >1.932 µmol/l may result in dementia and seizures, in addition to gastrointestinal signs. Chelation therapy with EDTA, D-penicillamine, or succimer (10 mg/kg orally q8h for 10 days; Ramsey et al., 1996) are specific therapies for intoxication, along with removal of the source of lead if appropriate.

Renal encephalopathy

Severe uraemia due to acute renal failure may result in seizures. Chronic renal failure more commonly causes mental dullness, weakness, muscle twitching and myoclonus. Treatment is aimed at monitoring blood pressure and maintaining hydration, acid–base status and electrolyte concentrations.

Thiamine deficiency

This is usually caused by a deficiency of dietary thiamine, through cooked food or a diet high in fish containing thiaminase. Clinical signs include signs of central vestibular disease, ataxia, ventroflexion of the head and neck, bilaterally dilated fixed pupils and seizures, stupor and coma. Thiamine hydrochloride (10–20 mg/kg i.v.) is used to treat signs and repeated intramuscularly or subcutaneously daily until improvement is noted.

Thyroid hormone

Hypothyroidism (myxoedema crisis) may result in depression, disorientation, stupor or coma, most commonly in the Dobermann. Serum cholesterol concentrations >25 mmol/l may occur. Abnormalities are reversible with thyroid supplementation. Respiratory support, glucocorticoids and intravenous L-thyroxine may be necessary in cases of coma (Kelly, 1989).

Hyperthyroidism may cause restlessness, hyperexcitability, circling and seizures. Rarely, lethargy may occur. Treatment with methimazole, surgery or radioactive iodine resolves these signs.

Acute vestibular or cerebellar signs

Signs of vestibular system dysfunction which occur regardless of lesion location include:

- Ataxia characterized by falling due to loss of balance
- Abnormal posture characterized by leaning, turning of the head, neck and body and/or rolling
- Head tilt. A head tilt exists when an imagined horizontal line running through both ears is tilted from the horizontal plane
- Ventral strabismus of the eye. The strabismus may not be noted until the head is elevated or returned to the horizontal plane
- Abnormal nystagmus.

Several techniques can be used to accentuate the clinical signs, for example blindfolding the animal may accentuate the ataxia, lifting the animal off the ground may increase the head tilt and rolling and placing the animal on its back may induce nystagmus.

Compulsive circling (associated with disease of the cerebral hemispheres and diencephalon) should not be attributed to disease of the vestibular system. With compulsive circling there is no ataxia, no loss of balance and no abnormal nystagmus.

Localizing signs of vestibular system dysfunction

Vestibular system dysfunction may result from disease of the inner ear (often termed peripheral vestibular disease) and medulla or cerebellum (often termed central vestibular disease). The location of the lesion may be determined by the presence of neurological deficits in addition to those listed above.

Ear

Disease of the inner ear alone results in only the signs listed above. Auditory dysfunction is rarely recognized. The animal falls towards the side of the lesion and has a head tilt and strabismus ipsilateral to the lesion. The direction of the nystagmus is usually horizontal or rotatory, with the slow phase directed towards the side of the lesion and unchanged when the position of the head is altered. If the middle ear is also affected, signs of CN VII dysfunction and Horner's syndrome may result. No postural reaction deficits occur.

Medulla/cerebellum

Disease of the medulla may cause changes in mental status. Hemiparesis and postural reaction deficits and dysfunction of CN V–XII may occur ipsilateral to the lesion. The direction of the nystagmus may be horizontal, rotatory or vertical and may change when the position of the head is altered.

Disease of the cerebellum may cause dysmetria and menace deficits ipsilateral to the lesion, and head and neck tremors.

Exceptions to rules of localization

Bilateral peripheral vestibular disease may result in a wide-based stance and swaying of the body. Often, no abnormal nystagmus or strabismus is noted. The animal is severely ataxic when blindfolded or when lifted off the ground.

Occasionally disease of specific sites within the cerebellum and medulla result in head tilt, strabismus and slow phase of the nystagmus directed away from the side of the lesion (paradoxical vestibular syndrome). The postural reaction deficits are ipsilateral to the lesion.

Causes and management of diseases of the vestibular system

Ear

Idiopathic labyrinthitis: Older dogs and cats of any age may be affected. CN VII dysfunction and Horner's syndrome do not occur. No abnormalities are found in blood, images of the bullae, deep otic examination, or thyroid testing. Antibiotics are recommended if a full work up for ear infection is not performed but are not necessary to treat labyrinthitis, which is presumed to be of viral origin. Spontaneous recovery is common.

Otitis interna/media: Images of the osseous bullae and/or deep otic examination may confirm middle ear disease. Treatment with cephalosporins, clindamycin, enrofloxacin or trimethoprim–sulphadiazine, with or without bulla osteotomy, is recommended.

Other causes: Polyneuropathy, tumours, nasopharyngeal polyps and trauma involving the inner ear may result in vestibular system dysfunction. Hypothyroidism may be associated with polyneuropathy, and occasionally vestibular signs resolve only after the institution of thyroid hormone supplementation. Aminoglycosides at high doses may result in deafness and signs of peripheral vestibular dysfunction.

Medulla/cerebellum

Infectious/inflammatory diseases: Canine distemper virus, Rocky Mountain spotted fever, *Toxoplasma*, *Neospora*, *Cryptococcus neoformans*, granulomatous meningoencephalomyelitis, feline infectious peritonitis, parasitic migration and other meningoencephalidites may result in vestibular system dysfunction.

Neoplasia: This may be suspected on the basis of CSF fluid abnormalities and images of the brain.

Toxicity: Metronidazole intoxication at doses greater than 30 mg/kg/day can result in an acute onset of vestibular system dysfunction with vertical nystagmus and, occasionally, seizures. Supportive care, requiring a week or more of hospitalization, results in recovery, although months may be required before all signs resolve. Recovery may be hastened by treatment with diazepam (Evans *et al.*, 2002).

Metabolic: Thiamine deficiency may result in vestibular system dysfunction. Intramuscular thiamine hydrochloride (10–20 mg/kg i.m., continued until signs improve) can resolve the signs.

Vascular: Infarction of the medulla or cerebellum may be suspected on the basis of CSF abnormalities and images of the brain.

Pelvic limb paresis and paralysis

Pelvic limb paresis and paralysis may result from a lesion between the third thoracic spinal cord segment and the first sacral spinal cord segment, as well as from diseases of peripheral nerve, muscle and neuromuscular junction.

Causes and management of diseases of the spinal cord

Intervertebral disc disease

Acute onset of neurological dysfunction and/or pain on palpation over the affected area may occur. Intervertebral disc protrusion/herniation may be confirmed by myelography, CT or MRI. Animals with pain and mild ataxia/paraparesis may be treated with strict cage confinement for 4 weeks. Animals with moderate paraparesis or paraplegia but with intact deep pain sensation (assessed by looking for conscious recognition of compression of digits with haemostats or bone with bone forceps) may be treated either with strict cage confinement or surgical decompression, although there is a higher rate of recovery in animals treated surgically. Animals initially managed with cage confinement that then deteriorate should be treated surgically, since this indicates further extrusion of the already-extruded disc. Animals with paraplegia and anaesthesia (i.e. lack of deep pain sensation) are a surgical emergency. If surgical decompression is performed within 24 hours of the onset of signs, there is an approximately 50% chance of significant recovery. These animals may be treated with methylprednisolone sodium succinate if seen within 8 hours of the onset of acute signs (30 mg/kg i.v.; then 15 mg/kg at 2 and 6 hours; then 2.5 mg/kg/h for 24–48 hours). However, there is considerable debate as to the efficacy of corticosteroids in this situation, surgical intervention is vital and potential adverse effects of high-dose corticosteroids should be considered.

Patients that are managed with cage confinement should initially be treated with analgesics. There is some evidence to suggest that the use of corticosteroids may be detrimental (Olby, 1999), and it is probably safer to use opioids initially followed by a longer course of non-steroidal anti-inflammatory drugs (NSAIDs). If corticosteroids are used, prednisolone can be given at a dose of 0.5 mg/kg orally twice daily for 3 days, followed by 0.5 mg/kg once daily for 3 days, followed by 0.5 mg/kg every other day for 3 days. In all cases, it is important to check neurological status regularly (at least twice daily), and if any worsening occurs surgery should be performed immediately.

Neoplasia
Neoplasia may result in a gradual or sudden onset of clinical signs. Imaging modalities confirm the presence and location of the mass. CSF rarely contains neoplastic cells; however examination of spinal fluid may raise suspicion of inflammatory disease. Biopsy yields a definitive diagnosis. Cats with lymphoma of the spinal cord frequently have multicentric disease, are frequently positive for feline leukaemia virus (FeLV) and often have lymphoblastic leukaemia on bone marrow aspiration (Spodnick et al., 1992). Signs due to spinal cord compression may respond to steroid therapy, and possibly decompressive surgery or radiation. Cage rest is recommended for neoplasia associated with vertebral body lysis, due to the risk of pathological fracture.

Discospondylitis
Fever, depression and pain over the affected area are common. Radiographs or bone scans may reveal lysis of the vertebral endplates; however, no abnormalities may be found early in the course of the disease. Culture of urine, blood or the affected disc may identify the causative organism. Treatment involves cage rest and antibiotics (cephalosporins, oxacillin, cloxacillin or tetracycline) for at least 6–8 weeks, although some recommend long-term therapy (Burkert et al., 2005).

Distemper, feline infectious peritonitis, mycotic/bacterial/protozoal myelitis
Diagnosis is aided by recognition of signs of systemic or ophthalmic disease, results of titres and CSF analysis. For viral infections, steroids may be temporarily palliative. Toxoplasmosis/neosporosis may be treated with clindamycin and trimethoprim–sulphadiazine (see below).

Trauma
Trauma, with or without vertebral body fracture or dislocation, may result in clinical signs of spinal cord dysfunction. Plain radiography or myelography must be performed with extreme caution if vertebral instability is suspected. Patients should be strapped to a rigid board during the initial investigation, to prevent excessive movement and worsening of spinal cord trauma. Sedation may be required if the patient struggles against the strapping. If possible, imaging should be performed with the animal conscious in order to maintain normal muscle tone and limit movement of the spinal column. If no deep pain sensation is present, myelography or CT may be considered in order to rule out complete spinal cord transection, which carries a hopeless prognosis.

Treatment involves cage rest, methylprednisolone sodium succinate within 8 hours of the onset of signs (30 mg/kg i.v; then 15 mg/kg at 2 and 6 hours; then 2.5 mg/kg/h for 24–48 hours), and surgical decompression and stabilization if marked spinal cord compression or vertebral column instability is present. An external splint applied from the scapulae to the base of the tail may be used to limit motion of the spinal column in cases of vertebral body fracture.

Fibrocartilaginous emboli
Signs in dogs commonly begin during a period of exercise; mild transient pain may be noted. Signs may progress over the first 12 hours and then stabilize. Hemiparesis/paralysis may occur. Myelography may reveal intramedullary swelling or may be normal. Methylprednisolone sodium succinate (30 mg/kg i.v.; then 15 mg/kg at 2 and 6 hours; then 2.5 mg/kg/h for 24–48 hours) may be given within 8 hours of the onset of signs. Supportive care should be provided. Severity of signs and prognosis vary with the extent and location of the cord infarct. Infarcts occurring within either the cervicothoracic or lumbosacral intumescences carry a more guarded prognosis. Recovery may take months and may be incomplete.

Causes and management of diseases of peripheral nerve, muscle and neuromuscular junction
Diseases of peripheral nerves and muscles commonly result in flaccid paresis or paralysis. Clinical signs include a short-strided gait, postural reaction deficits and diminished segmental reflexes. Neurogenic muscle atrophy is common.

Toxoplasmosis/neosporosis
In puppies, flaccid paralysis which progresses to rigid extension of the pelvic limbs occurs to such a degree that the joints are no longer able to flex, even under

general anaesthesia. Evidence of systemic disease may be recognized. Increased antibody titres occur. Trimethoprim–sulphadiazine (15 mg/kg q12h for 2 weeks) and clindamycin (10 mg/kg q12h for 8 weeks) may result in improvement of clinical signs, however, once hindlimb rigidity has developed, improvement will not occur with therapy. If only one limb is affected, amputation may be considered in these animals.

Aortic thromboembolism
Animals are in pain, limbs are cool, pulses are weak or absent and muscles are firm. Abdominal ultrasonography may identify a thrombus in the aorta. Analgesics, intravenous fluids, heparin, acepromazine and aspirin may be given. Thromboembolism has been associated with cardiomyopathy in cats and with protein-losing nephropathy in dogs (Flanders, 1986; Van Winkle et al., 1993).

Others
Hypoadrenocorticism and diabetes mellitus may cause hindlimb paresis in addition to signs of metabolic disease. Diabetic cats and dogs may have a plantigrade stance. Control of metabolic disease commonly results in resolution of neurological dysfunction. Early polyneuropathy or myasthenia gravis may result in signs of hindlimb paresis (see Episodic weakness/syncope).

Tetraparesis and paralysis

Tetraparesis and paralysis may result from peripheral nerve/muscle, cervical spinal cord and/or brainstem disease. Differentiating peripheral nerve and muscle disease from spinal cord and brainstem disease is essential to making the correct diagnosis. Disorders of the cervical cord typically result in spasticity and exaggerated segmental reflexes. Disorders of the peripheral nerve/muscle result in flaccidity, diminished segmental reflexes and rapidly progressing muscle atrophy (1–2 weeks).

Cervical cord and/or brainstem disease caudal to the thalamus
For discussions of intervertebral disc disease, neoplasia, discospondylitis, myelitis, trauma and fibrocartilagenous emboli see Pelvic limb paresis and paralysis, above.

Atlantoaxial subluxation
Neck pain and signs attributable to disease of cervical spinal cord segments 1–5 may occur in young small-breed dogs. Flexing the neck may result in pain, worsening of clinical signs and respiratory paralysis. Survey radiographs may reveal subluxation of the first and second cervical vertebrae (increased space between the dorsal arch of C1 and the ventral aspect of the dorsal spinous process of C2) and possible abnormalities of the dens. If possible, radiographs should be performed without general anaesthesia, to prevent loss of muscle tone that prevents excessive flexion and worsening of compression. Cage rest, corticosteroid therapy and external fixation with a neck brace may result in improvement. Surgical stabilization may ultimately be required.

Caudal cervical spondylomyelopathy ('wobblers')
This condition is most frequently seen in young Great Danes and in middle-aged Dobermanns. Signs of disease attributable to cervical spinal cord segment 6 to thoracic cord segment 2 are most common. Cord compression and instability are confirmed with myelography. Flexed, extended and traction views of the neck are useful. In the emergency situation, these animals may be treated in a manner similar to animals with intervertebral disc disease. Without surgery, many dogs will eventually show a progression of clinical signs.

Granulomatous meningoencephalomyelitis
CSF analysis may show increases in protein, mononuclear cells and non-degenerate neutrophils. Myelography may reveal an intradural/extramedullary or intramedullary lesion. Definitive diagnosis requires biopsy. Prednisolone at immunosuppressive doses (1 mg/kg q12h for 5 days; then 1 mg/kg q24h for 7 days; then 1 mg/kg q48h) may result in initial improvement in neurological signs. Other agents have also been used in combination with corticosteroids, including cytosine arabinoside and lomustine, and some cases may survive for up to 2 years, but ultimately progression is inevitable. Radiation therapy has also been used with some success.

Steroid-responsive meningitis
Signs of neck pain, fever, lethargy and neurological deficits attributable to disease of cervical spinal cord segments 1–5 may occur in young dogs. CSF analysis reveals marked increases in protein and in white blood cells, with non-degenerate neutrophils the most common cell type. Culture of the CSF is negative. Treatment with glucocorticoids (1 mg/kg prednisolone q12h for 3 days and then decreased over time to a dose necessary to control signs) is required for 2–4 weeks; relapse of clinical signs is common.

Peripheral nerve/muscle

Botulism
Signs of flaccid paralysis and hyporeflexia occur in dogs hours to days after ingesting preformed toxin. Cranial nerve deficits include decreased ability:

- To blink the eyelids
- To lift the upper lip
- To close the mouth
- To lap water or swallow.

Change in bark, regurgitation, megaoesophagus, decreased perineal reflex, faecal and urinary incontinence, and respiratory paralysis may occur. Botulism is suspected from the history, clinical signs and electrodiagnostic testing (decreased compound motor action potential following nerve stimulation). Toxin may be identified in food, serum, stomach contents or faeces early in the course of the disease. Supportive care is given, a gastrostomy tube is placed if needed and the animal is monitored for aspiration pneumonia and respiratory paralysis. Signs may resolve with supportive care within 2–3 weeks.

Acute polyradiculoneuritis and polyneuritis

Affected dogs may have been recently vaccinated or have a history of exposure to racoons. However, some dogs may have no history of exposure to either. Flaccid paralysis and hyporeflexia occur. Facial muscle paresis and a change in bark are common. Respiratory paralysis may occur. Interestingly, however, tail and neck motion, swallowing and faecal and urinary continence are often maintained. The animal may be hyperaesthetic to touch. CSF analysis may show an increase in protein and cells. Electromyography may reveal fibrillation potentials and positive sharp waves in the majority of muscles tested. Nerve conduction velocity is slow, and evoked potentials may be decreased in amplitude. Biopsy specimens of nerve root or nerve may show inflammatory cell infiltrates, demyelination and axonal loss. Prednisolone (1 mg/kg q12h for 1–2 weeks; then 1 mg/kg q24h for 1 month) may be given; however, there is controversy as to whether it has any effect on the progression of this disease. Supportive care to prevent and treat decubital ulcers and urinary tract infections and observation for respiratory muscle paresis should be performed. Recovery may take 6–8 weeks and may be incomplete. Signs may recur.

Tick paralysis

Some species of tick can cause signs of peripheral neuromuscular disease that start to develop several days following attachment of the tick. This disease is reported in the US and a more severe form occurs in Australia. In the US, *Dermacentor variabilis* and *D. andersoni* (the Rocky Mountain wood tick) are incriminated most often. Other species that occasionally cause paralysis are *Ixodes cornuatus* and *I. hirsti*. *Ixodes scapularis*, the principal vector of the agent of Lyme disease (*Borrelia burgdorferi*) in the northeast, midwest and southeast of the United States, can also cause tick paralysis in dogs. *Ixodes pacificus* has been incriminated in dogs in the Grass Valley area (Nevada Co.) of northern California. In Australia, especially along the east coast, *Ixodes holocyclus* is the most important species.

Affected dogs typically still have the tick attached. Flaccid paralysis and hyporeflexia occur. Nystagmus, change in voice, dysphagia, weakness of facial muscles and masticatory muscles, and respiratory paralysis may occur. Electrodiagnostic testing may show reduction in amplitude or absence of the compound motor action potential following nerve stimulation and a slow nerve conduction velocity. Removal of ticks results in resolution of clinical signs within 24–72 hours. Ticks may be hard to find, however, and whole-body shaving may be necessary.

Insulin-secreting tumours

Serum glucose concentrations <2.8 mmol/l may result in clinical signs. Flaccid paralysis, hyporeflexia, lethargy, bradycardia, muscle tremors, hypothermia, disorientation and seizures may occur. Electromyographic examination may show fibrillation potentials, positive sharp waves and complex repetitive discharges. Small quantities of food high in protein, fat and complex carbohydrates may be provided frequently. Diazoxide (10 mg/kg q12h) and prednisolone (0.5 mg/kg/day) may be given.

Tetanus

Tetanus is the continuous tonic contraction of a muscle due to rapidly repeated stimulation. The causative organism, *Clostridium tetani*, synthesizes a potent neurotoxin (tetanospasmin) following germination of spores under anaerobic conditions, typically after infecting a deep wound. The toxin then travels in a retrograde fashion along axons within a peripheral nerve into the central nervous system. Clinical signs occur due to the ability of the toxin to inhibit the release of neurotransmitters (glycine and GABA) from upper motor neurons and interneurons of the brain stem and spinal cord, resulting in a release of the lower motor neuron from inhibition. Clinical signs of generalized tetanus include extensor rigidity of appendicular muscles, risus sardonicus and trismus. Dyspnoea, dysphagia and urinary and faecal retention may occur. Focal tetanus occurs when rigid extension is limited to one limb or muscle group.

Treatment with penicillin G (20,000–100,000 IU/kg i.v. q6h) is recommended and, if a wound is identified, it should be debrided to remove *Clostridium tetani*. Tetanus antitoxin is given at 100–1,000 IU/kg i.v.; a small test dose may be given initially to observe for an anaphylactic reaction. The patient should be kept in a quiet environment with little stimulation. Diazepam and phenobarbital may be given to relax or calm the patient. Nursing care is essential to maintain hydration and nutrition until the patient is able to drink and eat without assistance. If paralysis of the intercostal muscles occurs, ventilatory support may be necessary.

Episodic weakness/syncope

Episodic weakness and collapse may occur due to neuromuscular or brain disease, syncope or metabolic disorders.

Neuromuscular disorders

Acquired myasthenia gravis

At least three clinical presentations may occur (Dewey *et al.*, 1997):

- Focal myasthenia gravis. Animals exhibit facial, pharyngeal and/or laryngeal muscle dysfunction without appendicular muscle involvement. Megaoesophagus, regurgitation and aspiration pneumonia may occur
- Generalized myasthenia gravis. Animals exhibit appendicular muscle weakness with a stiff, short-strided gait with or without signs of facial, pharyngeal and/or laryngeal muscle dysfunction. Strength may or may not return following periods of rest
- Acute fulminating myasthenia gravis. Signs include: a sudden, rapid progression of severe appendicular muscle weakness, resulting in recumbency which is unabated by rest; frequent regurgitation associated with megaoesophagus; respiratory difficulty; and facial, pharyngeal and/or laryngeal muscle dysfunction.

For diagnosis, blood acetylcholine receptor antibody concentrations may be elevated (>0.6 nmol/l in dogs and >0.3 nmol/l in cats). Edrophonium (0.1–0.2 mg/kg i.v.) may result in dramatic improvement in gait for 1–2 minutes. Pretreatment with atropine (0.02 mg/kg i.v.) is recommended. Compound action potentials recorded from the interosseous muscle may show a 10% or greater decremental response following repetitive stimulation (Hopkins, 1992).

Long-term management includes administration of oral pyridostigmine (0.2–2.0 mg/kg q8–12h); alternatively, in animals with significant dysphagia and regurgitation, neostigmine can be given intramuscularly (0.04 mg/kg q6–8h). Animals should be kept warm and exercise restricted. Animals with dysphagia and megaoesophagus should be fed from a height with the head and neck elevated for 10 minutes after eating. Aminoglycoside antibiotics should be avoided due to the possibility of neuromuscular blockade. Prednisolone may result in a rapid worsening of clinical signs and its use is contraindicated in the presence of aspiration pneumonia. However, in the authors' experience, prednisolone may improve pharyngeal dysfunction sooner than cholinesterase inhibitors alone. A starting dose of 0.5 mg/kg/day increased to 2 mg/kg/day over 1 week has been suggested when aspiration pneumonia is not present (Le Couteur, 1988). Additionally, treatment with azathioprine and mycophenylate mofetil has proven useful and may minimize side effects due to steroid administration.

Exertional rhabdomyolysis
Racing Greyhounds may present with scuffing of the nails of the hindlimbs, muscle pain, tachypnoea, collapse and hyperthermia within 72 hours of exercise. Increased creatine kinase, lactate dehydrogenase, aspartate aminotransferase, blood lactate and myoglobin may occur. Renal failure may also occur. Intravenous fluids, to treat shock and to aid in the excretion of myoglobin, cold water baths, pain medication and intravenous bicarbonate may be given.

Polymyositis
Dogs and cats of any age may present with generalized weakness which worsens with exercise (Evans *et al.*, 2004). The gait is stiff and short-strided and dysphagia, regurgitation, megaoesophagus, change in bark, painful appendicular muscles, fever and lethargy may occur. Increases in creatine kinase, aspartate aminotransferase, lactate dehydrogenase and antinuclear antibody may occur. Electromyography may reveal fibrillation potentials, positive sharp waves and bizarre high frequency discharges. Muscle biopsy reveals lymphoplasmacytic inflammation and muscle necrosis. Toxoplasmosis and neosporosis should be ruled out with titres and muscle biopsy. Prednisolone may be given (1 mg/kg q12h initially) and reduced to the lowest dose necessary to control signs. Pharyngeal and oesophageal muscle involvement may result in aspiration pneumonia.

Brain disease

Narcolepsy/cataplexy
Episodes last seconds to minutes and are marked by acute collapse, decreased muscle tone and rapid eye movement sleep. Episodes may be provoked by excitement, food or physostigmine (0.025–0.1 mg/kg i.v.). Minimizing excitement and giving imipramine hydrochloride (0.5–1 mg/kg orally q8h) may decrease the number of events.

Syncope
Syncope due to cardiovascular or respiratory disease occurs most commonly during periods of exercise or excitement.

Cardiovascular disease
Episodic weakness, ataxia, lethargy, dyspnoea and syncope may occur. Evidence of a heart murmur, irregular heart rate or rhythm, bradycardia or tachycardia, weak or irregular pulses, polycythaemia, heartworm infection and electrocardiographic abnormalities between or during events suggest cardiovascular disease as the cause.

Respiratory disease
Hypoxia, particularly if chronic, may result in syncope.

Metabolic disorders

Hyperthyroidism
Episodic weakness, decreased ability to jump, muscle tremors and ventroflexion of the neck may occur in addition to other signs of hyperthyroidism (Joseph and Peterson, 1992). Post-insertional trains of positive sharp waves are reported on electromyographic examination. Stress should be decreased and methimazole administered (10–15 mg/day orally divided q12h).

Hypoadrenocorticism
Episodic weakness, stiff, stilted hindlimb gait, muscle tremors, vomiting, anorexia, weight loss, dehydration, weak pulses and shock may occur. Intestinal parasites (whipworms in particular) may cause clinical signs mimicking those of an Addisonian crisis. Stress should be decreased; intravenous fluid support with 0.9% sodium chloride provided; and hypoglycaemia treated. Dexamethasone sodium phosphate (0.1–0.2 mg/kg i.v.) may be given until the diagnosis is confirmed (see Chapter 16).

Hyperkalaemia
Appendicular and neck muscle weakness, bradycardia, dysrhythmias, weak pulses, electrocardiographic abnormalities and hyporeflexia may occur when serum potassium is >6.5 mmol/l. Weakness resolves with treatment of hyperkalaemia.

Hypokalaemic myopathy
This is seen principally in cats. Ventroflexion of the neck, a stiff, short-strided gait, episodic weakness, pain on muscle palpation and respiratory muscle paresis/paralysis may occur. A serum potassium <3.5 mmol/l, increased creatine kinase, azotaemia and metabolic acidosis may be found. Electromyographic

examination may reveal fibrillation potentials and positive sharp waves. Mildly or moderately affected cats may be treated with oral potassium supplementation (5–8 mmol potassium q12–24h). Intravenous potassium infusion (CRI <0.5 mmol/kg/h) may be given to those with severe weakness and respiratory depression. Occasionally, hypomagnesaemia may accompany hypokalaemia and exacerbate the weakness. Weakness resolves with treatment of hypokalaemia and, if present, hypomagnesaemia.

Others

Other diseases which may present with episodic weakness include: mitochondrial myopathy of Clumber and Sussex Spaniels and Old English Sheepdogs; phosphofructokinase deficiency of English Springer Spaniels; panosteitis; hypertrophic osteodystrophy; polyarthritis; anaphylactic reactions; and the presence of a phaeochromocytoma. A good history is necessary to rule out epileptic activity as a cause for paroxysmal collapse.

References and further reading

Bagley RS (1996) Intracranial pressure in dogs and cats. *Compendium on Continuing Education for the Practicing Veterinarian* **18**, 605–621

Berendt M and Gram L (1999) Epilepsy and seizure classification in 63 dogs: a reappraisal of veterinary epilepsy terminology. *Journal of Veterinary Internal Medicine* **13**, 14–20

Braund KG (1994) *Clinical Syndromes in Veterinary Neurology, 2nd edn.* Mosby, St. Louis

Bunch SE (1995) Specific and symptomatic medical management of diseases of the liver. In: *Textbook of Veterinary Internal Medicine, 4th edn*, ed. SJ Ettinger and EC Feldman, pp. 1358–1371. WB Saunders, Philadelphia

Burkert BA, Kerwin SC, Hosgood GL, Pechman RD and Fontenelle JP (2005) Signalment and clinical features of diskospondylitis in dogs: 513 cases (1980–2001). *Journal of the American Veterinary Medical Association* **227**, 268–275

de Lahunta A (1983) *Veterinary Neuroanatomy and Clinical Neurology, 2nd edn.* WB Saunders, Philadelphia

Dewey CW, Bailey CS, Shelton GD, Kass PH and Cardinet GH III (1997) Clinical forms of acquired myasthenia gravis in dogs: 25 cases (1988–1995) *Journal of Veterinary Internal Medicine* **11(2)**, 50–57

Evans J, Levesque D, Knowles K, Longshore R and Plummer S (2002) The use of diazepam in the treatment of metronidazole toxicosis in the dog. *Journal of Veterinary Internal Medicine* **16**, 368

Evans J, Levesque D and Shelton GD (2004) Canine inflammatory myopathies: a clinicopathologic review of 200 cases. *Journal of Veterinary Internal Medicine* **18**, 679

Feldman EC (2005) Disorders of the parathyroid glands. In: *Textbook of Veterinary Internal Medicine, 6th edn*, ed. SJ Ettinger & EC Feldman, pp. 1508–1535

Flanders JA (1986) Feline aortic thromboembolism. *Compendium on Continuing Education for the Practicing Veterinarian* **8**, 473–484

Fortune JB, Feustel PJ, deLuna C, et al. (1995) Cerebral blood flow and blood volume in response to O_2 and CO_2 changes in normal humans. *Journal of Trauma* **39**, 463–471

Hopkins AL (1992) Canine myasthenia gravis. *Journal of Small Animal Practice* **33**, 477–484

Joseph RJ and Peterson ME (1992) Review and comparison of neuromuscular and central nervous system manifestations of hyperthyroidism in cats and humans. *Progress in Veterinary Neurology* **3**, 114–119

Kelly MJ (1989) Canine myxedema stupor and coma. In: *Current Veterinary Therapy X: Small Animal Practice*, ed. RW Kirk and JD Bonagura, pp. 998–1001. WB Saunders, Philadelphia

Le Couteur RA (1988) Disorders of peripheral nerves. In: *Handbook of Small Animal Practice*, ed. RV Morgan, pp. 299–318. Churchill Livingstone, New York

Muizelaar JP, Marmarou A, Ward JD et al. (1991) Adverse effects of prolonged hyperventilation in patients with severe head injury: a randomized clinical trial. *Journal of Neurosurgery* **75**, 731–739

O'Brien DP, Kroll RA, Johnson GC, Covert SJ and Nelson MJ (1994) Myelinolysis after correction of hyponatremia in two dogs. *Journal of Veterinary Internal Medicine* **8**, 40–48

Obrist WD, Langfitt TW, Jaggi JL, Cruz J and Gennarelli TA (1984) Cerebral blood flow and metabolism in comatose patients with acute head injury. Relationship to intracranial hyerptension. *Journal of Neurosurgery* **61**, 241–253

Olby N (1999) Current concepts in the management of acute spinal cord injury. *Journal of Veterinary Internal Medicine* **13**, 399–407

Oliver JE and Lorenz MD (1997) *Handbook of Veterinary Neurologic Diagnosis*. WB Saunders, Philadelphia

Podell M, Fenner WR and Powers JD (1995) Seizure classification in dogs from a nonreferral-based population. *Journal of the American Veterinary Medical Association* **206(11)**, 1721–1728

Ramsey DT, Casteel SW, Faggella AM et al. (1996) Use of orally administered succimer (meso-2,3-dimercaptosuccinic acid) for treatment of lead poisoning in dogs. *Journal of the American Veterinary Medical Association* **208(3)**, 371–375

Skippen P, Seear M, Poskitt K et al. (1997) Effects of hyperventilation on regional cerebral blood flow in head-injured children. *Critical Care Medicine* **25**, 1402–1409

Snyder JM, Shofer FS, Van Winkle TJ and Massicotte C (2006) Canine intracranial primary neoplasia: 173 cases (1986–2003). *Journal of Veterinary Internal Medicine* **20**, 669–675

Spodnick GJ, Berg J, Moore FM and Cotter SM (1992). Spinal lymphoma in cats: 21 cases (1976–1989). *Journal of the American Veterinary Medical Association* **200(3)**, 373–376

Troxel MT, Vite CH, Van Winkle TJ et al. (2003) Feline intracranial neoplasia: retrospective review of 160 cases (1985–2001). *Journal of Veterinary Internal Medicine* **17**, 850–859

Van Winkle TJ, Liu SM and Hackner SG (1993) Clinical and pathological features of aortic thromboembolism in 36 dogs. *Journal of Veterinary Emergency and Critical Care* **3**, 13–21

Walmsley GL, Herrtage ME, Dennis R, Platt SR and Jeffery ND (2005) The relationship between clinical signs and brain herniation associated with rostrotentorial mass lesions in the dog. *Veterinary Journal* **172**, 258–264

Wheeler S and Sharp N (1994) *Small Animal Spinal Disorders: Diagnosis and Surgery*. Mosby-Wolfe, London

10

Ophthalmological emergencies

Deborah C. Mandell

Introduction

Ocular emergencies can be intimidating and frustrating for veterinary surgeons. While most general practitioners do not have the equipment to perform thorough and detailed ophthalmic examinations or surgery (i.e. slit lamps, operating microscopes), the majority of ophthalmological emergencies can be treated successfully with the basic equipment available to every veterinary surgeon.

Many animals present to the emergency room because they have a painful eye or eyes. It is important to evaluate all structures of the eye in every animal that presents for an ocular emergency. It may be necessary to sedate animals with particularly painful eyes; topical anaesthesia, however, can often relieve enough discomfort to facilitate an ophthalmic examination. This examination should include the periorbital structures, conjunctiva, cornea, the anterior chamber, including the iris, the lens and the posterior chamber, including the vitreous and fundus. The pupillary light reflex, both direct and indirect, menace and dazzle should also be evaluated on initial examination.

This chapter discusses the diagnosis, treatment and prognosis of common ophthalmological emergencies. When a disease is not responding to treatment or when there are conflicting disease processes in the same eye, an ophthalmologist should always be consulted.

Glaucoma

Definition and causes
Glaucoma is an increase in intraocular pressure due to an obstruction of aqueous humour outflow from the ciliary body through the ciliary cleft. The causes are listed in Figure 10.1. Owners should be warned that glaucoma is usually a bilateral disease even if animals present with unilateral signs. Long-term medical therapy should be started in both eyes after stabilization of the acute stage.

Clinical signs
Clinical signs include buphthalmos (Figure 10.2), a painful, red eye, scleral injection, dilated pupil, negative menace response, absent pupillary light reflex, corneal oedema and possible decreased retinal vascularity. Breeds commonly affected with primary glaucoma include Cocker Spaniels, Poodles, Basset Hounds, Beagles and Samoyeds.

Primary
Primary open angle
Primary closed angle (goniodysgenesis)

Secondary
Uveitis [a]
Lens luxation [a]
Neoplasia [a]
Hyphaema
Cataracts – due to lens-induced uveitis or swelling of the lens

10.1 Causes of glaucoma. [a] Most common causes of glaucoma in cats.

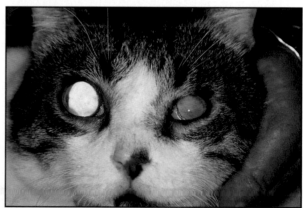

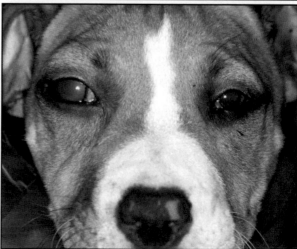

10.2 Glaucoma in a cat and a dog. Notice the buphthalmos and dilated pupil. The cat presented for a 2-day history of blindness, and had uveitis in the left eye. The dog presented with a 2-day history of right-sided blindness and blepharospasm.

Diagnosis

The intraocular pressure (IOP) should be measured using a Schiøtz or electronic tonometer (Figure 10.3). Normal IOP is 15–25 mmHg. If the IOP is greater than 35 mmHg, emergency treatment should be initiated.

One of the most important differential diagnoses of a dilated pupil with acute blindness is sudden acquired retinal degeneration syndrome (SARDS), in which the ocular examination and IOP will be normal. SARDS is usually bilateral and can present with concurrent signs such as polyuria, polydipsia and polyphagia. The cause is unknown and there is no treatment.

Treatment

The treatment for glaucoma consists of lowering the IOP to prevent permanent blindness by medically drawing fluid out of the vitreous chamber, by increasing drainage of aqueous humour and by decreasing aqueous production. Emergency treatment involves the use of agents that rapidly decrease intraocular pressure. Mannitol, an osmotic diuretic that draws water from the aqueous and vitreous into the vasculature, is given at a dose of 1 g/kg i.v. over 20–30 minutes. This therapy can lower the IOP within 1 hour. The dose can be repeated in 4 hours if the IOP does not decrease below 30 mmHg. The main side effect of mannitol is dehydration from the osmotic diuresis, thus it should not be given to patients in which dehydration could result in serious adverse consequences, for example animals with renal insufficiency. In addition to mannitol, pilocarpine drops (2%) can be instilled every 15–60 minutes for 3–4 hours. Pilocarpine acts as a parasympathomimetic, constricting the pupil and thus opening the drainage angle. Side effects such as bradycardia are usually not seen.

Carbonic anhydrase inhibitors (CAI) decrease the volume of aqueous produced. Oral CAIs are the mainstay of treatment of chronic glaucoma and should be

---

Tonometry is the indirect measurement of intraocular pressure. Techniques include digital palpation (gentle pressure exerted with finger) and/or indentation applanation tonometry.

Schiøtz tonometer

The most commonly used indentation tonometer is the Schiøtz tonometer, which consists of a corneal footplate, a plunger, a bracket to hold either a 7.5 g or a 10 g weight, and a recording scale. The footplate indents the cornea which moves the stylet. The scale reading is converted to mmHg using a conversion table.

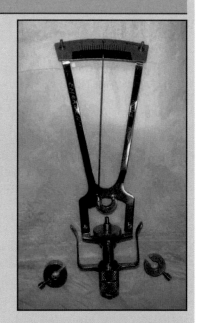

1. Topical anaesthetic (proparacaine) is placed in both eyes.
2. The animal is restrained so that the cornea is parallel to the floor/ceiling for an accurate reading. Typically, the animal is placed in dorsal recumbency or sternal with the head tilted back.
3. A 7.5 g or 10 g weight is placed on the tonometer.
4. The plunger is gently placed on the cornea, avoiding the third eyelid, and a reading is taken. This is repeated for two more readings to ensure an accurate and consistent reading.
5. The conversion table is then used to convert the reading to mmHg.
6. The readings can be repeated using a different weight to further ensure accuracy.
7. The intraocular pressure should be measured in both eyes.

Although the Schiøtz tonometer is the most inexpensive and can be easy to use, it does have limitations:

- The plunger must be cleaned periodically because accumulated debris can lead to an inaccurate reading
- The corneal footplate was designed for humans, so the curvature of the footplate may not match canine and feline corneas. Falsely low readings may result if the cornea is large
- Corneal disease results in inaccurate readings
- The Schiøtz cannot be used if the patient has had recent intraocular surgery.

Applanation tonometers

Applanation tonometers, which estimate IOP by measuring the force required to flatten (applanate) a small area of corneal surface, are inherently more accurate than the Schiøtz tonometer. They are easier to use but are much more expensive. The most common applanation tonometer in veterinary use is the Tonopen. It is a handheld, battery-operated instrument.

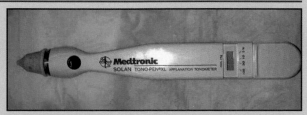

1. Topical anaesthetic is placed in both eyes.
2. A condom is placed on the probe of the tonometer.
3. The probe is gently tapped on the cornea three times. On each successful 'tap', a beep sounds, signalling that a reading was obtained.
4. An average reading is then shown on the display.

The applanation tonometer can be used with the animal in a normal standing position and can be used after intraocular surgery.

10.3 Intraocular pressure measurement. A Schiøtz tonometer is routinely used for measurement of IOP. An electronic applanation tonometer is more accurate and easier to use than the Schiøtz, but is more expensive.

started during emergency management of acute glaucoma. These drugs can decrease the IOP significantly, but side effects of the oral CAIs include anorexia, nausea, vomiting and central nervous system (CNS) sedation. The newer oral CAIs, such as dichlorphenamide, have fewer side effects. Topical CAIs (dorzolamide three times a day) can be used in the emergency setting and for chronic glaucoma, and they do not have such adverse side effects. Timolol maleate (0.25–0.5% twice a day), a topical beta blocker, can be used concurrently to further decrease the volume of aqueous fluid produced.

Latanoprost, a topical prostaglandin analogue, increases drainage of aqueous humour through an alternative route. It can rapidly decrease the IOP by 40–60% and is additive to the effects of mannitol. It should be used with caution in dogs with glaucoma secondary to anterior uveitis, because the drug causes miosis, which can be severe. Latanoprost is contraindicated for treatment of glaucoma secondary to lens luxation.

When glaucoma is secondary to another disease, the underlying disease such as lens luxation or uveitis must be treated as a priority. If primary glaucoma is diagnosed, an ophthalmologist should be consulted as long-term management will be required. The IOP should be measured every 4–6 months, and owners should monitor for recurrence of pain, blindness, buphthalmos or a dilated pupil.

Prognosis

If more than 24 hours have elapsed with an IOP above 50 mmHg, the prognosis for vision becomes poor due to damage to the retina and optic nerve. Anti-inflammatory doses of corticosteroids may improve optic nerve head oedema in acute glaucoma. Long-term prognosis for primary glaucoma is variable, depending on the length of time for which the medications control the IOP, but is usually poor. Most cases eventually become refractory to medical management and need definitive treatment to destroy the ciliary body such as enucleation, cyclocryotherapy, laser treatment or intravitreous gentamicin instillation.

Proptosis

Definition and causes

Proptosis is forward displacement of the globe, which can occur secondary to any blunt trauma to the head such as being hit by a car, or bite wounds (Figure 10.4). Brachycephalic breeds are predisposed because they have shallow orbits.

Clinical signs and management

Clinical signs and management depend on the cause of the proptosis and the degree of damage to the globe and extraocular structures. There are two options for therapy: enucleation or replacement with a temporary tarsorrhaphy. This decision is based on the severity of the proptosis. If the eye has ruptured, all of the extraocular muscles are ruptured and/or the extraocular muscles are necrotic or infected,

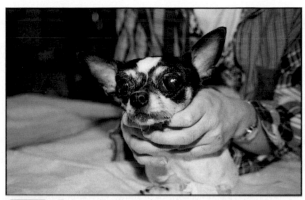

10.4 Traumatic bilateral proptosis secondary to a dog fight. One eye was enucleated and the other was replaced and a tarsorrhaphy performed.

the eye should be removed. If there is marked hyphaema, enucleation should also be considered. If the owner or veterinary surgeon is unsure whether the owner will be able to treat or monitor the eye, enucleation is usually the best option. Replacement can be attempted if the eye and extraocular muscles are relatively undamaged and few extraocular muscles have ruptured.

Replacement with temporary tarsorrhaphy

Although the eye should be replaced as soon as possible, if the animal has sustained significant head trauma, anaesthesia should be postponed until its condition is stable. Anaesthetic agents that increase IOP (e.g. ketamine) should be avoided. A topical sterile lubricant should be applied to the globe frequently to prevent desiccation.

Once the animal is anaesthetized, the surrounding area should be carefully clipped and aseptically scrubbed with chlorhexidine or betadine. A stay suture with 2–3 metric (2/0 or 3/0 USP) nylon should be placed in the upper and lower eyelids close to the lid margin. A lateral canthotomy is usually needed to facilitate replacement of the globe. Sterile lubricant is placed on the eye. While lifting out and up on the stay sutures, gentle pressure is placed on the eye to replace it into the orbit. A scalpel handle or other flat object can be used to apply pressure evenly. Once the eye is replaced, the stay sutures are crossed and held to prevent reproptosis. Tension-relieving sutures are then placed (Figure 10.5); 1.5 metric (4/0 USP) nylon can be used with pieces of a 3 or 5 French (Fr) red rubber catheter, intravenous tubing or rubber band as stents. A horizontal mattress suture is used and all sutures should be preplaced before tying. The suture should go through the stent, enter the lid 6–8 mm from the upper lid margin, exit through the Meibomian glands, then enter through the lower lid Meibomian glands, exit 6–8 mm from the lower lid margin and go through a second stent. The needle then goes back in the reverse direction and the suture is tied at the dorsal aspect. This suture pattern protects the cornea by everting the eyelids. The lateral canthotomy can then be sutured with 1–1.5 metric (4/0 or 5/0 USP) absorbable synthetic suture, e.g. Vicryl®. A small space should be left open medially to allow placement of medications.

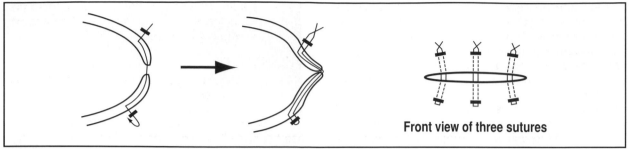

Front view of three sutures

10.5 Suture and stent placement for tarsorrhaphy. A 3–5 French red rubber catheter or rubber bands can be used as stents. The suture should go through a stent, enter 6–8 mm away from the upper lid margin, exit through the Meibomian glands, then enter the lower Meibomian glands, exit 6–8 mm away from the lower lid margin, then go through the stent. The needle then goes back in the reverse direction.

Aftercare

Aftercare consists of topical antibiotics (tobramycin or gentamicin 0.3% q4–6h) and topical atropine sulphate (1% q12h). Oral broad-spectrum antibiotics should also be used for 2 weeks. Anti-inflammatory doses of corticosteroids at a tapering dose over 3–5 days will decrease further damage to the optic nerve and decrease periorbital swelling. An Elizabethan collar must be worn at all times.

Frequent re-evaluations should be performed to make sure that the client is able to administer medications, the sutures are not abrading the cornea, the animal is not febrile and that there is no discharge crusted over the eye. The sutures are removed in 14 days. Once the sutures are removed, the cornea should be stained to check for ulcers and treated appropriately. Topical corticosteroids can be used (prednisolone acetate 1% q8h) if there is scarring with no corneal ulcer. When scarring is present with a corneal ulcer, a topical non-steroidal anti-inflammatory drug (NSAID), such as flurbiprofen (0.03% q8h), should be used instead.

The eye should be evaluated every 4–5 days for 2–3 weeks after suture removal to monitor for complications such as exposure keratitis. If the animal is lagophthalmic and has exposure keratitis, a partial permanent tarsorrhaphy may help.

Complications with replacement

Complications following replacement include infection, dorsolateral strabismus due to rupture of the medial rectus muscle, blindness and ulcerative or exposure keratitis with a resultant corneal ulcer. The dorsolateral strabismus may improve with time. Owners must be warned that enucleation may still be necessary.

Prognosis

Due to the stretching of the optic nerve, the prognosis for vision is poor but the prognosis for cosmetic repair is fair. A successful outcome is more likely if the proptosis is treated early and is evaluated frequently to circumvent complications. Brachycephalic breeds that require less force to proptose an eye have a better chance of regaining vision than dolichocephalic dogs or cats where a significant amount of force is necessary and more traumatic damage to the eye is likely to have occurred.

Enucleation

An ophthalmology or surgery text should be consulted for enucleation procedures.

Anterior uveitis

Definition

Uveitis is an inflammation of the iris and ciliary body. Many systemic disease processes manifest as uveitis in dogs and cats, and some examples are listed in Figure 10.6.

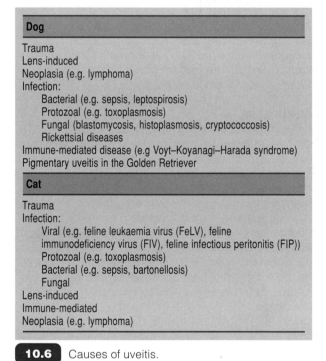

Dog
Trauma
Lens-induced
Neoplasia (e.g. lymphoma)
Infection:
Bacterial (e.g. sepsis, leptospirosis)
Protozoal (e.g. toxoplasmosis)
Fungal (blastomycosis, histoplasmosis, cryptococcosis)
Rickettsial diseases
Immune-mediated disease (e.g Voyt–Koyanagi–Harada syndrome)
Pigmentary uveitis in the Golden Retriever

Cat
Trauma
Infection:
Viral (e.g. feline leukaemia virus (FeLV), feline immunodeficiency virus (FIV), feline infectious peritonitis (FIP))
Protozoal (e.g. toxoplasmosis)
Bacterial (e.g. sepsis, bartonellosis)
Fungal
Lens-induced
Immune-mediated
Neoplasia (e.g. lymphoma)

10.6 Causes of uveitis.

Clinical signs

Clinical signs include blepharospasm, a miotic pupil due to ciliary spasm, pain, a red, inflamed, dull or 'fluffy' iris, aqueous flare, hypopyon or hyphaema, decreased IOP (<10 mmHg due to decreased aqueous production) and prolapsed nictitans.

Diagnosis

The diagnosis of anterior uveitis is based on clinical signs. Other differential diagnoses for patients presenting with a red painful eye include glaucoma and corneal ulceration. These diseases may not be mutually exclusive, for example uveitis can cause glaucoma, and trauma can cause both corneal ulcers and uveitis. Even if uveitis is suspected, the eye should still be stained with fluorescein, and IOP should be measured. As uveitis is often a manifestation of systemic disease a full and thorough general physical examination is also mandatory. Diagnostic tests should be geared towards identification of the underlying cause and can include any of the following: complete blood count; serum chemistry panel; urinalysis; toxoplasmosis titre and other infectious disease screening (depending on geographical location); and thoracic radiography. In the cat, feline leukaemia virus (FeLV)/feline immunodeficiency virus (FIV) and possibly feline infectious peritonitis (FIP) serology should also be performed. Vogt–Koyanagi–Harada (VKH) or uveodermatological syndrome is an immune-mediated disease associated with antibody production against melanocytes. It should be suspected in Japanese breeds of dog (e.g. Akita) presenting with uveitis (Figure 10.7).

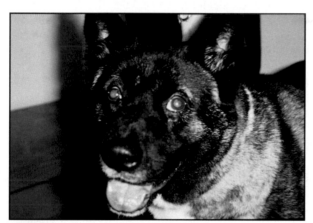

10.7 A 3-year-old Akita with a 5-day history of blindness. There was severe uveitis and retinal detachment. This dog had Vogt–Koyanagi–Harada syndrome.

Treatment

Topical atropine sulphate (1% q8–12h to maintain a dilated pupil) should be used to prevent the formation of synechiae. This will also improve the animal's comfort by paralysing the ciliary body (cycloplegia) and causing mydriasis. If secondary glaucoma is present, atropine is contraindicated, and adrenaline drops (1% q8h) can be used instead to dilate the pupil and decrease aqueous production. Adrenaline is contraindicated in animals predisposed to dysrhythmias. Alternatively, tropicamide, a short-acting mydriatic–cycloplegic drug, can be used. Topical corticosteroids (prednisolone acetate 1% q6h) are often necessary to decrease inflammation. In severe cases, systemic corticosteroids can be considered. Treatment of the underlying cause, if found, is also necessary. This may involve specific treatment for infectious or neoplastic disease or immunosuppressive therapy if an immune-mediated disease (e.g. VKH) is suspected. Lens-induced uveitis can be very severe and difficult to control. Any eye with uveitis should be rechecked in 4–5 days for progress.

Complications

Secondary complications include anterior or posterior synechia formation, glaucoma and cataracts. In cases involving either recurrent uveitis or multiple disease processes in the same eye, the animal should be referred to an ophthalmologist.

Prognosis

Many systemic disease processes have a fair to good short-term prognosis for control of uveitis but a poor long-term prognosis (e.g. FeLV/FIV infection). The prognosis can be good, however, when the underlying cause can be controlled (e.g. sepsis, rickettsial or immune-mediated diseases). Traumatic uveitis should respond to treatment and resolve within 1 week. A neoplastic cause can be challenging to rule out as diagnostic tests may initially be unremarkable. Neoplasia, especially lymphoma, may not be diagnosed until other clinical signs worsen, which may be many months later.

Corneal ulcers

Definition

Corneal ulcers are epithelial defects of the cornea, which are classified according to the layers that are affected. The most common causes of corneal ulcers are listed in Figure 10.8.

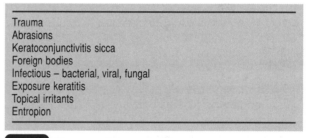

Trauma
Abrasions
Keratoconjunctivitis sicca
Foreign bodies
Infectious – bacterial, viral, fungal
Exposure keratitis
Topical irritants
Entropion

10.8 Causes of corneal ulcers.

Clinical signs and initial evaluation

Patients with corneal ulcers usually present with blepharospasm, ocular discharge, conjunctival hyperaemia and pain, causing photophobia and possibly a miotic pupil. Miosis may also occur secondary to concurrent uveitis. Corneal oedema and/or neovascularization may be found around the ulcer. A Schirmer tear test (Figure 10.9) should be performed on all eyes with corneal ulcers to rule out keratoconjunctivitis sicca (KCS) as the underlying cause. Normal tear production is 10–25 mm/min and less than 5 mm/min is highly suggestive of KCS. Fluorescein stain should be applied to characterize the ulcer. The eye should be thoroughly examined for any foreign body (under the nictitans and both eyelids).

Monitoring

For all ulcers, regardless of the treatment, owners should monitor the eye carefully. Urgent re-evaluation is warranted if: there is a discharge from the cornea; the animal starts to keep its eye closed; the eye appears red or pain recurs; the eye loses or changes shape; or the animal becomes lethargic or anorexic. Lagophthalmic breeds are very susceptible to central corneal ulcers. These ulcers can progress rapidly and require particularly careful monitoring.

The Schirmer tear test (STT) measures the amount of aqueous tears produced in 1 minute using a strip of 5 x 35 mm filter paper. Many ocular diseases can be secondary to decreased tear production (e.g. KCS) and thus the STT is an extremely important diagnostic tool in any ophthalmic emergency. Normal tear production in the dog is 10–25 mm/min. Dogs with KCS usually have a STT of <5 mm/min.

The most common Schirmer tear test (STT I) is performed in an unanaesthetized eye, before any medications are used. This measures the basal and reflex tear production. The STT II is used when the conjunctiva is anaesthetized and the nasal mucosa is irritated; it measures only basal tear production. The STT III is performed when the patient is looking into the sun.

The STT is easy to perform and can be done in most animals with minimal restraint. The strips now have a marker dye to show clearly the amount of tear production, and millimetre scale markings on them to facilitate the measurement. The strips should not be taken out of the package until the operator is ready to perform the test, and the test area of the strip should never be touched. For a valid reading, the STT I must be performed before any medications are placed in the eye.

1. While the test strip is still in the package, the strip is folded at the notch so that the end is perpendicular to the rest of the strip.

2. The folded part of the strip is placed in the ventrolateral conjunctival sac so that the notch rests at the eyelid margin.

3. The strip is held in place for 1 minute, and the tears produced flow down the test strip, moving the dye with them.

4. The eyelids are gently held closed to keep the strip in place.

5. The STT should be performed in both eyes.

10.9 Schirmer tear test.

Basic management

Topical corticosteroids are always contraindicated if the corneal epithelium is not intact. If severe uveitis accompanies the ulcer, topical NSAIDs (e.g. flurbiprofen q8h) or tapering doses of systemic corticosteroids can be used. If more than one topical eye medication is needed, a period of at least 5 minutes should be interposed between administration of different medications.

Superficial ulcers

Diagnosis

Superficial ulcers (Figure 10.10) are diagnosed based on fluorescein stain retention, and are relatively clear defects in the cornea.

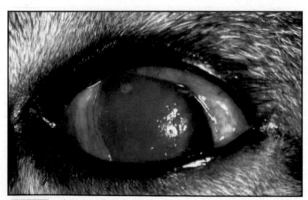

10.10 A superficial corneal ulcer affecting the majority of the cornea. This cat presented with a 1-day history of ocular discharge, blepharospasm and lethargy.

Treatment

Treatment includes topical antibiotics (triple antibiotic solution or fusidic acid 1% q6–8h is usually sufficient). Atropine sulphate (1% q12h) may also be used if a miotic pupil (due to ciliary spasm or iridocyclospasm) is present or the eye is painful. Ciclosporin (0.2–1%) should be started twice a day for 4 weeks if KCS is the initiating cause of the ulcer. If the ulcer was due to a topical irritant, such as a shampoo or soap, irrigation with copious amounts of sterile eye wash or saline is performed.

In cats, erythromycin or chloramphenicol 1% ointment (q6–8h) is preferred. The neomycin in triple antibiotic solutions or ointments can cause chemosis and severe irritation. Anaphylaxis to neomycin has been reported in a cat. Also, many corneal ulcers in cats have a viral aetiology, and an antiviral medication (trifluridine or vidarabine, if available, four or five times a day) can be included.

The eye should be re-stained after 4–5 days, at which time the ulcer should be healed. If not, an indolent or complicated ulcer should be suspected.

Prognosis

If there are no complications, the prognosis is excellent.

Indolent ulcers

Diagnosis

An indolent ulcer is a non-healing ulcer that occurs when the epithelium does not attach to the stroma due to an epithelial basement membrane or stromal defect. This type of ulcer is common in Boxer dogs. When the ulcer is stained with fluorescein, the stain extends further than the visible edges of the ulcer, demonstrating an area of epithelium that has not anchored to the stroma.

Treatment

A topical anaesthetic (proparacaine) is placed on the eye. A cotton swab (moistened with artificial tears or proparacaine) is used to debride the edges of the ulcer, creating a larger defect. Once the edges are debrided, a grid or punctate keratectomy is performed with a 20–25 gauge needle, avoiding going through the full thickness of the cornea (Figure 10.11). This aids healing and is thought to help the epithelium attach to the stroma. Topical antibiotics (tobramycin or gentamicin 0.3% q6h) and atropine sulphate (1% q12h) should then be started.

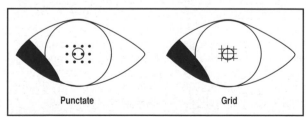

Punctate Grid

10.11 Punctate and grid keratectomy. After topical anaesthetic and debridement with a cotton swab, a 25 gauge needle is used to make punctate or grid marks on, not through, the corneal epithelium.

Prognosis

With treatment, the majority of indolent ulcers heal.

Deep corneal ulcer

Diagnosis

Deep corneal ulcers are also diagnosed based on fluorescein staining, although the defect may be appreciated on gross examination (Figure 10.12). Deep ulcers may not be as painful as superficial ulcers.

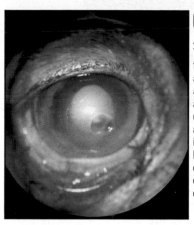

10.12 A deep ulcer. Treatment includes topical antibiotics, atropine sulphate and an anticollagenase (serum or acetylcysteine), if infected. Perforation can occur with restraint or if the animal rubs or scratches the eye.

Treatment

Therapy with topical antibiotics (tobramycin or gentamicin 0.3% q4–6h) and topical atropine sulphate (1% q6–12h) should be started. If the deep ulcer is infected or melting (Figure 10.13), then more aggressive treatment is needed. Gram-negative rods produce collagenases or proteases which can rapidly destroy (melt) the cornea. Topical broad-spectrum antibiotics (ciprofloxacin q2–3h) and topical atropine (q4–6h) should be started. A topical anticollagenase should also be added in patients with deep melting or infected ulcers (Figure 10.13). Autologous serum can be used, in which α-macroglobulin acts as the anticollagenase. Acetylcysteine, diluted to a 5% solution with artificial tears, may also be used. Anticollagenases should be instilled every 2–3 hours. If the animal is rubbing or scratching at the eye, an Elizabethan collar must be worn. For all deep ulcers, care must be taken to avoid excessive restraint of the patient, as this can lead to perforation (Figure 10.14). A conjunctival flap should be considered in any patient with a deep ulcer if it spans the majority of the stroma, or if it is progressing despite aggressive medical therapy.

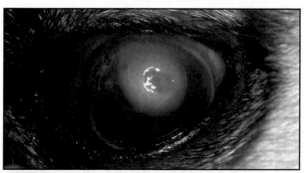

10.13 A melting ulcer. This pug had a 1-week history of blepharospasm and ocular discharge. The owners reported that the cornea became 'white' within the last 24 hours.

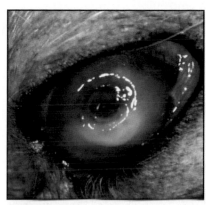

10.14 A perforated melting ulcer. This ulcer progressed to perforation within 12 hours.

Prognosis

With aggressive treatment the prognosis can be good. The eye should be monitored very carefully for the first 2–3 days, and then every 3 days for 2 weeks, to ensure that the ulcer continues to heal properly. A deep corneal ulcer can take up to 3 weeks to heal.

Descemetocele

Diagnosis

When Descemet's membrane (the corneal endothelium) protrudes through the ulcer, it looks clear, black or transparent (Figure 10.15) and does not retain fluorescein stain. In this case, the cornea is in imminent danger of perforation.

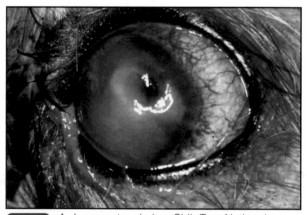

10.15 A descemetocele in a Shih Tzu. Notice the black bulging area in the centre of the ulcer. This area is only one cell layer thick. This is a surgical emergency and a conjunctival flap should be placed.

Treatment

A descemetocele is a true emergency. Topical antibiotics (tobramycin, gentamicin or ciprofloxacin 0.3% q2–3h) and topical atropine (q4–6h) should be started. An Elizabethan collar, cage rest and gentle restraint must be enforced. If the animal is struggling or resents restraint, medications should wait until after surgical repair as long as this can be performed immediately. The cornea can be sutured over the descemetocele, inverting the membrane if possible, with 0.3–0.7 metric (6/0 to 9/0 USP) absorbable synthetic suture, e.g. Vicryl®, in a simple interrupted or horizontal mattress pattern without penetrating full thickness through the cornea. Since the cornea is usually oedematous and weak, increased support and protection can be achieved with a conjunctival flap.

Prognosis
The prognosis is variable depending on the extent of corneal disease and the cause of the ulcer.

Iris prolapse

Diagnosis
The iris is visible protruding through the ulcer (Figure 10.16).

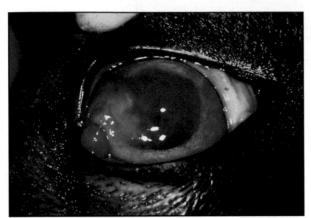

10.16 Iris prolapse. Notice the iris protruding through the edge of the ulcer. The exposed iris must be removed from the defect. The cornea can then be sutured closed with 0.3–0.7 metric (6/0 to 9/0 USP) Vicryl®. A conjunctival or third eyelid flap is then performed after reinflation of the anterior chamber with saline or air.

Treatment
Topical antibiotics (tobramycin or gentamicin 0.3% q4–6h) should be started. The iris must be removed from the ulcer. It can be freed from the edges of the cornea with an iris spatula or atraumatic forceps. The exposed iris can then be excised with tenotomy scissors. The cornea is sutured with 0.3–0.7 metric (6/0 to 9/0 USP) absorbable synthetic suture, e.g. Vicryl®, in a simple interrupted or horizontal mattress pattern without penetrating full thickness through the cornea. Placing a needle at the limbus, sterile saline or air can be used to reinflate the anterior chamber. A conjunctival flap is then performed. An Elizabethan collar should be worn at all times and oral and topical broad-spectrum antibiotics and topical atropine sulphate (1% q12h) should be administered.

Prognosis
The prognosis for vision is guarded. Frequent re-evaluations will determine whether the treatment is successful in sealing the cornea and preventing reperforation.

Corneal perforation

Diagnosis
Following corneal rupture or perforation, the cornea may seal with a fibrin clot (Figure 10.17) or continue to leak aqueous humour causing collapse of the anterior chamber. Clinical signs are similar to those for a corneal ulcer. If sealed, a fibrin clot may be visible on top of the cornea. A misshapen cornea or decreased depth of the anterior chamber may also be seen. If there is a leak, the fluorescein stain will form rivulets at the site of perforation (Seidel test).

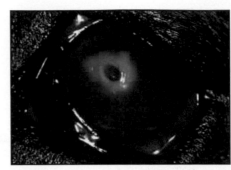

10.17 A perforated cornea that is sealed with a fibrin plug.

Treatment
Aggressive medical treatment with frequent topical antibiotics and atropine sulphate, and an Elizabethan collar as described above, can be attempted when there is a fibrin seal and the anterior chamber is intact. Systemic broad-spectrum antibiotics and NSAIDs should be added to help control infection and inflammation. The animal must be kept calm and ideally rested in a cage to help prevent the clot from dislodging and rupturing the eye.

When there is a leak, the corneal edges should be debrided and sutured with 0.3–0.7 metric (6/0 to 9/0 USP) absorbable synthetic suture, e.g. Vicryl®, in a simple interrupted or horizontal mattress pattern without penetrating full thickness through the cornea. The anterior chamber may require reinflation as described above. A conjunctival flap should then be performed.

Prognosis
If surgical repair can be performed and no complications are encountered, the prognosis for the eye is good but the prognosis for return of normal vision is guarded. If reparative surgery is not possible and the perforation is not sealed, enucleation may be appropriate.

Conjunctival flaps
For a detailed discussion on flap surgery, an ophthalmology text should be consulted. Conjunctival flaps provide support and protection to the damaged cornea. They provide fibroblasts to help seal the defect and a blood supply to deliver anticollagenases and antibiotics. Third eyelid flaps are technically an easy surgery, but they do not allow visualization of the cornea and monitoring of the ulcer and do not provide a blood supply to the defect. For this reason, most ophthalmologists do not recommend third eyelid flaps and prefer conjunctival flaps.

The two primary goals when performing conjunctival flaps are to make the flap as thin as possible and to have minimal tension on the flap. For pedicle flaps, the flap is started about 2 mm away from the dorsal limbus and extended using blunt dissection. As the flap is extended, care must be taken to keep it 'paper' thin. When the incisions are made perpendicular to the limbus, to mobilize the flap, it is important to ensure that the flap is wide enough to cover the defect (Figure 10.18). Once the flap can cover the defect with minimal to no tension, it is sutured on to the healthy cornea surrounding the ulcer with 0.3–0.5 metric (7/0 to 9/0 USP) absorbable synthetic suture, e.g. Vicryl®, in a simple interrupted pattern. The suture should penetrate about half the depth of the stroma (Figure 10.19). The part of the flap

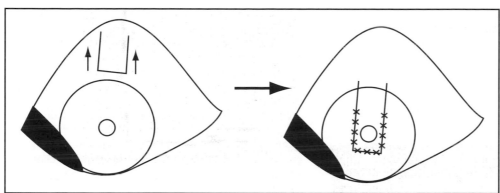

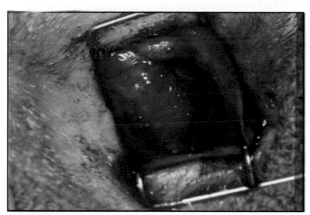

10.18 Pedicle flap placement. Starting 2 mm away from the dorsal limbus, the flap is extended using blunt dissection with tenotomy scissors. It can then be sutured on to the healthy cornea.

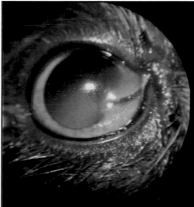

10.20 Corneal laceration in a cat. Notice the corneal oedema around the edges. All cases should be extensively evaluated for a foreign body. A twig caused the laceration in this cat.

10.19 Post-conjunctival flap placement. The flap is very thin and there is no tension on it. This helps ensure that the flap will not break down or cause pain.

connecting it to the conjunctiva is not sutured. Topical antibiotics (tobramycin or gentamicin 0.3% q4–6h) and topical atropine sulphate (1% q12h) should be used.

Monitoring
The owner must monitor for signs of discomfort, flap detachment, rupture of the eye or pain. The flap should be re-evaluated by the veterinary surgeon every week. The flap can simply be transected at its attachment to the conjunctiva after 4 weeks. Topical corticosteroids with antibiotics (neomycin–polymyxin–dexamethasone q6–8h) can then be used to decrease scar formation. Re-evaluations should be performed at 1 and 2 weeks post-detachment.

Corneal lacerations and foreign bodies

Diagnosis
The history and clinical signs are similar to those of corneal ulcers. Corneal lacerations (Figure 10.20) usually have oedema around the edges and may be difficult to distinguish from corneal ulcers. Lacerations can cause a descemetocele or iris prolapse and should be treated accordingly. All cases of corneal laceration should be extensively evaluated for ocular foreign bodies (Figure 10.21). Topical or general anaesthesia is usually necessary to perform a full evaluation and to prevent further damage. The area under and around the nictitans and under and at the margins of both eyelids should be carefully investigated; a magnifying lens

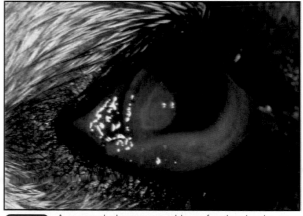

10.21 A corneal ulcer caused by a foreign body: a small piece of stick.

should be used to evaluate the cornea. If the laceration involves penetration of the eye (e.g. due to a cat claw) that touches or disrupts the anterior capsule of the lens, a very intense, severe anterior uveitis can ensue. This can be particularly difficult to treat.

Treatment
If the corneal laceration is not full thickness through the cornea, it should be treated as a deep corneal ulcer. If a corneal foreign body is present, gentle irrigation with sterile eyewash or saline may dislodge it. Alternatively, it can be dislodged using a 25 gauge needle, taking care not to push it further into the stroma. If the foreign body is lodged deeply in the cornea, an incision is made next to it using a no. 11 scalpel blade. The foreign body can then be pushed upward with the needle and removed.

If the cornea is perforated or has a full-thickness laceration, it should be sutured with 0.3–0.7 metric (6/0 to 9/0 USP) absorbable synthetic suture, e.g. Vicryl®, in a simple interrupted or horizontal pattern and then treated accordingly (see above). Topical antibiotics (ciprofloxacin 0.3% q4h) and atropine sulphate (1% q6–12h) should be used for 10–14 days. Broad-spectrum oral antibiotics should also be administered. NSAIDs should be added if a full-thickness corneal laceration is present. If the anterior lens capsule is disrupted, systemic anti-inflammatory doses of corticosteroids should be used instead of NSAIDs to control the inflammation. The lens may need to be removed if the animal is refractory to treatment.

Monitoring
The eye should be monitored for signs of suture breakdown/dehiscence and infection (i.e. discharge, redness and pain), with re-evaluations every 3–5 days for the first 1–2 weeks until it is healed. A conjunctival flap may be necessary if the cornea appears weak or unhealthy.

Prognosis
If the injury is uncomplicated, the prognosis is good. If the anterior lens capsule was damaged, the prognosis is guarded.

Lens luxation

Diagnosis
A lens luxation can be diagnosed based on the presence of an aphakic crescent (Figure 10.22), increased or decreased anterior chamber depth, abnormal iris movement, increased IOP and/or corneal oedema. The causes are listed in Figure 10.23. An anteriorly luxated lens can be an emergency due to the high possibility of secondary glaucoma. The IOP should therefore always be measured in these cases.

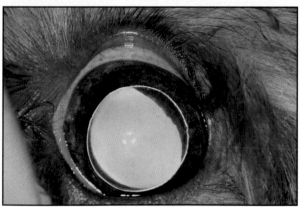

10.22 A luxated lens. Notice the aphakic crescent. The ideal treatment is surgical lens extraction, to avoid secondary complications of glaucoma, uveitis, vitreous liquefaction and cataracts.

Traumatic:	will see other evidence of trauma
Primary:	breeds predisposed include terriers
Secondary:	to glaucoma, neoplasia, uveitis

10.23 Causes of lens luxation.

Treatment
If IOP is increased, treatment with mannitol (1 g/kg over 20 minutes i.v.) is warranted. The ideal treatment is surgical lens extraction. An ophthalmology text or ophthalmologist should be consulted for lens extraction surgery. If surgery is not an option, the lens can be 'pushed' back into the vitreous using a short-acting mydriatic (tropicamide) followed by a miotic agent (pilocarpine) to keep it in the vitreous chamber. This treatment is not ideal, however, since the presence of the lens will lead to secondary vitreous liquefaction and intraocular disease.

Prognosis
As lens luxations can lead to glaucoma, uveitis, vitreous liquefaction and cataracts, the prognosis is guarded unless the lens luxation is diagnosed and treated early. Secondary glaucoma may still be a complication after lens extraction.

Hyphaema

Definition and causes
Hyphaema is blood in the anterior chamber; the most common causes are listed in Figure 10.24.

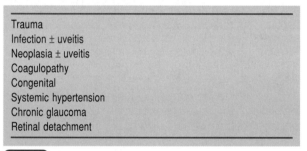

Trauma
Infection ± uveitis
Neoplasia ± uveitis
Coagulopathy
Congenital
Systemic hypertension
Chronic glaucoma
Retinal detachment

10.24 Causes of hyphaema.

Clinical signs
The clinical signs are dependent on the primary cause. Additional systemic signs of a coagulopathy, trauma or medical causes of uveitis may also be present.

Diagnosis
Diagnosis is based on direct visualization of blood in the anterior chamber (Figure 10.25). When no history or other signs of trauma are found, the diagnostic plan should proceed as with uveitis, and a full coagulation panel (platelet count, prothrombin time, partial thromboplastin time, fibrin split products and buccal mucosal bleeding time) should also be submitted.

Treatment
Treatment consists of treating the underlying cause if one is found. The use of topical corticosteroids or topical antibiotics has not been shown to be of benefit. There is controversy as to whether a mydriatic should be used in hyphaema. If there is no history of trauma, it can be difficult to rule out uveitis definitively, and then a mydriatic (atropine sulphate 1% q12h) is most appropriate. Secondary glaucoma should always be ruled out via tonometry before starting mydriatic therapy. IOP should be monitored during treatment.

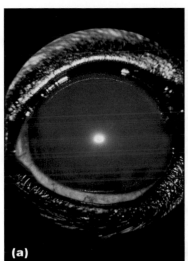

10.25
Hyphaema in **(a)** a dog and **(b)** a cat. Trauma, coagulopathy and neoplasia are the most common causes. The cat also had thrombocytopenia and mesenteric lymphadenopathy secondary to lymphoma.

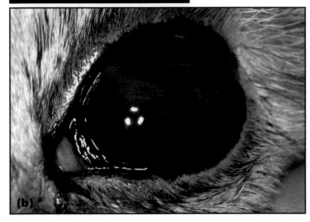

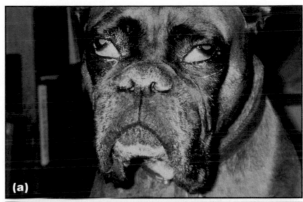

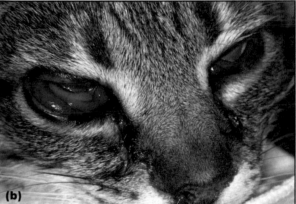

10.27 **(a)** Conjunctivitis in a 7-year-old Boxer, with ocular discharge and other signs of seasonal atopy, including pododermatitis and pruritus. **(b)** Conjunctivitis in a cat secondary to *Chlamydophila* infection.

Prognosis

The prognosis is variable depending on the underlying cause. If bleeding can be controlled the prognosis is good. If the haemorrhage is due to uveitis, the prognosis depends on the primary diagnosis.

Conjunctivitis

Definition and causes

Conjunctivitis is inflammation and/or infection of the conjunctiva. The most common causes are listed in Figure 10.26.

Bacterial
Viral, e.g. herpes (cats), distemper (dogs)
Chlamydophila infection (cats)
Corneal ulcers
Keratoconjunctivitis sicca
Allergy/atopy
Chemical irritants

10.26 Causes of conjunctivitis.

Clinical signs

Clinical signs include blepharospasm, ocular discharge, chemosis and conjunctival hyperaemia (Figure 10.27).

Diagnosis

The diagnosis is based on clinical signs. In cats, infectious conjunctivitis is more common than in dogs, and conjunctival scrapings and bacterial cultures should be submitted. In dogs, the two most common causes are allergic or non-infectious conjunctivitis and bacterial conjunctivitis secondary to KCS. Other signs of allergies (e.g. alopecia, pruritus) might be present in allergic conjunctivitis. A Schirmer tear test should be performed to rule out KCS. Other diagnostic tests including fluorescein stain, tonometry and FeLV/FIV serology (cats) may be indicated.

Treatment

The treatment is based on the underlying cause. The eye(s) should be irrigated with sterile eyewash. In cats, topical antibiotic ointment (tetracycline or erythromycin q6–8h) should be used. The antibiotic is then changed based on culture and sensitivity results. Topical antiviral ointment (vidarabine or trifluridine, if available, q2–4h) should be considered in cats with recurrent herpes conjunctivitis. In dogs, once bacterial conjunctivitis is ruled out (via cytology), topical corticosteroids with or without antibiotics (prednisolone acetate 1% q8h, neomycin–polymyxin–dexamethasone q6h) can be used. If KCS is the underlying cause, topical antibiotics should be started along with the treatment for KCS.

Prognosis

Many cases of allergic and viral conjunctivitis are recurrent. Owners should be warned of this because many get frustrated when the disease returns. An ophthalmologist should be consulted in recurrent or non-responsive cases.

Further reading

Bachrach A Jr (1992) Ocular emergencies. In: *Veterinary Emergency and Critical Care Medicine*, ed. RJ Murtaugh *et al.*, pp. 273–287. Mosby, St Louis

Collius BK and Moore CP (1999) Diseases and surgery of the canine anterior uvea. In: *Veterinary Ophthalmology, 3rd edn*, ed. KN Gelatt, pp. 755–795. Lippincott Williams & Wilkins, Baltimore

Gionfriddo JR (1995) Identifying and treating conjunctivitis in dogs and cats. *Veterinary Medicine* **90**, 242–253

Gionfriddo JR (1995) Recognizing and managing acute and chronic cases of glaucoma. *Veterinary Medicine* **90**, 265–275

Gionfriddo JR (1995) The causes, diagnosis, and treatment of uveitis. *Veterinary Medicine* **90**, 278–284

Glaze MB and Gelatt KN (1999) Feline ophthalmology. In: *Veterinary Ophthalmology, 3rd edn*, ed. KN Gelatt, pp. 997–1052. Lippincott Williams & Wilkins, Baltimore

Mandell DC and Holt E (2005) Ophthalmic emergencies. In: *Veterinary Clinics of North America: Small Animal Practice,* ed. KJ Drobatz, pp 455–480. WB Saunders, Philadelphia

Massa KL, Gilger BC, Miller TL and Davidson MG (2002) Causes of uveitis in dogs: 102 cases (1989–2000). *Veterinary Ophthalmology* **5**, 93–98

Morgan RV (1989) Vogt–Koyanagi–Harada syndrome in humans and dogs. *Compendium on Continuing Education for the Practicing Veterinarian* **11**, 1211–1218

Peiffer RL Jr and Petersen-Jones SM (1997) *Small Animal Ophthalmology: A Problem-Oriented Approach.* WB Saunders, London

Plunkett SJ (2000) Anaphylaxis to ophthalmic medication in a cat. *Journal of Veterinary Emergency and Critical Care* **10**, 169–171

Slatter D (1990) *Fundamentals of Veterinary Ophthalmology.* WB Saunders, Philadelphia

Strubbe DT and Gelatt KN (1999) Ophthalmic examination and diagnostic procedures. In: *Veterinary Ophthalmology, 3rd edn*, ed. KN Gelatt, pp. 427–466. Lippincott Williams & Wilkins, Baltimore

Whitley RD, Hamilton HL and Weigand CM (1993) Glaucoma and disorders of the uvea, lens and retina in cats. *Veterinary Medicine* **88**, 1164–1173

Whitley RD, Whitley EM and McLaughlin SA (1993) Diagnosing and treating disorders of the feline conjunctiva and cornea. *Veterinary Medicine* **88**, 1138–1149

Whitley RD and Gilger BC (1999) Diseases of the canine cornea and sclera. In: *Veterinary Ophthalmology, 3rd edn*, ed. KN Gelatt, pp. 635–673. Lippincott Williams & Wilkins, Baltimore

Wilkie DA (1993) Therapeutics in practice. Management of keratoconjunctivitis sicca in dogs. *Compendium on Continuing Education for the Practicing Veterinarian* **15**, 58–63

Willis AM, Diehl KA and Robbin TE (2002) Advances in topical glaucoma therapy. *Veterinary Ophthalmology* **5**, 9–17

11

Approach to gastrointestinal emergencies

Kate Murphy and Sheena M. Warman

Introduction

Animals with acute onset of gastrointestinal (GI) signs and/or abdominal pain present certain diagnostic and therapeutic challenges to the veterinarian. Immediate and aggressive therapy may be required and a frequent dilemma for the practitioner is the decision as to whether the patient requires conservative medical management or surgery. Further, the practitioner must decide if the surgery should be performed immediately or after a period of medical stabilization. This chapter will concentrate on the diagnostic approach to patients presenting with gastrointestinal signs, the diagnostic tests available for abdominal disease and the management of the non-surgical abdomen. Chapter 12 will discuss management of the surgical abdomen.

Diagnostic approach

History and physical examination

Triage is essential when animals are presented in an emergency, allowing assessment of the major body systems with identification of any life-threatening abnormalities, and implementation of any urgent stabilization measures if necessary. As soon as the patient is stable, a full history (Figure 11.1) should be obtained and a complete physical evaluation performed. Although the patient may be presenting with an acute problem, it is essential that historical questioning establishes whether this may be a chronic problem with acute decompensation. Information regarding the age and sex of the patient might refine the differential diagnoses, e.g. young patients are more likely to have viral or parasitic causes of gastroenteritis, or to have ingested a foreign body. Linear foreign bodies are particularly common in young cats and it is important to check under the tongue for trapped material such as string. Pyometra, pancreatitis and diabetic ketoacidosis (DKA) should be considered in older dogs with vomiting and/or diarrhoea. Hyperthyroidism, DKA and chronic renal failure deserve consideration in geriatric cats. Other potential causes of an acute gastrointestinal presentation include toxin access and non-GI disease, e.g. acute urethral obstruction or hypoadrenocorticism.

Physical examination (see Chapter 1) should be complete, starting with assessment of major body systems (cardiovascular, respiratory and central nervous systems) and then assessing all body systems with a strong focus on abdominal palpation (Figure 11.2). The hydration status of the patient should be assessed and, if indicated, fluid therapy can be initiated after collection of blood samples and/or urine for analysis.

Vaccination and worming status

Sex and neutering status

Previous medical/surgical conditions, e.g. chronic pancreatitis, previous abdominal surgery

Primary complaint

Medications, e.g. ibuprofen, paracetamol

Toxin access, e.g. lead, ethylene glycol

Progression of illness

Systemic manifestations of disease:

> Differentiate vomiting and regurgitation – vomiting is associated with retching and abdominal contractions, regurgitation is passive. Note that patients can have both

> Establish nature of diarrhoea, e.g. small or large intestinal, presence of fresh blood or melaena

> Abnormal behaviour, e.g. 'praying' stance consistent with cranial abdominal pain

> Cover all body systems, e.g. appetite, weight, polyuria/polydipsia, respiratory signs

11.1 History checklist.

Visual evaluation for evidence of abdominal distension or bruising

Abdominal auscultation for increased borborygmi (acute enteritis, acute obstruction) or decreased borborygmi (peritonitis, ileus, chronic obstruction, abdominal effusion)

Four-quadrant approach to abdominal palpation to ensure full evaluation. Elevation of forelegs may aid detection of cranial abdominal abnormalities

Assess for organomegaly, masses, foreign body, intussusception, mesenteric lymphadenopathy

Assess for pain:

> Focal – small intestinal obstruction (foreign body, intussusception), mild pancreatitis, gastrointestinal ulceration

> Regional – moderate/severe pancreatitis, cholecystitis, pyometra, pyelonephritis

> Diffuse – diffuse gastroenteritis, peritonitis, referred spinal pain

Assess for fluid – ballottement, presence of fluid thrill

Rectal examination, assess faecal character

Assess urogenital tract

11.2 A guide to the physical examination of patients with gastrointestinal emergencies.

Vascular access and the principles of fluid therapy are covered in Chapters 2 and 4 and will be discussed in this chapter with respect to symptomatic treatment.

Clinical signs

The typical signs of gastrointestinal disease include regurgitation, vomiting, diarrhoea, weight loss, variable appetite and abdominal pain. The major differential diagnoses for acute presentations of regurgitation, vomiting, diarrhoea and abdominal pain are detailed in Figures 11.3, 11.4, 11.5 and 11.6.

Type	Selected causes
Intraluminal oesophageal obstruction	Foreign body, stricture
Oesophagitis	Secondary to vomiting, reflux under anaesthesia, ingestion of caustic/irritant or scalding substance, spontaneous, gastric reflux secondary to hiatal hernia
Megaoesophagus	Idiopathic, focal or generalized myasthenia gravis, secondary causes (myopathy, neuropathy/junctionopathy, toxic, hypoadrenocorticism, hypothyroidism, other miscellaneous causes)
Extraluminal oesophageal obstruction	Cranial mediastinal mass, persistent right aortic arch, neoplasia
Mural oesophageal disease	Oesophageal diverticulum, gastro-oesophageal intussusception, hiatal hernia, primary neoplasia, *Spirocerca lupi* granuloma (not endemic in UK)

11.3 Differential diagnosis of regurgitation.

Type	Selected causes
Gastric	Gastritis, gastric ulceration, neoplasia, foreign body, motility disorder
Intestinal	Inflammatory bowel disease, foreign body, intussusception, ileus, neoplasia
Non-gastrointestinal, intra-abdominal	Pancreatitis, pancreatic neoplasia, (cholangio)hepatitis, biliary obstruction or rupture Pyometra, (pyelo)nephritis, urinary obstruction, prostatitis
Metabolic/endocrine	Hypoadrenocorticism, renal failure, diabetic ketoacidosis, hyperthyroidism, hypercalcaemia, hepatic encephalopathy, sepsis
Drugs	Erythromycin, chemotherapy, digoxin
Toxins	Ethylene glycol, strychnine
Dietary	Indiscretion, intolerance
Neurological	Vestibular disease, inflammatory or neoplastic central nervous system disease, elevated intracranial pressure
Infectious	Parvovirus, distemper, infectious canine hepatitis, leptospirosis, feline infectious enteritis, salmonellosis, parasites

11.4 Differential diagnosis of acute vomiting.

Type	Selected causes
Acute small intestinal diarrhoea	
Dietary	Indiscretion, intolerance
Parasitic	Roundworms, hookworm, *Giardia*, coccidia
Viral	Parvovirus, coronavirus
Bacterial	*Salmonella, Campylobacter*
Intestinal	Obstruction (foreign body, intussusception), inflammatory bowel disease, haemorrhagic gastroenteritis, neoplasia
Non-intestinal intra-abdominal	Infectious canine hepatitis, (cholangio)hepatitis, canine distemper
Metabolic/endocrine	Hypoadrenocorticism, acute renal failure (e.g. leptospirosis), hepatic disease
Acute large intestinal diarrhoea	
Dietary	Indiscretion, intolerance
Parasitic	Hookworms, *Giardia*, coccidia, whipworms
Bacterial	*Salmonella, Campylobacter, Clostridium perfringens*
Intestinal	Obstruction (foreign body, intussusception), inflammatory bowel disease, haemorrhagic gastroenteritis, neoplasia
Non-intestinal intra-abdominal	Pancreatitis

11.5 Differential diagnosis of acute small and large intestinal diarrhoea.

Type	Selected causes
Gastrointestinal	Gastric dilatation (± volvulus), ulceration, obstruction, foreign body Small intestinal obstruction, foreign body, enteritis, ulceration Large intestinal disease
Urinary	Bladder or urethral obstruction/rupture, acute renal ischaemia/infection
Genital	Pyometra, metritis, uterine torsion, dystocia Prostatitis, prostatic abscess, testicular torsion (abdominal)
Hepatobiliary	Hepatic lobe torsion, haematoma, abscess, cholangiohepatitis Biliary obstruction/rupture, inflammation, cholelithiasis
Pancreatic	Pancreatitis, abscess, necrosis
Splenic	Neoplasia, torsion, infarction, splenitis
Lymphatic	Lymphadenitis
Mesenteric	Volvulus, herniation, thrombosis
Peritoneum	Peritonitis (septic, uroperitoneum, bile), haemoperitoneum
Body wall/skin	Hernia, penetrating injury, panniculitis
Referred pain	Spinal pain (intervertebral disc disease, discospondylitis, neoplasia, fracture/luxation), pelvic trauma

11.6 Differential diagnosis of abdominal pain.

Clinical pathology

An emergency database (packed cell volume (PCV), total solids (TS) or total protein (TP), glucose and urea estimation, electrolytes, and evaluation of a blood smear) should be performed in all clinically ill emergency patients (see Chapter 1). A minimum database that includes haematology, biochemistry and urinalysis should be submitted in all emergency patients with GI signs, to aid in early diagnosis and appropriate treatment including fluid therapy. For a full description of the laboratory evaluation of gastrointestinal, pancreatic and hepatic disease, the reader is referred to the *BSAVA Manual of Canine and Feline Clinical Pathology* and the *BSAVA Manual of Canine and Feline Gastroenterology*. Tests which are particularly useful for patients with gastrointestinal disease include:

- Routine haematology including smear assessment:
  - Inflammatory leucogram with inflammatory/ infectious disease
  - Elevation of red cell parameters with haemoconcentration
  - Eosinophilia with gastrointestinal parasites
  - Lymphopenia with lymphangiectasia or stress
  - Lack of a stress leucogram with lymphocytosis, eosinophilia and an inappropriately normal neutrophil count with hypoadrenocorticism
- Total protein, albumin, urea, creatinine, alanine aminotransferase (ALT), alkaline phosphatase (ALP) (and gamma-glutamyl transferase (GGT) in cats), bilirubin, sodium, potassium and chloride:
  - Panhypoproteinaemia (decreased albumin and globulin) most suggestive of protein-losing enteropathy (PLE), but hypoalbuminaemia alone may be seen with PLE
  - Hyperglobulinaemia seen in cats with feline infectious peritonitis (FIP) and lymphocytic cholangitis
  - Elevations in urea and creatinine suggest either prerenal azotaemia (dehydration, hypovolaemia), renal disease or postrenal azotaemia. Concurrent measurement of the urine specific gravity, urine volume and serum calcium and phosphorus will help to identify the underlying cause. Elevation in blood urea alone can occur with gastrointestinal bleeding. An increased serum urea:creatinine ratio may be helpful in non- or mildly azotaemic patients to support a suspicion of gastrointestinal haemorrhage although the authors do not use this ratio. Low blood urea is associated with hepatic dysfunction, particularly portosystemic shunts
  - Elevations in ALT, ALP, GGT and bilirubin suggest hepatic disease. If GGT is normal and ALT and ALP are increased in a cat, hepatic lipidosis is an important differential
  - Hyponatraemia and hyperkalaemia are typical of primary hypoadrenocorticism, although the classic electrolyte changes are not always present. This pattern of electrolyte abnormalities can also be seen with severe secretory intestinal disease, e.g. salmonellosis and *Trichuris* infection, and some other less common diseases, e.g. pseudoaddison's in late pregnancy
- Amylase and lipase can aid the diagnosis of pancreatitis if increased more than two to five times the upper normal limit. However they are neither sensitive nor specific, especially in cats
- Urinalysis: specific gravity, dipstick and sediment analysis
- Faecal analysis
  - Routine parasitology
  - Viral (e.g. enzyme-linked immunosorbent assay (ELISA) or polymerase chain reaction (PCR) for parvovirus, electron microscopy for some viruses, viral isolation techniques)
  - Microbiological culture.

Additional blood tests may include:

- Adrenal function: ACTH stimulation test
- Gastrointestinal function: serum folate and cobalamin
- Pancreatic function: serum pancreatic lipase (PLI). PLI is a more sensitive and specific indicator of pancreatic inflammation than are amylase and lipase, and the test is available for both dogs and cats
- Hepatic function:
  - Serum bile acids
  - Blood ammonia.

Abdominal imaging

Survey radiographs of the abdomen (lateral and ventrodorsal views) are indicated in animals presenting with acute vomiting, diarrhoea or abdominal pain. Ventrodorsal radiographs should only be performed once the patient has a stable cardiovascular system. Survey radiographs may show:

- Decreased serosal detail:
  - Loss of intra-abdominal fat, e.g. cachexia
  - Free peritoneal fluid/ascites, e.g. peritonitis (septic/non-septic), haemoabdomen
  - Localized loss of detail in the right cranial quadrant ± lateral displacement of the duodenum can be consistent with pancreatitis (see Figure 12.2)
- Organomegaly
- Mass
- Gaseous GI tract distension:
  - Gastric dilatation (± volvulus) (see Figure 12.6)
  - Ileus (generalized small intestinal distension)
  - Focal bowel loop distension – normally fluid filled, particularly if secondary to intestinal obstruction, but can be gas filled
  - As a guide, the maximum normal width of a loop of intestine (from serosal surface to serosal surface) should be less than 1.6 times the height of L5 (at the narrowest point of L5 on a lateral radiograph) (Graham *et al.*, 1998)
- Other evidence of full or partial GI obstruction, e.g. 'gravel' sign, plicated small intestine
- Radiodense foreign bodies

- Abnormalities of the diaphragm or body wall, e.g. ruptured diaphragm, hernia
- Free air/pneumoperitoneum (see Figure 12.3):
  - Hollow viscus rupture
  - Non-surgical causes of pneumoperitoneum, e.g. recent (<18 days) abdominal surgery, possibly open-needle abdominocentesis
  - Occasionally pneumothorax/pneumomediastinum results in pneumoretroperitoneum or, very rarely, pneumoperitoneum.

Radiographs of the thorax (right and left lateral and dorsoventral) are indicated in any patient where neoplastic disease is suspected, as part of a screen for metastatic disease. In addition, in patients with regurgitation or suspected oesophageal disease, plain radiography may be useful for identifying gross dilation of the oesophagus (Figure 11.7) and to evaluate for evidence of aspiration pneumonia. If plain radiographs are inconclusive, a barium swallow may be helpful to identify structural oesophageal lesions or motility abnormalities. The reader is referred to Chapter 12 for indications for surgical exploration of the abdomen.

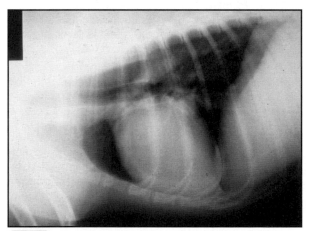

11.7 Radiograph showing gross dilation of the oesophagus with air.

Abdominal ultrasonography is an extremely useful imaging modality in patients with acute abdominal disease. It is more sensitive than radiography for detecting small volumes of abdominal fluid (<4 ml/kg) and helps to characterize lesions in solid tissues. Small volumes of fluid are seen most readily around the apex of the urinary bladder or between liver lobes in the cranioventral abdomen. Ultrasonography can also prove very helpful in diagnosing certain conditions, e.g. pancreatitis (Figure 11.8) and intussusceptions.

The *BSAVA Manual of Canine and Feline Gastroenterology* and the *BSAVA Manual of Small Animal Diagnostic Imaging* should be consulted for a full description of the application of radiography and ultrasonography in abdominal imaging.

Endoscopy

Endoscopy can be used for both diagnostic and therapeutic purposes. In emergency patients, it is a useful technique for aiding removal of oesophageal or gastric foreign bodies and, in stabilized critically ill patients, it can be used to facilitate gastrostomy tube placement.

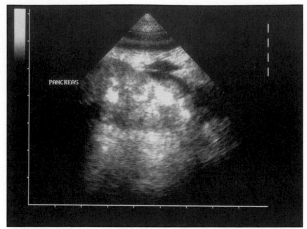

11.8 Ultrasonographic image showing severe pancreatitis with several hyperechoic foci within the pancreatic parenchyma.

Endoscopy is also an excellent minimally invasive diagnostic technique for evaluating mucosal lesions (Figure 11.9) in the gastrointestinal tract. The oesophagus can be examined with endoscopy but biopsies are difficult because of the tough nature of the mucosa. Gastric and intestinal biopsy specimens should be collected and submitted for histopathology even if the tissue looks grossly normal. Due to the superficial nature of endoscopic biopsy specimens, deeper lesions can be missed and full-thickness biopsies may be required if a diagnosis is not reached. Endoscopy does not permit examination of the whole intestinal tract, and therefore lesions may be missed. The *BSAVA Manual of Canine and Feline Gastroenterology* contains a chapter on gastrointestinal endoscopy to which the reader is referred for further information.

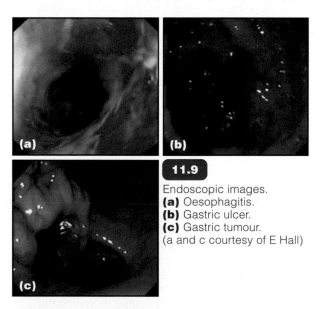

11.9 Endoscopic images.
(a) Oesophagitis.
(b) Gastric ulcer.
(c) Gastric tumour.
(a and c courtesy of E Hall)

Abdominocentesis

If free abdominal fluid is suspected based upon physical examination and/or diagnostic imaging, abdominocentesis should be performed to obtain fluid for biochemical and cytological analysis. Blind abdominocentesis is most successful in patients with large volumes of fluid. In those with smaller effusions, the chances of fluid retrieval can be increased using ultrasound-guided aspiration. If either of these techniques is unsuccessful, but the presence of fluid is still suspected, diagnostic peritoneal lavage should be performed. Contraindications to abdominocentesis include severe coagulopathy or thrombocytopenia, marked distension of an abdominal viscus, severe organomegaly and previous abdominal surgery which may have resulted in adhesions of the bowel to the body wall.

Abdominocentesis is performed using either a single centesis or a four-quadrant approach (increasing the chances of fluid retrieval if the procedure is performed without ultrasound guidance) (Figure 11.10).

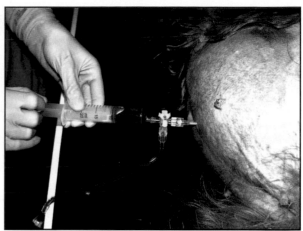

1. The patient is usually restrained in right lateral recumbency.
2. The abdomen is clipped and prepared as for a sterile surgical procedure.
3. Sites for placement of the needles are shown in Figure 11.11. Either a hypodermic needle or over-the-needle catheter may be used.
4. The first needle is placed in the ventral aspect of the right cranial quadrant:
   - Minimizes the risk of splenic or bladder penetration
   - Fluid tends to pool in this area as a result of gravity and diaphragmatic movement.
5. The needle can be left open (open-needle abdominocentesis) or attached to a syringe (closed-needle abdominocentesis):
   - Open-needle centesis is more likely to result in fluid flow as suction with a syringe will tend to draw the omentum or viscera on to the needle. It may result in small volumes of air entering the abdominal cavity and this should be taken into account when interpreting subsequent abdominal radiographs
   - The needle can be twisted gently to try to encourage fluid flow
   - With open-needle abdominocentesis, the needle should be left in place for 1–2 minutes. If no fluid is obtained, then gently aspirate with a syringe (Figure 11.12).
6. If no fluid is obtained following gentle aspiration, the procedure can be repeated in the other three sites; right caudal, left cranial (risk of splenic penetration), left caudal.
7. False-positive results can be obtained if the needle punctures the bladder, spleen or gastrointestinal tract.
8. If blood is aspirated, stop the aspiration, place the blood into a glass tube and observe for clot formation. Blood from the abdominal cavity will not clot, whereas blood from a vessel or organ will clot.

11.10 Abdominocentesis.

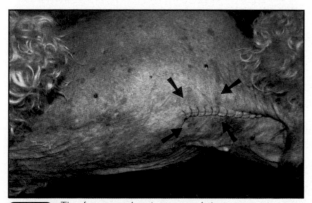

11.11 The four-quadrant approach to abdominocentesis. Arrows show suitable positions for needle insertion.

11.12 Gentle aspiration of an abdominal effusion using a syringe and over-the-needle catheter.

Diagnostic peritoneal lavage

Diagnostic peritoneal lavage (DPL; Figure 11.13) should be performed if abdominocentesis has not yielded fluid, but suspicion for the presence of abdominal fluid or inflammation remains high. DPL can detect small volumes of fluid (1–4.4 ml/kg) and is also a useful technique in patients suspected of having peritonitis, but where abdominal fluid has not yet formed in detectable volumes or is sequestered by the omentum.

DPL can be performed using specialized peritoneal dialysis catheters or a modified over-the-needle catheter. The authors fenestrate the over-the-needle catheter with a scalpel blade to create additional

1. The patient is restrained in lateral or dorsal recumbency. Sedation can be used if needed. The urinary bladder should be emptied.
2. The abdomen is clipped and prepared for a sterile surgical procedure.
3. If using an over-the-needle catheter, a stab incision is made in the skin and then the catheter is inserted through the abdominal wall caudal to the umbilicus. The catheter is aimed caudally towards the pelvis and once the abdominal wall is penetrated, the catheter is slid off the stylet into the abdomen and the stylet is removed.
4. If using a DPL catheter, the needle stylet is introduced as above and the J-wire is fed through the stylet into the abdomen. The stylet is removed, leaving the guidewire in place. The dialysis catheter is then placed over the guidewire into the abdomen and the wire removed.
5. Warm isotonic crystalloid is then infused using gravity flow/gentle injection into the abdomen. A total volume of 10–20 ml/kg is infused.
6. The animal is gently rolled from side to side to distribute the fluid, ideally with the dialysis catheter still *in situ*. If the catheter becomes displaced during the procedure then a right quadrant tap can be performed using a blind technique.
7. Fluid is then allowed to drain into a sterile container. It is not unusual to retrieve only a very small proportion of the infused volume. This cannot be used for quantitative analysis because the dilution factor is unknown. However, cytological analysis can be very helpful, particularly if degenerate neutrophils or bacteria are identified.

11.13 Diagnostic peritoneal lavage.

163

Parameter	Transudate	Modified transudate	Exudate
Total protein (g/l)	<25	>25	>30
Total nucleated cell count (x10⁹/l)	<1	<7	>7
Cell types	Mesothelial cells and macrophages	Mesothelial cells, macrophages, few neutrophils ± small lymphocytes	Neutrophils and macrophages

11.14 Classification of abdominal fluids based on cytology and total protein content.

drainage holes. The catheter should be fenestrated whilst on the metal stylet; V-shaped incisions are made to create fenestrations in a spiral pattern around the catheter. Care should be taken to ensure that fenestrations are not made directly opposite each other (which would weaken the catheter) and it is also important that no burrs remain which could impair entry and exit of the catheter. The holes should not extend beyond 50% of the circumference of the catheter or there is a risk of breakage at this weak point.

Peritoneal fluid analysis

Peritoneal fluid analysis is an essential part of the evaluation of the patient with acute abdomen, and can assist in making the decision as to whether surgery is appropriate. The fluid should be collected into an EDTA tube (cytology) and two plain tubes (biochemistry and bacteriology). The fluid should be assessed as follows:

- Gross appearance (including odour): clear, serosanguineous, haemorrhagic, purulent, chylous
- PCV measurement. The abdominal fluid from a patient with simple acute haemoabdomen will have a PCV close to circulating PCV. In patients where the abdominal fluid has a lower PCV (often in the 4–12% range) there may be a component of haemorrhage but another concurrent cause for the abdominal fluid should also be sought
- Total solids on refractometer or total protein measured on biochemistry analyser
- Total nucleated cell count
- Cytology (direct smear or spun sediment)
- Additional biochemical tests as indicated (e.g. creatinine, potassium, amylase, lipase, bilirubin, lactate, glucose)
- Culture when indicated (high numbers of neutrophils in the fluid, bacteria).

The reader is referred to the *BSAVA Manual of Canine and Feline Clinical Pathology* for a detailed description of fluid analysis. Classification of abdominal fluid into transudates, modified transudates and exudates is shown in Figure 11.14.

Management of specific medical conditions

Oesophageal

Regurgitation

Regurgitation is a passive event and results in expulsion of undigested food and/or mucus. It is a sign of oesophageal disease and can be complicated by the development of aspiration pneumonia. The differential diagnoses of regurgitation are discussed in Figure 11.3. Diagnosis is based upon the history and physical examination. Oesophageal dilation may be evident on plain thoracic radiographs, but in some cases contrast studies (e.g. barium swallow with fluoroscopy) will be needed to diagnose oesophageal motility abnormalities. Thoracic radiographs should be evaluated for evidence of aspiration pneumonia. Further investigation of regurgitation may include oesophagoscopy to assess for structural lesions or blood tests for myasthenia gravis (acetylcholine receptor antibody titres), hypothyroidism and hypoadrenocorticism.

Treatment of regurgitation involves management of the underlying condition if this is possible (e.g. medical treatment of hypothyroidism, hypoadrenocorticism, myasthenia gravis, polymyositis, oesophagitis; ligation and resection of a vascular ring anomaly). For cases of idiopathic megaoesophagus/oesophageal dysmotility and whilst treating the underlying condition, the treatment aims include:

- Elevated feeding – aim to maintain the gravitational effect for 10–15 minutes after eating
- Modify the texture of the food to find the ideal consistency for that patient, e.g. meatballs, liquid diet
- Feed a high-calorie diet in small frequent meals (four to six times daily)
- Pro-kinetic drugs have variable benefit but may be of more use in cats than dogs
- Treatment of aspiration pneumonia if present with broad-spectrum intravenous antibiotics, intravenous fluid therapy, nebulization and coupage
- If the patient is unable to maintain their body weight, consider placement of a gastrostomy tube for feeding. This will not prevent aspiration pneumonia as saliva can still be inhaled, but will allow nutritional support.

Oesophagitis

Oesophagitis can occur secondary to acid reflux (anaesthesia, vomiting, hiatal hernia), or following ingestion of irritant substances. Clinical signs of oesophagitis include hypersalivation, anorexia, regurgitation and odynophagia (pain on swallowing). Oesophagoscopy demonstrates the presence of mucosal erosions and ulceration and is useful to evaluate for secondary complications such as stricture formation.

Treatment includes the use of mucosal protectants such as sucralfate, and drugs to reduce acid production (e.g. a proton pump inhibitor). If oesophagitis occurs secondary to vomiting, it should also be managed with anti-emetic therapy and treatment of the primary cause. The severity of the oesophagitis determines the nutritional plan. With mild cases, food should be withheld for 24–48 hours and then small frequent meals of a low-fat diet introduced. If the oesophagitis is severe, oral feeding may not be tolerated for several days and placement of a gastrostomy tube should be considered to allow delivery of adequate nutrition. Most cases will improve with medical management, but some may develop a stricture necessitating further treatment (balloon dilation, bougienage). Some patients unfortunately do not respond to treatment.

Gastric/intestinal

Acute vomiting

The differential diagnoses of acute vomiting are detailed in Figure 11.4. A thorough history and physical examination are essential parts of the investigation of acute vomiting and a minimum database (including electrolytes) should be performed to evaluate for systemic/metabolic causes of vomiting. Abdominal radiography and ultrasonography can be useful to rule out obstruction and foreign bodies, to assess the presence of gastrointestinal lesions and to evaluate for extra-intestinal causes of vomiting e.g. pancreatitis. Gastroduodenoscopy is useful to assess the presence of mucosal lesions, neoplastic disease and foreign bodies. However in some patients further laboratory evaluation or exploratory laparotomy may be indicated based on early findings.

Management of the acutely vomiting patient should include:

- Treatment of the underlying cause
- Supportive care. The majority of cases of acute vomiting are secondary to dietary indiscretion and should resolve with symptomatic therapy:
  - Intravenous fluid therapy
  - Nil by mouth for 24 hours
  - Small volumes of water can then be offered and, if tolerated, a highly digestible, low-fat diet can be introduced in small amounts fed frequently
- If vomiting is unresponsive to symptomatic therapy or is severe, then anti-emetic therapy should be used. Anti-emetics should only be used once obstructive disease has been excluded
- Antiparasitic therapy should be considered if gastrointestinal parasitism (*Giardia*, ascarids, *Trichuris vulpis*) is a possible cause of the vomiting.

Gastric ulceration

Gastric ulceration can occur secondary to a number of events including:

- Drug administration (non steroidal anti-inflammatory agents (NSAIDs), corticosteroids)
- Hypotension, shock, sepsis
- Mast cell tumour, gastrinoma
- Renal and hepatic disease
- Gastric foreign body
- Gastric wall neoplasia.

Clinical signs usually include vomiting and the presence of 'coffee grounds' or fresh blood suggestive of gastric bleeding. Melaena can also be present. If the patient loses a significant amount of blood acutely, systemic signs of acute blood loss will be seen. The minimum database may reveal evidence of blood-loss anaemia (which, if chronic, may be microcytic and hypochromic) and serum proteins may also be decreased. Systemic bleeding disorders can result in gastric bleeding and should be excluded by checking platelet numbers, performing a buccal mucosal bleeding test and evaluating clotting times (prothrombin time (PT), activated partial thromboplastin time (APTT)). Abdominal radiography and ultrasonography may yield useful information. Gastroscopy allows evaluation of mucosal lesions and biopsy specimen collection for histopathology. In some cases it can be difficult to differentiate grossly between gastric ulcers (see Figure 11.9b) and gastric tumours (see Figure 11.9c). Deep biopsy specimens from the edge of the lesion are required but misdiagnosis remains a possibility if the specimens reflect surface inflammation and not deeper tumour infiltration.

Treatment includes use of H_2 antagonists or proton pump inhibitors in combination with a mucosal protectant, e.g. sucralfate. In a recent study, Bersenas *et al.* (2005) have shown that proton pump inhibitors and famotidine are most effective at suppressing acid secretion. If NSAID administration causes ulceration, misoprostol could be used to protect against further ulceration. Intravenous fluids should be given until oral therapy is tolerated, and prokinetics and/or anti-emetics may be needed. If blood loss has been severe, treatment with whole blood products or haemoglobin-based oxygen carrier solutions should be considered. Occasional severely affected animals may require surgical resection of deep focal ulcers, especially if there is any evidence of perforation.

Acute small bowel diarrhoea

The differential diagnoses for acute small bowel diarrhoea are detailed in Figure 11.5. A thorough history and physical examination are important and the clinician should try to characterize the diarrhoea as small or large intestinal in nature, or both. Small bowel diarrhoea is recognized by the production of large volumes of watery or soft stool. Straining with production of small volumes of faeces or mucus is more consistent with large bowel diarrhoea (colitis, see below). Haemorrhage, if originating in the small intestine where the blood will be digested before it reaches the colon, is manifested by the presence of dark brown or black stool (melaena). Haemorrhage that occurs in the colon will be manifested in the faeces as undigested, red blood. When patients are presented with diarrhoea, systemic disease should be excluded using a minimum database. If the patient is clinically stable then a symptomatic approach can be used for initial management of acute diarrhoea:

- Withhold food for 24 hours; allow free access to water so long as there is no vomiting
- Reintroduce food as small, frequent feeds of a low-fat, easily digestible diet

- Gradually reintroduce the normal diet once the signs have resolved
- Oral rehydration solutions can be used to address fluid losses
- If the patient is not regularly wormed, consider treatment for giardiasis and trichuriasis with fenbendazole
- Anti-secretory drugs and motility modifiers (e.g. loperamide, diphenoxylate, butylscopolamine) are not favoured by the authors as they make assessment of response to treatment difficult.

In patients with more severe systemic signs (e.g. haemorrhagic diarrhoea, shock, painful abdomen) the following should also be considered:

- Intravenous fluid therapy including management of electrolyte and acid–base abnormalities
- Further diagnostics including blood tests, abdominal imaging (see above)
- Intravenous antibiotics, particularly if there is haemorrhage or evidence of sepsis.

Haemorrhagic gastroenteritis
Haemorrhagic gastroenteritis is caused by acute loss of integrity of the gut mucosa. *Clostridium perfringens* has been implicated as a causal agent. It is reported typically to affect small-breed, middle-aged dogs but can be seen at any age and in any sized dog. Clinical signs include acute vomiting, progressing to haemorrhagic diarrhoea, dehydration and potentially shock. Septic shock can be seen due to translocation of bacteria across the compromised mucosa. The diarrhoea contains fresh blood and sloughed intestinal mucosa. Diagnosis is based upon the history and physical examination and can be assisted by some classical laboratory features. The PCV in these patients is generally >60% with normal or high total solids initially. Albumin will typically drop once treatment is started. Faecal cytology may show clostridial spores and assays are available for faecal clostridial enterotoxin. Treatment includes:

- Intravenous fluid therapy with an isotonic replacement solution. The rates should be appropriate to the patient's cardiovascular status. Monitor PCV and total solids to guide therapy. Colloidal support may be needed in some cases
- Potassium supplementation of the fluids may be required and ideally should be based upon serum potassium levels
- Broad-spectrum intravenous antibiotics:
  - Penicillin or metronidazole to treat possible clostridia and reduce risk of sepsis following translocation of anaerobic bacteria
  - Amoxicillin/clavulanate, ampicillin or second-generation cephalosporin to reduce risk of sepsis from Gram-negative bacteria if GI integrity is severely compromised
- Nil by mouth until vomiting is controlled and then introduce water and diet as for treatment of acute diarrhoea.

Canine parvovirus infection
Parvovirus is an important cause of severe viral enteritis. There are two strains of canine parvovirus. CPV-1 causes myocarditis, pneumonitis and gastroenteritis in very young puppies and CPV-2 causes classical parvovirus enteritis. Clinical signs occur 5–12 days after infection (faecal–oral route) and certain breeds (Dobermanns, Rottweilers, Pit Bull Terriers and Labrador Retrievers) appear more susceptible. The virus replicates in the intestinal crypts and clinical signs vary but include lethargy, anorexia, vomiting (possibly haematemesis) and diarrhoea beginning 24–48 hours after the initiation of vomiting. The diarrhoea can be haemorrhagic and profuse. Short-term severe protein-losing enteropathy can develop. Parvovirus can also cause bone marrow suppression resulting in neutropenia and an increased risk of sepsis. Dogs may present with signs of septic shock.

Diagnosis is made based on history (vaccination status), physical findings and additional laboratory analysis. Neutropenia with GI signs can be seen with parvovirus but also with salmonellosis or other severe infections. There may be biochemical changes such as hypokalaemia, prerenal azotaemia, increased liver enzymes and bilirubin, and hypoglycaemia. Disseminated intravascular coagulation (DIC) can develop. Abdominal imaging is indicated to exclude GI obstruction, however be aware that parvovirus can result in ileus with intestinal gas and fluid accumulation. Confirmation of the diagnosis is via faecal ELISA for CPV-2 even if the dog no longer has diarrhoea. The ELISA may be negative early in the disease or after 10–14 days of infection. Additional faecal tests such as PCR are available.

Treatment is supportive:

- Intravenous fluids to correct fluid and electrolyte imbalance. Potassium supplementation is indicated. Supplement fluids with dextrose if the patient is hypoglycaemic and consider plasma or colloids if the oncotic pressure decreases
- Antibiotics should be given to neutropenic, non-pyrexic dogs, e.g. amoxicillin/clavulanic acid or a first-generation cephalosporin. If the patient is showing signs of septic shock, broad-spectrum parenteral antibiotic cover should be provided. Clavulanate-potentiated penicillins provide good broad-spectrum coverage whereas first-generation cephalosporins have poor activity against anaerobes and Gram-negative organisms. Metronidazole can be used to improve anaerobe cover. Increased Gram-negative coverage can be provided by a second-generation cephalosporin, aminoglycoside (if renal function is adequate and hydration normal) or a fluoroquinolone (although this may be avoided in dogs less than 1 year of age). It should be noted that in recent years, resistance to first-generation cephalosporins in Gram-negative organisms has become more common, and knowledge of local resistance patterns may influence the choice of antibiotic. Further combinations are discussed in the section on Symptomatic management

- Anti-emetics to control vomiting; a constant rate infusion of metoclopramide is often effective and also has a prokinetic effect
- Gastric protectants if there is gastrointestinal haemorrhage or oesophagitis
- Recombinant feline interferon-omega may reduce mortality in dogs with parvovirus
- Colony stimulating factor (G-CSF) can be used to increase neutrophil numbers but may not affect outcome
- Nutrition is essential and parenteral nutrition may need to be considered if the vomiting is intractable. The enteral route should be used as soon as vomiting is controlled.

Feline parvovirus/panleucopenia

Feline parvovirus or feline infectious enteritis (FIE) is seen in unvaccinated cats and in locations with high population density. Clinical signs are similar to those in dogs and diagnosis is based upon history, physical examination, presence of neutropenia and faecal ELISA. There is cross-reaction between feline and canine parvoviruses so the same ELISA can be used. Treatment priorities are the same as in the dog.

Acute colitis

Colitis is a frequent presentation to general practitioners. The differential diagnoses of acute large bowel diarrhoea are listed in Figure 11.5. Clinical signs of large intestinal diarrhoea include increased frequency, small volumes of faeces, urgency, tenesmus, mucus and fresh blood. Acute colitis is often self-limiting. Diagnosis is based upon history and physical findings, which may be normal. Rectal examination should be performed. Faecal examination for parasites and clostridial spores is indicated. Further investigation should be performed if the patient is refractory to therapy or has more chronic signs.

Symptomatic therapy for colitis is as follows:

- Withhold food for 12–24 hours
- Antiparasitic drugs if the patient is not regularly wormed
- Use of a fibre-supplemented diet has been recommended to provide short-chain fatty acids as fuel for the colonocytes
- Antibiotics should not be used in all cases but if clostridial disease is suspected then amoxicillin, metronidazole or tylosin would be suitable
- Sulfasalazine (and other immunosuppressants) should be reserved for chronic cases.

Extra-intestinal

Hepatic encephalopathy

Hepatic encephalopathy (HE) is a term used to describe a myriad of neurological signs which result from impaired hepatic clearance of metabolic products from the GI tract. Dogs and cats with HE may have congenital or acquired portosystemic shunts (PSS), cirrhosis/fibrosis or acute hepatic failure. Several factors are implicated in the development of these signs including ammonia, mercaptans and altered neurotransmitters. There is a species difference in the signs seen:

- Dog: depression, stupor, coma, blindness, ataxia, occasionally seizures
- Cat: aggression, seizures, blindness, ataxia, hypersalivation, discoloured iris (copper-coloured).

In addition, these patients may have GI signs, poor growth (congenital PSS), polyuria/polydipsia (dogs), lower urinary tract signs due to the presence of urate calculi, renomegaly and occasionally coagulopathy.

Diagnosis is based upon history and physical examination but is greatly assisted by laboratory analysis. Elevated fasting ammonia or bile acids suggests hepatic dysfunction but if these are unremarkable, measurement of postprandial samples may increase sensitivity for detection of disease. Haematology and biochemistry may show other changes consistent with hepatic dysfunction (microcytosis, anaemia, hypoalbuminaemia, low urea, hypocholesterolaemia, possibly hypoglycaemia and possibly abnormal liver enzymes). Coagulation times should be assessed before any invasive procedures. Abdominal imaging (ultrasonography, scintigraphy) can help to confirm a diagnosis of congenital PSS and with acquired liver disease may indicate the need for hepatic biopsy.

The treatment aims for a patient with HE are to:

- Maintain fluid and electrolyte balance:
  - Potassium should be closely monitored as hypokalaemia may contribute to worsening of signs of HE
  - Fluids containing lactate should be used with caution as lactate is metabolized in the liver
  - Consider blood products if the patient is coagulopathic
- Decrease absorption and production of ammonia and other toxins in the gastrointestinal tract:
  - Lactulose is an osmotic laxative agent which acidifies the colon and decreases absorption of ammonium ions. It decreases the quantity of ammonia-producing bacteria in the gut and hastens gut transit time so that there is less time for absorption of toxins. Lactulose can be given orally or, in severe cases, as a retention enema
  - Antibiotics with activity against colonic bacteria, thereby decreasing ammonia production, and with systemic activity as these patients are at increased risk for bacteraemia (e.g. ampicillin (enterally/ parenterally), neomycin (enterally) or metronidazole (enterally/parenterally))
- Decrease protein content of the diet whilst maintaining high biological value protein. Commercial diets are recommended for use.
- Decrease precipitating factors: control constipation and GI haemorrhage.

If patients have exhibited seizure activity, antiepileptic medication should be started. Phenobarbital should be used cautiously and at reduced doses in patients with hepatic insufficiency. Alternatives include potassium bromide in dogs with intermittent seizure activity and propofol infusions in dogs or cats with status epilepticus. For further details see Chapter 9.

Hepatic lipidosis (feline)

Hepatic lipidosis is a serious complication that usually occurs secondary to other disease in the cat. It is typically seen in obese cats with a recent stressful event which has resulted in inappetance/anorexia. There is massive accumulation of fat in the cytoplasm of the hepatocytes, associated with acute hepatic failure. Cats present with a history of anorexia, vomiting and icterus. They may have signs consistent with concurrent pancreatitis and diabetes mellitus.

Laboratory features include increased bilirubin, ALT and ALP concentrations, but normal/mildly increased GGT concentration. Ammonia and pre- and postprandial bile acids can also be increased. There may be coagulation abnormalities. Ultrasonography of the liver reveals diffuse hyperechogenicity of the parenchyma and generalized hepatomegaly. A fine needle aspirate can be diagnostic, but if not biopsy should be considered. Treatment includes:

- Intravenous fluids to correct fluid and electrolyte imbalances. Potassium supplementation is likely to be needed and blood glucose, phosphate and other electrolytes should be monitored and managed as indicated. Phosphate can decrease as part of refeeding syndrome 12–72 hours after initiating feeding, and if hypophosphataemia is severe this could cause haemolytic anaemia
- Treat any underlying cause
- Nutritional support:
  - Naso-oesophageal tube feeding can be used for temporary support until the cat is stable enough for anaesthesia to place an oesophagostomy or gastrostomy tube, as tube feeding may be required for 4–6 weeks
  - The diet should contain high-quality protein (unrestricted quantity unless hyperammonaemic) with addition of taurine 500 mg/day, carnitine 150–500 mg/day and thiamine 100–200 mg/day
- Anti-emetics can be used if the cat is vomiting, e.g. metoclopramide
- Prokinetics can be used if there is delayed gastric emptying
- Parenteral vitamin K1 can be used if the cat has a coagulopathy
- Additional therapy might include gastric protectants/antacids and appetite stimulants such as cyproheptadine
- Hepatic encephalopathy may be present in severe cases and should be managed with lactulose and antibiotics.

Acute pancreatitis

Acute pancreatitis was classically thought of as a canine disease but is now not an uncommon diagnosis in cats. Clinical signs vary in their severity between cases but include vomiting (dogs > cats), cranial abdominal pain (dogs > cats) and sometimes diarrhoea. Cats are more variable in their presentation and typically will have weight loss, lethargy, anorexia, dehydration and may be hypothermic. Physical examination may reveal abdominal pain particularly in the cranial quadrants and in some patients a mass is palpated.

Body temperature may be elevated (more common in dogs) or decreased (more common in cats). Cardiovascular abnormalities suggestive of hypovolaemic or distributive shock may be seen. If the pancreatic swelling causes biliary obstruction, icterus may develop. These patients are at risk of developing DIC.

The diagnosis of pancreatitis is challenging. History, physical examination and minimum database may be non-specific. Elevations in amylase and lipase concentrations can be useful in the dog (though not the cat) but they are not elevated in all cases and can be increased by some drugs and in patients with renal or gastric disease. Hypocalcaemia and hypoglycaemia are also reported in cats with acute pancreatitis. Radiography may provide some suggestions of pancreatitis (loss of serosal detail, lateral displacement of the duodenum). Abdominal ultrasonography performed by a competent ultrasonographer is more sensitive than radiography in detecting changes consistent with pancreatitis which include:

- Increased size of the pancreas
- Heterogenous parenchyma
- Fluid accumulation around the pancreas
- Hyperechoic fat in the peripancreatic area
- Pain on ultrasonography of the pancreatic area.

Abdominocentesis could also be performed as discussed earlier in this chapter and generally shows a non-septic exudate. Measurement of species-specific blood pancreatic lipase levels (canine or feline pancreatic lipase immunoreactivity, PLI) has greatly assisted the diagnosis of pancreatitis.

Treatment of pancreatitis includes:

- Intravenous fluid therapy to treat shock (if present) and replace maintenance requirements and losses
- Nil by mouth until vomiting has stopped for at least 12 hours, then reintroduce small volumes of water. If this is tolerated a low-fat diet fed in small frequent meals can be started.
  Considering the risk of hepatic lipidosis, different recommendations are made in cats and feline patients should be fed a low-fat diet as soon as possible and if necessary via assisted feeding
- Analgesia for abdominal pain. Opiates are generally recommended and if the pain is refractory, local analgesia or constant rate infusions can be added
- Anti-emetics can be used to control vomiting
- Antibiotics are generally not recommended in dogs unless there is evidence of sepsis or a high risk of bacterial translocation from the gut. Antibiotics are used more commonly in cats due to concerns about ascending infection via the common pancreatic/bile duct
- Colloidal support ideally in the form of plasma can be helpful in patients with severe pancreatitis and secondary complications associated with DIC
- If prolonged starvation is needed due to intractable vomiting, additional nutritional support should be considered. Enteral feeding

could be performed via a jejunostomy tube. In cats, naso-oesophageal feeding is commonly started, to minimize the risk of hepatic lipidosis. Some patients will tolerate trickle-feeding with electrolyte and glutamine solutions before they will tolerate food. If enteral nutrition is not possible and the patient has been starved for more than 3–4 days, partial or total parenteral nutrition should be considered
- If an underlying cause is identified this should be treated specifically
- Surgery is generally not indicated unless there is evidence of a pancreatic abscess, to facilitate placement of a feeding tube, to relieve obstruction of the common bile duct or to debride the pancreas.

Patients with acute pancreatitis can develop acute renal failure, DIC, acute respiratory distress (ARDS, aspiration pneumonia) and diabetes mellitus.

Causes of peritoneal effusion

Haemoabdomen
Abdominal haemorrhage can result from trauma or from rupture of intra-abdominal neoplasms, e.g. splenic haemangiosarcoma. It can also be associated with coagulopathies and liver disease, particularly in cats. The peripheral PCV will be normal until there is redistribution of fluid into the vascular space. Total solids (protein) may be decreased at presentation.

If bloody fluid is collected by abdominocentesis, diagnostic samples should be collected initially and no attempt should be made to 'drain' the abdomen. The PCV of the fluid should be measured and compared to the PCV of the circulating blood. The fluid should be observed for clotting. Free fluid collected from the peritoneal cavity should not clot, however blood collected from an inadvertent centesis of an organ/vessel will clot, assuming no coagulopathy is present. If the PCV of the fluid is similar to the circulating PCV, assessment of the patient's coagulation status should be considered as this suggests recent haemorrhage. If the haemorrhage stops and the patient receives fluid therapy, then the relationship between the circulating PCV and the fluid PCV will be altered. The fluid PCV will remain the same but the circulating PCV will decrease due to the dilutional effect of fluid therapy.

Peritonitis

Septic peritonitis
Septic peritonitis is the presence of suppurative inflammation in the abdominal cavity. A diagnosis of septic peritonitis can be made if the abdominal fluid contains degenerate neutrophils and intracellular bacteria (Figure 11.15). Typically the fluid is an exudate but modified transudates can occur. The most common cause of septic peritonitis is rupture/perforation of the gastrointestinal tract.

If the clinician suspects septic peritonitis, fluid should be submitted for aerobic and anaerobic culture. Abdominal fluid glucose and lactate have been

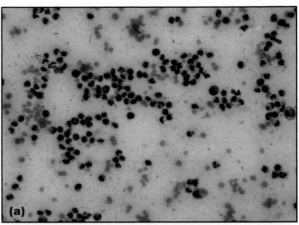

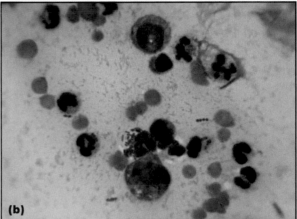

11.15 Microscopic images of a septic peritoneal effusion in a dog. **(a)** X40 lens. **(b)** X100 oil immersion lens. (Courtesy of K Papasouliotis)

evaluated and are useful in distinguishing between septic and non-septic peritonitis. An abdominal fluid glucose <2.8 mmol/l has been shown to be 100% specific for septic peritonitis (Bonczynski *et al.*, 2003) in a small group of clinical patients. Lactate concentration >5.5 mmol/l in the abdominal fluid is consistent with septic peritonitis.

Non-septic peritonitis
Non-septic peritonitis is the presence of neutrophilic inflammation in the peritoneal cavity without intracellular bacteria, and can be caused by inflammatory processes such as pancreatitis, hepatitis, prostatitis, neoplasia, intestinal obstruction, a sequestered or 'walled off' septic process, or previous antibiotic therapy of a patient with septic peritonitis. Neutrophil morphology is variable and degenerative changes may be present. Measurement of abdominal fluid amylase and lipase can be helpful in diagnosing pancreatitis in challenging cases; however pancreatitis could be primary or secondary to septic peritonitis. In the cat, feline infectious peritonitis (FIP) should always be considered as a possible cause of a non-septic exudate or modified transudate.

Bile peritonitis
Biliary rupture can result from trauma, cholelithiasis, neoplasia or necrotizing cholecystitis. Bile leakage can result in abdominal effusion, pain and icterus. These signs can be delayed for 7–10 days after rupture of the

biliary system. Abdominocentesis yields a modified transudate which progresses to an exudate. Generally bile peritonitis is sterile, however if the bile is infected then a septic exudate will develop and the prognosis is more guarded. Grossly the fluid is yellow–brown to green in colour. Microscopic assessment can reveal bilirubin crystals. Measurement of total bilirubin concentrations in the fluid and peripheral blood is useful. Higher bilirubin concentration in the abdominal fluid compared to blood confirms bile peritonitis and is an indication for exploratory laparotomy.

Uroabdomen

Uroabdomen results from rupture of the urinary tract. Urine can accumulate in the peritoneal and/or retroperitoneal cavities. The nature of the fluid changes with time, severity of the leakage, and the presence or absence of infection; the fluid can be a transudate, modified transudate or an exudate. Cytology is consistent with inflammation. Measurement of creatinine and potassium in both the fluid and serum can be diagnostic of uroabdomen, with higher concentrations in the abdominal fluid compared to serum. A false-positive diagnosis of uroabdomen could be obtained in an azotaemic patient with an abdominal effusion related to other disease; in these patients rapid administration of intravenous fluids can result in decrease of serum potassium and creatinine (dilutional) whilst the abdominal fluid levels are unchanged.

Chyloabdomen

Chyloabdomen is an unusual finding in an emergency patient. Diagnostic features include a milky/strawberry milkshake gross appearance, with total protein count similar to serum and higher triglycerides in the fluid than in serum. Causes include trauma, neoplasia, idiopathic and FIP.

Non-gastrointestinal causes of abdominal effusion

It should be noted that right-sided cardiac failure, e.g. due to pericardial disease, or dilated cardiomyopathy can result in an abdominal effusion. These patients may also exhibit discomfort on palpation of the cranial abdomen which may be secondary to hepatic engorgement. The presence of hepatojugular reflux can be useful to demonstrate the presence of right-sided cardiac disease. Other non-gastrointestinal causes of a transudative abdominal effusion include vascular occlusion by thrombi or neoplasms, portal hypertension, and hypoproteinaemia.

Symptomatic management

Figure 11.16 gives suggested doses of the commonly used drugs discussed below.

Acid blockers

Drugs that block secretion of gastric acid are an important element of treatment of oesophageal and gastric ulceration. Two classes of drugs are available: histamine (H_2) receptor antagonists and proton pump inhibitors. There are no veterinary licensed products in the UK.

Drug	Dosage
Antacid	
Cimetidine	5–10 mg/kg orally or i.v. q6–8h
Famotidine	0.1–0.5 mg/kg orally or i.v. q12h
Nizatidine	1–3 mg/kg s.c., i.m. or i.v. q8h
Ranitidine	1–2 mg/kg orally or i.v. q8–12h 0.5–2 mg/kg orally q12h (cat)
Antibiotic	
Amoxicillin (± clavulanate)	20 mg/kg orally q8–12h 20 mg/kg i.v. q8h
Erythromycin	Antibiotic 10 mg/kg orally q8h Prokinetic 1 mg/kg orally q8h
Metronidazole	10–20 mg/kg orally or i.v. q8–12h Higher doses (>50 mg/kg/day) may be associated with central vestibular signs
Oxytetracycline	10–20 mg/kg orally q8h
Tylosin	10 mg/kg orally q8–12h
Anti-emetic	
Chlorpromazine	0.2–0.4 mg/kg s.c. q8h
Metoclopramide	0.2–0.5 mg/kg orally or s.c. q8h or 1–2 mg/kg/24h i.v. as a CRI
Ondansetron	0.5–1.5 mg/kg i.v. q6h 0.5–1 mg/kg orally q12–24h
Antiparasitic	
Fenbendazole	50 mg/kg orally q24h for 3–5 days as broad-spectrum anthelminthic. See formulary for specific guidelines
Hepatic encephalopathy treatment	
Ampicillin	10 mg/kg orally q8h
Lactulose	1–15 ml orally q8h (dog) 0.25–1 ml orally q8h (cat) Lactulose enema 20 ml/kg of 30% solution
Mucosal protectant	
Sucralfate	1 g per 30 kg orally q8h (dog) 250 mg/cat orally q8h
Proton pump inhibitor	
Omeprazole	0.7 (0.2–1) mg/kg slow i.v. or orally q24h for dogs

11.16 Dose rates for commonly used drugs for treatment of gastrointestinal problems.

There are four available H_2 antagonists; in the UK the most commonly used are cimetidine and ranitidine. Both can be given orally or parenterally. Ranitidine has some benefits over cimetidine in that it has an additional prokinetic effect and does not have hepatic side effects. Rapid intravenous administration of ranitidine can result in cardiac dysrhythmias. Rebound acid secretion after withdrawal of these drugs is highest with cimetidine.

Proton pump inhibitors (PPIs) such as omeprazole irreversibly bind the proton pump and therefore are potent inhibitors of acid secretion. They can be administered once daily. Acid secretion is progressively blocked and reaches maximal activity after approximately 5 days. Therapeutic effects persist for several days after cessation of therapy. Omeprazole is available in capsules (contain enteric coated granule; must not be crushed) and as an intravenous preparation, and is recommended in cases of confirmed gastric ulceration or oesophagitis as it is the most effective drug for increasing gastric pH.

Misoprostol is a synthetic prostaglandin analogue which inhibits gastric acid secretion and increases epithelial cell turnover. It can prevent and promote healing of gastric and duodenal ulcers, particularly those associated with NSAID use. It must not be used in pregnant animals, and pregnant staff or owners should not handle the drug.

Analgesia

Analgesia is important in patients with abdominal pain and should not be overlooked. Patients (especially cats) may not always show classical signs of pain and therefore the clinician should remain aware of the likelihood that pain may be present in certain conditions, for example pancreatitis. Analgesia helps to reduce morbidity and mortality in many diseases. Treatment of the underlying cause of the pain will be the most effective management, but in the short term analgesia should be provided. If the patient is hypoperfused, if there is questionable renal function or if gastrointestinal ulceration is suspected, then NSAIDs should be avoided. Opioid analgesia is appropriate, and suitable drugs include pethidine, buprenorphine, methadone and morphine. The reader is referred to the *BSAVA Manual of Anaesthesia and Analgesia* and Chapter 22 in this manual for further information about analgesia.

Antibiotics

If septic peritonitis is suspected or diagnosed, antibiotic therapy should be started as soon as samples have been collected for culture. Broad-spectrum (Gram-positive and Gram-negative, aerobes and anaerobes), bactericidal intravenous antibiotics should be used. These are also indicated in patients with a high risk of bacterial translocation across the gastrointestinal mucosa, e.g. gastrointestinal obstruction or ulceration. Suitable broad-spectrum antibiotic combinations include:

- Penicillin and fluoroquinolone
- First-generation cephalosporin and fluoroquinolone
- Second-generation cephalosporin
- Metronidazole can be added to any of the above regimes to provide increased anaerobic coverage.

Aminoglycosides or third-generation cephalosporins may be required to treat some infections of enteric origin, as bacteria exhibiting broad-spectrum antimicrobial resistance are being isolated from small animal patients with increasing frequency. Use of these drugs should be reserved for patients with a culture confirming they are required or for patients with severe sepsis that are not responding to the combinations suggested above.

Antibiotics may also be considered in animals with acute infectious (bacterial) diarrhoea due to *Salmonella* or *Campylobacter*, severe haemorrhagic diarrhoea (increased risk of sepsis secondary to mucosal ulceration), immunosuppression (e.g. parvovirus infection) and in patients with aspiration pneumonia secondary to oesophageal disease. *Clostridium perfringens* and *C. difficile* have been associated with severe diarrhoea and in particular have been linked to haemorrhagic gastroenteritis (HGE). Metronidazole is one of a number of antibiotics which are recommended for treating both clostridial species and should be considered in patients with HGE.

Antidiarrhoeals

Symptomatic management of diarrhoea (GI rest and introduction of a bland, easily digestible low-fat diet) is often all that is needed to resolve acute small bowel diarrhoea. In some situations additional therapy may be required although infectious and obstructive disease must be excluded before these are introduced.

Opioids (loperamide or diphenoxylate) increase intestinal transit time and reduce intestinal fluid loss by increasing segmental contraction. Antispasmodics (butylscopolamine) may reduce discomfort and pain associated with acute GI disease but could potentiate ileus by reducing gut motility. Intestinal protectants/adsorbents (kaolin and pectin, activated charcoal, bismuth) have been used for many years in general practice to treat acute diarrhoea but their efficacy is unproven.

Sulfasalazine is a combination of 5-aminosalicylic acid (5-ASA) and sulphapyridine. 5-ASA is the active ingredient. It has anti-inflammatory activity in the colon and is used for the treatment of chronic colitis. Side effects are uncommon but can include keratoconjunctivitis sicca, vomiting, allergic dermatitis and cholestatic jaundice.

Anti-emetics

Anti-emetics are indicated in patients with protracted vomiting causing fluid and electrolyte imbalances. They should not be used in patients with potential gastrointestinal obstruction, toxin ingestion (because they may prevent elimination of the toxin) or severe hypotension. Anti-emetics may act via peripheral or central mechanisms. Metoclopramide is the most commonly used anti-emetic. It has a central anti-emetic action in the chemoreceptor trigger zone and also a peripheral prokinetic effect which can reduce emesis by increasing lower oesophageal sphincter tone and gastric emptying. In acutely vomiting patients, intravenous administration is recommended and the authors frequently use a constant rate infusion (CRI) as an alternative to intermittent administration. Metoclopramide CRI is particularly useful in patients with GI ileus and persistent vomiting, e.g. those patients recovering from parvovirus infection or abdominal surgery. The central nervous system (CNS) side effects of metoclopramide appear to be less common if the drug is given by CRI. Metoclopramide is a light-sensitive formulation and therefore infusion bags should be covered to protect the drug from breakdown. It has been suggested that this is not an effective anti-emetic in cats but our experience is that it can be a useful drug in this species.

Alternative anti-emetics include ondansetron and phenothiazines. Ondansetron is generally more effective when used pre-emptively in situations where vomiting is expected, e.g. following chemotherapy. It is effective in dogs but due to expense is usually reserved for refractory cases. Phenothiazines (e.g. chlorpromazine) are effective broad-spectrum anti-emetics but can also cause hypotension due to their vasodilatory effects. They should therefore be reserved for those patients whose fluid deficits have been corrected. They have a number of potential drug interactions and the reader is advised to consult a formulary before using these drugs.

Antiparasitics

The gastrointestinal tract is susceptible to infection by a number of parasites including nematodes and cestodes. Infection with some species can result in acute and severe gastrointestinal signs. Whipworm (*Trichuris vulpis*) infection can result in inflammation, haematochezia and protein-losing enteropathy and, in extreme situations, can produce electrolyte abnormalities that mimic hypoadrenocorticism. Roundworms, e.g. *Toxocara canis/cati* and *Toxascaris leonina* can be associated with severe gastrointestinal signs particularly in puppies and kittens. Hookworm (*Ancylostoma* spp) infection can cause severe potentially fatal gastrointestinal blood loss. Diagnosis of these infections should be confirmed with faecal analysis prior to treatment. Fenbendazole is effective against all of these helminths.

Antiprotozoals

Protozoal infections, e.g. *Giardia*, *Cryptosporidium* and *Tritrichomonas foetus* (cats) can cause GI signs but generally these cause chronic rather than acute disease.

Fluid therapy

Fluid therapy is discussed in more detail in Chapter 4 of this manual. In health, the GI tract absorbs approximately 99% of the fluid presented to it. There is a massive flux of fluid into the GI tract each day (oral fluid intake 30–50 ml/kg, secretions into the GI tract 70 ml/kg). When GI disorders occur it is common for there to be significant fluid loss from, or sequestration of fluid within, the tract. This fluid loss or sequestration can result in marked electrolyte abnormalities. The cause and effect of fluid loss/sequestration is dependent upon the area of the GI tract affected. Vomiting or gastric outflow obstruction will result in loss of acid-rich fluid and chloride and therefore the development of a systemic metabolic alkalosis, hypochloraemia and hypokalaemia. Losses secondary to diarrhoea contain large amounts of potassium and bicarbonate and can result in metabolic acidosis and hypokalaemia. Patients with diarrhoea can also lose significant quantities of protein into the gut and become hypoalbuminaemic; this should also be considered when planning fluid therapy.

The aims of fluid therapy should be correction of volume loss, electrolytes and acid–base balance. The route and rate of administration and the type of fluid are chosen based upon the patient's history, physical examination and electrolyte/acid–base status. Anaemia, hypoalbuminaemia and ongoing fluid losses will all influence the fluid choice. Oral fluid therapy may be suitable for patients with mild diarrhoea but for the majority of patients with severe signs, intravenous administration is appropriate.

The rate of administration of the intravenous fluids will be influenced by the patient's status. Rapid administration is recommended in patients with severe hypovolaemia/shock and consideration should be given when obtaining intravenous access to catheter gauge and length and the need for multiple catheters. Bolus administration is recommended in these patients. A 10–20 ml/kg bolus is given over 10–20 minutes and the response assessed by measurement of physical parameters; the bolus can be repeated if needed. Losses due to dehydration can be replaced more gradually, usually over 24–36 hours.

Most patients will respond to crystalloid administration, however if there is marked hypoalbuminaemia or severe hypovolaemia, colloids may be considered often in addition to appropriate crystalloid therapy. In patients with severe anaemia either a blood product or a haemoglobin-based oxygen-carrying solution may be considered. If the patient is hypokalaemic or anorexic then potassium supplementation of the fluids is indicated (see Chapter 4).

Acid–base status can be evaluated with blood gas analysis and treatment adjusted accordingly. If acid–base status is normal or there is a mild metabolic acidosis, lactated Ringer's or Hartmann's is an appropriate choice of fluid. Severe acidosis (pH <7.1) may require treatment with sodium bicarbonate, although in most cases appropriate fluid therapy will correct the acidosis. Patients with metabolic alkalosis can be treated with Ringer's solution or 0.9% sodium chloride supplemented with potassium. If a patient has hepatic dysfunction, it is sometimes recommended that lactate-containing fluids should be avoided since lactate requires hepatic metabolism.

Mucosal protectants

Mucosal protectants aid the barrier function of the oesophagus and stomach when mucosal deficits are present. They can act as cytoprotective agents, chemical diffusion barriers or both. Sucralfate is an orally administered complex of aluminium hydroxide and sucrose octasulphate available as both tablets and a suspension. It binds to gastro-oesophageal erosions/ulceration and forms a barrier to gastric acid penetration, thus aiding healing. In the acid environment the sucrose is released and cross-polymerizes proteinaceous exudates over ulcers. Sucralfate also has a number of other properties which may increase its clinical benefits. It is not licensed for veterinary use in the UK. The aluminium component can interfere with absorption of some orally administered drugs such as fluoroquinolones and possibly cimetidine, and therefore it is recommended that such drugs are administered at least 2 hours before sucralfate administration. There is some controversy regarding the necessity to separate administration of antacids and sucralfate and the reader is referred to the *BSAVA Manual of Canine and Feline Gastroenterology* for more information.

Other mucosal protectants include aluminium or magnesium hydroxide, calcium carbonate, sodium bicarbonate, misoprostol and bismuth salts.

Nutrition

Nutrition is a vital part of the management of patients with gastrointestinal disease and in some diseases, e.g. parvovirus, early enteral nutrition has been associated with lower morbidity. The enteral route should be used whenever possible and the patient's individual signs determine the level of the feeding within the GI tract, e.g. patients with oesophageal diseases may be fed via a gastrostomy tube (surgically or endoscopically placed), while those with gastric disease might require jejunostomy tube feeding. Parenteral (partial or total) feeding should be considered in patients that are unable to tolerate enteral feeding, but enteral feeding should be restarted as soon as possible. Nutritional support of the critical patient is discussed in more detail in Chapter 23.

Prokinetics

Prokinetics can stimulate motility in part of or the entire GI tract. These drugs are indicated when there is a need to improve motility in patients with ileus, once electrolyte abnormalities have been corrected and GI obstruction excluded. The most commonly used prokinetics are metoclopramide, H_2 antagonists (ranitidine) and erythromycin.

References and further reading

Beal MW (2005) Approach to the acute abdomen. *Veterinary Clinics of North America: Small Animal Practice* **35**, 375–396

Bersenas AME, Mathews KA, Allen DG and Conlon PD (2005) Effects of ranitidine, famotidine, pantoprazole, and omeprazole on intragastric pH in dogs. *American Journal of Veterinary Research* **66**, 425–431

Bischoff MG (2003) Radiographic techniques and interpretation of the acute abdomen. *Clinical Techniques in Small Animal Practice* **18**, 7–19

Boag A and Hughes D (2004) Emergency management of the acute abdomen in dogs and cats 1. Investigation and initial stabilisation. *In Practice* **26**, 476–483

Bonczynski JJ, Ludwig LL, Barton LJ, Loar A and Peterson ME (2003) Comparison of peritoneal fluid and peripheral blood pH, bicarbonate, glucose, and lactate concentration as a diagnostic tool for septic peritonitis in dogs and cats. *Veterinary Surgery* **32(2)**, 161–166

Cruz-Arámbulo R and Wrigley R (2003) Ultrasonography of the acute abdomen. *Clinical Techniques in Small Animal Practice* **18**, 20–31

Graham JP, Lord PF and Harrison JM (1998) Quantitative estimation of intestinal dilation as a predictor of obstruction in the dog. *Journal of Small Animal Practice* **39**, 521–524

Hall EJ, Simpson JW and Williams DA (2005) *BSAVA Manual of Canine and Feline Gastroenterology, 2nd edn.* BSAVA Publications, Gloucester

Lee R (1995) *BSAVA Manual of Small Animal Diagnostic Imaging.* BSAVA Publications, Gloucester

Mazzaferro EM (2003) Triage and approach to the acute abdomen. *Clinical Techniques in Small Animal Practice* **18**, 1–6

Villiers E and Blackwood L (2005) *BSAVA Manual of Canine and Feline Clinical Pathology, 2nd edn.* BSAVA Publications, Gloucester

Walters JM (2003) Abdominal paracentesis and diagnostic peritoneal lavage. *Clinical Techniques in Small Animal Practice* **18**, 32–38

Walters PC (2000) Approach to the acute abdomen. *Clinical Techniques in Small Animal Practice* **15**, 63–69

12

Acute abdominal and gastrointestinal surgical emergencies

David Holt and Dorothy Brown

Introduction

Abdominal and gastrointestinal surgical emergencies include a diverse group of conditions that can be challenging to diagnose and manage successfully. Initially, the animal must be carefully evaluated and appropriate resuscitative measures commenced. Once a diagnosis is made, resuscitation is continued to stabilize the animal prior to anaesthesia. Emergency surgery requires a complete exploratory procedure, critical evaluation of tissue viability and exacting surgical technique for best results. Adept postoperative management, including diligent monitoring and an index of suspicion for potential complications, is vital.

Initial examination and resuscitation

Dogs and cats frequently present for emergency evaluation because of acute vomiting or regurgitation, with or without diarrhoea. Each animal must be carefully evaluated to determine if it has a true emergency problem requiring extensive resuscitation, diagnostic investigation and emergency surgery. A rapid initial examination should be performed at presentation to evaluate the animal's degree of dehydration and hypovolaemia, and exclude imminently life-threatening conditions, including severe aspiration pneumonia, shock and sepsis. An initial emergency database, performed on blood withdrawn during catheter placement, includes measurement of packed cell volume (PCV), total solids (TS), blood urea nitrogen (BUN – Azo strip test), blood glucose and serum electrolytes. Initial resuscitation is started based on this information, and then a thorough history is obtained and a complete physical examination performed.

History obtained from the owner should include questions on: the animal's vaccinations; worming history; previous medical conditions; the possibility of foreign body ingestion; the recent ingestion of rubbish, refuse or a fatty meal; and possible exposure to toxins (heavy metals including lead, ethylene glycol) or medications (corticosteroids, non-steroidal anti-inflammatory drugs (NSAIDs), paracetamol). It is important for the veterinarian to try to distinguish between vomiting and regurgitation from the history. Vomiting is characterized as an active retching process with repeated contractions of the abdominal muscles. Regurgitation is often more passive with owners reporting that the animal 'opens its mouth and the food falls out'; this tends to indicate oesophageal rather than gastric or small

intestinal disease. Finally, the veterinarian should perform a systems review, questioning the owner about other clinical signs that might indicate an underlying disease process. For example, polydipsia and polyuria might indicate renal disease, pyometra, diabetes mellitus, hypercalcaemia or hepatic disease.

Abdominal and gastrointestinal emergencies include a great range of conditions from oesophageal foreign bodies through peritonitis and rectal prolapse. Physical examination findings vary depending on the nature of the presenting emergency. During physical examination, the veterinarian focuses on:

- The degree of hypovolaemia (loss of intravascular volume, indicated to an extent by the animal's mucous membrane colour, capillary refill time, heart rate and pulse quality) and dehydration (the loss of interstitial fluid, indicated by changes in skin turgor and mucous membrane dryness)
- The possibility of a linear foreign body trapped under the tongue of the animal
- A thorough auscultation of the heart and lungs to rule out underlying cardiac disease, which might affect fluid therapy and anaesthesia, and to evaluate for the possibility of aspiration pneumonia occurring secondary to vomiting or regurgitation
- Abdominal palpation to evaluate for:
  - Generalized abdominal distension with free gas or fluid
  - Hepatic, gastric, intestinal, or splenic distension or malposition
  - Urinary bladder distension (indicating possible obstruction) or absence (indicating possible urinary leakage)
  - The presence of a palpable foreign body or intussusception
  - The presence of pain (indicating possible pancreatitis or peritonitis)
  - If possible, the animal's forelimbs are held off the ground during palpation to allow the cranial abdominal contents to slide caudal to the last ribs
- Rectal examination to evaluate the rectum, anal sacs, urethra, vagina, distal uterus and cervix, and to obtain a faecal sample for evaluation for parasites and pathogenic bacteria
- A thorough palpation of peripheral lymph nodes and evaluation of the skin for the presence of masses which might be histamine-secreting mast cell tumours.

The nature and urgency of further diagnostic testing is determined by the findings on physical examination. Further evaluation may be necessary, including: a complete blood count; serum biochemistry and electrolyte analysis; serum amylase, lipase and trypsin-like immunoreactivity levels; coagulation testing; blood typing and cross-matching; plain and contrast abdominal radiographs; and abdominal ultrasound evaluation with guided peritoneal fluid aspiration and analysis. If diarrhoea is present, animals should be tested for parvovirus with a commercial enzyme-linked immunosorbent assay (ELISA) kit. Faecal flotation and zinc sulphide sedimentation tests are used to test for helminths, coccidia and *Giardia*. Gram staining of faecal samples helps to identify *Campylobacter*, *Salmonella* and clostridia.

Resuscitation and evaluation of the animal's response to initial treatment continues during the diagnostic process. Animals with acute abdominal and gastrointestinal crises often exhibit signs of hypovolaemia in addition to dehydration. Large amounts of fluid are lost in vomitus and diarrhoea. Additional fluid is sequestered in distended, inflamed, non-motile intestines. Rupture of the gastrointestinal tract leads to the release of gastric acid, pepsin, pancreatic enzymes, bile and bacteria into the peritoneal cavity. This in turn leads to severe local or diffuse peritoneal inflammation and the loss of massive amounts of fluid and protein into the peritoneal cavity. Diaphragmatic lymphatics that normally return peritoneal fluid to the circulation become plugged with fibrin. Fluid losses are often accompanied by dangerous electrolyte and acid–base abnormalities. The severe inflammation and absorption of bacteria and bacterial toxins, notably endotoxin, activate the body's multiple inflammatory, coagulation, fibrinolytic and immunological cascades, leading to the 'systemic inflammatory response syndrome' (SIRS).

Treatment should begin immediately in unstable shock patients. In animals with no previous history of heart disease, no respiratory abnormalities and no murmur evident on initial examination, a bolus of up to 50–100 ml/kg of balanced electrolyte solution may be administered intravenously in the first 60 minutes (see Chapter 4). Two large-bore intravenous catheters are inserted and, prior to fluid therapy, blood is obtained for an initial database. Where possible, urine is obtained before aggressive fluid therapy is begun. Evidence of isosthenuria (urine specific gravity (USG) 1.007–1.015) in the presence of dehydration indicates poor renal function. Azotaemia (prerenal, renal or postrenal) can be confirmed by a high BUN measured by Azo strip test or identified on a serum biochemical screen. A blood smear should be made to provide an indication of the white blood cell and platelet counts.

The PCV and TS are usually increased in non-anaemic animals that are dehydrated, but should be interpreted in light of clinical findings. For example, an animal with a 'normal' initial PCV may actually be quite anaemic following rehydration. Animals with acute haemorrhage may have a normal PCV at presentation. In dogs with an acute haemorrhagic crisis, the PCV at presentation may be maintained in the

normal range by splenic contraction. TS, however, drops very quickly and is a better early indicator of the severity of blood loss. As intravenous fluids are given, both the PCV and TS may drop to dramatically low values. Blood transfusion is usually required if the PCV rapidly drops below 25% and blood products may need to be administered rapidly in anaemic, hypovolaemic patients (see Chapter 14). Colloids (plasma, hetastarch, dextran, albumin) should be considered in cases with low total protein levels (less than 40 g/l). Synthetic haemoglobin solutions may be considered as a source of both colloid and oxygen-carrying capacity (see Chapter 14).

Serum electrolytes should be measured, and blood gas analysis should be performed. Since severe electrolyte and acid–base disturbances can occur with vomiting and diarrhoea, these tests provide valuable information and help determine the appropriate fluid for resuscitation. Animals vomiting gastric contents secondary to a pyloric obstruction will lose sodium, potassium and chloride, and have a metabolic alkalosis. For these animals, 0.9% sodium chloride supplemented with potassium is the ideal replacement fluid. Hyperkalaemia associated with hyponatraemia should increase suspicion of hypoadrenocorticism (Addison's disease). Animals vomiting secondary to small intestinal obstruction will lose not only sodium, potassium and chloride, but also bicarbonate, and their acid–base status can be more variable.

Patient evaluation and diagnostic investigation

Results from a complete blood count and serum biochemical analysis including amylase and lipase, although not always immediately available, often indicate potential underlying metabolic diseases or inflammatory conditions (see Chapter 11).

Radiographs

Additional diagnostic tests, such as radiographs, are obtained depending on the results of the physical examination. Plain abdominal radiographs are indicated in animals with abdominal pain or persistent vomiting. Plain cervical and thoracic radiographs should be made to evaluate the oesophagus for foreign bodies in animals presenting with regurgitation. Radiographs should be critically evaluated for evidence of gastrointestinal obstruction, foreign bodies, pancreatitis, masses, and the presence of free air or fluid in the peritoneal cavity. Radiographic signs of obstruction include the presence of gas or fluid-distended small bowel loops (Figure 12.1). Severe generalized intestinal gas distension can be associated with a mesenteric volvulus. Decreased radiographic contrast in the right cranial abdomen, displacement of the stomach to the left, widening of the angle between the pyloric antrum and the duodenum, displacement of the duodenum to the right and static gas in the duodenum are all radiographic signs associated with pancreatitis (Figure 12.2). Evidence of free gas in the abdominal cavity without prior abdominocentesis or surgery indicates intestinal perforation or the presence

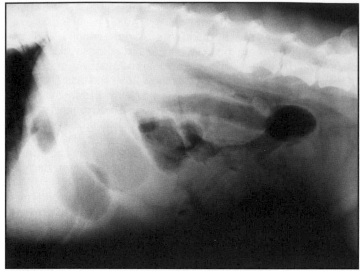
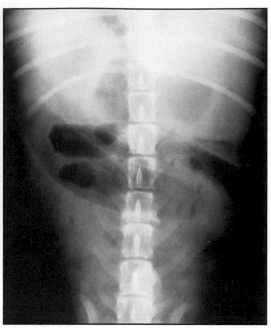

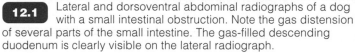

12.1 Lateral and dorsoventral abdominal radiographs of a dog with a small intestinal obstruction. Note the gas distension of several parts of the small intestine. The gas-filled descending duodenum is clearly visible on the lateral radiograph.

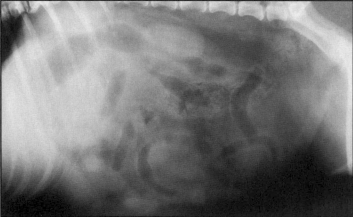
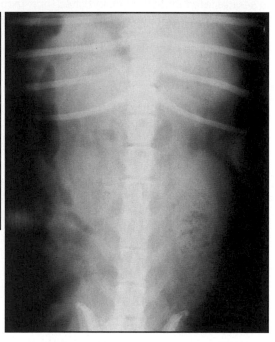

12.2 Lateral and dorsoventral abdominal radiographs of a dog with pancreatitis. Radiographic signs suggestive of pancreatitis include: increased soft tissue opacity and decreased abdominal detail in the right cranial abdomen; a static, gas-filled descending duodenum; displacement of the pyloric antrum to the left; and displacement of the duodenum to the right, producing a widened angle between the stomach and the duodenum. (Courtesy of Dr HM Saunders, University of Pennsylvania School of Veterinary Medicine)

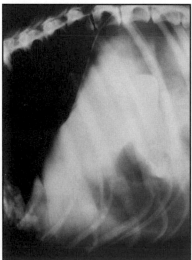

12.3 Lateral radiograph of a dog with gastric perforation, illustrating free gas in the peritoneal cavity. Note the diaphragm outlined clearly by the lungs cranially and the free peritoneal gas caudally.

of gas-forming organisms in the abdominal cavity, and is an indication for immediate laparotomy. The free gas often accumulates caudal to the diaphragm, outlining the crura of the diaphragm clearly (Figure 12.3). Loss of abdominal detail due to fluid should prompt abdominal paracentesis and peritoneal fluid analysis.

Contrast radiographs

Contrast radiographs should be made if gastric or intestinal obstruction is suspected but not definitive on plain abdominal radiographs; 5–10 ml/kg body weight of a 25% liquid barium suspension is given. Iodine-based contrast agents (iohexol, 2–5 ml/kg orally) may be considered if intestinal perforation is suspected, because of concerns that barium may worsen peritonitis if it leaks from the gastrointestinal tract. However, radiographs obtained using iodine-based contrast agents may be difficult to interpret because of dilution of the contrast agent. If barium is used and perforation of the intestine has occurred, rapid surgical intervention may prevent any worsening of peritonitis that might occur due to leakage of barium into the peritoneal cavity.

Abdominal paracentesis

Abdominal paracentesis is performed if peritoneal fluid is detected on physical examination or there is loss of detail on plain abdominal radiographs. The ventral abdomen is clipped and prepared as for aseptic surgery. An ultrasound-guided tap is performed with a 20–22 gauge needle. Retrieved fluid should be examined microscopically for evidence of degenerate neutrophils and the presence of intracellular bacteria. Peritoneal fluid glucose and lactate levels should be compared to those of the peripheral blood. A peritoneal fluid glucose concentration 1.1 mmol/l lower than that of the peripheral blood, or a peritoneal fluid lactate level 2 mmol/l higher than that of peripheral blood, is diagnostic for peritonitis. Creatinine and bilirubin levels may also be measured in the peritoneal exudate or lavage fluid. Values for bilirubin, creatinine and amylase that exceed corresponding serum levels indicate biliary leakage, urinary tract leakage or pancreatitis, respectively.

Diagnostic peritoneal lavage

In some cases, peritoneal fluid is present but cannot be recovered by paracentesis, presumably because the needle becomes plugged with omentum. In this situation, diagnostic peritoneal lavage is indicated. The bladder is expressed and the ventral abdomen is prepared aseptically. An over-the-needle catheter or dialysis catheter is introduced into the abdomen 2 cm caudal to the umbilicus, and 10–20 ml/kg of warm, balanced electrolyte solution is rapidly infused through the dialysis catheter. The fluid is distributed by abdominal massage, and then collected. Only a few millilitres of fluid may be retrieved. In normal animals, lavaged fluid leucocyte counts before surgery are usually less than 10^6 cells/l. After uncomplicated intra-abdominal surgery, lavaged fluid neutrophil numbers generally increase to 10^7 cells/l or fewer. Toxic, degenerate neutrophils with intracellular bacteria indicate septic peritonitis, and are an indication for immediate exploratory laparotomy. Contraindications for peritoneal lavage include dyspnoea, diaphragmatic hernia and severe organomegaly.

Abdominal ultrasonography

Abdominal ultrasonography can be used to evaluate the abdominal organs, especially when free peritoneal fluid makes radiographic interpretation difficult. Particular attention should be paid to the pancreas in animals with abdominal pain. The spleen and liver should be carefully evaluated for possible neoplasms or ruptured haematomas in cases of haemoperitoneum, and for evidence of splenic torsion or thrombosis. The biliary tree, urogenital tract (especially the prostate or uterus) and mesenteric lymph nodes are carefully evaluated.

Other tests

In animals with respiratory difficulty, thoracic radiographs will help to confirm suspected aspiration pneumonia secondary to vomiting. Arterial blood gas analysis will indicate the severity of hypoxia, and a transtracheal or endotracheal wash will provide important information on the type and antibiotic sensitivities of bacteria associated with the pneumonia. Further evaluation of the vomiting animal could include adrenocorticotrophic hormone (ACTH) stimulation tests for hypoadrenocorticism, endoscopy and gastrointestinal biopsies (see Chapter 11).

Exploratory laparotomy

Complete stabilization of the animal with an acute abdominal crisis may not be possible until the underlying cause is treated. In many cases, this requires abdominal surgery. Indications for exploratory abdominal surgery include:

- Free gas visible in the peritoneal cavity of an animal that has not had recent (within 3–4 weeks) abdominal surgery
- Gastric dilatation–volvulus
- Gastrointestinal foreign body, obstruction (including intussusception), linear foreign body
- Gastric haemorrhage not responding to medical management
- Intracellular bacteria and degenerate neutrophils on a peritoneal lavage or tap
- Bilirubin or creatinine levels in the peritoneal fluid greater than those in the serum
- Animals with abdominal haemorrhage that fail to stabilize or remain stable after initial resuscitation
- Splenic torsion
- Mesenteric volvulus
- Pyometra/prostatic abscessation
- Penetrating abdominal injury (gunshot, impalement).

Oesophagus

Oesophageal foreign bodies

Oesophageal foreign bodies should be suspected in any animal presenting with a history of regurgitation, or in cases where the owner cannot clearly distinguish between regurgitation and vomiting. Other clinical signs may include gagging, salivation, anorexia and lethargy. Most animals with complete or near complete obstruction regurgitate food shortly after eating, although they may be able to retain water. Animals may also be dyspnoeic and cough, and be variably depressed secondary to aspiration pneumonia. Occasionally, animals may have partial oesophageal obstruction and remain reasonably bright, yet regurgitate after large meals. Oesophageal perforation may occur with sharp foreign bodies. Even relatively blunt bony foreign bodies can cause oesophageal muscle spasm and mucosal necrosis. Necrosis may extend through the entire oesophageal wall causing mediastinitis, pleuritis and pyothorax. It is important to note that although pneumomediastinum and pneumothorax may develop secondary to oesophageal perforation, these are not consistent radiographic findings and cannot be relied upon to rule in or rule out this diagnosis.

Foreign bodies tend to lodge at points of oesophageal narrowing, which include the thoracic inlet, heart base and the lower oesophageal sphincter. In animals with a suspected oesophageal foreign body, the mouth and pharynx should be evaluated and the neck thoroughly palpated. The thorax should be carefully auscultated for crackles or wheezes that indicate aspiration pneumonia. Most foreign bodies are radio-opaque and can be visualized on plain cervical and thoracic radiographs (Figure 12.4). Thoracic radiographs are also evaluated for changes compatible with pneumonia. Non-radio-opaque foreign bodies require a positive-contrast oesophagram using a sterile, water-soluble iodinated contrast agent for visualization.

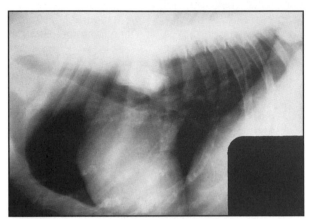

12.4 Lateral thoracic radiograph of a dog illustrating a thoracic oesophageal body present over the heart base. (Courtesy of Dr Colin Harvey, University of Pennsylvania School of Veterinary Medicine)

Foreign body removal should be immediate to minimize the chance of perforation, and is performed using the simplest means possible. The animal is placed under general anaesthesia and a cuffed endotracheal tube is placed to protect the airway. The area under the tongue is carefully evaluated for a thread or line in animals with a needle or hook lodged in the oesophagus. A flexible fibreoptic endoscope or rigid scope and long, blunt-ended forceps are used to remove most foreign bodies. Either type of scope must give the veterinary surgeon the ability to insufflate air to dilate the oesophagus around the foreign body. This must be done with extreme care, and with close monitoring of the animal's blood pressure and ease of ventilation. Insufflation of the oesophagus in an animal with an undiagnosed oesophageal perforation can lead to tension pneumothorax and an immediate life-threatening drop in both haemoglobin oxygen saturation and blood pressure. Removal of radio-opaque foreign bodies under fluoroscopic guidance is also reported.

Once the oesophagus has been carefully dilated around the foreign body, the object is grasped with the forceps and rotation is attempted. Often, the foreign body can be carefully withdrawn. However, if it is firmly lodged, excessive traction should not be applied as this may cause or worsen a perforation. An attempt should be made gently to push foreign bodies into the stomach if they cannot be removed. This technique is most applicable to large cartilage foreign bodies that break off into small pieces when grasped with forceps, and occasionally extremely large oesophageal hair balls in cats. A large-diameter, well lubricated stomach tube is used to push the foreign body distally. Once in the stomach, bones will generally be digested. Hair balls

should be surgically removed. The oesophagus is inspected with the endoscope after foreign body removal. Clean lacerations that do not extend through the full thickness of the oesophageal wall (as judged by gently pushing the tip of a forceps against the laceration through the endoscope) can be left to heal by epithelialization. Full-thickness tears or areas of necrotic oesophagus require immediate surgical management.

Surgery is indicated when a foreign body cannot be retrieved or advanced into the stomach; when there is concern that forceps extraction might lacerate the oesophagus and other intrathoracic structures; and when the oesophagus is perforated.

The cervical oesophagus is accessed via a ventral midline incision in the neck. The ventral sternohyoideus and sternothyroideus muscles are separated on the midline and the oesophagus is located on the left of the trachea. For foreign bodies lodged at or cranial to the heart base, a right third or fourth intercostal thoracotomy provides the best exposure of the oesophagus. For foreign bodies lodged caudal to the heart base, a left eighth intercostal thoracotomy is used. Although foreign bodies in the distal oesophagus can occasionally be retrieved by manipulation through a gastrotomy incision, this approach is not generally recommended. The foreign body is located by palpation. Fish hooks can be difficult to feel in the thoracic oesophagus and occasionally an assistant must locate the hook using an endoscope via the mouth while the thorax is open. A longitudinal oesophagotomy is performed (Figure 12.5) and the foreign body is removed. The oesophageal wall opposite the incision is checked for perforation, and the incision is closed with a single layer of interrupted, appositional sutures. The authors prefer 1.5–2 metric (3/0 or 4/0 USP) monofilament suture material. The oesophagus lacks a serosal covering, necessitating careful apposition of the oesophageal layers to prevent dehiscence. Factors inherent in oesophageal surgery which may predispose to dehiscence are impairment of its intramural blood supply, tension and motion at the anastomosis site, lack of omentum, general debilitation of the patient and movement of food and saliva across the oesophageal anastomosis. All tissues must be handled extremely gently. The areas are lavaged thoroughly. Omental, diaphragmatic and pericardial grafts have been used to reinforce the anastomosis. Nutrition is increasingly demonstrated to be vital to wound healing and the ability to fight infection. In the nutritionally compromised

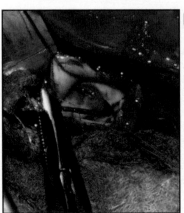

12.5

Longitudinal oesophagotomy performed in the thoracic oesophagus to remove an embedded fish hook. Stay sutures are used to retract the oesophageal wall. The incision is closed with a single layer of simple interrupted sutures of 2 metric polydioxanone (PDS).

patient, consideration should be given to the insertion of a gastrostomy tube via a flank laparotomy at the time of oesophageal surgery.

After uncomplicated endoscopic foreign body removal, food is withheld for at least 12–24 hours followed by introduction of small amounts of soft food or a slurry. The major complication is mediastinitis due to oesophageal perforation, which is manifested by fever, reluctance to eat and widening of the mediastinum on a dorsoventral thoracic radiograph. The diagnosis is confirmed by repeat oesophagoscopy or a contrast oesophagram using a water-soluble, iodinated contrast agent. Surgical repair of the perforation and thoracic drainage via chest tubes are indicated. Uncommonly, animals may develop oesophageal stricture, with recurring signs of regurgitation, up to several weeks following endoscopic removal of a foreign body.

Oesophageal perforation

Oesophageal perforation may occur as a sequel to chronic foreign body obstruction, ingestion of a sharp foreign body or foreign body removal, direct cervical or thoracic trauma, penetrating bite wounds, neoplasia or oesophagoscopy. Clinical signs of obstruction may or may not be present. Pleuritis, mediastinitis, abscessation, broncho-oesophageal fistulation or cervical cellulitis may occur. Perforation should be suspected in patients with a history of oesophageal obstruction and depression, fever, elevated white blood cell count, cough, dyspnoea or a cervical soft tissue swelling. Diagnosis is by oesophagoscopy or contrast radiography using soluble iodine-based agents. Treatment is initially aimed at stabilizing the potentially septic patient with volume support and intravenous broad-spectrum, bactericidal antibiotics. Leakage from the cervical oesophagus is treated by establishing drainage, controlling the infection and repairing the oesophagus. Thoracic oesophageal perforation requires exploratory thoracotomy, removal of infected debris and repair of the damaged area. The chest cavity is thoroughly lavaged and drained via chest tubes.

Stomach

Gastric dilatation–volvulus

Gastric dilatation–volvulus (GDV) syndrome is a range of conditions that includes:

- Gastric dilatation without rotation of the stomach
- Gastric dilatation–volvulus
- Chronic intermittent volvulus with little, if any, dilatation.

Although large-breed, deep-chested dogs are 'classically' affected, these conditions can occur in smaller breeds of dogs and have been reported in cats. The exact aetiology of the disease is uncertain and is probably multifactorial. Clinical signs in dogs with GDV include retching (non-productive), abdominal distension, weakness and collapse. These clinical signs are not specific for the condition and could be associated with other diseases including ruptured splenic haemangiosarcoma or haematoma, splenic torsion, mesenteric volvulus or peritonitis. Physical

examination findings vary depending on the severity of the GDV and the associated circulatory collapse, but often include pale mucous membranes, a rapid heart rate, weak, thready pulses and a distended, often tympanic, abdomen.

The basis for a rational, effective treatment plan is a thorough understanding of the pathophysiology of GDV. Distension of the stomach with food and swallowed air compresses the portal vein and caudal vena cava. This compression, which leads to decreased venous return to the heart and, in turn, decreased cardiac output, can occur with gastric dilatation only and does not require volvulus. The decrease in cardiac output can be profound, and has been estimated to be 50% of normal in experimental canine models with intragastric pressures approximating those seen in spontaneous cases. This decrease in cardiac output leads to decreased tissue perfusion affecting all organs, including the heart. Myocardial ischaemia is one of the main factors cited in the genesis of dysrhythmias seen in dogs with GDV. Decreased perfusion to a distended or twisted stomach often leads to gastric necrosis and then reperfusion injury. Many dogs with GDV are endotoxaemic, presumably because a compromised gastrointestinal mucosal barrier leads to endotoxin absorption into the portal blood and mesenteric lymphatic system.

It is vital to correct the GDV animal's perfusion deficits before anaesthesia and surgery. A rational treatment plan for GDV therefore includes:

- Rapid intravascular volume expansion
- Gastric decompression
- Differentiation of gastric dilatation from GDV
- Surgery once the animal is stable, to reposition the stomach, assess gastric and splenic viability, and fix the pyloric antrum to the right abdominal wall to prevent recurrence of volvulus
- Careful monitoring postoperatively for complications, including aspiration pneumonia.

Fluids for resuscitation must be administered through cephalic or jugular catheters, as fluid administration through saphenous catheters will be ineffective because the caudal vena cava is obstructed. Two large-bore (16–18 gauge) catheters are generally placed in the cephalic veins. Balanced electrolyte solutions are administered at 60–90 ml/kg in the initial hour of treatment (see Chapter 4). Hypertonic saline/ dextran solutions can also be used initially (5 ml/kg i.v. administered over 5–10 minutes), but must be followed by crystalloids at shock doses to maintain the increase in perfusion. Clinical and laboratory parameters, ideally including blood lactate concentrations, are monitored to determine the response to therapy. Once resuscitation is underway, the stomach is decompressed by carefully passing an orogastric tube. The tube must not be forced into the stomach as rupture of the twisted distal oesophagus may occur. If passage of the tube is not possible, the stomach is trocharized. The abdomen is carefully palpated to determine the optimum site for trocharization, to avoid perforation of the spleen. Radiographs, including a right lateral view, are made to differentiate dilatation from volvulus. In a normal animal in right lateral recumbency, the pylorus lies on the 'down' side of the abdomen, contains no gas and, therefore, is unlikely to be visible radiographically. In many dogs with GDV, the pylorus moves away from the right side of the abdomen and so, in right lateral recumbency, the pylorus will be on the 'up' side of the abdomen, contain gas, and, therefore, be visible as a separate gas-filled structure dorsal to the rest of the stomach (Figure 12.6).

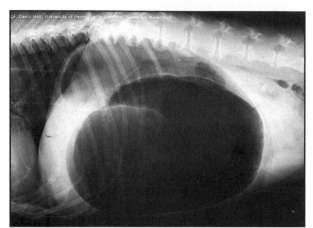

12.6 Right lateral radiograph of a dog with gastric dilatation–volvulus. Note the appearance of the pylorus in the craniodorsal abdomen as a gas-filled structure.

Anaesthesia is commenced only after the animal has been stabilized (see Chapter 21). At surgery, the stomach is decompressed, de-rotated and replaced in a normal position. In most dogs, the pylorus rotates from its normal position on the right side of the abdomen, passing between the fundus of the stomach and the ventral body wall to end up either on the left side of the abdomen (180-degree volvulus), dorsal to the rest of the stomach (270-degree volvulus) or towards the right side of the abdomen (360-degree volvulus). The surgeon, standing on the right side of the dog, locates the duodenum and traces it to the pylorus. The pylorus is then gently pulled back into a normal position with one hand, while the other hand gently pushes the remainder of the stomach dorsally to facilitate de-rotation. The spleen is exteriorized and examined for viability, venous or arterial thrombosis, and short gastric vessel rupture. A splenectomy is performed if necessary. The remainder of the abdomen is explored, and then the stomach is re-examined for necrosis, particularly along the greater curvature. As a guide, areas of the stomach that are discoloured dark purple or grey–green, feel paper thin, or do not bleed when incised, must be removed. If there is doubt concerning the viability of an area it should be removed. Stay sutures are placed in healthy stomach and the necrotic area is resected in stages. The edges of the remaining stomach are examined to ensure they are bleeding and viable. A simple continuous Lembert pattern in the submucosa is initially used to close the stomach. A simple interrupted or continuous Lembert pattern is then used to close the muscularis and serosa. Alternatively, the stomach may be closed with a surgical stapling device (e.g. TA-90, 4.8 mm staple cartridge, US Surgical) reinforced with a continuous Lembert inverting pattern, oversewing the staple line.

Many procedures have been described to 'pexy' or fix the pyloric antral region of the stomach to the right body wall. The aim is to create a permanent adhesion between the antral region of the stomach and the right body wall to prevent recurrence of volvulus. All of the various techniques work well when performed properly. In straightforward cases, an incisional gastropexy is performed. A 5–8 cm incision is made in the transverse abdominus muscle just caudal to the last rib on the right body wall. A matching, partial-thickness incision is made in the seromuscular layers of the pyloric antrum. The edges of the body wall and pyloric incisions are sutured to each other using polydioxanone (PDS) or polypropylene suture (Figure 12.7). The abdomen is lavaged with large volumes of a warm, balanced electrolyte solution and closed in a routine manner.

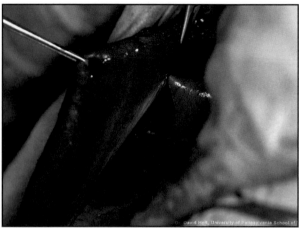

12.7 Incisional gastropexy with the cranial aspect of the incisions in the body wall and pyloric antrum sewn together.

Gastric outflow enhancing procedures have been performed in an attempt to decrease recurrence of gastric dilatation or GDV. Pyloromyotomy and pyloroplasty have been described. However, gastric outflow obstruction is not thought to play a major role in the pathogenesis of GDV. These procedures have not been shown to decrease recurrence, and have been associated with higher immediate postoperative complication rates and therefore *are not indicated*.

Postoperatively, GDV patients require extensive treatment and monitoring. Crystalloid and sometimes colloid fluid administration is continued, with fluid administration rates based on clinical (mucous membrane colour, capillary refill time, heart rate, pulse quality, urine output, blood pressure) and laboratory (PCV, TS, serum electrolyte concentrations, lactate concentration) parameters. Colloids (plasma, hetastarch, human serum albumin) are necessary in some cases with hypoalbuminaemia due to dilution, loss into the gastrointestinal system, or leak into the interstitium secondary to systemic inflammation.

Cardiac dysrhythmias often develop in the first 24–48 hours postoperatively. They are not necessarily associated with a poorer prognosis, but should prompt the veterinarian to re-evaluate the animal's perfusion status, serum electrolytes and oxygenation. When the dysrhythmia is intermittent and not affecting tissue perfusion, no specific anti-dysrhythmic therapy is required. Anti-dysrhythmic therapy is started if the dysrhythmias are associated with a decrease in tissue perfusion, have a rate greater than 160–180 per minute, or are associated with severe, potentially life-threatening cardiac electrical conduction disturbances ('R on T' phenomenon). One or two lidocaine boluses of 1–2 mg/kg are administered to convert the heart to a sinus rhythm, and an infusion of lidocaine is started (50–70 µg/kg/min).

Other complications in the postoperative period include aspiration pneumonia, gastric necrosis, disseminated intravascular coagulation and systemic inflammation/sepsis. Any postoperative GDV dog that becomes febrile should be carefully evaluated for possible gastric necrosis and peritonitis. However, it is often possible to overlook aspiration pneumonia in this situation, as the focus has been on the abdomen during the animal's hospitalization. Many GDV dogs present with a history of retching and vomiting that predisposes them to 'silent' episodes of aspiration and subsequent pneumonia. Thoracic radiographs are made and evaluated for alveolar changes. Treatment of aspiration pneumonia (see Chapter 7) includes oxygen supplementation, nebulization, coupage and, initially, broad-spectrum, bactericidal antibiotics administered intravenously. Culture and sensitivity results from an endotracheal or transtracheal wash should direct antibiotic therapy when they are available.

Gastric foreign bodies

Most gastric foreign bodies are not true emergencies. However, needles should be removed as soon as possible to prevent migration or perforation. Coins which may contain zinc are removed to prevent haemolytic anaemia. In most cases, this is readily accomplished using a flexible endoscope. Recently, several cases have been reported in which ingestion of a hydrophilic adhesive product ('Gorilla Glue') resulted in severe gastric distension and clinical signs. The product expands on contact with gastric fluids, often encompassing and distending the entire stomach. Removal of this material through a large gastrotomy should be performed as an emergency procedure.

Gastric ulceration

Gastric ulceration and severe haemorrhage are frequently associated with the ingestion of NSAIDs. Other causes of gastric ulcers include gastric neoplasia, mast cell tumours, gastrin-secreting tumours and exogenous corticosteroids. Surgery is considered for those cases with massive haemorrhage in which medical therapy fails. The animal is stabilized with transfusions of red blood cells. Rapid endoscopy is useful preoperatively to differentiate focal bleeding amenable to surgical treatment from diffuse gastric haemorrhage, and intraoperatively to pinpoint the site of the gastric haemorrhage for the surgeon, as this may not be apparent externally. Gastric lavage may be necessary to remove blood clots and allow endoscopic visualization of the gastric mucosa.

Small intestine

Intestinal luminal obstruction: foreign bodies and masses

Intraluminal intestinal obstruction is one of the most common indications for laparotomy in dogs and cats, and is most frequently a result of foreign body ingestion. Clinical signs associated with small intestine obstruction vary with the location, duration and severity of the obstruction. Vomiting, anorexia, depression and abdominal tenderness are common. Vomiting may be frequent and even projectile with a complete proximal obstruction, or more sporadic and less profuse with a distal or partial obstruction.

The classic radiographic sign of mechanical obstruction is the presence of multiple loops of gas-dilated small intestine of varying diameters (see Figure 12.1). In animals with complete obstruction, intestinal distension can be severe, particularly if the obstruction is distal. Radiographic changes associated with partial obstruction are less severe and may not be distinguishable from those of gastroenteritis or ileus.

Contrast radiography is frequently used to provide a definitive diagnosis of intestinal obstruction. Most proximal small intestinal obstructions will be evident within 6 hours after administration of barium suspension; up to 24 hours may be necessary to highlight distal obstructions. Ultrasonography provides a more rapid method of diagnosis but has false-positive and -negative rates of 6% and 15%, respectively.

Once a mechanical intestinal obstruction is diagnosed and the animal is stabilized, an exploratory laparotomy is performed and the entire gastrointestinal tract is thoroughly examined. If a foreign body is found and the bowel is relatively healthy, the object is removed through a longitudinal, antimesenteric enterotomy slightly aboral to the obstruction (Figure 12.8). If the bowel wall is necrotic, or if the obstruction is caused by a mass, intestinal resection and anastomosis are performed (Figure 12.9).

Prognosis is usually good after foreign body removal. Resection of non-neoplastic or benign neoplastic masses generally has a better prognosis than resection of malignant neoplasms. Prognosis is usually poor if gross metastases are present at surgery, and life expectancy may be limited to a few months.

Intestinal incarceration and strangulation

Intestinal incarceration is an unnatural displacement and entrapment of the intestine. With the exception of intussusception (discussed separately below), it is reported infrequently in the dog. Entrapment usually occurs within traumatic body wall hernias; entrapments in omental tears, congenital hernias, mesenteric rents or subsequent to duodenocolic ligament ruptures have also been reported.

The intestinal lumen may become constricted, resulting in clinical and radiographic signs of obstruction. If intestinal blood vessels are also compressed and arterial inflow is inhibited, mucosal degeneration may result in translocation of bacteria and endotoxin into the blood stream and peritoneal cavity. Therefore, unlike simple luminal obstruction, incarceration can rapidly progress to strangulation with subsequent intestinal ischaemia and septic or endotoxic shock.

Surgical procedure	Suture material	Suture pattern	Technical considerations
Enterotomy	Synthetic absorbable monofilament • 2 metric for dogs • 1.5 metric for cats	Single layer simple interrupted appositional sutures	
Small intestinal resection and anastomosis		Single layer simple interrupted appositional sutures	Options for managing disparity between luminal diameters of bowel: • Sutures on the larger lumen side can be spaced farther apart than those of the smaller side • The intestine with the smaller lumen can be transected at an angle to create a larger luminal diameter • The intestine with the smaller lumen can be spatulated to create a larger luminal diameter • The luminal diameter of the larger segment can also be reduced by oversewing with a simple interrupted Lembert suture pattern
Colonic resection and anastomosis		Single layer simple interrupted appositional sutures	To equalize the lumen sizes in an ileo- or jejunocolonic anastomosis: 1. Oversew the colonic segment using a simple interrupted Lembert suture pattern to slightly invert the colonic mucosa 2. Incise the antimesenteric border of the jejunum to widen its lumen 3. Proceed with anastomosis
Enteroplication	Synthetic absorbable or non-absorbable monofilament • 2 metric for dogs • 1.5 metric for cats	Simple interrupted sutures placed midway between the mesenteric and antimesenteric borders	• Adjoining segments of intestine are placed side by side in a series of gentle loops to avoid kinking or sharp bends • Complete plication of the jejunum and ileum is recommended because intussusception tends to recur at sites away from the initial lesion • Plication of the duodenum is not necessary since intussusception in this area is rare
Colopexy	Synthetic non-absorbable monofilament • 3 metric for dogs • 2 metric for cats	Simple interrupted sutures placed between the antimesenteric surface of the descending colon and the left ventrolateral abdominal wall	Sutures pass through the colonic submucosa

12.8 Recommendations and considerations for surgical procedures used in the treatment of intestinal emergencies. (1.5 metric = 4/0 USP; 2 metric = 3/0 USP; 3 metric = 2/0 USP)

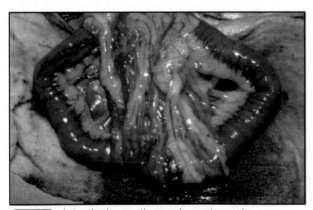

12.9 Intestinal resection and anastomosis completed. The anastomosis site has been wrapped in omentum.

Clinically, animals with strangulation exhibit severe abdominal pain, shock, unexpectedly severe systemic signs or poor response to stabilization. Treatment of intestinal incarceration includes stabilization of the animal and correction of the intestinal displacement and the initiating cause, with or without intestinal resection (Figure 12.8). Surgery should not be delayed if strangulation or necrosis is suspected. The prognosis for intestinal incarceration depends on the degree of vascular compromise and the resulting systemic inflammatory response. If extensive areas of the bowel are affected and the host immune response has been triggered, the prognosis is guarded to poor. If there is minimal vascular compromise and the animal's cardiovascular parameters are stable, the prognosis is good.

Linear foreign bodies

Linear foreign bodies (thread, nylon stocking, rope, string, carpet, etc.) produce a unique form of intestinal obstruction. The foreign body typically anchors itself around the base of the tongue or at the pylorus. Peristaltic waves carry the remainder of the foreign body aborally, and the intestines progressively gather into accordion-like pleats along the object. As peristalsis continues, the object becomes taut and embedded into the mesenteric side of the intestinal lumen. Untreated, the intestine becomes devitalized, eventually developing multiple full thickness perforations of its mesenteric border.

Linear foreign bodies are reported more frequently in cats than dogs. Vomiting, anorexia and depression are the most common clinical signs for both species. Bowel obstruction caused by linear foreign bodies tends to be incomplete, and vomiting may not be as severe or frequent as that seen with complete obstruction. Diagnosis may be delayed because of the non-specific nature of the clinical signs.

The linear foreign body is attached around the base of the tongue in as many as 50% of affected cats, though it may be difficult to see once it becomes embedded in the soft tissues. Linear foreign bodies are rarely discovered under the tongues of dogs during physical examination. On plain abdominal radiographs, the small bowel appears plicated, and is gathered in the cranial to mid-ventral abdomen instead of being dispersed uniformly throughout. Gas collects in small, eccentrically-located intraluminal bubbles instead of normal curvilinear columns. After contrast medium administration, pleating becomes more obvious, and the foreign body may appear radiolucent. After barium passes into the colon, the foreign body may retain the barium and become more apparent.

Cats that are clinically stable, have no evidence of peritonitis, and present soon after ingestion of lingually-anchored foreign bodies have been successfully managed without surgery. After being freed from around the tongue, the string may pass through the gastrointestinal tract in several days. Conservative management is not described in the dog; most linear foreign bodies in this species are lodged in the pylorus and, since 40% of such dogs have peritonitis at the time of surgery, immediate surgical intervention is recommended.

Delay in surgical removal may result in serious morbidity because of development of perforations, peritonitis and sepsis; therefore, surgical removal of string foreign bodies is considered the safest treatment for most animals. At laparotomy, the foreign body is typically removed through multiple enterotomies (see Figure 12.8). An enterotomy incision is made midway along the site of the obstruction and the string is located and grasped. The anchored portion under the tongue or in the pylorus can then be cut without losing control of the foreign body. The foreign body is gently retracted to remove as much as possible. Removal of its entire length may however require multiple enterotomies. It is important not to pull too vigorously on the foreign body, as this may cause perforation of an already compromised intestinal wall. Perforations of the mesenteric border of the plicated bowel may not become apparent until the tension on the string is released and the plications relax. Even then, this area of the bowel can be difficult to evaluate due to the presence of mesenteric fat. Large sections of the intestine may have multiple mesenteric perforations, necessitating resection.

A single enterotomy catheter technique has been described in cats. A 1 cm incision is made in the antimesenteric border of the proximal duodenum. The foreign body is grasped through this incision, cut at its anchor point, and then tied to a segment of rubber or silicone catheter or tubing. The catheter is inserted distally into the intestines with the attached string, and the enterotomy is closed. The catheter is then milked aborally through the intestines and out to the anal orifice, carrying the foreign body with it. Because linear foreign bodies in dogs tend to be wider in diameter (e.g. fabric, carpet, plastic, tights), it is unlikely that this technique would be useful in this species.

Prognosis following uncomplicated linear foreign body removal in cats is good. Intestinal perforations, which are uncommon in cats, are more likely to be associated with death after surgery. The prognosis for dogs is more guarded. The probability of peritonitis and death is nearly double that reported in cats.

Intussusception

Intussusception is the invagination of one portion of the gastrointestinal tract into the lumen of an adjoining segment. Affected animals are often less than 1 year of age. The condition may be associated with enteritis secondary to parasites, viruses, linear foreign bodies, intestinal masses or previous abdominal surgery; in older animals, it is often associated with neoplasia.

Clinical signs are those of bowel obstruction, including vomiting, diarrhoea, depression and anorexia. Clinical signs vary with the level and completeness of the obstruction. Animals with duodenojejunal or proximal jejunal intussusception often have frequent vomiting. Animals with ileocolic intussusception vomit less frequently and may have a more chronic history of tenesmus and haematochezia.

In affected dogs, a cylindrical mass in the cranial to mid-abdomen is often palpable. On plain radiographs, a mass effect or accumulation of gas proximal to the intussusception may be noted. Intussusception can be differentiated from other causes of intestinal obstruction with contrast studies or ultrasonography. On ultrasonography, an intussusception appears as a series of concentric rings in the transverse image or parallel lines in a longitudinal image, reflecting the folded layers of the intestinal wall.

Surgical reduction or resection is usually required to correct intussusceptions. During surgery, the entire gastrointestinal tract is carefully examined, since multiple intussusceptions can occur simultaneously. Manual reduction can be attempted if the visible enteric vessels are patent and the bowel wall does not look ischaemic. Resection and anastomosis (see Figure 12.8) are required when the lesion cannot be reduced, the involved bowel is necrotic or underlying neoplasia is suspected.

After surgery, animals should be tested and treated for endoparasites and any underlying predisposing conditions (e.g. viral enteritis). Prognosis for animals that have received appropriate supportive care and have undergone uncomplicated reduction or resection of a small intestinal intussusception is good. Recurrence rates range from 6–27%. Recurrences are usually noted within 3 days but have been reported up to 3 weeks after surgery. When the cause of the intussusception is not definitively addressed at surgery (i.e. neoplasia or foreign body) enteroplication (see Figure 12.8) can decrease this recurrence rate. When used in cases of ongoing enteritis (viral, parasitic, etc.), complete plication of the jejunum and ileum is recommended because intussusception tends to recur at sites away from the initial lesion or proximal to areas of limited enteroplication. Plication of the duodenum is not necessary since intussusception in this area is rare.

Mesenteric volvulus

Mesenteric volvulus is a rare and usually fatal condition in which the bowel twists on its mesenteric axis, resulting in strangulating mechanical obstruction of the small intestines and compression of the cranial mesenteric artery and its branches. With a mesenteric volvulus, the thin-walled veins and lymphatics become obstructed first, resulting in oedema formation and vascular engorgement of the bowel wall. Eventually, the cranial mesenteric artery and its branches are obstructed, leading to ischaemic necrosis of the distal duodenum, jejunum, ileum, caecum, ascending colon and proximal descending colon.

The cause of mesenteric volvulus is unknown, although it has been reported in association with other diseases, including lymphocytic–plasmacytic enteritis, ileocolic carcinoma, gastrointestinal foreign bodies, recent gastrointestinal surgery, blunt abdominal trauma, GDV and exocrine pancreatic insufficiency. The disease tends to occur in young adult, male, large-breed dogs. German Shepherd Dogs and possibly English Pointers may be predisposed. It has also been reported in a cat.

Clinical signs are peracute to acute, with rapidly progressive abdominal distension and haematochezia reported most frequently. Vomiting secondary to obstruction and pain has also been reported in some animals. Diagnosis can be challenging because the clinical signs are non-specific and the condition is rapidly progressive. In general, if an animal presents in shock with gaseous abdominal distension that is not relieved by appropriate placement of an orogastric tube, mesenteric volvulus should be suspected and surgery, if it is to be performed, should not be delayed by diagnostic tests.

Abdominal radiographs may initially be unremarkable. With progression of the disease, gaseous distension of the entire intestinal tract is noted. The stomach and descending colon are usually not dilated. The uniform and extensive nature of the small intestine distension and normal position of the stomach help differentiate this condition from a simple mechanical obstruction of the small bowel or GDV. Unfortunately, once the diagnosis becomes clear on radiographs, most of the intestinal tract is ischaemic and necrotic, and the animals are destined to die or be euthanased. De-rotation and re-oxygenation of the bowel may actually increase the severity of the systemic response through reperfusion injury.

Unless recognition and treatment of the condition are immediate or the volvulus is only partial, prognosis for recovery is grave. The vast majority of dogs succumb to the cascade of vascular obstruction, intestinal ischaemia, and circulatory, endotoxic and cardiogenic shock (Figure 12.10).

Trauma

Penetrating abdominal injury may cause direct perforation of the bowel. Blunt trauma may result in acute intestinal tears or in ischaemic necrosis and eventual perforation secondary to vascular compromise. Both types of trauma may lead to development of septic peritonitis; however, in cases of blunt trauma, the diagnosis is often delayed for several days.

Volvulus	Surgical intervention	Prognosis
Gastric	• De-rotation of the stomach • Resection of non-viable stomach • Splenectomy if necessary • Gastropexy	Good
Splenic	• Splenectomy • The twisted organ pedicle should not be untwisted prior to resection • Prophylactic gastropexy in the stable patient	Good
Liver lobe	• Liver lobectomy • The twisted organ pedicle should not be untwisted prior to resection	Good
Mesenteric	• Intraoperative euthanasia is usually indicated due to extensive bowel necrosis • De-rotation in the rare case that the bowel is not completely necrotic	Grave
Caecocolic	• Replacement of the bowel into its normal location • Resection of non-viable tissue • Colopexy	Guarded

12.10 Types of abdominal organ volvulus necessitating emergency surgical intervention.

Clinical signs may include abdominal pain, vomiting, bloody stools, lethargy, anorexia or shock. Clinical findings and results of blood tests are not good predictors of intraperitoneal injury. Blunt probing of the wound can also be inaccurate. On abdominal radiographs, animals with a penetrating gastrointestinal wound may have free gas within the abdominal cavity if the omentum did not seal the leak. Analysis of fluid obtained by abdominal paracentesis and/or lavage is important for early recognition of intra-abdominal injury. If an adequate amount of fluid cannot be obtained by paracentesis, peritoneal lavage should be performed. Exploratory laparotomy is indicated if bacteria or vegetative matter are seen on cytology, or if neutrophils are degenerate and significantly increased in number. If results of abdominal fluid cytology are normal but intestinal damage is still a concern, radiographs and peritoneal lavage can be repeated at a later time, or an exploratory laparotomy can be performed.

The surgical management of small bowel perforations depends on the size, location and number of perforations, as well as the vascular supply to the involved bowel segment(s). Small defects in an otherwise healthy segment of bowel may be amenable to debridement and primary closure (see Figure 12.8). Large defects or those involving non-viable bowel segments require intestinal resection and anastomosis. The prognosis for traumatic intestinal wounds depends largely on the duration and extent of damage.

Large intestine

Intussusception

Severe colonic obstruction can occur secondary to intussusception. On plain radiographs, a mass effect or accumulation of gas proximal to the intussusception may be noted. Confirmation of the diagnosis through a contrast study is most quickly attained via a barium enema. Surgical treatment involves reducing the intussusception. In situations where this is not possible, the affected area of bowel is resected and the ends anastomosed (see Figure 12.9). This often involves resection of the ileum and anastomosing a jejunal segment of bowel to a colonic segment of bowel (Figure 12.11).

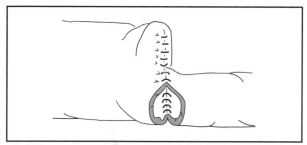

12.11 Diagrammatic representation of anastomosis of the small intestine to the large intestine. The large intestine has been oversewn so that its lumen approximates the size of the small intestine. The front is still to be sutured.

Caecocolic volvulus

Caecocolic volvulus has been reported infrequently in both dogs and cats. Clinical signs include vomiting, tenesmus, diarrhoea and shock. Radiographs reveal severely dilated loops of bowel in the caudal abdomen. Surgery involves replacement of the bowel into its normal location and resection of non-viable tissue. Colopexy (see Figure 12.8) may prevent recurrence. The prognosis for this condition is guarded, as at least 50% of the animals reported with this condition died in spite of intensive treatment (see Figure 12.10).

Perforation

Perforation of the colon is a true emergency because of the high colonic bacterial content. Untreated, colonic perforations are rapidly fatal. Perforation occurs secondary to penetrating trauma, rupture of colonic neoplasms or, rarely, from foreign bodies. Leakage may also be seen at biopsy sites following surgical biopsy of the colon. Due to the high colonic bacterial load and poor healing of the colon, surgical full-thickness colon biopsy should only be undertaken if considered to be absolutely essential. Perforation has also been associated with corticosteroid administration in animals with intervertebral disc prolapse.

The diagnosis is initially one of peritonitis, based on the clinical signs of shock, abdominal distension and pain, and a peritoneal tap or lavage showing severe peritonitis, with degenerate neutrophils and intracellular bacteria. Emergency fluid resuscitation, antibiotics and laparotomy are indicated. At surgery, the affected area of colon is packed off and either debrided and sutured or resected. Treatment for peritonitis is discussed later in this chapter.

Pancreas

Emergency surgery of the pancreas is usually limited to abscess drainage or removal. Abscesses are diagnosed by ultrasonographic evaluation of the pancreas. They appear as large, hypoechoic areas within the inflamed pancreas. Aspiration of pus from a cavity within the pancreas is an indication for surgical exploration. The surgeon should be thoroughly familiar with the anatomy of the pancreas, its blood supply and the pancreatic and common bile ducts, to avoid damaging vessels supplying the duodenum and stomach, the pancreatic papillae or the common bile duct. If the abscess is thick-walled and well delineated, it may be treated by closed-suction drainage. A balloon catheter (such as a Foley) is placed through the body wall and into the abscess cavity. The abscess cavity is thoroughly drained and flushed repeatedly at surgery. The abscess is then drained for 5–10 days postoperatively. Alternatively, the affected area of the pancreas is opened, debrided and flushed. Omentum is then packed into the cavity. The surgeon should strongly consider placing a jejunostomy tube to allow for postoperative enteral nutrition. This measure is controversial in human medicine and controlled clinical trials of its use in veterinary medicine are lacking. However, one of the authors has had some success with its clinical use. The abdomen is generously lavaged with warm, balanced electrolyte solution. Open peritoneal drainage is considered in cases with severe peritonitis associated with pancreatitis (see Peritonitis, below).

Biliary surgery

True surgical emergencies of the biliary tract are usually associated with leakage of bile, which can occur secondary to trauma, cholelithiasis, necrotizing cholecystitis or gall bladder infarction. Penetrating trauma (gunshot, arrow or stab wounds) can damage any part of the biliary system and cause leakage from hepatic ducts, the common bile duct or the gall bladder. Choleliths generally cause biliary obstruction, but can occasionally perforate the common bile duct. Gall bladder infarction has been seen in dogs with increasing frequency at our clinic in recent years. The gall bladder undergoes transmural coagulative necrosis with minimal associated inflammation. In some cases, thrombi are found in vessels supplying the gall bladder. This condition has been associated with underlying diseases including hypothyroidism and hyperadrenocorticism, and has been seen in conjunction with biliary mucoceles and occasionally choleliths.

Clinical signs are variable and depend somewhat on the underlying cause of the disease. In cases of biliary leakage secondary to trauma, the clinical signs may reflect bile peritonitis or may be associated with other injuries, such as severe haemorrhage or bowel perforation, caused by the inciting trauma. Animals with cholelithiasis and gall bladder necrosis frequently have non-specific clinical signs, including vomiting, anorexia and diarrhoea. Icterus is not a consistent clinical sign. Levels of serum liver enzymes and bilirubin are variably elevated. Plain abdominal radiographs show a loss of detail in the cranial abdomen and may reveal radio-opaque choleliths. Abdominal ultrasonography allows visualization of the liver and gall bladder, and allows the clinician to sample and subsequently analyse small amounts of peritoneal effusion. Bilirubin levels that are higher in peritoneal fluid than in the serum are an indication for exploratory laparotomy.

Stabilization of the animal with bile peritonitis is discussed in more detail in the peritonitis section. Evaluation of a preoperative coagulation screen is mandatory, as the absence of bile in the digestive tract often prevents adequate emulsification of dietary fats and the absorption of fat-soluble vitamins, including vitamin K. Vitamin K is administered by subcutaneous injection and plasma is made available if necessary to supplement blood clotting factors. At surgery, a complete exploratory laparotomy is performed. Careful evaluation of each liver lobe, the hepatic and common bile ducts and gall bladder is vital, although often made difficult by omental and visceral adhesions. Rupture of a hepatic duct is managed by ligating the duct; collateral drainage of bile from the affected liver lobe will develop. Choleliths that have perforated the common bile duct are removed. Often, the opening in the common bile duct must be enlarged to facilitate removal. The duct is then sutured closed with fine (0.7–1 metric; 5/0 or 6/0 USP) synthetic absorbable suture material over a stent placed through the major duodenal papilla up the common bile duct. If suturing the duct is not possible or results in duct stenosis, the common bile duct is ligated proximal to the leaking area and a cholecystoduodenostomy or -jejunostomy is performed. In cases of necrotizing cholecystitis, the duodenum is opened and the common bile duct is catheterized and flushed to ensure patency of the biliary tree. The gall bladder is then dissected free of the right medial and quadrate liver lobes, the cystic duct and artery are ligated using transfixation sutures, and the gall bladder is removed.

Peritonitis

The peritoneum is a serous membrane lining the abdominal cavity and reflected around the abdominal organs. In the normal animal, a small amount of fluid separates the parietal and visceral peritoneal layers and decreases friction between the abdominal contents. Fluid (or contamination) disperses rapidly throughout the peritoneal cavity. Fluid in the peritoneal space drains via diaphragmatic lymphatics to sternal and mediastinal lymph nodes and the thoracic duct.

Peritonitis is defined as any inflammatory process involving the peritoneum. In most cases, peritonitis occurs as a sequela of another disease process, and can be aseptic or septic. Aseptic peritonitis may be secondary to foreign bodies (surgical sponges), ruptured neoplasms, chemical agents such as pancreatic enzymes, bile or urine (although these can contain bacteria) or stomach or proximal duodenal contents, in which bacterial concentrations are low. Primary peritonitis occurs most commonly in cats, especially those with coronavirus infection (feline infectious peritonitis – FIP).

Septic peritonitis results from bowel perforation distal to the duodenum, penetrating wounds, surgical contamination or extension of a urogenital infection (ruptured pyometra or prostatic abscess). The peritoneum is exposed to large numbers of usually Gram-negative organisms as well as chemical bowel contents. Endotoxin is liberated and produced as bacteria grow in the peritoneal exudate.

Chemical injury results in inflammation of the peritoneum. Vasodilation and increased vascular permeability initially result in loss of isotonic fluid into the peritoneal cavity. As vascular permeability increases, albumin is lost into the peritoneal space. Given the large peritoneal surface area, fluid and protein loss can be massive. Diaphragmatic lymphatics, which normally return peritoneal fluid to the systemic circulation, become overloaded and plugged with fibrin. Concurrent vomiting and diarrhoea exacerbate fluid loss. Fluid loss decreases circulating blood volume and results in decreased cardiac output and poor tissue perfusion, which in turn results in cellular hypoxia and anaerobic cellular metabolism. Cellular energy depletion causes loss of cell membrane integrity, cell death and, eventually, organ failure.

Different aetiological agents cause some variation in the pathophysiology of chemical peritonitis. For example, uroperitoneum rapidly causes a life-threatening hyperkalaemia. This should be initially treated by a slow intravenous injection of calcium gluconate (a functional antagonist of potassium) at a dose of 50 mg/kg. Although it does not lower serum potassium, it returns membrane excitability to normal for approximately 20–30 minutes. Regular insulin (0.2–0.5 IU/kg) and glucose (1–2 g/IU of insulin) can also be administered intravenously. Animals with uroperitoneum are often also severely acidotic. Sodium bicarbonate can be administered (1–2 mmol/kg i.v.) to correct acidosis (see Chapter 5). Bile, although usually sterile, can cause permeability changes in the intestinal wall, allowing transmural bacterial migration. Gastric and pancreatic secretions are more irritating than bile, and produce a rapid and severe peritonitis.

In septic peritonitis, bacteria are initially rapidly opsonized by white blood cells or absorbed by diaphragmatic lymphatics. Haemoglobin and mucus enhance the virulence of intraperitoneal organisms. Bacterial synergism, wherein the virulence of the total bacterial load is greater than the sum of the individual organisms, occurs. Bacterial destruction liberates endotoxins, exotoxins and proteases. Endotoxin and cell membrane damage both activate the arachidonic acid pathways, generating prostaglandins and leucotrienes. The complement, clotting and fibrinolytic systems are also activated. Macrophages are stimulated to release tumour necrosis factor, stimulating the release of other inflammatory cytokines. Ongoing absorption of bacteria and toxins and generation of inflammatory mediators results in sepsis or SIRS.

Systemically, the animal responds to these profound changes by attempting to maintain perfusion to the heart and brain. Hypotension stimulates the carotid baroreceptors; subsequent inhibition of vagal tone and sympathetic stimulation should increase heart rate and cause peripheral vasoconstriction. In practice, many animals with peritonitis have at least a phase of peripheral vasodilation due to SIRS. This occurs for several reasons, including decreased vasopressin levels, increased nitric oxide synthesis, opening of cellular potassium channels, and secondary to a lack of adenosine triphosphate (ATP), acidosis and increased cellular lactate concentrations. Opening of cellular potassium channels allows potassium to escape from the smooth muscle cells of the arterial walls, hyperpolarizing them and preventing vasoconstriction.

Peritonitis may be difficult to diagnose. The clinical signs are largely non-specific. Depression and diffuse abdominal pain are often present, to a degree greater than that usually seen following abdominal surgery or trauma. Most animals splint their abdominal wall at the slightest touch. Vomiting is also a prominent sign of peritonitis. Peritoneal inflammation often causes a paralytic ileus and intestinal dilation, in addition to the effusion. In septic peritonitis, fever and leucocytosis are not consistent findings. Animals with peritonitis may have a leucocytosis with a left shift or a neutropenia. In uroperitoneum, elevations in BUN, serum creatinine and potassium are detected. Serum alkaline phosphatase, alanine aminotransferase and total bilirubin levels are usually elevated in cases of bile peritonitis. Abdominal radiographs may show free gas or a lack of intestinal detail and a ground glass appearance from free fluid in the abdominal cavity. Recovery and examination of peritoneal exudate is extremely valuable in the diagnosis of peritonitis. Abdominocentesis is performed with ultrasound guidance, and if this does not yield fluid, peritoneal lavage should be considered. Degenerate neutrophils with intracellular bacteria indicate septic peritonitis. Creatinine, potassium and bilirubin levels may also be measured on the peritoneal exudate.

A low peritoneal fluid glucose concentration (≤ 2.8 mmol/l) and a high peritoneal lactate concentration (>5.5 mmol/l) have been reported to be specific indicators of septic peritonitis in veterinary patients; however, sensitivity with this test was low, resulting in a large number of false-positives. In a more recent study, peripheral blood and peritoneal fluid glucose and lactate concentrations were compared. Peritoneal fluid glucose concentrations that were 1.1 mmol/l lower than those in the serum, and peritoneal lactate concentrations 2 mmol/l higher than those in the peripheral blood, were 100% sensitive and specific for a diagnosis of peritonitis in dogs.

Aggressive patient stabilization is required prior to anaesthesia and surgery. Intravenous fluids are administered at shock doses. Capillary refill time, heart rate, arterial blood pressure, urine output and central venous pressure are monitored to assess the response to therapy. Plasma or synthetic colloids (e.g. hydroxyethyl starch, dextran) are often required because of the massive loss of albumin into the peritoneal cavity. The choice of fluid type and electrolyte supplementation is based on the results of sequential electrolyte and blood gas measurements.

Broad-spectrum, bactericidal antibiotics are administered intravenously as soon as the diagnosis of peritonitis is made. Antibiotics effective against Gram-positive and -negative, aerobic and anaerobic bacteria are recommended. A combination of a penicillin or first-generation cephalosporin with an aminoglycoside or fluoroquinolone antibiotic is usually effective. Cefazolin (20 mg/kg i.v. q6h) should be used in preference to cephalothin, which does not reach adequate tissue levels in dogs. In animals without renal disease, amikacin should be administered once daily at 15 mg/kg i.v., as the single high dose is more effective and less nephrotoxic than multiple smaller doses. Metronidazole (10 mg/kg orally or i.v. q8h) may be added for additional anaerobic coverage. Penicillins, cephalosporins and aminoglycosides all reach intraperitoneal levels equivalent to their serum levels.

High-dose corticosteroid administration in septic shock has largely been abandoned after human clinical trails showed that corticosteroids were associated with a higher mortality. However, there is emerging evidence that a subset of patients with peritonitis and sepsis have poor adrenal function, and these patients may benefit from physiological doses of glucocorticoids and mineralocorticoids. NSAIDs are also controversial in the treatment of septic shock. In experimental septic shock models demonstrating therapeutic benefit, the NSAID (aspirin, indomethacin, phenylbutazone, flunixin meglumine) had to be administered prior to the onset of shock. Potential side effects of NSAIDs include gastrointestinal haemorrhage (especially if administered in conjunction with corticosteroids), nephrotoxicosis and blood dyscrasias. Potential benefits include improved cardiac index, increased blood pressure, decreased microvascular damage and permeability and improved survival.

One of the most important aspects of treating peritonitis is prompt removal of the inciting cause. While the animal should be stabilized before anaesthesia and surgery, the underlying source must be addressed to resolve the peritonitis. Exploratory laparotomy is mandatory to treat the source of the peritonitis, remove peritoneal contamination and exudate, and provide a route for enteral nutrition. A large ventral midline incision is used for exposure. A complete exploratory laparotomy is performed. The source of the peritonitis is identified and isolated from the remainder of the abdomen using moistened laparotomy sponges. In animals with generalized peritoneal contamination, the authors prefer to lavage the peritoneal cavity with a large volume of warm sterile saline before proceeding with definitive treatment. The fluid is immediately aspirated from the peritoneal cavity.

Definitive treatment of peritonitis often involves resection and anastomosis of damaged bowel. Omental wrapping or serosal patching is recommended to reinforce anastomoses in the face of peritonitis. Serosal patching is a technique in which loops of healthy bowel are loosely sutured to the bowel adjacent to the anastomosis (Figure 12.12). The serosal surfaces of the healthy bowel are then in contact with the anastomosis site allowing a reinforcing fibrin seal to form.

Few animals with peritonitis will eat voluntarily, and many vomit during the postoperative period, so mechanisms for nutritional support should be considered during surgery. Placement of a gastrostomy or jejunostomy tube should be considered unless it interferes with repair of the leaking intestine.

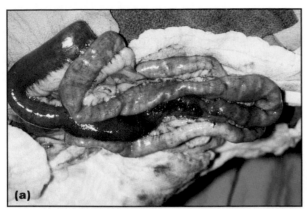

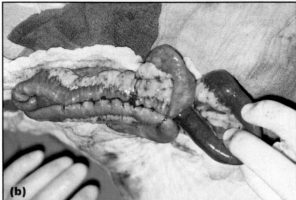

12.12 Serosal patching. **(a)** Two healthy loops of small intestine are brought alongside the loop of bowel to be patched. Sutures are placed between the mesenteric sides of the normal and affected intestine loops. **(b)** The antimesenteric surfaces of the two healthy loops of intestine are apposed with single interrupted sutures, covering the affected area with bowel. Please note: this procedure should only be performed to reinforce healthy bowel. Patching does not remove the need for accurate assessment of bowel viability and resection of unhealthy bowel.

The peritoneal cavity should be thoroughly lavaged with a large volume of warm, sterile, balanced electrolyte solution to remove bacteria and debris. The volume of fluid required varies from 500 ml in a cat to several litres in a large dog. All lavage fluid must be aspirated. Lavage with inadequate aspiration merely spreads bacteria throughout the peritoneal cavity, and sequesters them from phagocytosis.

The addition of antiseptics to the lavage fluid has been controversial, and is currently not recommended. Several human studies have concluded that there is no benefit to adding povidone–iodine to lavage fluid. Experimental studies have shown that 2 ml/kg of povidone–iodine (10% solution, 1% available iodine) instilled into the peritoneal cavity of dogs with peritonitis is lethal. Intraperitoneal povidone–iodine also decreases the neutrophil percentage and increases bacterial numbers in the peritoneal cavity in rats with experimental peritonitis. The addition of antibiotics to peritoneal lavage fluid is also debated. Most studies indicate that this treatment is not beneficial in patients receiving appropriate parenteral antibiosis.

Contamination often remains within the peritoneal cavity even after extensive debridement and lavage. The veterinary surgeon must decide which cases require postoperative peritoneal drainage. Local peritoneal drainage is important when the inflammation is confined to a specific area of the peritoneal cavity. Drainage tubes, with or without suction, can be used in such cases; examples include prostatic and pancreatic abscesses. Ideally, drain exit points should be covered with a sterile dressing. Drainage tubes were, until recently, considered ineffective for draining the entire peritoneal cavity, as they were thought to be rapidly sealed by fibrin and omentum. The presence of drains, which are effectively foreign bodies, resulted in increased bacterial translocation and histological inflammation in an experimental peritonitis model. In spite of this, draining the peritoneal cavity with closed suction drains has been described in clinical cases of peritonitis in dogs and cats, with similar results to open drainage. Drains are placed in the cranial, and sometimes caudal, abdomen (Figure 12.13).

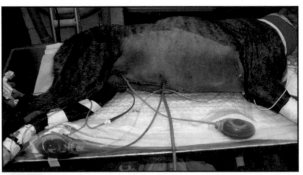

12.13 Two closed suction drains, one placed in the cranial abdomen and one placed in the caudal abdomen, used to drain the peritoneal cavity after surgery for septic peritonitis.

Open peritoneal drainage is accomplished by incompletely closing the abdominal incision. The falciform ligament is removed, and the linea is sutured with a continuous monofilament suture leaving a gap of 2–4 cm between the wound edges (Figure 12.14). The wound is bandaged using a sterile dressing of gauze impregnated with petroleum jelly, covered by sterile towels. This primary dressing is covered with a layer of

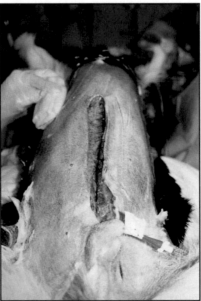

12.14

Open peritoneal drainage. The linea alba is sutured approximately 3 cm apart with non-absorbable material. This open incision is then covered with a sterile bandage that will require changing every 6–12 hours.

thick, absorbent material, a layer of conforming, stretchable gauze bandage, then adhesive tape. The dressing usually requires changing every 6 hours initially, as fluid from the peritoneum soaks through. Bandage changes are performed under sterile conditions with the animal sedated. Fibrous adhesions, which may entrap peritoneal exudate, are gently freed. There are no exact criteria to help the clinician judge either which cases of peritonitis require open abdominal drainage, or when to close the open incision. In general, the incision is closed when drainage has decreased and the peritoneum appears grossly healthy at bandage changes. This generally occurs 3–5 days after the initial surgery. Closure should be performed as a complete laparotomy, and the peritoneal cavity examined for any evidence of residual infection.

Haemoperitoneum

Haemoperitoneum is the abnormal accumulation of blood in the peritoneal space and is a common diagnosis in small animal emergency practice. Neoplasia and trauma are the most common causes of haemoperitoneum. Definitive diagnosis is made by retrieval of a sample of the peritoneal fluid for analysis. Abdominocentesis using 'blind' or ultrasound-guided techniques will reveal the presence of a sanguineous non-clotting peritoneal fluid. If the blood retrieved by abdominocentesis forms clots, inadvertent splenic or vascular penetration should be suspected.

Regardless of the cause of haemoperitoneum, circulatory support is often necessary. The rate and composition of intravenous fluids is tailored to each individual animal, and packed red cell or whole blood transfusions may be required. By increasing intra-abdominal pressure, abdominal bandages can be helpful for short-term stabilization to help attenuate or arrest intra-abdominal haemorrhage. Although high intra-abdominal pressures may be reached by these means, it is unlikely that arterial haemorrhage will be stopped using an abdominal bandage. Increasing intra-abdominal pressure for prolonged periods of time can have serious consequences for liver, renal and other abdominal organ blood flow; the long-term use of tight abdominal bandages is, therefore, not recommended. Surgical therapy is aimed at resection or control of the bleeding focus, removal of any devitalized tissue and biopsy of additional sites of suspicion.

Neoplastic haemoperitoneum

Neoplasia is the most common cause of non-traumatic haemoperitoneum and is common in dogs with splenic malignancy. It has also been reported in association with primary and metastatic hepatic, renal and adrenal malignancies. The majority of splenic malignancies metastasize to the liver and, occasionally, to the lungs. Haemangiosarcoma, in particular, can be identified at multiple sites within the body (spleen, liver, lungs and right atrial appendage). A systematic abdominal ultrasound examination, which can be helpful despite peritoneal fluid, should aid in the diagnosis. Thoracic radiographs should also be made in left and right lateral and dorsal recumbency to assess for gross

metastatic disease. If further information about the heart is needed, echocardiography should be performed. Ultrasonographic visualization of the right atrial appendage, however, may be very difficult in the absence of a pericardial effusion. Failure to identify areas of suspicion on radiographs or ultrasonography does not rule out metastatic disease. With this in mind, surgery is often approached as an excisional biopsy procedure that may also return cardiovascular stability. However, surgical exploration could uncover findings (e.g. multiple haemorrhaging hepatic masses) that will make proceeding further with surgery an untenable option (Figure 12.15).

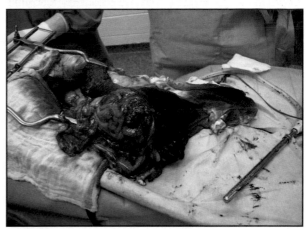

12.15 Haemorrhagic splenic mass responsible for haemoperitoneum. Note the presence of multiple masses in the omentum, suggesting local metastatic disease.

Resection of the affected organ or organ part should be carried out as efficiently as possible once the location of the haemorrhage has been identified. In the case of a splenic mass, complete splenectomy is usually the quickest and safest choice even if the disease is limited to just one pole. If the haemorrhagic focus is confined to one or two liver lobes, partial hepatectomy can be considered. Unilateral nephrectomy may be needed if a lesion is present in only one kidney. This procedure is well tolerated in dogs and cats when the remaining kidney has normal function. Although definitive information regarding relative renal function is usually not known for patients undergoing urgent surgery for haemoperitoneum, normal function may be implied if only one kidney contains tumour and the other is grossly normal, and if urine specific gravity, serum creatinine and BUN were all normal preoperatively. If the haemorrhagic focus is in another abdominal organ, resection should be carried out if it is feasible. If multiple liver lobes contain bleeding foci, if both kidneys are actively haemorrhaging or if multiple other sites are bleeding, surgical therapy may be impossible and intraoperative euthanasia is the only reasonable option. If metastatic disease is present throughout the peritoneal cavity, but only one site is actively bleeding, the veterinarian and clients have to choose between securing a diagnosis, in the hope that medical treatment will be possible, and intraoperative euthanasia. The long-term prognosis for these patients depends upon the tumour type and its biological behaviour.

Splenic and liver lobe torsion

Splenic and liver lobe torsion are rare conditions associated with haemorrhagic peritoneal effusion. Clinical features of both diseases are inconsistent and non-specific. Splenic torsion is often suspected on the basis of abdominal radiographs and may be further suspected or confirmed by abdominal ultrasound examination. Liver lobe torsion may be a difficult diagnosis to make without exploratory laparotomy. Treatment for both conditions is resection. The twisted organ pedicle should not be untwisted prior to resection (see Figure 12.10). There are reports of GDV occurring in dogs with prior splenic torsions, so if the animal is stable, a prophylactic gastropexy may be indicated following removal of the spleen. The prognosis for surgical treatment of these conditions is generally good.

Trauma

Both blunt and penetrating abdominal trauma can result in intra-abdominal haemorrhage. Usually, the most rapid haemorrhage to follow accidental trauma comes from a laceration or rupture of a major vessel or parenchymatous organ (liver, spleen or kidney). Bleeding from these structures can be rapidly fatal. Other traumatic lesions that cause haemoperitoneum may have less damaging haemodynamic effects but can be equally life threatening if left undiagnosed. Such conditions include rupture of the urinary bladder, ureteric rupture or avulsion, urethral rupture, gall bladder rupture and intestinal mesenteric avulsion. Despite all these possibilities, traumatic haemoperitoneum is often minor, self-limiting and of no long-term significance.

Postoperative management and monitoring

Diligent postoperative care and monitoring are essential for successful treatment of gastrointestinal emergency cases. The goal of postoperative management is to maintain adequate tissue perfusion, and to anticipate and monitor for potentially life-threatening complications. Although the conditions discussed in this chapter are diverse and cases will vary in severity, postoperative complications following laparotomy may include hypovolaemia due to haemorrhage or fluid losses from the intravascular space, respiratory dysfunction (e.g. aspiration pneumonia, acute respiratory distress syndrome), cardiac dysrhythmias (especially in dogs with GDV), renal failure and sepsis. Frequent clinical, electronic and laboratory monitoring is vital in critical cases to evaluate cardiac function, perfusion, pulmonary gas exchange and renal function. The reader is referred elsewhere in the Manual for a more detailed discussion of these methods of monitoring.

Further reading

Anderson SA, Lippincott CL and Gill PJ (1992) Single enterotomy removal of gastrointestinal linear foreign bodies. *Journal of the American Animal Hospital Association* **28**, 487–490

Basher AW and Fowler JD (1987) Conservative versus surgical management of gastrointestinal linear foreign bodies in the cat. *Veterinary Surgery* **16**, 135–138

Bellah JR (1983) Colonic perforation after corticosteroid and surgical treatment of intervertebral disk disease in a dog. *Journal of the American Veterinary Medical Association* **183**, 1002–1003

Bentley AM, O'Toole TE, Kowaleski MP, Casale SA and McCarthy RJ (2005) Volvulus of the colon in four dogs. *Journal of the American Veterinary Medical Association* **227**, 253–256

Bonczynski JJ, Ludwig LL, Barton LJ, Loar A and Peterson ME (2003) Comparison of peritoneal fluid and peripheral blood pH, bicarbonate, glucose, and lactate concentration as a diagnostic tool for septic peritonitis in dogs and cats. *Veterinary Surgery* **32(2)**, 161–166

Brockman DJ, Mongil CM, Aronson LR and Brown DC (2000) A practical approach to hemoperitoneum in the dog and cat. *Veterinary Clinics of North America: Small Animal Practice* **30**, 657–668

Cairo J, Font J, Gorraiz J, Martin N and Pons C (1999) Intestinal volvulus in dogs: a study of four clinical cases. *Journal of Small Animal Practice* **40**, 136–140

Carberry CA and Flanders JA (1993) Cecal-colic volvulus in two dogs. *Veterinary Surgery* **22**, 225–228

Conzemius MG, Sammarco JL, Holt DE and Smith GK (1995) Clinical determination of preoperative and postoperative intra-abdominal pressures in dogs. *Veterinary Surgery* **24**, 195–201

Crawshaw J, Berg J, Sardinas JC *et al.* (1998) Prognosis for dogs with nonlymphomatous, small intestinal tumors treated by surgical excision. *Journal of the American Animal Hospital Association* **34**, 451–456

Downs MO, Miller MA, Cross AR *et al.* (1998) Liver lobe torsion and liver abscess in a dog. *Journal of the American Veterinary Medical Association* **212**, 678–680

Evans K, Hosgood G, Boon GD and Kowalewich N (1991) Hemoperitoneum secondary to traumatic rupture of an adrenal tumor in a dog. *Journal of the American Veterinary Medical Association* **198**, 278–280

Evans KL, Smeak DD and Biller DS (1994) Gastrointestinal linear foreign bodies in 32 dogs: a retrospective evaluation and feline comparison. *Journal of the American Animal Hospital Association* **30**, 445–450

Farrow CS (1997) The obstructive bowel pattern: an inconsistent radiographic sign of obstruction. *Canadian Veterinary Journal* **38**, 309–310

Feeney DA, Klausner JS and Johnston GR (1982) Chronic bowel obstruction caused by primary intestinal neoplasia: a report of five cases. *Journal of the American Animal Hospital Association* **18**, 67–77

Felts JF, Fox PR and Burk RL (1984) Thread and sewing needles as gastrointestinal foreign bodies in the cat: a review of 64 cases. *Journal of the American Veterinary Medical Association* **184**, 56–59

Gaskell CJ, Pass MA and Biery DN (1973) Intestinal obstruction in a dog due to incarceration of small intestine in a coccygeal fracture. *Journal of Small Animal Practice* **14**, 101–105

Graham JP, Lord PF and Harrison JM (1998) Quantitative estimation of intestinal dilation as a predictor of obstruction in the dog. *Journal of Small Animal Practice* **39**, 521–524

Harvey HJ and Rendano VT Jr (1984) Small bowel volvulus in dogs: clinical observations. *Veterinary Surgery* **12**, 91–94

Hassinger KA (1997) Intestinal entrapment and strangulation caused by rupture of the duodenocolic ligament in four dogs. *Veterinary Surgery* **26**, 275–280

Holt DE, Mehler, S. Mayhew PD and Hendrick MJ (2004) Canine gall bladder infarction: 12 cases (1993–2003). *Veterinary Pathology*, **41**, 216–218

Hosgood G, Bunge M and Dorfman M (1992) Jejunal incarceration by an omental tear in a dog. *Journal of the American Veterinary Medical Association* **200**, 947–950

Huber E (1994) Caecal and colonic volvulus in a dog. (French) *Schweizer Archiv fur Tierheilkunde* **136**, 352–354

Kantrowitz B and Biller D (1992) Using radiography to evaluate vomiting in dogs and cats. *Veterinary Medicine* **87**, 806–813

Kolata RJ and Johnston DE (1975) Motor vehicle accidents in urban dogs: a study of 600 cases. *Journal of the American Veterinary Medical Association* **167**, 938–941

Lamb CR and Mantis P (1998) Ultrasonographic features of intestinal intussusception in 10 dogs. *Journal of Small Animal Practice* **39**, 437–441

Levitt L and Bauer MS (1992) Intussusception in dogs and cats: a review of thirty-six cases. *Canadian Veterinary Journal* **33**, 660–664

Lewis DD and Ellison GW (1987) Intussusception in dogs and cats. *Compendium on Continuing Education for the Practicing Veterinarian* **9**, 523–535

Manczur F, Voros K, Vrabely T *et al.* (1998) Sonographic diagnosis of intestinal obstruction in the dog. *Acta Veterinaria Hungarica* **46**, 35–45

Matushek KJ and Cockshutt JR (1987) Mesenteric and gastric volvulus in a dog. *Journal of the American Veterinary Medical Association* **191**, 327–328

McAnulty JF and Smith GK (1986) Circumferential external counterpressure by abdominal wrapping and its effect on simulated intra-abdominal hemorrhage. *Veterinary Surgery* **15**, 270–274

McConkey S, Briggs C, Solano M and Illanes O (1997) Liver torsion and associated bacterial peritonitis in a dog. *Canadian Veterinary Journal* **38**, 438–439

Mehler SJ, Mayhew PD, Drobatz KJ and Holt DE (2004) Risk factors associated with mortality in extrahepatic biliary tract surgery in dogs: 60 cases (1988–2002). *Veterinary Surgery* **33**, 644–649

Millis DL, Nemzek J, Riggs C and Walshaw R (1995) Gastric dilatation-volvulus after splenic torsion in two dogs. *Journal of the American Veterinary Medical Association* **207**, 314–315

Mongil CM, Drobatz KJ and Hendricks JC (1995) Traumatic hemoperitoneum in 28 cases: a retrospective review. *Journal of the American Animal Hospital Association* **31**, 217–222

Mueller MG, Ludwig LL and Barton LJ (2001) Use of closed-suction drains to treat generalized peritonitis in dogs and cats: 40 cases (1997–1999). *Journal of the American Veterinary Medical Association* **219(6)**, 789–794

Neath PJ, Brockman DJ and Saunders HM (1997) Retrospective analysis of 19 cases of isolated torsion of the splenic pedicle in dogs. *Journal of Small Animal Practice* **38**, 387–392

Nemzek JA, Walshaw R and Hauptman JG (1993) Mesenteric volvulus in the dog: a retrospective study. *Journal of the American Animal Hospital Association* **29**, 357–362

Oakes MG, Lewis DD, Hosgood G and Beale BS (1994) Enteroplication for the prevention of intussusception recurrence in dogs: 31 cases (1978–1992). *Journal of the American Veterinary Medical Association* **205**, 72–75

Prymak C, McKee LJ, Goldschmidt MH and Glickman LT (1988) Epidemiologic, clinical, pathologic, and prognostic characteristics of splenic hemangiosarcoma and splenic hematoma in dogs: 217 cases (1985). *Journal of the American Veterinary Medical Association* **193**, 706–712

Rosenthal RE, Smith J, Walls RM *et al.* (1987) Stab wounds to the abdomen: failure of blunt probing to predict peritoneal penetration. *Annals of Emergency Medicine* **16**, 172–174

Shaiken, L (1999) The radiographic appearance of linear foreign bodies in cats. *Veterinary Medicine* **94**, 417–422

Shealy PM and Henderson RA (1992) Canine intestinal volvulus. A report of nine new cases. *Veterinary Surgery* **21**, 15–19

Sonnenfield JM, Armbrust LJ, Radlinsky MA *et al.* (2001) Radiographic and ultrasonographic findings of liver lobe torsion in a dog. *Veterinary Radiology and Ultrasound* **42**, 344–346

Spencer CP and Ackerman N (1980) Thoracic and abdominal radiography of the trauma patient. *Veterinary Clinics of North America: Small Animal Practice* **10**, 541–559

Stevenson S, Chew DJ and Kociba GJ (1981) Torsion of the splenic pedicle in the dog: a review. *Journal of the American Animal Hospital Association* **17**, 239–244

Stickle RL (1989) Radiographic signs of isolated splenic torsion in dogs: eight cases (1980–1987). *Journal of the American Veterinary Medical Association* **194**, 103–106

Swann HM and Brown DC (2001) Hepatic lobe torsion in 3 dogs and a cat. *Veterinary Surgery* **30**, 482–486

Tomlinson J and Black A (1983) Liver lobe torsion in a dog. *Journal of the American Veterinary Medical Association* **183**, 225–226

Toombs JP, Caywood DD, Lipowitz AJ and Stevens JB (1980) Colonic perforation following neurosurgical procedures and corticosteroid therapy in four dogs. *Journal of the American Veterinary Medical Association* **177**, 68–72

Vinayak A and Krahwinkel DJ (2004) Managing blunt trauma-induced hemoperitoneum in dogs and cats. *Compendium on Continuing Education for the Practicing Veterinarian.* **26**, 276–291

Westermarck E and Rimaila-Parnanen E (1989) Mesenteric torsion in dogs with exocrine pancreatic insufficiency: 21 cases (1978–1987). *Journal of the American Veterinary Medical Association* **195**, 1404–1406

Wilson GP and Burt JK (1974) Intussusception in the dog and cat: a review of 45 cases. *Journal of the American Veterinary Medical Association* **164**, 515–518

Wolfe DA (1977) Recurrent intestinal intussusceptions in the dog. *Journal of the American Veterinary Medical Association* **171**, 553–556

Wright JF and Berman E (1973) Intestinal torsion in the cat. *Feline Practice* **3**, 42–43

13

Haematological emergencies

Susan G. Hackner

Anaemia

Anaemia is defined as a decrease in the red blood cell mass, occurring due to decreased production, increased destruction (haemolysis) or loss (haemorrhage) of red blood cells. The consequences of anaemia are tissue hypoxia and, ultimately, death. Successful management depends on a systematic diagnostic approach and timely, effective intervention.

Approach in the emergency situation

Anaemic patients are usually presented for progressive weakness, which may culminate in collapse. The duration of clinical signs ranges from peracute to chronic. The patient in an anaemic crisis requires urgent intervention (Figure 13.1), with an initial goal of stabilization of life-threatening clinical signs. The primary survey of the emergency patient is an initial rapid assessment of vital organ systems to determine if a life-threatening situation exists. Pallor is the hallmark sign of anaemia, and should be differentiated from pallor associated with hypoperfusion by determination of clinical perfusion parameters and the packed cell volume (PCV). Patients in an anaemic crisis are moribund or extremely depressed, with marked

---

1. Primary survey
2. Establish vascular access
3. Collect pretreatment samples:
   - Minimum database (PCV/TP)
   - Blood smear
   - EDTA plasma (for later CBC, reticulocyte count, platelet count, blood typing, immune testing)
   - Serum (for later chemistry profile and/or serological testing)
   - In-saline agglutination test, if haemolysis suspected
   - Citrated plasma, if bleeding suspected (for later coagulation testing)
4. Initiate therapy to stabilize the patient:
   - Support of airway and/or breathing, if indicated
   - Fluid therapy to maintain adequate perfusion
   - Control of haemorrhage, if present
   - Blood transfusion, if indicated
5. Secondary survey:
   - Complete history
   - Thorough physical examination
6. Diagnostic work up (see text)
7. Specific therapy (see text)

13.1 Emergency approach to the anaemic patient.

---

pallor, tachypnoea, tachycardia and bounding pulses. If the anaemia is due to severe blood loss, signs of hypoperfusion predominate.

Venous access is achieved by placement of a large-bore peripheral catheter, ideally the largest-bore catheter possible, in case aggressive fluid therapy is warranted. In large dogs with evidence of hypoperfusion, two catheters may be required. Blood is collected from the catheter for a minimum database, including a PCV and total solids (TS) or total protein (TP) (see Chapter 1). Samples should be collected prior to initiating therapy, to determine baseline results before treatment changes the laboratory parameters. In addition to the minimum database, other samples obtained at this time should include a blood smear, an in-saline agglutination test, blood typing, and serum, EDTA and citrated plasma samples for later laboratory testing.

Following the collection of blood samples, therapy should be initiated to stabilize the patient. In severe anaemia, blood transfusion is usually required. The decision to transfuse should be based on the patient's clinical signs rather than simply on the PCV. Animals with chronic anaemia may tolerate remarkably low PCVs with few clinical signs. Conversely, patients acutely affected by moderate anaemia may be extremely decompensated if concurrent hypoperfusion or hypoxaemia exacerbate tissue hypoxia.

Selection of blood components is based on the PCV and TP (see Chapter 14). If only the PCV is low, packed red blood cells should be transfused. If both PCV and TP are decreased, whole blood transfusion is indicated. If only packed cells are available, synthetic colloid solutions can be used instead of plasma to provide colloidal support during resuscitation. All cats must be blood typed prior to transfusion to avoid potentially fatal transfusion reactions. As a general guide, whole blood is transfused at a dose of 20 ml/kg in the dog, and 10–15 ml/kg in the cat. In patients that are not in shock, the recommended transfusion rate is 5 ml/kg/h for dogs, and 3 ml/kg/h for cats. In the hypovolaemic patient, this rate can be substantially increased depending on individual needs. Slower transfusion rates (1–2 ml/kg/h) are recommended in patients with significant concurrent cardiac disease, hypertension or hyperviscosity disorders. Blood transfusion is generally sufficient for the initial stabilization of the anaemic patient, unless ongoing haemorrhage is present. All patients should be closely monitored during and following resuscitation for changes in PCV and perfusion parameters.

Following initial stabilization, the secondary survey includes a complete history and thorough physical examination. A diagnostic plan is formulated to determine the cause of the anaemia. Following PCV/TP assessment, laboratory testing should begin with blood smear examination, a complete blood count (CBC) and a reticulocyte count.

Clinical and laboratory assessment

History and physical examination
The signalment of the patient may be informative. Young animals are more likely to have congenital disease or blood loss due to parasites, whereas older animals are at greater risk of malignancies. The history should include a detailed enquiry into vaccines, medications, diet, travel and past illnesses. Vaccination and drug therapy may predispose to immune-mediated disease, marrow suppression or thrombopathia. Dietary indiscretion (onions, zinc) may result in haemolysis. Travel to certain locations might alert the clinician to the possibility of tick-borne disease or red cell parasites. Previous bleeding episodes should increase the suspicion that haemorrhage is the likely cause of the current anaemia, and the owner should be questioned regarding the presence of melaena, haematuria or epistaxis. Since many anaemic cats have viral disease, detailed questions should be asked about serological testing and exposure to other cats.

Animals with acute onset of haemolysis or bleeding will develop clinical signs at a higher PCV than animals with a gradual onset of anaemia due to decreased erythropoiesis. Physical examination should include a thorough search for any evidence of haemorrhage: evaluation of the body cavities, examination of the skin, mucous membranes and joints, as well as rectal and fundic examinations. The clinician should also actively seek evidence of neoplasia, infectious disease or immune-mediated disease (arthritis, uveitis, glomerulonephritis or cutaneous lesions). Icterus may be due to haemolysis or to hepatic or biliary disease. Splenomegaly may be due to haemolysis, neoplasia, infectious disease, torsion or extramedullary haemopoiesis. Fever may result from infectious disease, neoplasia or acute immune-mediated haemolysis.

Packed cell volume and total solids/total protein
A decreased PCV confirms anaemia. Typically, a concurrent decrease in TP suggests blood loss, whereas a normal TP suggests haemolysis or decreased red cell production. In dogs with acute blood loss (for example following trauma), the PCV may be normal or increased due to splenic contraction and because fluid shifts have not yet occurred. Thus, in dogs that have sustained trauma, a decreased TP is an important early clue to active haemorrhage. Splenic contraction does not occur in cats. The plasma should be examined for evidence of haemolysis or icterus.

Blood smear examination
Blood smear examination using a Romanowsky-type stain (e.g. Diff-Quik) is probably the single most useful tool for evaluating anaemia in the emergency setting. It permits evaluation of the regenerative response (in

dogs) and frequently indicates the cause of the anaemia (Figure 13.2). If the anaemia is judged to be non-regenerative, erythrocyte morphology may indicate the aetiology, e.g. microcytosis in animals with iron deficiency. If haemolysis is suspected, erythrocytes may show oxidative damage (Heinz bodies, eccentrocytes), evidence of immune-mediated destruction (spherocytes), physical damage (schistocytes) or parasites.

Abnormality	Interpretation
Polychromasia	Regeneration
Macrocytosis	Regeneration; dyserythropoiesis; feline leukaemia virus infection; breed-associated (Poodles)
Microcytosis	Iron deficiency; copper deficiency; portosystemic shunt; breed-associated (Akitas)
Hypochromia	Iron deficiency; copper deficiency
Nucleated red blood cells	Regeneration; lead toxicity; splenic disease; haemangiosarcoma; corticosteroid therapy; systemic stress (cats)
Spherocytosis	Immune-mediated haemolytic anaemia; other haemolytic anaemias
Schistocytosis	Microangiopathy (haemangiosarcoma; disseminated intravascular coagulation; dirofilariasis; myelofibrosis; glomerulonephritis)
Heinz bodies	Oxidative red cell injury; may be normal in cats
Eccentrocytosis	Onion toxicity
Codocytosis	Iron deficiency; hepatic disease; post-splenectomy
Parasitic inclusions	Babesiosis, haemobartonellosis, distemper inclusion bodies

13.2 Common erythrocyte abnormalities observed on blood smear examination.

It is important to realize that regeneration cannot be accurately assessed on blood smear examination in cats. Due to the different forms of reticulocytes in cats (see below), the absence of identifiable reticulocytes in this species does not exclude regeneration. Conversely, evidence of any degree of reticulocytosis on blood smear examination in a cat probably indicates an acute and profound regenerative response.

If the patient is bleeding, smear examination is vital to make an immediate assessment of platelet numbers and morphology. In addition, evaluation of leucocytes is informative with regard to white cell numbers and proportions, and may indicate the presence of a left shift, morphological/neoplastic changes or parasites. Approximately 18–51 leucocytes per X10 objective field indicates a normal total white cell count.

Complete blood count
The CBC determines absolute cell numbers and red cell parameters. Cell types are distinguished based on a size threshold. In cats, there is often considerable overlap between erythrocyte and platelet volumes, and automated cell counters cannot resolve the cells into two distinct populations, resulting in inaccuracy of automated platelet counts.

Reticulocyte count

A reticulocyte count should be performed in all anaemic patients, providing accurate quantification of the regenerative response. Reticulocyte counts are performed by vital staining that allows visualization of ribosomes. Usually, a few drops of blood are mixed with an equal volume of 0.5% new methylene blue in physiological saline; 1000 red blood cells are counted and the percentage of reticulocytes is recorded.

Counting of reticulocytes is simple in the dog, as there is essentially only one type of reticulocyte. The cat, however, has two types of reticulocytes: aggregate reticulocytes, in which the organelles are coalesced into aggregates; and punctate reticulocytes, in which the organelles are present as small particles. Aggregate forms are released from the marrow and, after approximately 12 hours, develop into punctate forms that persist in the circulation for 10–12 days. Aggregate forms therefore indicate active regeneration, whereas punctate forms indicate recent, cumulative regeneration. Since punctate forms are not recognizable on routine staining, the degree of regeneration may be underestimated in cats. If both forms are counted and not distinguished, active regeneration may be overestimated.

The degree of reticulocytosis must be interpreted relative to the degree of anaemia, by calculation of the absolute reticulocyte count (number per litre of blood) or a corrected reticulocyte count (%). In dogs, an absolute reticulocyte count $>60 \times 10^9/l$ is evidence of regeneration. In cats, $>50 \times 10^9/l$ aggregate reticulocytes is considered regenerative. The corrected reticulocyte count is calculated by the formula:

Corrected reticulocyte % =

(Observed reticulocyte count) x $\dfrac{\text{PCV of the patient}}{\text{Mean normal PCV}}$

Mean normal PCV is considered to be 45% for the dog and 37% for the cat. A corrected reticulocyte count above 1% indicates active erythropoiesis.

Saline agglutination test

Evaluation for autoagglutination is performed by mixing a drop of blood (fresh or anticoagulated with EDTA) with an equal or greater volume of saline on a glass slide. Macroagglutination can be visualized grossly. Microscopic evaluation of a fresh wet mount will allow detection of microagglutination and differentiation from rouleaux formation. Autoagglutination, if present, should persist following washing of the cells three times in saline. If agglutination is present, this provides strong evidence for immune-mediated haemolytic anaemia, however it is present in only a relatively small percentage of cases.

Diagnostic approach

The essential first step of diagnosis in the anaemic patient is to determine the mechanism of the anaemia: decreased erythropoiesis, haemolysis or haemorrhage (Figure 13.3).

Haemolysis

Antibody-mediated:
 Immune-mediated haemolytic anaemia
 Neonatal isoerythrolysis
 Transfusion reaction
Toxic:
 Zinc toxicity
 Oxidative injury (onions, paracetamol (acetaminophen), propylthiouracil, methylene blue, DL-methionine, lead, cephalosporins, fenbendazole, dapsone, gold salts, phenacetin, modified live-virus vaccine)
 Copper toxicosis
Infectious:
 Erythroparasites
  Babesiosis (*Babesia canis, B. gibsoni*)
  Haemobartonellosis (*Haemobartonella canis, Mycoplasma haemofelis*)
  Cytauxoonosis (*Cytauxoon felis*)
  Ehrlichiosis (*Ehrlichia canis*)
 Viral
  Feline leukaemia virus
  Feline immunodeficiency virus
Microangiopathic:
 Disseminated intravascular coagulation
 Splenic torsion
 Haemangiosarcoma
 Vena caval syndrome
Congenital:
 Pyruvate kinase deficiency (Basenji, Beagle, West Highland White Terrier, Abyssinian cats)
 Phosphofructokinase deficiency (English Springer Spaniel, American Cocker Spaniel)
 Congenital porphyria
 NADH methaemoglobin reductase deficiency
 Vitamin B_{12} deficiency (Giant Schnauzer)
Miscellaneous:
 Hypophosphataemia
 Snake bites

Haemorrhage

 Trauma/surgery
 Bleeding disorders
 Ectoparasites
 Gastrointestinal (endoparasites, ulceration, neoplasia)
 Neoplasia (haemangiosarcoma, others)

Decreased erythropoiesis

Extra-marrow disease:
 Anaemia of chronic disease/inflammation
 Renal failure
 Endocrine disease (hypoadrenocorticism, hypothyroidism)
 Feline leukaemia virus
Intra-marrow disease:
 Myeloaplasia
 Drug-associated (chemotherapy, oestrogen, phenylbutazone, griseofulvin, trimethoprim–sulphadiazine, thiacetarsamide, quinidine, chloramphenicol)
 Infectious (feline leukaemia virus, canine enrlichiosis, parvovirus)
 Idiopathic aplastic anaemia
 Haematopoietic malignancy
 Myelodysplasia
 Myelofibrosis
Nutritional:
 Iron deficiency
 Inadequate protein intake

13.3 Causes of anaemia.

Regenerative *versus* non-regenerative

The most important question is to determine whether the anaemia is regenerative or non-regenerative by performing a reticulocyte count or, in the emergency setting, examination of a blood smear. On a routinely stained smear, reticulocytes (the only reliable indicator of regeneration) are seen as larger, more basophilic erythrocytes, resulting in anisocytosis and polychromasia (Figure 13.4). Nucleated red blood cells are not a reliable indicator of erythroid hyperplasia, as they may be present in numerous conditions in spite of a quiescent marrow (e.g. some neoplasms, lead toxicity, splenic disease).

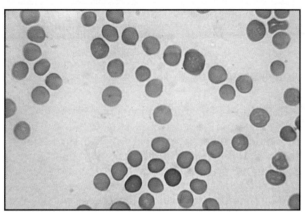

13.4 Regenerative anaemia in a dog with immune-mediated thrombocytopenia, showing anisocytosis and polychromasia (Diff-Quik®).

In general, the presence of regeneration indicates that either haemolysis or haemorrhage is the cause of the anaemia, whereas the absence of regeneration suggests that the cause is decreased erythropoiesis. There are, however, three important exceptions:

- Acute haemorrhage or haemolysis of less than 2–4 days' duration, as there has been insufficient time for bone marrow response
- Concomitant disease that precludes an appropriate bone marrow response, e.g. renal failure
- Immune-mediated haemolytic anaemia where the immune response is targeted to the red cell precursors (Figure 13.5).

Therefore, if the anaemia is regenerative, the next step is to determine if it is due to haemolysis or to haemorrhage. If the anaemia is non-regenerative, decreased erythropoiesis should not be assumed.

Regenerative	Non-regenerative
Haemolysis Haemorrhage	Decreased erythropoiesis Peracute haemolysis/haemorrhage Haemolysis/haemorrhage with concurrent disease precluding regeneration Immune-mediated destruction of erythrocyte precursors

13.5 Regenerative *versus* non-regenerative anaemia.

Haemolysis *versus* haemorrhage

Several clinical clues are available to differentiate haemolysis from haemorrhage (Figure 13.6). Blood loss is not always obvious, so a careful search must be made for evidence of haemorrhage. In some patients, haemorrhage and haemolysis occur simultaneously. The serum protein concentration is generally normal with haemolysis and decreased with haemorrhage. There are, however, exceptions: patients with concomitant haemolysis and protein loss (e.g. protein-losing nephropathy) or those with pre-existing hyperglobulinaemia. Haemoglobinaemia and haemoglobinuria indicate haemolysis. Splenomegaly and icterus usually suggest haemolysis, but are neither consistent nor specific findings.

Clinical feature	Haemorrhage	Haemolysis
Evidence of bleeding	Common	Rare
Serum protein	Low to normal	Normal to high [a]
Haemoglobinaemia/uria	No	Common
Icterus	No [a]	Common
Splenomegaly	No [a]	Common

13.6 Clinical features to assist in differentiating haemorrhage from haemolysis. [a] Exceptions can occur in the presence of concurrent or associated disease.

Having determined the mechanism of the anaemia, a comprehensive list of differential diagnoses can be constructed, and further diagnostic testing allows determination of the specific cause (see Figure 13.3).

Haemorrhagic anaemia

Acute haemorrhage is treated by arresting the bleeding and restoring the circulating blood volume. Significant blood loss may occur internally into the pleural cavity, the peritoneal cavity, the retroperitoneal space, the fasciomuscular planes and the gastrointestinal tract. Large volumes of blood can accumulate in the intestines for several days before melaena becomes evident. When haemorrhage is identified without evidence of trauma, it is important to determine whether the bleeding is due to local factors or a systemic bleeding disorder, based on the history or the presence of multiple sites of bleeding. Where doubt exists, haemostasis should be tested.

Patients with chronic blood loss generally do not become emergencies until they are severely anaemic due to depletion of iron stores. Since younger animals have smaller stores, they become anaemic more readily than adults, usually from endo- and ectoparasitism. The anaemia is variably regenerative and is usually microcytic and hypochromic. Thrombocytosis may be present. Chronic blood loss in the adult is usually into the gastrointestinal tract. Even when parasites are identified in the adult, additional testing is indicated to eliminate the possibility of an additional cause of haemorrhage (e.g. neoplasia, ulceration).

Haemolytic anaemia

Haemolytic anaemia is common in dogs, often occurring acutely. Most haemolysis is extravascular, with erythrocyte destruction occurring in the spleen and liver. Splenomegaly is frequently present. Intravascular haemolysis is less common and results in haemoglobinaemia and haemoglobinuria, which may cause acute nephrosis. With either process, the rate of erythrocyte destruction may exceed the rate of hepatic clearance, resulting in hyperbilirubinaemia and icterus. The absence of hyperbilirubinaemia, however, does not exclude haemolysis.

The evaluation of patients with haemolytic anaemia should always include a blood smear examination and a saline agglutination test. In cats, viral serology is imperative. Morphological abnormalities highly suggestive of a particular aetiology are frequently detectable on smear examination. These include spherocytes, Heinz bodies, eccentrocytes, erythroparasites and schistocytes (see Figure 13.2).

There are numerous causes of haemolytic anaemia (see Figure 13.3), which can be divided into the following major categories:

- Immune-mediated
- Toxic
- Infectious
- Microangiopathic
- Congenital
- Miscellaneous.

The most common are briefly discussed below.

Immune-mediated haemolytic anaemia

Immune-mediated haemolytic anaemia (IMHA) is the most common cause of haemolysis in dogs. Haemolysis is usually extravascular, but may be intravascular. IMHA may be primary (idiopathic) or secondary to drug administration (e.g. sulphonamides), live-virus vaccination, neoplasia (especially lymphoma and haemangiosarcoma), tick-borne disease (babesiosis, ehrlichiosis), dirofilariasis or bacterial infection (e.g. leptospirosis). It may be accompanied by other immune-mediated processes such as immune-mediated thrombocytopenia or systemic lupus erythematosus (SLE).

The onset of signs is usually acute. Splenomegaly is common, as are icterus and fever. The anaemia is usually regenerative, and neutrophilia occurs frequently. Up to 33% of cases have reticulocytopenia, which may indicate recent haemolysis or the destruction of red cell precursors in the bone marrow. Thrombocytopenia may be present due to antibody-mediated destruction or as a result of consumption (thrombosis or disseminated intravascular coagulation (DIC)).

Diagnosis of IMHA requires elimination of other causes of haemolysis and demonstration of immune-mediated erythrocyte injury. Spherocytosis is the most reliable feature of IMHA in canine patients (Figure 13.7). Autoagglutination is the next most convincing evidence, but is not always present. A positive direct Coombs' test supports the diagnosis, but a negative test does not rule out IMHA. When spherocytosis is not convincing, and autoagglutination and Coombs' testing are negative, a saline fragility test may help to document erythrocyte injury.

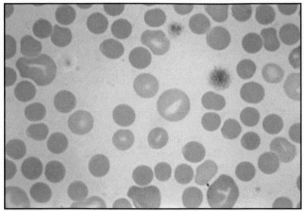

13.7 Spherocytosis is recognized by the presence of many small round erythrocytes that lack central pallor. The finding of large numbers of these cells is highly suggestive of immune-mediated haemolytic anaemia. (Courtesy of Dr Patricia McManus, University of Pennsylvania)

If the anaemia is non-regenerative, recognition of spherocytes is an important clue to the presence of immune-mediated anaemia. Bone marrow examination, usually reveals a distinct maturation block at one stage of erythroid development, with an absence or paucity of later stages. Erythrophagocytosis may be evident. Immune-mediated pure red cell aplasia can also occur due to destruction of stem cells. Diagnosis of immune-mediated anaemia in these cases can be difficult, and response to therapy provides important information. In cases of non-regenerative immune-mediated anaemia, a longer period should be anticipated for a response to therapy (weeks to months).

Once a diagnosis of IMHA is made, a thorough search for underlying causes or systemic immune-mediated disease should begin. In addition to a CBC, biochemical profile and urinalysis, diagnostic tests could include radiology/ultrasonography, an anti-nuclear antibody test (ANA) and serology for tick-borne diseases and occult dirofilariasis. Tests for infectious diseases should be chosen based on the geographical location and travel history.

IMHA is uncommon in the cat. Since recognition of spherocytes is difficult in the cat, the saline fragility test can be used to detect erythrocyte injury. Infection with *Mycoplasma haemofelis* is frequently associated with IMHA. A direct association between feline leukaemia virus (FeLV) and IMHA is equivocal, but concurrent disease occurs relatively commonly, and cats with IMHA should be evaluated for viral disease.

Treatment of IMHA includes the elimination of any underlying cause, adequate immunosuppression and appropriate supportive care. Glucocorticoids are the backbone of immunosuppressive therapy, and should be initiated without delay, following diagnosis and testing for underlying neoplasia. Glucocorticoid therapy can be initiated with prednisolone (1–2 mg/kg q12h orally or s.c. for animals <10 kg and 15 mg/m^2 q12h for animals >10 kg) or dexamethasone (0.1–0.3 mg/kg i.v. q12h). The use of gastrointestinal protectants (H$_2$-receptor antagonists) is recommended. When tick-borne disease is possible, doxycycline should be administered (5–10 mg/kg q12–24h orally or i.v.).

Most patients with regenerative IMHA respond to glucocorticoid therapy within 5–7 days. Response to therapy is evaluated based on the haematocrit, which depends on the balance between cell destruction and bone marrow regeneration. The need for adjunctive therapy with more potent immunosuppressive agents in the acute scenario remains unclear, as their efficacy has yet to be firmly established in small animals. These drugs are generally reserved for those patients with intravascular erythrocyte destruction, autoagglutination, severe hyperbilirubinaemia or unrelenting aggressive haemolysis. Several adjunctive immunosuppressive drugs may be considered. Ciclosporin (3–7 mg/kg q12h in dogs; 4–6 mg/kg orally q12h in cats) is an attractive option for adjunct immunosuppression in the acute scenario, as it acts rapidly and does not induce myelosuppression. A newer alternative in the dog is mycophenolate (10–15 mg/kg q12h orally or i.v.). While reports of efficacy are lacking, clinical experience with this drug has been encouraging. Cyclophosphamide (200 mg/m^2 total dose i.v. or orally once or divided over 3–4 consecutive days) may be used but, due to the potential for myelosuppression, it should be avoided, or used only as a last resort, in patients without a regenerative response. Rapid responses to human intravenous immunoglobulin (0.5–1.5 g/kg i.v. as a single infusion) have been described in dogs. The drug is expensive, but has not been associated with significant adverse effects, and can be used together with other immunosuppressive therapy. Experience in small animal patients, however, is limited, so it is difficult to give firm recommendations for use.

The guidelines for blood transfusion are no different from those for other forms of anaemia. There is no basis for the statement that transfusion is contraindicated in this disease. Intravenous fluid therapy is indicated in severely affected patients to prevent blood stasis, minimize hypercoagulability (thromboembolism and DIC) and to ensure adequate diuresis in patients with intravascular haemolysis.

IMHA is a potentially hypercoagulable state; the risk of thrombosis is exacerbated by stasis, immobility, vascular catheterization, inflammation associated with the systemic inflammatory response syndrome (SIRS) and corticosteroid therapy. The risk of thromboembolism in the individual patient, however, is difficult to determine objectively. A recent study suggested significantly improved survival in dogs that received antiplatelet therapy with ultra low-dose aspirin at 0.5 mg/kg q24h orally (Weinkle *et al.*, 2005). The benefit:risk ratio of this practice may support its routine use. More aggressive antithrombotic therapy with anticoagulants may be indicated in more severely affected patients (those with autoagglutination or massive unrelenting haemolysis), or in the presence of a second disease process that predisposes to hypercoagulability (see below). The benefits of anticoagulation in these patients, however, remain undocumented, as do established protocols for such drugs (see below).

Corticosteroids are continued at the initial dosage until the haematocrit begins to increase, usually a minimum of 2–3 weeks. They are then gradually tapered over subsequent months. The addition of other immunosuppressive agents may provide a synergistic effect,

and facilitate tapering of corticosteroids. In the dog, azathioprine is most commonly prescribed (2.2 mg/kg q24h for small- and medium-sized dogs, and 1.5 mg/kg q24h for larger dogs). As azathioprine can lead to bone marrow suppression in some individuals, regular (every 2–4 weeks) monitoring of CBC is recommended in patients receiving azathioprine, especially if daily dosing is continued for a prolonged period. If the haematocrit decreases with tapering of the corticosteroid, other immunosuppressive agents can be substituted, such as cyclophosphamide (200 mg/m^2 divided over 3–4 consecutive days weekly), ciclosporin (3–7 mg/kg q12h orally) or mycophenolate (10–15 mg/kg q12h orally or i.v.). In feline patients that do not respond adequately to corticosteroids, or relapse with dose tapering, adjunctive therapy with ciclosporin is recommended (4–6 mg/kg q12h orally). Vincristine (0.025 mg/kg i.v. weekly) has also been described for this use. Azathioprine should not be used in cats.

The prognosis for animals with IMHA is variable. A poorer prognosis is associated with intravascular haemolysis, severe hyperbilirubinaemia and neoplasia. Thromboembolic complications, particularly pulmonary thromboembolism, are relatively common. A small proportion of cases may have protracted disease that precludes discontinuation of corticosteroids. Relapse is possible.

Zinc toxicity

Zinc toxicity should be considered in any patient that has acute haemolytic anaemia without autoagglutination or morphological abnormalities on the blood smear (Figure 13.8). Ingestion of some coins (e.g. UK pound coins, US pennies), zinc nuts or bolts or topical skin protectants can result in toxic concentrations of zinc, causing severe intravascular haemolysis and gastrointestinal irritation. Acute renal failure can result from massive haemoglobinuria. A tentative diagnosis is based on a history of exposure, and foreign objects in the gastrointestinal tract can often be demonstrated radiographically. Since the mere presence of metal-dense foreign bodies does not confirm zinc toxicity, diagnosis requires the presence of convincing clinical signs or an elevated blood zinc concentration. Due to the high mortality associated with zinc toxicity, these patients constitute serious emergencies and treatment should not be delayed pending the results of zinc concentrations.

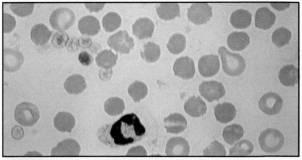

13.8 Small erythrocytes that have sustained intravascular membrane damage may occasionally be mistaken for spherocytes, for example in this case of zinc intoxication. (Courtesy of Dr Patricia McManus, University of Pennsylvania)

Treatment of zinc toxicity begins with patient stabilization, followed by removal of the suspect object via endoscopy or laparotomy. Appropriate fluid therapy is given based on perfusion parameters and renal function, and packed red blood cells should be transfused if necessary. Treatment with H_2-receptor antagonists (cimetidine, famotidine) is recommended to decrease 'leaching' of zinc from the source prior to removal. Chelation therapy with calcium ethylenediamine tetra-acetic acid (CaEDTA) should be initiated (25 mg/kg diluted in 5% dextrose, s.c. q6h). Since CaEDTA can be nephrotoxic, careful attention should be paid to dosing and adequate fluid therapy. The duration of chelator therapy remains unclear, as serum zinc concentrations may take 2–21 days to decline following removal of the object. Where feasible, the decision should be based on normalization of the serum zinc concentration. The prognosis for complete recovery is good with timely and aggressive intervention.

Oxidative injury

Oxidative injury causes denaturation of haemoglobin resulting in Heinz body formation, or oxidation of haem iron resulting in methaemoglobinaemia. Heinz bodies lead to altered erythrocyte deformability and shortened survival. Heinz bodies usually appear within 24 hours of exposure, with haemolysis occurring after several days.

The most common cause of Heinz bodies in the dog is the ingestion of onions (raw, cooked or dehydrated). Haemolysis occurs approximately 5 days after ingestion. Heinz bodies in the dog are usually small, occur in multiples and are readily identified with reticulocyte staining. When large they may be seen as clear 'blebs' protruding from the cell surface. Eccentrocytes – erythrocytes with the haemoglobin displaced to one side and a clear zone on the other side – frequently accompany Heinz bodies in the dog (Figure 13.9).

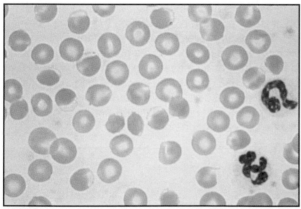

13.9 Eccentrocytes and Heinz bodies in a dog, caused by the ingestion of onions. (Courtesy of Dr Patricia McManus, University of Pennsylvania)

Feline haemoglobin is highly sensitive to oxidative denaturation, and Heinz body formation is common in the cat (up to 96% of erythrocytes in normal cats). Heinz bodies can accompany numerous feline primary diseases, including lymphoma, hyperthyroidism and diabetes mellitus. Commercial cat foods containing propylene glycol are associated with susceptibility to oxidative injury, but do not generally cause clinical anaemia. A variety of other agents may induce Heinz body formation and severe anaemia in cats (see Figure 13.3). Heinz bodies in the cat are usually single, may project from the membrane and are best visualized with one of the reticulocyte stains. Diagnosis of overt Heinz body anaemia requires visualization of relatively large Heinz bodies in many erythrocytes, with convincing evidence of haemolysis.

Treatment of Heinz body anaemia includes removal of the causative toxin or treatment of the underlying disease, blood transfusion where indicated and supportive care.

Erythroparasites

Mycoplasma haemofelis (previously *Haemobartonella felis*) can cause acute anaemia, especially in cats with an underlying immunosuppressive infection such as FeLV or feline immunodeficiency virus (FIV). Diagnosis requires identification of ring or rod forms of the organism on erythrocytes on blood smear examination (Figure 13.10) or polymerase chain reaction (PCR) to confirm the presence of parasite DNA. Identification of the parasite may require examination of a smear on several consecutive days. Ring forms consist of a fine basophilic ring with a clear centre. Rod forms are observed on the periphery of the cell. Since the organisms are epicellular, they can be easily dislodged or washed off the cells in EDTA. Identification is thus best achieved by examination of a fresh blood smear. Prolonged alcohol fixation decreases the displacement of organisms during staining. The disease is treated with tetracycline (20 mg/kg orally q8h) or doxycycline (5 mg/kg orally q12h) for 2–3 weeks. Concurrent corticosteroid therapy has been advocated, since an immune-mediated process is likely. Supportive care and specific therapy for concurrent disease are intuitive.

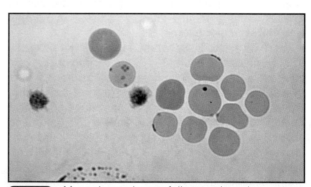

13.10 *Mycoplasma haemofelis* organisms in a cat (Diff-Quik®). Note the difference between the peripherally located *M. haemofelis* organisms and the larger, refractile, centrally located Howell–Jolly body in one cell.

Haemobartonella canis is rare, usually only occurring in splenectomized, severely debilitated or immunosuppressed dogs. Organisms are readily seen as chains across the surface of the red cell. Spherocytosis is common, indicating an immune-mediated pathophysiology. Treatment should consist of tetracyclines, using the same regimen as for the cat. Corticosteroids can be added to the regimen if response to antibiotics alone is inadequate.

The tick-transmitted protozoans, *Babesia canis* and *Babesia gibsoni*, cause haemolytic anaemia in dogs. The clinical manifestations range from acute disease with severe intravascular haemolysis to subacute or chronic disease with mild or moderate anaemia. Immune-mediated haemolysis appears to occur frequently, and dependent on geographical location, concurrent infection with *Ehrlichia canis* is common. Complicated cases of babesiosis may manifest as DIC, respiratory distress syndrome or SIRS. Diagnosis of babesiosis requires identification of intra-erythrocytic pyriform bodies on blood smear examination (Figure 13.11). Since parasitized erythrocytes tend to 'sludge' in the capillaries, diagnostic yield is best on an ear-stick blood smear. When infection is suspected, but organisms cannot be found, serological or PCR testing is indicated. Diagnostic work up should also include evaluation for IMHA and serological testing for ehrlichiosis. Treatment includes appropriate supportive therapy and specific antiparasitic drugs, such as diminazene aceturate and imidocarb diproprionate. Tetracyclines have limited efficacy.

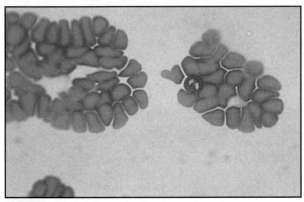

13.11 *Babesia canis* piroplasms in a dog (Diff-Quik®).

Congenital disorders
Inherited enzyme deficiencies are rare, but may mimic IMHA. Phosphofructokinase (PFK) deficiency has been described in English Springer and American Cocker Spaniels. Chronic mild to moderate anaemia occurs, with superimposed episodes of intravascular haemolysis precipitated by vigorous exercise or panting, due to the sensitivity of these erythrocytes to alkalaemia. These dogs present at a young age with acute intravascular haemolysis, a strong regenerative response and spontaneous recovery. If immunosuppressive therapy is initiated, recovery may be erroneously ascribed to the drug. Diagnosis of PFK deficiency is made via enzyme assay performed by specialized laboratories.

Pyruvate kinase (PK) deficiency has been described in Basenjis and Beagles. It is characterized by chronic severe haemolysis and moderate to severe anaemia, usually first recognized at 3–6 months of age. The haematocrit slowly declines over the following 1–3 years. Typically, the anaemia is initially highly regenerative, but terminal myelofibrosis may develop. Diagnosis is presumptive based on elimination of other causes, and confirmed via enzyme assay by specialized laboratories.

Microangiopathy
Microangiopathic haemolytic anaemia results from mechanical fragmentation of erythrocytes. Causes include splenic torsion, haemangiosarcoma, DIC and caval syndrome associated with heartworm disease. Erythrocyte fragmentation is recognized by finding schistocytes (sheared erythrocytes) on blood smear examination. Ordinarily, anaemia is subclinical, but in severe cases overt anaemia develops (e.g. in splenic torsion and caval syndrome).

Decreased erythropoiesis
Decreased erythropoiesis can be caused by extra-marrow or intra-marrow disease (see Figure 13.3). Anaemia is caused by extra-marrow disorders if a systemic disease selectively depresses erythropoiesis. The anaemia is generally mild (haematocrit range 25–35% in dogs and 20–25% in cats) and because the anaemia develops slowly, clinical signs of the underlying disease usually predominate. Intra-marrow disease, such as myeloaplasia (aplastic anaemia), myelodysplasia, myeloproliferative disorders and myelofibrosis, results from injury to the stem cells and/or marrow microenvironment. Depending on the course of the disease, variable cytopenias are observed. Acute disease is usually characterized by granulocytopenia and thrombocytopenia, with mild to non-existent anaemia. Chronic marrow disease is characterized by moderate to severe anaemia, with variable degrees of leucopenia and thrombocytopenia.

Evaluation of patients with non-regenerative anaemia includes investigation into possible drug exposure, a CBC to determine other blood cell counts, evaluation for systemic disease, serological testing for FeLV and FIV in the cat and for ehrlichiosis in the dog, and bone marrow examination. The bone marrow aspirate may reveal evidence of neoplasia or dysplasia, and allows estimation of cellularity. Immune-mediated non-regenerative anaemia, in which the cell targeted by the immune system is a red cell precursor, may also be identified on marrow examination. A core bone marrow biopsy, however, is required to determine fully the degree of cellularity or fibrosis, and to assess maturation sequences accurately.

Treatment for non-regenerative anaemia depends on the cause, but may include blood transfusion and/or the administration of colony stimulating factors.

Bleeding disorders

Bleeding disorders are classified as primary (platelet or vascular disorders) or secondary (coagulation factor disorders). They can be inherited or acquired.

Approach in the emergency situation
Bleeding disorders should always be considered life threatening. Even the stable patient with a bleeding disorder can decompensate rapidly and without pre-emptive signs. Animals in haemorrhagic crisis usually show typical signs of hypovolaemic shock. The rapid establishment of a diagnosis and institution of rational therapy can represent a major challenge.

Blood samples should be collected prior to initiating therapy, and should include a minimum database, a blood smear, and EDTA and citrated plasma for later laboratory testing. The minimum database usually reveals a decreased PCV and TP. In canine acute haemorrhage, the PCV may be normal or elevated due to compensatory splenic contraction, but the TP may be low, reflecting blood loss. A blood smear should be examined, with emphasis on platelet numbers and morphology and the presence of schistocytes. Depending on the findings in the individual patient, further testing may include a CBC, chemistry profile, screening coagulation tests, immune and/or serological testing.

Stabilization of the bleeding patient requires control of haemorrhage and blood volume replacement. The most life-threatening problem in these animals is shock, so initial therapy should involve aggressive fluid replacement (crystalloid with or without synthetic colloids) until blood is available. There is no justification for withholding fluid therapy in the anaemic patient. Fluid therapy will not alter the absolute red cell mass, and hypoperfusion will only exacerbate tissue hypoxia.

Animals should be kept quiet and unstressed, subcutaneous injections should be avoided and venipunctures performed only when required for platelet enumeration. Following venipuncture, the site should be held off with firm manual pressure for 5 minutes. An intravenous catheter can usually be safely placed and used to collect all other blood samples (including regular PCV monitoring). Patients should be closely monitored for evidence of ongoing haemorrhage, including evaluation of perfusion, respiratory rate and effort, mucous membrane colour, neurological status and PCV/TP.

Once the patient has been stabilized, three initial questions must be answered:

- Is the bleeding due to local factors or does the animal have a generalized haemostatic abnormality?
- If a systemic bleeding disorder does exist, what is the nature of the haemostatic defect?
- Is the defect congenital or acquired?

This is generally achieved based on the history, physical examination and screening laboratory tests.

Pathophysiology

Traditionally the haemostatic system has been divided into three major parts: primary haemostasis, secondary haemostasis and fibrinolysis. Newer models of haemostasis have been proposed (Hoffman, 2003) that may provide a better model for the complex interaction between the components of the haemostatic system including the vascular endothelium. However, for the purpose of clinical patient evaluation the traditional approach is adequate and is described below.

Primary haemostasis

Primary haemostasis involves interactions between the vessel wall and the platelets, terminating in the formation of a primary haemostatic plug, which constitutes a temporary seal over the injured vessel. At the site of vascular injury, platelets adhere to the subendothelial collagen, mediated by von Willebrand factor (vWF) and membrane glycoproteins. Following adherence, the platelets undergo conformational changes and release bioactive substances that stimulate platelet aggregation. These aggregated platelets constitute the primary haemostatic plug and expose platelet phospholipid (platelet factor 3) that plays an important role in secondary haemostasis. Defects in primary haemostasis may be due to platelet or vascular disorders. Platelet disorders can be quantitative (thrombocytopenia) or qualitative (thrombopathia). Vasculopathies may lead to excessive fragility or abnormal interaction with platelets.

Secondary haemostasis

Secondary haemostasis involves the formation of fibrin by the sequential activation of the coagulation factors, in and around the primary haemostatic plug. All coagulation factors are produced in the liver, with the exception of factor VIII. Vitamin K is required for the activation of factors II, VII, IX and X, as well as protein C. Classically, two pathways of coagulation activation are recognized: an intrinsic and an extrinsic pathway. The intrinsic pathway is surface-activated and operates strictly with components present in the blood, whereas the extrinsic pathway requires tissue factor for activation. These two pathways converge in a final common pathway of fibrin formation. Defects of secondary haemostasis may include quantitative or qualitative coagulation factor disorders.

Fibrinolysis

The fibrinolytic system consists of plasminogen and all substances that convert it to its active form, plasmin. Plasmin is responsible for dissolution of the fibrin clot. Dissolution of fibrinogen and fibrin results in the production of various fragments, or fibrin split/degradation products (FSP/FDPs). These FSPs have anticoagulant activity by interfering with platelet function and inhibiting thrombin. They are ultimately removed from the circulation by the liver (half-life approximately 9–12 hours). Excessive fibrinolysis and generation of FSPs can occur in conditions such as DIC and hepatic disease, and may contribute to a bleeding tendency. D-dimers represent the breakdown products of cross-linked fibrin and are a more specific measure of active coagulation and fibrinolysis.

Clinical and laboratory assessment

Following initial stabilization, the first step is to determine whether the haemorrhage is due to a systemic bleeding disorder. A bleeding disorder must then be categorized as a defect of primary or secondary haemostasis. The history and physical examination often provide important clues, but definitive classification requires laboratory testing.

History

A detailed history is vital. Severe inherited disorders are generally apparent within the first 6 months of life. Milder forms may not be diagnosed until surgery, trauma or concurrent disease precipitate excessive bleeding. Certain inherited disorders are breed-related, for example von Willebrand's disease (vWD) in the Dobermann. It is important to ascertain whether previous bleeding episodes have occurred in the patient, or in family members. The history should include detailed enquiries about previous illnesses and medications. Live-virus vaccines and certain drugs may cause thrombocytopenia 3–10 days post-treatment. Specific enquiries about the environment and patient behaviour may reveal the potential of exposure to toxins or trauma. Some animals with bleeding disorders are presented for apparently unrelated disease; for example, shifting leg lameness may result from recurrent haemarthrosis, and acute blindness may be due to hyphaema.

Physical examination

Evaluation of the distribution, extent and nature of current haemorrhage requires careful examination of all body systems, including the skin, mucous membranes, eyes and joints, as well as the urine and faeces. The nature of the haemorrhage helps to characterize the haemostatic defect (Figure 13.12). Defects of primary haemostasis are characterized by petechiation/ecchymosis and spontaneous bleeding from mucosal surfaces, including epistaxis, gingival bleeding, haematuria, melaena and ocular haemorrhage. Platelet and vascular abnormalities generally cannot be distinguished from each other on physical examination alone. Defects of secondary haemostasis are usually characterized by single/multiple haematomas and bleeding into subcutaneous tissue, body cavities, muscles or joints. Some acquired abnormalities, such as DIC, defy this classification because multiple haemostatic defects are present. Likewise, vWD usually has the characteristics of a primary haemostatic defect, but in its most severe form may mimic a secondary haemostatic disorder.

The physical examination should also aim to identify any evidence of concurrent disease, such as neoplasia, infectious or immune-mediated disease. This requires examination for masses, organomegaly, lymphadenopathy, uveitis, chorioretinitis, mucocutaneous lesions and arthropathy.

Screening coagulation tests

Laboratory tests are essential to confirm and characterize the haemostatic defect (Figures 13.13 and 13.14). These tests should be performed and interpreted carefully, together with the clinical findings. Blood samples should be collected via atraumatic venipuncture prior to the initiation of therapy. The jugular vein should be avoided where possible in patients with a suspected coagulation disorder as application of sufficient pressure to stop bleeding may be difficult. The common screening tests are discussed below; for normal values see Figure 13.15.

Platelet enumeration/estimation: Quantitative platelet disorders are detected via a platelet count. This should be performed in all patients with a suspected bleeding disorder. Samples for platelet counting should be collected (via rapid and clean venipuncture) in EDTA and analysed within 12 hours of collection, either manually (by haemocytometer) or by an automated cell counter. Both techniques are reliable for canine blood. In cats there is considerable overlap between erythrocyte and platelet volumes, resulting in erroneous results from automated cell counters. Feline platelets should therefore be enumerated manually.

Disorders of primary haemostasis	Disorders of secondary haemostasis
Petechiae common	Petechiae rare
Haematomas rare	Haematomas common
Bleeding often involves mucous membranes	Bleeding into muscles and joints common
Bleeding usually at multiple sites	Bleeding frequently localized
Prolonged and repeated bleeding from cuts (rebleed)	Bleeding may be delayed in onset

13.12 Clinical features helpful in differentiating between primary and secondary haemostatic abnormalities.

Process	Screening test	Component/factors evaluated
Primary haemostasis	Platelet enumeration Platelet estimation [a]	Platelet numbers Platelet numbers
	Bleeding time (BT) [a]	Platelet numbers and function, vascular integrity
Secondary haemostasis	Activated clotting time (ACT) [a]	Intrinsic and common pathways: factors XII, XI, IX, VIII, X, V, II and fibrinogen
	Partial thromboplastin time (PTT) [b]	As with ACT, but more sensitive
	Prothrombin time (PT) [b]	Extrinsic and common pathways: factors III, VII, X, V, II and fibrinogen
	Thrombin time (TT)	Terminal common pathway: fibrinogen quantity and quality
Fibrinolysis	Fibrin split products (FSPs) [b]	Products of fibrinolysis
	D-dimers [b]	Products of fibrinolysis, specific for lysis of cross-linked fibrin

13.13 Screening tests for the evaluation of haemostasis ([a] in-house tests; [b] in-house testing options available).

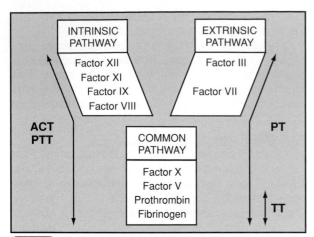

13.14 Factors evaluated with the screening coagulation tests (ACT, activated clotting time; PTT, partial thromboplastin time; PT, prothrombin time; TT, thrombin time).

Variable	Dog	Cat
Platelet count (x 10⁹/l)	180–500	200–600
Buccal mucosal bleeding time (minutes)	1.7–4.2	1.4–2.4
Cuticle bleeding time (minutes)	2–8	2–8
Activated clotting time (seconds)	60–110	50–75
Prothrombin time (seconds)	7–10	9–12
Partial thromboplastin time (seconds)	9–12	15–21
Fibrin split products (mg/l)	<10	<10
D-dimers (µg/l)	<250	<250

13.15 Normal values for screening coagulation tests. Normal values for prothrombin time and partial thromboplastin time are laboratory and technique dependent. Normal values for in-house coagulometers are provided by the manufacturer.

Examination of a blood smear allows rapid estimation of platelet numbers. This is essential in the emergency setting where automated counts may not be available, and in cats where automated counts are usually inaccurate. Smear examination also serves to verify the findings of automated counters. Approximately 11–25 platelets per high-power field (hpf) is considered normal, although individuals of some breeds (notably Cavalier King Charles Spaniels and Greyhounds) normally have a lower number of larger platelets. Spontaneous bleeding may occur when the platelet count is lower than 3–4/hpf. Platelet clumping at the feathered edge of the smear may result in artefactually low estimates and counts. Large platelets (macroplatelets or 'shift' platelets) generally indicate megakaryocytic hyperplasia (a regenerative response). The blood smear should be examined for schistocytes (fragmented erythrocytes), which suggest microangiopathic haemolysis and DIC.

Bleeding time: The bleeding time is the duration of haemorrhage resulting from infliction of a small standardized injury involving microscopic vessels. The buccal mucosal bleeding time (BMBT) is considered the most reliable and reproducible method. Cats usually require light sedation. The patient is restrained in lateral recumbency and a strip of gauze is tied around the maxilla to fold up the upper lip, tightly enough to cause moderate mucosal engorgement. A two-blade, spring-loaded device is used to make two 1 mm deep incisions in the mucosa of the upper lip. The incisions should be made at a site devoid of visible vessels and inclined so that the blood flows towards the mouth. Shed blood is carefully blotted with filter paper, taking extreme care not to disturb the incision sites. The time from incision to cessation of bleeding is measured. The cuticle bleeding time – the duration of bleeding after the tip of the dermis of the nail has been severed by a guillotine-type nail clipper – is far less reliable and reproducible.

The bleeding time reflects *in vivo* primary haemostasis. It may be prolonged by thrombocytopenia, thrombopathia or vascular anomalies and its measurement is indicated in patients with a suspected primary haemostatic defect when the platelet count is adequate. This test is unnecessary if the patient is thrombocytopenic.

Activated clotting time: The activated clotting time (ACT) is a simple screening test for the intrinsic and common pathways. Blood (2 ml) is drawn into a prewarmed (37°C) commercial tube containing diatomaceous (Fuller's) earth, which serves as a chemical activator of factor XII. The first few drops of blood are discarded because of the possible presence of tissue factor. The sample is mixed by inversion and then placed into a 37°C heat block or water bath for 50 seconds. It is inverted every 10 seconds, observed for clot formation and replaced. The ACT is the time interval to first clot formation. It is prolonged by severe abnormalities of the intrinsic and/or common pathways. It is a relatively insensitive, but easily performed, test. Severe thrombocytopenia (<10 x 10⁹/l) causes mild prolongation of the ACT (10–20 seconds). Similarly, hypofibrinogenaemia and some thrombopathias may result in ACT prolongation.

Partial thromboplastin time: The partial thromboplastin time (PTT) tests the intrinsic and common pathways. Usually, at least one factor must be decreased to below 30% of normal concentration before prolongation occurs. This test is more sensitive than the ACT and is not affected by primary haemostatic disorders. Samples for coagulation testing should be collected into plastic or siliconized glass tubes with 3.8% citrate as an anticoagulant at a ratio of 1:9 with the blood sample. If samples cannot be analysed within 12 hours, the plasma should be separated and frozen. Factor deficiencies may be differentiated from the effects of an anticoagulant, such as heparin, by repeating the PTT following dilution of the abnormal plasma 1:1 with normal plasma. Correction of the test indicates a factor deficiency, whereas failure to correct suggests the presence of an anticoagulant.

A patient-side coagulometer (e.g. SCA 2000®) is an alternative to conventional laboratory PTT determination in the emergency setting. While the methodology allows for testing of both whole blood with no anticoagulant and citrated blood, the latter is preferable with respect to sensitivity and specificity. Using citrated whole blood, reported sensitivity for diagnosis of PTT prolongation is 100%, with a specificity of approximately 83% (Tseng *et al.*, 2001). As such, it is an excellent screening test for abnormalities of the intrinsic and common pathways. False-positives, however, do occur. A prolonged PTT on the SCA should, therefore, be validated via conventional laboratory testing. For whole blood with no anticoagulant, reported sensitivity and specificity are 86.7% and 88.9%, respectively (Tseng *et al.*, 2001).

Prothrombin time: The prothrombin time (PT) tests the extrinsic and the common pathways. As such, it is the principal test of the extrinsic pathway. Because of the short half-life of factor VII, this test is very sensitive to vitamin K deficiency or antagonism. It is less sensitive to heparin than is the PTT. Sample collection and handling are as for the PTT.

As with PTT testing, a patient-side coagulometer (e.g. SCA 2000®) is an alternative to conventional laboratory testing. Using citrated whole blood, reported sensitivity and specificity for diagnosis of PT prolongation are 85.7% and 95.5%, respectively. That is, the test will not detect all anomalies of the extrinsic system, and a small number of false-positives occur. Abnormal results that do not correlate with clinical findings should be verified via conventional testing. Using blood with no anticoagulant, sensitivities are similar, but the test is significantly less specific.

Thrombin time: The thrombin time (TT) determines the reactivity of fibrinogen to exogenous thrombin. It assesses the conversion of fibrinogen to fibrin (the common pathway) and bypasses all other steps. It may be prolonged by hypofibrinogenaemia (<1 g/l), by dysfibrinogenaemia or by substances that inhibit thrombin, such as heparin or FSPs. Sample collection and handling are as for the PT and PTT.

Fibrin split products/fibrin degradation products: FSPs are the end products of fibrinolysis, and are generated when fibrinogen, soluble fibrin or cross-linked fibrin is lysed. They are commonly quantified via a commercial kit. Elevated concentrations of FSPs imply increased fibrinolysis, commonly due to DIC, but are not specific for the syndrome. Hepatic disease may also result in enhanced fibrinolysis and reduced clearance of FSPs. False elevations occur when fibrinogen is not clotted by thrombin and remains in solution, for example in patients on heparin therapy or those with dysfibrinogenaemia.

D-dimers: D-dimers are unique FSPs that are formed when cross-linked fibrin is lysed by plasmin. In contrast to FSPs, which indicate only the activation of plasmin, D-dimers indicate the activation of thrombin and plasmin, and are specific for active coagulation and fibrinolysis.

D-dimers are a sensitive test for DIC and are probably superior to traditional FSP assays for this purpose. However, they are not always elevated in patients with DIC, and elevated D-dimers are certainly not specific for DIC. They should be considered an ancillary diagnostic test, with the diagnosis of DIC relying on the appropriate constellation of clinical findings and abnormal results of haemostatis testing.

Disorders of primary haemostasis

The causes of primary haemostatic disorders are listed in Figure 13.16. An algorithmic diagnostic approach to patients with disorders of primary haemostasis is outlined in Figure 13.17.

Quantitative platelet disorders (thrombocytopenia)

Decreased production:
Drug-induced (oestrogen, chloramphenicol, cytotoxics)
Immune-mediated megakaryocytic hypoplasia
Viral (FeLV)
Chronic rickettsial disease
Oestrogen-secreting neoplasm
Myelophthisis (myeloproliferative disease)
Myelofibrosis
Cyclic thrombocytopenia (*Ehrlichia platys*)
Radiation
Idiopathic bone marrow aplasia

Increased destruction:
Immune-mediated (IMTP)
    Primary
        Idiopathic
        Evan's syndrome (IMHA and IMTP)
        Systemic lupus erythematosus
    Secondary
        Drugs
        Live-virus vaccination
        Tick-borne disease
        Neoplasia
        Bacterial infection
Non-immune
    Drug-induced
    Ehrlichiosis
    Rocky Mountain spotted fever
    Dirofilariasis

Consumption/sequestration:
Disseminated intravascular coagulation
Microangiopathies
Sepsis
Vasculitis
Splenic torsion, hypersplenism
Hepatic disease
Heparin-induced
Profound acute haemorrhage
Haemolytic uraemic syndrome

Qualitative platelet disorders (thrombopathia)

Inherited:
Von Willebrand's disease (numerous dog breeds)
Canine thrombopathia (Basset Hound)
Canine thrombasthenic thrombopathia (Otterhound)

Acquired:
Drug-induced (e.g. NSAIDs, synthetic colloid solutions, antibiotics, heparin)
Uraemia
Hepatic disease
Pancreatitis
Myeloproliferative disorders
Dysproteinaemia (e.g. myeloma)

Vascular disorders

Inherited:
Ehlers–Danlos syndrome

Acquired:
Vasculitis
Hyperadrenocorticism

13.16 Causes of disorders of primary haemostasis.

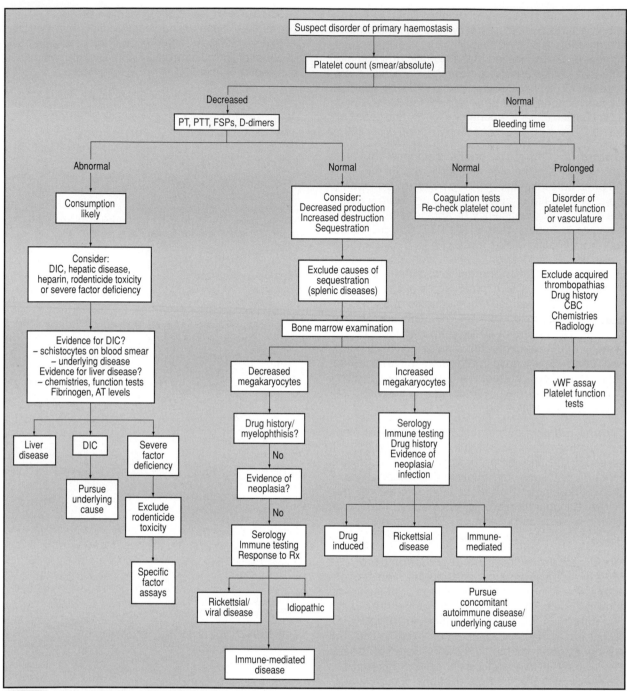

13.17 Approach to the diagnosis of disorders of primary haemostasis (DIC, disseminated intravascular coagulation; AT, antithrombin; vWF, von Willebrand factor).

Thrombocytopenia

Thrombocytopenia is the most common primary haemostatic defect and may be due to decreased platelet production or increased destruction, consumption or sequestration. Spontaneous bleeding generally does not occur until platelet counts are lower than approximately 40 x 10⁹/l, unless another concomitant bleeding disorder exists. Many animals tolerate lower counts without evidence of haemorrhage.

The secondary haemostatic mechanisms should be evaluated in all thrombocytopenic animals to exclude DIC or other combined defects, which are consistent with consumption or sequestration. If these are normal, a bone marrow aspirate or biopsy is indicated to evaluate platelet production. A CBC may show evidence of other cytopenias. Megakaryocytic hypoplasia can result from numerous conditions. In the absence of a compatible drug history or evidence of myelophthisis on bone marrow examination, further testing should include investigation into potential neoplastic, infectious or immune-mediated aetiologies. Oestrogen-secreting tumours, chronic rickettsial disease (*Ehrlichia canis*) and viral infections such as FeLV and FIV should be considered where appropriate. Immune-mediated megakaryocytic hypoplasia can present a diagnostic dilemma, which is usually resolved by exclusion of other differentials and evaluation of the response to immunosuppressive therapy.

Normal or increased numbers of megakaryocytes in thrombocytopenic patients indicate increased platelet destruction, consumption or sequestration. Some common causes of platelet consumption and sequestration include DIC, sepsis, vasculitis and splenic torsion, which can usually be excluded based on clinical findings. As a general rule, most causes of consumptive thrombocytopenia lead to a mild or moderate decrease in circulating platelet numbers. Splenic torsion is an exception, occasionally causing a severely decreased platelet count. DIC may also occasionally result in profound thrombocytopenia, but is then associated with concomitant anomalies in secondary haemostasis.

Immune-mediated thrombocytopenia (IMTP) is a common cause of severe thrombocytopenia in the dog. Diagnosis of IMTP is based on exclusion of other causes of thrombocytopenia. Tick-borne diseases may be diagnosed by examination of an ear-stick blood smear (*E. canis* morulae or *Babesia canis* trophozoites) or serologically (ehrlichiosis, Rocky Mountain spotted fever). A negative titre, however, does not exclude tick-borne disease and should be repeated in 10–14 days. IMTP may be idiopathic, may be associated with other autoimmune processes, such as IMHA or SLE, or may develop secondary to drug administration (notably sulphonamides), live-virus vaccination, neoplasia (especially lymphoid) and infection. Suspicion of IMTP should prompt a thorough search for underlying disease. In addition to a CBC, chemistry and urinalysis, diagnostic testing could include radiology/ultrasonography, a direct Coombs' test, an antinuclear antibody (ANA) test, Baermann faecal examination for *Angiostrongylus vasorum* and serology for tick-borne diseases and occult dirofilariasis.

Management of IMTP includes treatment of any underlying cause, adequate immunosuppression and appropriate supportive care. Glucocorticoids are the backbone of immunosuppressive therapy: either prednisolone (1–2 mg/kg q12h for animals <10 kg and 15 mg/m^2 q12h for animals >10 kg) or dexamethasone (0.1–0.2 mg/kg i.v. q12h). The use of gastrointestinal protectants (H$_2$-antagonists and/or sucralfate) is recommended. When tick-borne disease is possible, doxycycline should be administered (10 mg/kg q24h orally or i.v.). Response to glucocorticoid therapy generally requires 2–7 days. Vincristine (0.01–0.025 mg/kg i.v.) has been advocated in dogs with IMTP and megakaryocytic hyperplasia to cause a more rapid increase in platelet numbers. Improved responses have been documented in dogs using vincristine, compared with prednisolone alone, but are not universal. Anecdotal reports of rapid responses to human intravenous immunoglobulin (0.5–1.5 g/kg as a single infusion) have been described in dogs and a cat. Several aspects of this drug make its use in IMTP very appealing. Responses appear to be rapid (1–2 days) thus decreasing the potential for fatal haemorrhage. It can be administered together with other immunosuppressive drugs, and has not been associated with adverse effects. The drug is expensive, however, and veterinary experience is limited. It is difficult, therefore, to give evidence-based recommendations for its use.

Thrombocytopenic patients can deteriorate rapidly due to massive haemorrhage (most commonly in the gastrointestinal tract) or due to haemorrhage into a vital organ (e.g. lungs or brain). Patients should be hospitalized until platelet counts are above 50 x 10^9/l and bleeding has ceased. Thereafter, platelet counts should be regularly monitored. When these are within the reference range, the prednisolone dose is decreased by approximately 25%. The dose is then decreased gradually over 3–6 months, with close monitoring of platelet counts.

Relapses of thrombocytopenia with decrease of the prednisolone dose are unpredictable and not uncommon. Periodic monitoring of the platelet count is therefore essential. If relapse occurs, the prednisolone dose should be increased temporarily and another immunosuppressive drug added to the therapeutic regimen. Options in the dog include: azathioprine (2.2 mg/kg/day orally); ciclosporin (3–7 mg/kg q12h in dogs); mycophenolate (10–15 mg/kg q12h); cyclophosphamide (200 mg/m^2 weekly, divided over 3–4 days); or danazol (5 mg/kg orally q12h). Ciclosporin is used in the cat (4–6 mg/kg q12h). Splenectomy is generally reserved for patients that have splenomegaly and exhibit refractory IMTP. Prior to splenectomy, it is crucial to ascertain (via bone marrow examination) that the spleen is not a significant source of extramedullary haemopoiesis.

Thrombopathia
Vascular disorders are a relatively uncommon cause of bleeding. In patients with clinical evidence of a primary haemostatic disorder and normal platelet numbers, a platelet function defect is likely. A prolonged bleeding time in a patient with adequate platelet numbers generally confirms thrombopathia. The patient's drug history should be carefully appraised, as drugs are frequent causes of thrombopathia. Numerous diseases can precipitate platelet dysfunction, including uraemia, hepatic disease, pancreatitis, myeloproliferative disorders and myeloma. If no obvious cause of thrombopathia can be found, a hereditary disorder is suspected. Von Willebrand's disease is the most common. von Willebrand factor can be assayed for confirmation. Other thrombopathias require specific platelet function testing, performed by specialized laboratories.

Control of haemorrhage in a dog with vWD includes administration of von Willebrand factor (vWF) in plasma products, and desmopressin acetate (DDAVP). Cryoprecipitate is the ideal plasma product, as it contains relatively large quantities of vWF. If this is not available, fresh frozen plasma may be used. DDAVP (1 µg/kg s.c.) may have a positive clinical effect, but a limited duration of action. It can be administered during a bleeding crisis or 20–30 minutes prior to an anticipated trauma such as surgery. Efficacy can be determined by repeating the BMBT 30–60 minutes after administration.

Disorders of secondary haemostasis
Figure 13.18 lists the causes of disorders of secondary haemostasis (coagulopathies) in small animals. Figure 13.19 outlines an algorithmic approach to these patients.

Inherited
Deficient factor:
    I: Hypo/dysfibrinogenaemia (St Bernard, Borzoi)
    II: Hypoprothrombinaemia (Boxer)
    VII: Hypoproconvertinaemia (Beagle, Malamute)
    VIII: Haemophilia A (numerous dog breeds, mongrels, cats)
    IX: Haemophilia B (numerous dog breeds, British Shorthair cats)
    X: Stuart Prower trait (Cocker Spaniel)
    XI: Plasma thromboplastin antecedent deficiency (Springer Spaniel, Great Pyrenees)
    XII: Hageman factor deficiency (numerous dog breeds, cats)

Acquired
Vitamin K deficiency/antagonism
Hepatic disease
Disseminated intravascular coagulation
Circulating anticoagulants (e.g. heparin)

13.18 Causes of disorders of secondary haemostasis.

Defects of secondary haemostasis may be hereditary or acquired. Hereditary coagulopathies are quantitative disorders of specific coagulation factors, usually noted in purebred dogs. Acquired disorders include vitamin K deficiency or antagonism, hepatic disease, DIC and the presence of anticoagulants (e.g. heparin). These conditions tend to affect multiple factors in both the intrinsic and extrinsic pathways. Factor VII has the shortest half-life (4–6 hours) so prolongation of the PT may precede PTT prolongation in early vitamin K deficiency or early acute hepatic failure. Conversely, the PTT alone may be prolonged with chronic hepatic disease, DIC or heparin therapy.

Anticoagulant rodenticide toxicity
The most common cause of vitamin K deficiency is the ingestion of anticoagulant rodenticides. Synthesis of vitamin K-dependent factors occurs in the liver. Vitamin K is an essential cofactor for carboxylation of

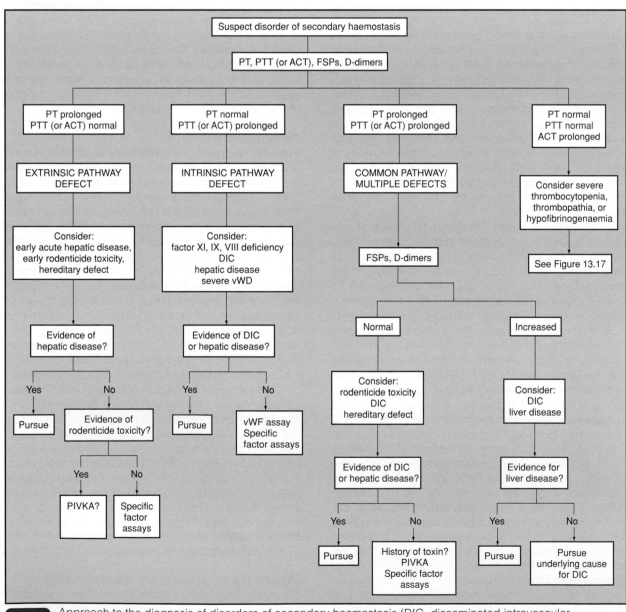

13.19 Approach to the diagnosis of disorders of secondary haemostasis (DIC, disseminated intravascular coagulation; vWF, von Willebrand factor; vWD, von Willebrand's disease; PIVKA: test for proteins induced by vitamin K absence/antagonism).

these proteins, rendering them functional. During this reaction, vitamin K is converted to an epoxide metabolite, which is recycled back to vitamin K. Anticoagulant rodenticides interfere with this recycling, resulting in rapid depletion of vitamin K and subsequent inability to produce functional clotting factors.

Clinical signs of a secondary haemostatic disorder generally occur 2–3 days following ingestion. Prolongation of the PT occurs first, but by the time haemorrhage is evident, the PT, PTT and ACT are usually all prolonged. FSP, D-dimer and fibrinogen concentrations are generally normal. The platelet count is usually normal, but may be decreased by consumption during bleeding. Toxicological testing for specific rodenticides or for proteins induced by vitamin K antagonism (PIVKA) is not usually helpful in the emergency situation, but may serve to confirm an uncertain diagnosis.

Vitamin K1 is essential to management. Improved coagulation, however, requires the synthesis of new factors, which commonly takes up to 12 hours. Emergency needs for clotting factors can be met only by transfusion of plasma (recommended dose 9 ml/kg). Fresh whole blood (20 ml/kg), or packed red blood cells with plasma, are indicated when anaemia is present. The half-life of transfused clotting factors is relatively short, thus plasma transfusion should be repeated after approximately 6 hours. Parenteral administration of vitamin K1 (5 mg/kg q12h) is recommended for initial therapy, ideally subcutaneously or intramuscularly using a small-gauge needle. The intravenous route should be avoided, due to the potential for anaphylaxis. After 24 hours, if the patient is not vomiting, vitamin K1 therapy is administered orally (0.25–2.5 mg/kg daily in warfarin exposure, 2.5–5.0 mg/kg for long-acting rodenticides).

Vitamin K1 has no effect on toxin elimination. Therapy must be maintained until the toxin has been metabolized, with varying durations depending on the type of rodenticide. If the anticoagulant is known to be warfarin, 1 week of therapy is usually sufficient. If the anticoagulant is unknown or a second-generation rodenticide, oral vitamin K1 should be continued for at least 3–4 weeks. The PT must be evaluated 48–72 hours after cessation of therapy. If it is prolonged, therapy should be reinstituted for an additional 2 weeks and the PT again re-evaluated after discontinuation.

Hepatic disease

Severe hepatocellular damage results in variable factor deficiencies and/or abnormalities in vitamin K metabolism. Both quantitative and qualitative platelet disorders may occur. FSPs and D-dimers may be elevated, and antithrombin and fibrinogen concentrations may be reduced. Excessive fibrinolysis can result from reduced clearance of plasminogen activators and reduced synthesis of fibrinolytic inhibitors. Differentiation from DIC is sometimes impossible based on coagulation testing alone, and depends on clinical findings, serum chemistry and liver function testing. Patients with hepatic failure frequently have gastrointestinal bleeding, resulting in a 'protein meal' that may precipitate hepatic encephalopathy. Bleeding tendencies must be corrected before pursuing a hepatic biopsy or

other invasive procedures. Transfusion of fresh frozen plasma can temporarily offset factor deficiencies. Vitamin K1 may be beneficial in some patients; efficacy should be ascertained by repeating coagulation tests at least 12 hours after initiating therapy.

Disseminated intravascular coagulation

DIC refers to the intravascular activation of haemostasis with resultant microcirculatory thrombosis. Exaggerated consumption of platelets and coagulation factors results in defective haemostasis and a bleeding tendency. Fibrinolysis of microthrombi generates FSPs, further exacerbating the bleeding disorder. Consumption of the natural anticoagulants can precipitate a thrombotic tendency.

DIC occurs secondary to a wide variety of underlying diseases, including sepsis, severe infections (viral, bacterial, parasitic and protozoal), neoplasia, shock, heat stroke, haemolysis, pancreatitis, severe hepatic disease, trauma and tissue necrosis. Three basic 'trigger' mechanisms have been proposed:

- Activation of the extrinsic coagulation pathway by tissue factor released during cell injury
- Contact activation of the intrinsic coagulation pathway via endothelial damage and exposure of the subendothelial matrix
- Direct activation of coagulation factors by certain enzymes (for example, trypsin in pancreatitis).

Numerous factors can act as 'enhancers' of DIC. Acidosis and hypoxia increase endothelial damage and inhibit antithrombin. Vascular stasis decreases the removal of activated coagulation factors and exacerbates local acidosis and hypoxia. The functional capacity of the mononuclear phagocytic system and the liver may be overwhelmed, hindering the removal of endotoxins, FSPs, enzymes and immune complexes.

The clinical manifestations of DIC vary depending on the inciting cause, the ability to replace depleted factors and platelets, the concentrations of natural anticoagulants and the efficacy of clearance of activated factors and FSPs. DIC may be subclinical, mild or severe, and acute or chronic. It may manifest as multiple organ failure due to microvascular thrombosis or as bleeding due to consumption of coagulation factors and platelets. Microthrombosis leads to ischaemia, which can manifest as renal failure, respiratory insufficiency, hepatic failure, neurological signs or gastrointestinal disorders. Bleeding tendencies may manifest as prolonged bleeding from venipuncture sites, petechiae, ecchymoses, epistaxis, gastrointestinal haemorrhage and/or haematoma formation.

The diagnosis of acute fulminant DIC is usually easily made, while chronic or subclinical DIC may prove more difficult. The laboratory findings are extremely variable. Thrombocytopenia is almost invariably present but may be mild. Relative changes may be undetected unless a recent platelet count is available for comparison. The PT, and more often the PTT, may be prolonged, but both may be normal if compensatory factor production is adequate. Significant elevations of FSPs or D-dimers are highly suggestive of DIC, but are non-specific. Schistocytes on the blood smear are significant, but are not invariably present and may occur with other conditions. Antithrombin levels are decreased in 85% of dogs with DIC. Fibrinogen concentrations are usually low, but may be normal or increased because fibrinogen is an acute phase reactant. Diagnosis of DIC, therefore, requires careful consideration of both the clinical and the laboratory findings, with no single finding being pathognomonic.

The treatment of DIC is fourfold:

- Correction of the underlying cause
- Optimization of perfusion via fluid therapy
- Prevention of secondary complications
- Control of the haemostatic defects.

Correction of the underlying cause must be the primary focus because, until it is removed, haemostatic activation will continue. In some cases, removal of the inciting cause is impossible or unfeasible. Fluid therapy is essential to remove activated clotting and fibrinolytic factors from the microcirculation and to maintain adequate tissue perfusion, thereby alleviating vascular stasis, tissue hypoxia and acidosis. The prevention or control of secondary complications includes: correction of acid–base and electrolyte disorders; supplemental oxygen therapy where indicated; maintenance of adequate perfusion to prevent renal and gastrointestinal ischaemia; and the prevention of secondary sepsis.

Control of the haemostatic defects of DIC can be attempted via blood product transfusion and heparinization. Plasma administration provides antithrombin and replaces depleted coagulation factors. If the patient is actively bleeding, fresh whole blood can replace red blood cells, coagulation factors and platelets. The adage that the administration of blood products to a patient in DIC 'adds fuel to the fire' has not proven to be true. In fact, experimental studies have shown that the administration of antithrombin is an effective therapy. The use of heparin in the treatment of DIC remains somewhat controversial. In theory, heparin acts to inhibit coagulation, thereby decreasing the rate of consumption of coagulation factors. The primary mechanism of action of heparin is via potentiation of antithrombin activity, thus inhibiting the activity of thrombin and other factors. Therefore, heparin is not effective unless adequate concentrations of antithrombin are present. The optimal dose of heparin is unclear, and most recommended doses are anecdotal. In mild cases of DIC, mini- or low-dose unfractionated heparin (5–10 or 75–200 IU/kg s.c. q8h) is generally recommended. In moderate to severe cases, intermediate or high doses (300–500 or 750–1000 IU/kg s.c. q8h) may be necessary.

Monitoring of patients on heparin therapy is difficult. When unfractionated heparin is used, ideally the PTT should not exceed 1.5–2 times the pre-treatment value. The PTT indicates the risk of haemorrhage and not the adequacy of anticoagulation. The PTT, therefore, may be normal in an adequately heparinized patient. It may be impossible to ascertain whether increased PT/PTT is due to heparinization or to changes in the basal coagulation status.

Hypercoagulation and thrombosis

Thrombosis is the deposition of a thrombus within the vasculature, resulting in tissue ischaemia. Fragmentation of the thrombus produces emboli that can obstruct remote sites. The term thromboembolism (TE) is used inclusively to refer to thrombosis and/or embolism. TE can be characterized as arterial (aortic, cerebral, myocardial) or venous (pulmonary, portal, vena caval). Hypercoagulability or thrombophilia is the propensity for thrombosis.

Pathophysiology

Thrombosis depends on three major risk factors (Virchow's triad): changes in the vessel wall (vascular injury); impairment of blood flow (stasis); and alterations in blood constituents to promote coagulation (hypercoagulability). Vascular injury leads to the exposure of subendothelial components, resulting in platelet adhesion and activation of the coagulation system. Factors resulting in vascular injury include trauma, catheterization, inflammation, neoplastic invasion, parasitic damage and plaque deposition (atherosclerosis, amyloidosis). Vascular stasis retards the removal of activated coagulation factors and causes local hypoxia and vascular injury. Stasis results from hypovolaemia, shock, cardiac insufficiency, blood vessel compression, immobility and hyperviscosity. True hypercoagulability refers to a change in the coagulation system that can be caused by: platelet hyperaggregability; excessive activation or decreased removal of coagulation factors; deficiencies of natural anticoagulants (antithrombin, protein C); or defective fibrinolysis.

Hyperaggregability of platelets increases thrombotic risk. Platelet aggregation is controlled by the interaction between platelets and the vascular endothelium. Platelets produce and release various pro-aggregating substances (including thromboxane A_2 and adenosine diphosphate), while the endothelium releases several inhibitors of platelet aggregation, notably prostacyclin. Disturbance in this balance can promote thrombosis. There is no correlation between thrombocytosis and hypercoagulation.

The coagulation system is finely regulated by three principal mechanisms: antithrombin; protein C; and the fibrinolytic system. These mechanisms operate to prevent thrombus formation in normal circumstances, and to limit and localize the formation of the haemostatic plug. If one or more of these mechanisms fail, thrombosis is favoured.

Antithrombin is synthesized primarily in the liver. It binds to and neutralizes thrombin (factor IIa) and factors IXa, Xa, XIa and XIIa. The rate of neutralization is markedly increased by heparin. Antithrombin deficiency may result from decreased production, increased loss or consumption. Decreased production of antithrombin can occur with hepatic failure, but thrombosis generally does not result because coexisting factor deficiencies favour haemorrhage. A similar situation occurs with protein-losing enteropathies. In contrast, protein-losing nephropathies permit selective loss of smaller plasma proteins such as antithrombin, creating an imbalance that favours hypercoagulability. DIC results in increased antithrombin consumption.

Protein C is a vitamin K-dependent natural anti-coagulant that inactivates factors Va and VIIIa, suppressing thrombin production. The role of protein C deficiency in thrombosis in small animal patients remains unclear.

The fibrinolytic system is extremely important in the pathophysiology of TE. In a normal animal, thrombi lyse spontaneously within hours. The presence of persistent TE therefore implies defective fibrinolysis. Studies in humans have shown defective fibrinolysis to be a contributing mechanism in all of the hypercoagulable states. The fibrinolytic system consists of plasminogen and the activators that convert plasminogen to plasmin. Plasmin causes dissolution of the fibrin clot. There are two physiological plasminogen activators, tissue-type plasminogen activator (t-PA) and urokinase (UK), and numerous inhibitors of these activators. Hypofibrinolysis can occur due to decreases in plasminogen or plasminogen activators, or due to increases in inhibitors. The most common mechanism appears to be an increase in plasminogen activator inhibitor (PAI-1).

Aetiology

The term 'hypercoagulable states' in small animals refers to acquired disorders in patients with underlying systemic disease known to be associated with an increased risk of thrombosis. In these diseases, the pathogenesis is generally multifactorial and complex. Inherited hypercoagulable states have not been reported in animals. While hypercoagulability represents a risk for TE, the actual incidence is variable and unpredictable. A single disease associated with hypercoagulability is unlikely to result in TE unless it is combined with another hypercoagulable state or thrombophilic condition. Retrospective studies of postmortem examinations in dogs and cats with pulmonary TE have shown that a large proportion of patients had more than one condition potentially predisposing to hypercoagulability (64% and 47%, respectively).

Numerous conditions have been associated with TE in dogs and cats (Figure 13.20). The likelihood of TE in patients with these conditions appears to be increased when the disease is severe, when a second hypercoagulable condition is present, and when other factors that promote thrombosis are present (such as hypoperfusion, dehydration, immobility, venous catheterization, tissue injury and inflammatory cytokines). For these reasons, TE is most commonly seen in the critical patient.

Most hypercoagulable states can result in arterial or venous thrombosis. There are, however, exceptions. Atherosclerosis is almost exclusively an arterial event, whereas IMHA is largely associated with venous thrombosis.

Clinical signs

The clinical signs of TE depend on the site of the TE, the function of the ischaemic organ, the degree of vascular compromise and the ability of collateral circulation to compensate for the insult. Clinical signs vary from mild subclinical effects to life-threatening complications. Manifestations of pulmonary thromboembolism (PTE) range from mild acute tachypnoea, to severe dyspnoea and death. Embolization of the central nervous system ('stroke') can cause a variety of acute neurological signs. Emboli related to cardiac disease in cats frequently lodge in the aortic bifurcation. Signs are peracute and the affected limb is painful, cool, paretic, pale and pulseless. In contrast, aortic TE in dogs varies from peracute to chronic, and chronic cases may show only lameness or paresis. Clinical myocardial infarction manifests as dysrhythmias or functional compromise. Visceral arterial thrombosis causes acute abdominal pain, vomiting, diarrhoea and/or haematochezia. Renal TE may cause abdominal pain, haematuria and/or vomiting. None of these signs is specific for TE. Diagnosis, therefore, frequently relies on a suspicion of TE and exclusion of other causes.

Diagnosis

The diagnosis of TE should include:

- Exclusion of other potential causes of the clinical signs
- Confirmation of the presence of a thrombus/embolus
- Laboratory evaluation of hypercoagulation
- Identification of underlying systemic disorders.

Depending on the site of TE, diagnosis can be difficult. Perhaps the most important aspect in diagnosis is an index of suspicion. In order to make a diagnosis of TE, it must be on the list of differentials. TE should be included in the differential diagnoses for dyspnoea, abdominal effusion, intestinal compromise, acute abdomen, haematuria, hindlimb lameness/paresis/paralysis and acute neurological signs. Since signs of TE are non-specific, and confirmation is frequently elusive, exclusion of other possible causes for the signs is an important diagnostic step.

Confirmation of the presence of a thrombus/embolus depends on the site, but generally relies on imaging studies. PTE can be confirmed via scintigraphy, spiral computed tomography (CT) or angiography. Cerebral TE may be evident on magnetic resonance imaging (MRI). Aortic, caval or visceral thrombosis may be detectable via ultrasonography and Doppler studies. In some situations, imaging studies may not be feasible, due to limited availability or

Renal disease (nephrotic syndrome, protein-losing nephropathy)

Cardiac disease (vegetative endocarditis, heartworm disease, cardiomyopathy)

Neoplasia (carcinomas and sarcomas)

Acute pancreatic necrosis

Immune-mediated haemolytic anaemia

Hypercortisolism (hyperadrenocorticism, chronic corticosteroid therapy)

Atherosclerosis (hypothyroidism)

Diabetes mellitus

Sepsis

Protein-losing enteropathy (rarely)

Major trauma

13.20 Conditions associated with thromboembolism in dogs and cats.

patient instability. In such cases, diagnosis rests on exclusion of other causes, documentation of hypercoagulability (where possible) and evidence of the presence of an underlying disease process predisposing to thrombosis.

The presence of hypercoagulability neither confirms nor predicts TE. It merely indicates that it is possible and, together with other compatible findings, enables the clinician to build a case for a diagnosis. Laboratory confirmation of hypercoagulability, however, is difficult. The routine coagulogram is not helpful in identifying hypercoagulation. There is little evidence for a relationship between thrombocytosis, shortened bleeding times, shortened PT and PTT and a thrombotic tendency. Routine screening coagulation tests, therefore, are generally normal in the hypercoagulable patient. When thrombosis has occurred, screening tests may show evidence of consumption (e.g. thrombocytopenia, prolonged PTT).

D-dimers have proven clinical utility in the diagnosis of TE in humans. Since D-dimers are specific for active coagulation and fibrinolysis, they are useful for detecting TE, but not thrombotic risk. The half-life of D-dimers, however, is short (approximately 5 hours). As such, they are most useful for detection of acute TE. They are also not specific for TE, with elevated concentrations being found in dogs with neoplasia, hepatic disease, renal failure, cardiac failure, internal haemorrhage, DIC and following surgical procedures. However, D-dimers in human patients have a high negative predictive value for TE, and are extensively employed as a screening test for PTE. They are considered most useful to rule out TE in patients deemed to have a low clinical probability. The utility of D-dimers in small animal patients is less clear, but may be similar. Sensitivities of 89–100% have been reported in dogs, using the standard ELISA test, a latex bead agglutination test (Accuclot D-dimer®, Sigma), and a canine-specific point-of-care test (AGEN canine D-dimer test®, Sigma). Reported specificity is approximately 70%. When semi-quantitative methods have been employed, specificity approaches 90%, with strong positive results (>1000 µg/l on latex agglutination) occurring only in patients with TE and with haemoabdomen. Based on the available data in dogs, it appears that TE can be considered unlikely if the D-dimer test is negative and clinical suspicion is low. TE is not, however, excluded by a negative D-dimer, especially if the time period from the event to presentation is prolonged. A positive test should always be interpreted in the light of other clinical findings. If these support TE, further testing is indicated. A strong positive test, in the absence of intracavitary haemorrhage, is highly suggestive of TE.

Significant hyperfibrinogenaemia can indicate hypercoagulability, but occurs in few of the hypercoagulable states (e.g. some cases of pancreatitis and sepsis). The majority of patients with TE do not have hyperfibrinogenaemia. Similarly, assay of antithrombin concentration or activity may be useful. Low concentrations of antithrombin have been correlated with thrombotic risk when antithrombin deficiency is the primary mechanism for thrombosis (e.g. protein-losing nephropathy). Antithrombin levels may also be decreased as a result of consumption during massive TE. Normal antithrombin levels do not exclude hypercoagulability. Thromboelastography (TEG) has been described in small animals for the assessment of overall hypercoagulability, and experience is encouraging. Few institutions, however, offer TEG, and further studies are needed to fully elucidate its clinical utility.

Since TE occurs almost exclusively secondary to one or more underlying conditions, any suspicion of TE should prompt a thorough search for these conditions (see Figure 13.20). While their presence does not confirm TE, it provides further support for the diagnosis of TE when a definitive diagnosis is not possible. Knowledge of any predisposing disease is also essential in clinical management.

Treatment

Therapy should include:

- Support of the affected organ system/s
- Prevention of thrombus propagation and recurrence
- Possibly removal of the thrombus/embolus.

A relatively small percentage of TE events are immediately fatal. Even in patients with disturbed fibrinolysis, some degree of reorganization and lysis occurs in the days following the event. Therefore, if the patient can be supported through the compromise, and further exacerbations can be prevented, survival is possible. In some cases, however, compromise may be so extreme that adequate support is not possible, or thrombi may persist for extended periods. In such cases, pharmacological or mechanical thrombolysis may be indicated.

Prevention of propagation and recurrence of thrombi

Thrombi tend to propagate, and this can result in further compromise. Furthermore, the patient with TE is always at risk for additional TE episodes. Management, therefore, should be focused on prevention, using anticoagulants and/or antiplatelet drugs. Traditionally, anticoagulants have been recommended to prevent venous thrombosis, and antiplatelet drugs to prevent arterial thrombosis. This was based largely on observations that arterial thrombi contain large numbers of platelets, whereas venous thrombi are composed predominantly of red cells in a fibrin matrix. Recent evidence in human patients has revealed that early venous thrombi are indeed platelet-rich, and that patients with venous TE have lower morbidity and mortality when antiplatelet drugs are added to the regimen. As such, there is an indication for the use of adjunctive antiplatelet therapy together with anticoagulants in patients with venous thrombosis. Furthermore, since most hypercoagulable states can result in either venous or arterial thrombosis in an unpredictable fashion, the concurrent use of anticoagulants and antiplatelet drugs has merit.

Anticoagulants: Unfractionated heparin is the cornerstone of anticoagulant therapy. Low-molecular-weight heparins (LMWH) offer significant advantages.

However, since experience in veterinary patients is limited, unfractionated heparin remains the most frequently used drug for initial management of TE in dogs and cats.

Unfractionated heparin is composed of mucopolysaccharides of varying molecular weights. The primary mechanism of action is the potentiation of antithrombin activity, leading to the inactivation of thrombin (factor IIa), and factors Xa, IXa, XIa and XIIa. Of these, thrombin and factor Xa are the most responsive to inhibition. The relative effect of heparin on these factors is dependent on its molecular size. Smaller heparin molecules are unable to catalyse thrombin inhibition. These molecules, however, are effective in catalysing the inhibition of factor Xa. Other effects of heparin include induction of decreased blood viscosity, decreased platelet function and increased vascular permeability. These effects contribute to the haemorrhagic risk.

The anticoagulant effects of a standard dose of heparin vary widely among patients. Heparin may be poorly absorbed from subcutaneous sites, and plasma clearance is variable and unpredictable. Higher-molecular-weight species are cleared more rapidly than lower-molecular-weight species, resulting in varied anticoagulant activity over time. In addition, some patients appear to have heparin resistance, requiring larger doses to achieve a therapeutic effect. It has been shown in human patients that, unless a prescriptive normogram is used, many patients receive inadequate heparinization in the initial 24–48 hours of therapy, resulting in an increased incidence of recurrent TE. Successful heparin therapy necessitates monitoring the anticoagulant response, and titrating the dose to the individual patient. Anticoagulant response can be monitored by measuring the plasma heparin concentration or the PTT. The therapeutic range of heparin is a concentration of 0.3–0.7 IU/ml by anti-factor Xa assay. The turnaround time of this assay, however, can make it impractical for clinical monitoring of the TE patient. Monitoring of the PTT is more feasible. Target ranges quoted in the veterinary literature are based on human studies, and appear to be excessive for dogs. Until further data is available, the author uses a target PTT range of 1.5–2.0 times the baseline.

It is impossible to give evidence-based recommendations for heparinization in small animals. There are exceedingly few studies, and most quoted doses are anecdotal. It would appear prudent, therefore, to utilize protocols established in human patients and in animal models, and to monitor PTT values and/or heparin concentrations closely. That is, to initiate heparin therapy with an intravenous bolus, followed by continuous-rate intravenous infusion. Studies in humans have demonstrated no increase in major bleeding, compared to subcutaneous administration. The author uses an extrapolation of this protocol in dogs (Figure 13.21). Because antithrombin is required for heparin effect, concurrent plasma transfusion is recommended in patients with documented or suspected antithrombin deficiency.

Subcutaneous administration of unfractionated heparin is not recommended for initial therapy. While this protocol can produce PTT values within target ranges, they are rarely achieved rapidly. The use of subcutaneous heparin in patients with acute TE should be reserved for those patients in which therapy with intravenous heparin is not feasible. Published doses vary enormously. A small number of canine studies have shown marked individual variability in response, emphasizing the importance of monitoring. The author uses a dose of 200 IU/kg s.c. q6h, with adjustments based on regular PTT determinations. There is evidence that PTT results do not reliably correlate with plasma heparin concentrations in cats. For this reason, it is prudent to evaluate plasma heparin concentrations intermittently in cats on heparin therapy.

LMWHs are manufactured from unfractionated heparin to yield smaller molecules. They differ from unfractionated heparin in several important respects: superior subcutaneous bioavailablility; a prolonged half-life; predictable clearance; and predictable antithrombotic effects. This allows once or twice daily dosing in humans, with treatment based on body weight and without laboratory monitoring. Their onset of action is rapid, with peak effects generally seen at 2–4 hours. LMWHs have little anti-IIa activity, and cannot be monitored via PTT. Anticoagulant efficacy is monitored via an anti-factor Xa assay.

An intravenous bolus of unfractionated heparin of 80–100 IU/kg is administered, followed by a continuous rate infusion of 18 IU/kg/h. PTT is evaluated 6 hours after initiation of therapy. The PTT is compared with the mean value of the normal range for that laboratory, or to the pretreatment value for that patient.
Adjustments are as follows:

PTT	Dose change (IU/kg/h)	Additional action	Next PTT
<1.2 x mean normal (baseline)	+4	Repeat bolus of 80 IU/kg	6 hours
1.2–1.5 x mean normal (baseline)	+2	Repeat bolus of 40 IU/kg	6 hours
1.5–2.0 x mean normal (baseline)	0	0	6 hours for first 24 hours, then daily
2.0–3.0 x mean normal (baseline)	-2	0	6 hours
>3.0 x mean normal (baseline)	-3	Stop infusion for 1 hour	6 hours

13.21 Protocol for intravenous unfractionated heparin infusion in dogs.

Experience with LMWH in small animals is limited. They therefore cannot be recommended as first choice in the initial therapy of TE. They can be considered, however, when intravenous heparin infusion is not feasible. In this role, subcutaneous therapy with LMWH is likely to be preferable to intermittent subcutaneous unfractionated heparin. Based on current knowledge, the author recommends a starting dose of dalteparin of 150 IU/kg s.c. q8–12h in the dog, and 100 IU/kg s.c. q8h in the cat. A suggested starting dose of enoxaparin is 1 mg/kg s.c. q12h. Regardless, it is imperative that anticoagulant efficacy is monitored until an effective dose is established for that patient. The target therapeutic range is a plasma anti-factor Xa concentration of 0.3–0.7 IU/ml. Monitoring can begin as early as 24 hours after initiation of therapy. Samples should be collected just prior to injection, and 3–4 hours following injection, to determine peak effect and duration. Dose and frequency are adjusted accordingly. Once an effective protocol is established for the patient, continued monitoring appears unnecessary, except for patients in renal failure.

Antiplatelet drugs: Aspirin is the only widely used antiplatelet drug in small animals. It acetylates cyclooxygenase, thus preventing the formation of thromboxanes and prostaglandins (including prostacyclin). The effect on platelets is irreversible whereas the effect on endothelial prostacyclin production is reversible. Effective antiplatelet therapy with aspirin, therefore, depends on using an ultra low dose that affects the platelets irreversibly, but allows the endothelial cells to recover. In dogs, ultra low-dose aspirin (0.5 mg/kg orally q24h) has been shown to be effective in decreasing platelet aggregation. In cats, a dose of 81 mg/cat q72h has been traditionally used. More recently, a study of aortic TE in cats revealed no statistical difference in outcome between traditional and low-dose (5 mg/cat q72h) aspirin, but there were fewer gastrointestinal effects with the low-dose protocol.

Thrombolysis

Thrombolytic agents (streptokinase (SK), urokinase, tissue plasminogen activator (t-PA)) are plasminogen activators that result in the production of plasmin, and subsequent dissolution of the fibrin thrombus. Advantages of thrombolytic therapy include rapid clot lysis and improved perfusion. These must be carefully weighed against the risk of massive haemorrhage, which is appreciable. The goal of thrombolytic therapy is to restore circulation rapidly, in such a manner that the procedure is clinically beneficial, and the risks of therapy justifiable. Thrombolytic therapy, therefore, is reserved for patients with life-threatening TE who are unlikely to survive without rapid reperfusion, or those with persistent TE that is significantly affecting function. Anticoagulant therapy, with intravenous unfractionated heparin or subcutaneous LMWH, is recommended following thrombolysis. Contraindications for thrombolytic therapy include: active internal bleeding; hypertension; recent (within 2–3 weeks) surgery or organ biopsy; and gastrointestinal ulceration.

Veterinary experience with thrombolytic agents is limited, making evidence-based recommendations for their use exceedingly difficult. Risk-to-benefit ratios have not been investigated, and safe and effective protocols are not established. There is a small number of reports involving the use of thrombolytics in animals. In one report, SK was used successfully in four dogs with non-pulmonary TE. In that report, the treatment protocols varied tremendously: loading doses of 5200–18,000 IU/kg were administered intravenously over 30 minutes once or three times. Maintenance doses ranged from 2083–9000 IU/kg/h, infused for 3–10 hours per day. The use of SK has been reported in cats with aortic TE, using a loading dose of 90,000 IU over 20–30 minutes, followed by a maintenance dose of 45,000 IU/h for 3 or more hours. Most cats had evidence of thrombus dissolution, but bleeding complications were common, and mortality high.

t-PA offers theoretical advantages over SK and, in humans, has proved superior. The successful use of t-PA has been described in a dog with aortic thrombosis. The author has used t-PA (together with heparin) with some success in a small number of dogs with PTE. Bolus intravenous injections of 1 mg/kg are given over 15–20 minutes every 1–3 hours until there is clinical evidence of improvement, then repeated thereafter as needed. Studies in human patients indicate that a single infusion of t-PA over 90 minutes may be superior to intermittent bolus injections. This remains to be evaluated in animals. Experience with t-PA in cats with aortic TE has not been encouraging. While thrombolysis generally occurred, approximately 50% of patients died during therapy, most deaths resulting from reperfusion injury.

Ongoing therapy

Initial therapy should be continued until the patient is stabilized, followed by a transition to longer-term therapy prior to hospital discharge. Longer-term anticoagulant therapy is aimed at preventing recurrent TE, and is addressed below. It should be continued until the risk of TE is considered sufficiently decreased. In patients with short-term reversible causes, such as pancreatitis, therapy for 1–2 weeks following clinical recovery is likely to be adequate. In patients with ongoing risk, such as IMHA, anticoagulant therapy is continued until the patient is weaned off corticosteroids. Indefinite therapy is recommended in patients with recurrent TE, or TE complicating malignancy or cardiac disease.

Prevention

The morbidity and mortality rates of TE are substantial. Moreover, diagnosis is difficult, and treatment of TE is not invariably successful. This makes prevention imperative in the patient at risk. Prevention should address all aspects of Virchow's triad. This includes:

- Minimizing vascular stasis by maintaining adequate perfusion
- Minimizing vascular injury by the appropriate handling of venous catheters
- Altering the haemostatic system via the appropriate use of drugs.

Antithrombotic drugs are indicated when there is significant risk of TE. Assessment of TE risk in veterinary patients remains largely subjective. Understanding the risk factors in patient groups and in individual patients forms the basis for risk determination. The most convincing evidence of risk is a prior TE event. In many patients, multiple risk factors are present, and the risks are cumulative. Such a situation therefore should prompt consideration of prophylaxis. The author considers severe IMHA, severe acute pancreatitis and sepsis to be indications for anticoagulant therapy. Risk stratification, however, is subjective, and based on the severity of disease and concomitant risk factors. Nephrotic syndrome is associated with a significant risk of TE, and determination of antithrombin level may provide objective evidence of risk. Risk may also be estimated by the severity of renal protein loss, the existence of potentially contributing factors and any history of prior TE events. Patients with uncomplicated hyperadrenocorticism or diabetes mellitus appear to have a low incidence of TE, and the need for prophylactic drugs in these patients is doubtful. The risk increases, however, when another thrombophilic condition is added, such as hypertension, protein-losing nephropathy or surgery.

The choice of anticoagulant for PTE prophylaxis depends on the anticipated duration of therapy, and the compliance and finances of the owner. Options include subcutaneous unfractionated heparin, warfarin and LMWH. Prophylaxis is usually initiated with low-dose, subcutaneous, unfractionated heparin. In human patients, small fixed doses are used. This protocol does not require laboratory monitoring, and has been shown to reduce the rate of fatal PTE by two thirds. Recommended doses of unfractionated heparin for prophylaxis in small animals range from 100–200 IU/kg s.c. q8–12h. These doses seem unlikely to result in major haemorrhage, but efficacy rates have yet to be assessed.

Warfarin is most commonly used for long-term outpatient TE prophylaxis. It is an oral vitamin K antagonist, thus inhibiting the activation of vitamin K-dependent factors. Due to the half-lives of these factors, the anticoagulant effect of warfarin is not immediate. During the first 24–48 hours of therapy, only factor VII and protein C are significantly affected. Inhibition of protein C leads to a thrombotic tendency, before other factors are inhibited. For these reasons, heparin therapy should always overlap warfarin for at least the first 2 days, and until therapeutic levels of warfarin are achieved. Warfarin is initiated at a dose of 0.05–0.1 mg/kg orally q24h in the dog and the cat. A therapeutic range is generally achieved within 5–7 days. Therapy is monitored by use of the PT, and the calculated international normalization ratio (INR). The therapeutic range for warfarin is an INR of 2.0–3.0. Due to the risk of haemorrhage, and the influence of diet, comorbidity and administration of other drugs, close continued monitoring of warfarin therapy on an outpatient basis is essential.

LMWHs are an attractive alternative to warfarin. They are less frequently associated with haemorrhage and, after the initial establishment of an effective dose, do not require ongoing monitoring. Since their onset of action is rapid, unfractionated heparin can be discontinued when LMWH therapy is initiated. These benefits contribute to offsetting the costs of these drugs. Until effective dosing protocols are established in small animals, however, initial dose adjustments based on anti-Xa assay are mandatory (see above).

Antiplatelet drugs are indicated as adjunctive therapy in most cases of TE prophylaxis. In diseases associated almost exclusively with arterial thrombosis (e.g. atherosclerosis) or where anticoagulant therapy is not feasible or is deemed excessive, sole therapy with aspirin has merit. A recent retrospective study indicated improved outcomes in dogs with IMHA when ultra low-dose aspirin (with or without heparin) was included in the treatment regimen.

References and further reading

Catalfamo JL and Dodds WJ (1988) Hereditary and acquired thrombopathias. *Veterinary Clinics of North America: Small Animal Practice* **18**, 185–193

Fogh JM and Fogh IT (1988) Inherited coagulation disorders. *Veterinary Clinics of North America: Small Animal Practice* **18**, 231–243

Giger U (1992) The feline AB blood group system and incompatability reactions. In: *Kirk's Current Veterinary Therapy XI*, ed. RW Kirk and JD Bonagura, pp. 470–474. WB Saunders, Philadelphia

Giger U (1998) Emergency management of the bleeding patient: plasma and platelet transfusions, vitamin K and DDAVP. *Proceedings of the Sixth International Veterinary Emergency and Critical Care Symposium*, 205–206

Hackner SG (2000) Hypercoagulation: Introduction and perspective. *American College of Veterinary Emergency and Critical Care Postgraduate Course*, 8–15

Hackner SG (2004) Intravenous immunoglobulins in the therapy of immune-mediated hematologic disorders. *Proceedings of the Tenth International Veterinary Emergency and Critical Care Symposium*, 343–347

Hackner SG (2004) Pulmonary thromboembolism: The current state of affairs – I Etiology, pathophysiology and diagnosis. *Proceedings of the Tenth International Veterinary Emergency and Critical Care Symposium*, 610–614

Hackner SG (2004) Pulmonary thromboembolism: The current state of affairs – II Treatment and prevention. *Proceedings of the Tenth International Veterinary Emergency and Critical Care Symposium*, 615–620

Harvey JW (1995) Methemoglobinaemia and Heinz-body haemolytic anemia. In: *Kirk's Current Veterinary Therapy XII*, ed. JD Bonagura, pp. 437–442. WB Saunders, Philadelphia

Hoffman M (2003) Remodelling the blood coagulation cascade. *Journal of Thrombosis and Thrombolysis* **16**, 17–20

Jain NC (1993) Erythrocyte physiology and changes in disease. In: *Essentials of Veterinary Haematology*, ed. NC Jain, pp. 133–158. Lea and Febiger, Philadelphia

Johnson LR, Lappin MR and Baker DC (1999) Pulmonary thromboembolism in 29 dogs: 1985–1995. *Journal of Veterinary Internal Medicine* **13**, 338–345

Jordan HL, Grindem CB and Breitschwerdt EB (1993) Thrombocytopenia in cats: a retrospective study of 41 cases. *Journal of Veterinary Internal Medicine* **7**, 261–265

LaRue MJ and Murtaugh RJ (1990) Pulmonary thromboembolism in dogs: 47 cases (1986–1987). *Journal of the American Veterinary Medical Association* **197**, 1368–1372

Lewis DC and Meyers KM (1996) Canine idiopathic thrombocytopenic purpura. *Journal of Veterinary Internal Medicine* **10**, 207–218

Rackear DG (1988) Drugs that alter the haemostatic mechanism. *Veterinary Clinics of North America: Small Animal Practice* **18**, 67–77

Ramsey CC, Burney DP, Macintire DK and Finn-Bodner S (1996) Use of streptokinase in four dogs with thrombosis. *Journal of the American Veterinary Medical Association* **209**, 780–785

Rozanski EA, Callan MB, Hughes D, Sanders N and Giger U (2002) Comparison of platelet count recovery with use of vincristine and prednisone or prednisone alone for treatment for severe immune-mediated thrombocytopenia in dogs. *Journal of the American Veterinary Medical Association* **220**, 477–481

Stewart AF and Feldman BF (1993) Immune-mediated haemolytic anemia. Part II: clinical entity, diagnosis and treatment theory. *Compendium on Continuing Education for the Practicing Veterinarian* **15**, 1479–1491

Stokol T (2003) Plasma D-dimer for the diagnosis of thromboembolic disorders in dogs. *Veterinary Clinics of North America: Small Animal Practice* **33**, 1419–1435

Stone MS and Cotter SM (1992) Practical guidelines for transfusion therapy. In: *Kirk's Current Veterinary Therapy XI*, ed. RW Kirk and JD Bonagura, pp. 475–479. WB Saunders, Philadelphia

Thompson MF, Scott-Moncrieff JC and Hogan DF (2001) Thrombolytic therapy in dogs and cats. *Journal of Veterinary Emergency and Critical Care* **11**, 111–121

Troy GC (1988) An overview of haemostasis. *Veterinary Clinics of North America: Small Animal Practice* **18**, 5–20

Tseng LW, Hughes D and Giger U (2001) Evaluation of a point-of-care coagulation analyzer for measurement of prothrombin time, activated partial thromboplastin time, and activated clotting time in dogs. *American Journal of Veterinary Research* **62(9)**, 1455

Weinkle TK, Center SA, Randolph JF *et al.* (2005) Evaluation of prognostic factors, survival rates, and treatment protocols for immune-mediated hemolytic anemia in dogs: 151 cases (1993–2002). *Journal of the American Veterinary Medical Association* **11**, 1869–1874

Weiser MG (1995) Erythrocyte responses and disorders. In: *Textbook of Veterinary Internal Medicine IV*, ed. S. Ettinger, pp. 1864–1891. WB Saunders, Philadelphia

Weiser G (1995) Haematologic technology for diagnosing anemias. In: *Kirk's Current Veterinary Therapy XII*, ed. JD Bonagura, pp. 437–442. WB Saunders, Philadelphia

14

Transfusion medicine

Gillian Gibson

Introduction

Interest in veterinary transfusion medicine has been growing over the past few decades, in line with the advancing capabilities of general practitioners and speciality referral hospitals in managing critically ill and emergency patients. Recent changes in the guidance provided by the RCVS and in drug legislation are likely to lead to further development of transfusion medicine and animal blood banking within the UK.

As all blood must be sourced from healthy donors, this is leading to an increased need for donor animals. A practice can increase its donor pool by actively recruiting suitable candidates, and screening for blood type in advance of need. Client evenings or veterinary staff visits to breed or training club meetings, information displays in reception areas, and local newspaper articles can increase public awareness about the need for canine and feline donors, and often lead to people volunteering their animal for donation. Volunteer-based donor schemes rely on the altruism of the pet owner, with direct rewards usually being a bag of pet food or toys for the donor. Currently there are no commercial animal blood banks in the UK. Historically, whole blood (drawn directly from the donor with the use of an anticoagulant) has been used in veterinary medicine, and is usually administered to the recipient within hours of donation. However, with increased need for and use of blood coupled with limited supply, administration of blood components (packed red cells, plasma) is a more economical use of this resource.

Knowledge and practice of appropriate blood collection, processing, storage and administration methods are essential to ensure the safety of the donor and the recipient, as well as to maximize the use of limited clinical resources.

Donor selection

Canine blood donors

Canine donors should be healthy, well tempered, large-breed dogs weighing at least 25 kg to allow collection of blood in standard human collection bags. Many blood donor programmes set an age limit of 1–8 years, with use of dogs older than the age limit at the discretion of the veterinary surgeon after careful evaluation of the donor. The dogs should receive routine veterinary preventative health care, including vaccination according to practice protocols. They should not be receiving any medication at the time of donation with the exception of flea preventive, routine worming medication or heartworm preventative (location specific). As blood is most frequently obtained from the jugular vein, consideration should be given to the conformation of the dog and venous access. It is preferable to use dogs that will remain still with minimal restraint during the blood collection procedure, avoiding sedation and possible adverse consequences of its use. Any dog that has previously received a transfusion may have developed alloantibodies against differing blood types and is therefore unsuitable as a donor. Some programmes exclude bitches which have previously whelped litters due to similar concerns.

Pre-donation tests for canine donors include determination of blood type (at a minimum, DEA 1.1 status), yearly haematology and general biochemistry profiles, as well as screening for infectious diseases endemic to the region or to geographical locations in which the animal previously lived. Infectious disease agents of concern, which have the potential to be transmitted by blood transfusion, include *Babesia*, *Leishmania*, *Ehrlichia*, *Anaplasma*, *Neorickettsia*, *Brucella canis*, *Trypanosoma cruzi*, *Bartonella vinsonii* and *Mycoplasma haemocanis*. The decision about which donors to test for these diseases, as well as the frequency of testing and retesting, depends on the risk of infection for that particular donor. The cost of testing should be considered; however, the safety of the blood transfusion is paramount, and appropriate testing of a donor should not be compromised for financial reasons. In the UK, exclusion of dogs that have travelled outside the UK currently avoids the need for exhaustive infectious disease testing. However, periodic review of this policy will be important, as the prevalence of infectious disease may increase with greater pet travel.

Feline blood donors

Feline donors should be clinically healthy cats between the ages of 1 and 8 years, receiving routine veterinary preventative health care. They should weigh at least 4 kg. Unlike canine donors, cats usually require sedation for the donation; however, they should still be of an agreeable temperament to allow transportation to the veterinary surgery and handling for administration of the sedative. Given the problems with naturally occurring alloantibodies in cats (see Feline blood types) it is essential that all feline donors as well as recipients be blood typed prior to collecting blood to prevent incompatibility of mismatched transfusions. To ensure that feline donors are in good health, haematology, serum biochemistry and infectious disease screening for feline leukaemia virus (FeLV) (serology), feline immunodeficiency virus (FIV) (serology) and *Mycoplasma haemofelis* (polymerase chain reaction (PCR)) are evaluated each year. Cats that are positive for infectious diseases should not be used as donors. Furthermore, to have confidence in the maintenance of a negative disease status, it is preferable to use only cats that are confined to living indoors.

Given the need for sedation in donor cats, and the stringent requirements for prevention of infectious disease transmission, it is often difficult to develop a large pool of feline donors. Some larger veterinary facilities choose instead to house a colony of disease-free donor cats which, after a period of service, are re-homed as pets and allowed to lead an indoor or outdoor lifestyle as their owner prefers. Veterinary surgeons in the UK seeking to establish a donor colony should consult the Home Office and RCVS regarding the legal requirements.

Testing for the presence of other infectious disease agents such as *Bartonella* should be considered, and is recommended by some haematologists. Screening healthy donor cats for *Cytauxzoon felis*, *Ehrlichia*, *Anaplasma* and *Neorickettsia* may be warranted if these agents are endemic in the area. Controversy remains over testing donor cats for feline coronavirus, as many clinically healthy cats can have positive titres yet never develop clinical feline infectious peritonitis (FIP), and transmission of clinical disease via blood transfusion has not yet been documented. Despite the lack of documentation of transmission of clinical disease, enough concern exists about possible transmission from seropositive donors that some institutions prefer to use donors who are negative for coronavirus. *Toxoplasma gondii* screening antigen, antibody or DNA tests are not recommended, as healthy cats may have positive test results, which are not necessarily a concern for the safety of the blood transfusion.

General considerations

In addition to the yearly comprehensive health examinations, a complete donor history, physical examination and packed cell volume (PCV) or haemoglobin (Hb) level should be performed prior to every donation, to safeguard the health and confirm the suitability of the donor.

Blood types

Red blood cell types are determined by species-specific, inherited antigens present on the cell surface. Blood type incompatibility is observed clinically as transfusion reactions or neonatal isoerythrolysis, the occurrence and severity of which is variable between individuals and species. The frequency of canine and feline blood types varies with geographical location and breed. Although the published population incidence of various blood types may offer the verterinary surgeon guidance, it is based on surveys with limited animal numbers and may not be applicable to the individual animal in question.

Canine blood types

Many systems are used to describe the blood groups of dogs; however, the dog erythrocyte antigen (DEA) nomenclature is most widely in use in the current literature. Typing antisera exist for 6 DEAs (1.1, 1.2, 3, 4, 5 and 7). For all of the DEA groups, a dog may be positive or negative. The DEA 1 group has at least two subtypes, DEA 1.1 and 1.2. A third subtype, DEA 1.3, has been described but not yet extensively evaluated due to lack of typing antisera. A dog may be positive for only one of these DEA 1 subtypes, or it may be negative for all three.

The relevance of blood type is related to its antigenic potential. The most antigenic blood type is DEA 1.1; however there are no naturally occurring alloantibodies against DEA 1.1. As such, most dogs will not experience a severe transfusion reaction from a first transfusion of DEA 1.1-incompatible blood. However, sensitization occurs in DEA 1.1-negative dogs that receive DEA 1.1-positive cells. Antibodies (strong haemolysins and agglutinins) are produced which can cause an acute haemolytic transfusion reaction following repeated antigen exposure (e.g. a second transfusion with DEA 1.1-positive blood). Additionally in some of these dogs a delayed haemolytic transfusion reaction may occur more than 9 days after the first transfusion, as antibody production increases. Production of antibodies to other red cell antigens may develop in a sensitized recipient as early as 4 days after transfusion, emphasizing the importance of crossmatching donor and recipient samples prior to a second blood transfusion.

The significance of transfusion incompatibility associated with red cell antigens DEA 3, 5 and 7 varies, depending on the clinical consequences of a mistyped transfusion, as well as the prevalence of these antigens in the dog population. Sensitization to these antigens or the presence of naturally occurring alloantibodies may result in a delayed transfusion reaction involving sequestration and loss of transfused red blood cells. Prevalence studies in the US report a low incidence of both DEA 3 and 5, with naturally occurring alloantibodies documented in 10% and 20% of dogs negative for these types respectively. DEA 7-negative dogs may experience delayed transfusion reactions as a consequence of transfusion with DEA 7-positive blood. Considering that approximately 50% of dogs are positive for this antigen, the presence of this alloantibody, although of weak titre, may be significant with regard to the possibility of a transfusion reaction.

Most dogs are DEA 4-positive. There is no known naturally occurring alloantibody to this antigen, and in many instances its transfusion significance is minor. However, a recent report of a DEA 4-negative dog, sensitized by previous transfusion, experiencing an acute haemolytic transfusion reaction after administration of DEA 4-positive blood, suggests that more investigation into the significance of this antigen is necessary.

Blood typing is based on an agglutination reaction. Most antigens are detected by visualizing a haemoagglutination reaction in response to polyclonal or monoclonal antibodies. When using these antibodies, agglutination detects the presence of the particular red cell antigen being tested, and the dog is then considered positive for that antigen. Lack of haemoagglutination in response to the antibody indicates that the dog is negative for the test antigen.

As DEA 1.1 is the most antigenic blood type, it is strongly advised that the DEA 1.1 status of both the donor and recipient is determined prior to transfusion, or that only DEA 1.1-negative donors are used. DEA 1.1 testing can be performed by a variety of methods, either at a reference laboratory or using an in-house card test kit. Typing for antigens other than DEA 1.1 requires the use of polyclonal antisera, available from only a few specialized blood service laboratories. Ideally donors should be negative for DEA 1.1, 1.2, 3, 5 and 7. However, the cost involved in typing for these antigens must be weighed against the low risk of a transfusion reaction after the first transfusion to a recipient typed only for DEA 1.1. As a general rule, DEA 1.1-negative dogs should only receive DEA 1.1-negative blood, and DEA 1.1-positive dogs may receive either DEA 1.1-negative or -positive blood. Subsequent potential incompatibilities to known or as yet undetermined antigens in animals who receive repeated transfusions should be identified on a crossmatch.

The card test kits for DEA 1.1 use whole blood and the test is completed within 2 minutes. Blood typing cannot be performed easily in animals with autoagglutination, because a false-positive or undeterminable blood type will result. If in-saline autoagglutination is present, the cells should be washed to assess for persistence. If the results of the typing are unclear, the recipient is considered to be DEA 1.1-negative until the autoagglutination resolves and an attempt can be made to type a repeat blood sample.

Weak positive results should be interpreted cautiously, as occasionally false-positive results to DEA 1.1 occur when testing DEA 1.2-positive dogs. Such a dog is actually DEA 1.1-negative; however, the weak positive result may lead the clinician to classify the dog as DEA 1.1-positive. The clinical implication of this false-positive result is that a DEA 1.1-negative dog may be administered DEA 1.1-positive red cells, resulting in sensitization of the recipient to DEA 1.1 and an increased risk of experiencing an acute haemolytic transfusion reaction upon repeated exposure to DEA 1.1 positive cells.

Furthermore, care should also be taken when typing severely anaemic dogs. The prozone effect may prevent proper agglutination of blood from a DEA 1.1-positive dog with the DEA reagent. Due to the low number of red blood cells, the quantity of antigen is reduced compared to the amount of antibody present in the reagent, consequently cross-linking between cells (agglutination reaction) may not occur. In this circumstance, it may be helpful to centrifuge the patient's whole blood test sample, and remove one drop of the plasma to increase the relative concentration of red blood cells. The red cells and plasma are then remixed prior to performing the card test with the modified whole blood sample. Finally, inaccurate results may occur if a patient has recently received a transfusion (prior to sampling for blood type determination).

Given these potential pitfalls with in-house blood typing, although it is advisable to determine the blood type of a dog prior to transfusion, in the emergency situation it may be necessary to assume that the patient is DEA 1.1-negative and use only a DEA 1.1-negative donor. This practice would prevent the administration of DEA 1.1-positive cells to a DEA 1.1-negative recipient. Using donors of previously determined known blood types is then of utmost importance. Patients should always be sampled prior to transfusion so blood typing can be performed at a later time point.

Feline blood types

Blood groups in cats are described by the A–B system, which includes three blood types: A, B and AB. The blood types are inherited as a simple dominant trait, with A being dominant over B. Genotypically type A cats are either homozygous *a/a* or heterozygous *a/b*; whereas type B cats are homozygous *b/b*. Type AB is a rare blood type in which a third allele is present, recessive to the *a* allele but dominant to the *b* allele, leading to expression of both A and B antigens. Mating studies have shown that type AB is not simply the result of mating a type A to a type B cat, but rather the type A cat must carry the rare allele for type AB blood. However this genetic pattern has not applied in all AB cats, and there is likely to be more than one mechanism for inheritance of this blood type.

Typing of cats prior to transfusion is imperative. In cats, naturally occurring alloantibodies are present in the plasma. These alloantibodies are isoagglutinins against the red blood cell antigen that is not present in that individual cat (i.e. type A cats have alloantibodies against the B antigen and vice versa). These antibodies are found in all type A and B cats after 2 months of age and their formation does not require prior exposure through transfusion or pregnancy. These antibodies may cause a potentially fatal immediate transfusion reaction and are also responsible for neonatal isoerythrolysis. Therefore, **all donor and recipient cats must be blood typed** prior to transfusion, even in an emergency situation. The risk of a transfusion reaction is greatest if a type B cat is given type A blood, as almost all type B cats have high titres of anti-A antibodies that result in rapid intravascular haemolysis (with complement activation) of the donor red blood cells. Signs of an acute haemolytic transfusion reaction may occur after a B cat has received as little as 1 ml of type A blood. Initially the cat may appear either depressed or agitated with bradycardia, apnoea or hypopnoea; it may also vocalize, salivate, urinate and defecate (signs typical of an anaphylactic reaction). If cats survive this initial phase, they may become tachycardic and tachypnoeic, and haemolysis and haemoglobinuria may become evident. Type A cats generally have weak anti-B antibodies, that are usually of a low titre. The transfusion reaction if a type A cat receives type B blood is usually less severe, resulting in accelerated destruction of the red blood cells primarily due to extravascular haemolysis. The clinical signs observed in these patients are usually milder, and most often recognized by a rapid drop in PCV within days after a transfusion. Thus, type A cats must only receive type A blood and type B cats must only receive type B blood. The rarer type AB cats do not possess either alloantibody. Type AB cats should ideally receive type AB blood, but when that is not available type A blood is the next best choice.

The presence of naturally occurring alloantibodies may cause neonatal isoerythrolysis in type A and AB kittens born to a type B queen, due to the ingestion of colostral anti-A alloantibodies in the first few days of life. Clinical signs of neonatal isoerythrolysis may develop within hours to days of colostrum ingestion, and include anaemia, haemoglobinaemia, jaundice, and in some cases death as a consequence of red cell haemolysis. Knowledge of the blood type of breeding cats and offspring, and removal and foster nursing of at-risk kittens for the first 2–3 days of life can prevent this transfer of colostral antibody and subsequent neonatal isoerythrolysis.

Breeds with a documented increased prevalence of type B compared to the non-pedigree cat population include: British Shorthair, Devon Rex, Persian, Somali, Abyssinian, Himalayan, Birman, and Scottish Fold. Previous prevalence reports from the US and UK suggest that the majority of domestic non-pedigree cats are type A (92.1–98.2%); however, recent studies indicate that the prevalence of type B is increasing.

Blood typing can be performed by several methods, including tube and slide agglutination assays, gel column and card methods. Blood typing by these methods indicates agglutination in the presence of A or B cells, determining the blood type as type A or B. The simplest in-house method available is the use of a blood typing agglutination test card with monoclonal anti-A antibodies and *Triticum vulgaris* lectin as the B agglutinin (Figure 14.1), although alternative in-house testing methods are being evaluated. Agglutination with both antigens A and B determines that the cat is type AB. Autoagglutination must be excluded prior to typing, and as in dogs false results may occur in anaemic cats.

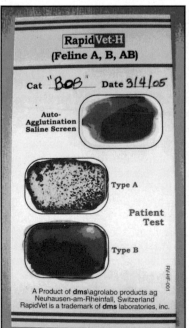

14.1

Feline blood type card – agglutination in the Patient Test Type A well identifies the cat as having type A blood. (Courtesy of dms laboratories, inc.).

Occasionally type AB cats may not be correctly identified, as only a weak agglutination reaction may occur in the A well. Although type AB cats are rare, this error could lead to misinterpretation of the result as type B, with the potential for administration of a mismatched transfusion (type B blood to a type AB cat). When using the card method, it has been recommended to confirm AB or B typing results with either alloantibody or crossmatch testing, or using an alternative typing method at a commercial laboratory.

Crossmatching

Crossmatching is performed to determine the serological compatibility between the patient and the donor red blood cells. Crossmatching in dogs should be performed whenever:

- The recipient has been previously transfused more than 4 days prior, even if a DEA 1.1-negative donor was used
- There has been a history of a transfusion reaction
- The recipient's transfusion history is unknown
- The recipient has been previously pregnant.

Crossmatching allows detection of previous sensitization, but does not prevent new sensitization from occurring. Once the recipient receives a transfusion and 4–5 days elapse, crossmatches must be repeated as the recipient may no longer be compatible with the same donors.

The major crossmatch is an assessment of the compatibility, as assessed by agglutination, between the donor RBCs and patient plasma/serum. The minor crossmatch assesses the interaction between the donor plasma/serum and patient RBCs. Minor crossmatch incompatibilities are less frequently the cause of haemolytic transfusion reactions and are mostly of concern when large volumes of plasma are to be administered. Patient autoagglutination or haemolysis may result in incompatibility and a control should be run with the patient RBCs and patient serum (Figure 14.2). Some animals may have antibodies at too low a level to be detected by crossmatch and may then experience a mild haemolytic reaction despite an apparently compatible result.

Cats should have a crossmatch performed if they require more than one transfusion, as previously transfused blood (even though it was the same A–B type) may induce antibody production against RBC antigens separate from the A–B blood group system. If the donor or recipient blood type is unknown, a crossmatch must be performed. A recently detected novel red cell antigen causing crossmatch incompatibility in a type A cat has prompted a recommendation that crossmatching may be necessary prior to even a first blood transfusion in cats.

Despite using blood products from a crossmatch-compatible donor, it is still possible for a patient to experience a haemolytic or non-haemolytic transfusion reaction, and recipient monitoring during and after administration of blood products is essential.

Standard crossmatch procedure

1. Collect blood into an EDTA tube from recipient and donor. Alternatively for the donor sample, a segment of anticoagulated blood from the donor blood tubing may be used.

2. Centrifuge tubes to settle the red blood cells, remove the supernatant and transfer to a clean, labelled glass or plastic tube.

3. Wash the red blood cells three times with a normal saline solution, discard the supernatant after each wash.

4. Re-suspend the washed red blood cells to create a 3–5% solution by adding 0.2 ml of red blood cells to 4.8 ml of normal saline (or 1 drop RBC:20 drops saline).

5. For each donor prepare three tubes labelled as major, minor and recipient control.

6. Add to each tube 1 drop of the appropriate 3–5% red blood cells and 2 drops of plasma according to the following:
   - Major crossmatch = donor red blood cells + recipient plasma
   - Minor crossmatch = recipient red blood cells + donor plasma
   - Recipient control = recipient red blood cells + recipient plasma.

7. Incubate the tubes for 15 minutes at room temperature. (Ideally the crossmatch procedure should also be performed at 4 and 37°C.)

8. Centrifuge the tubes at 1000 x g for approximately 15 seconds to allow the cells to settle.

9. Examine the samples for haemolysis (reddening of the solution).

10. Gently tap the tubes to resuspend the cells, examine and score the tubes for agglutination as follows:
    - 4+ one solid aggregate of cells
    - 3+ several large clumps/aggregates of cells
    - 2+ medium sized clumps/aggregates of cells, clear background
    - 1+ small/microscopic aggregates of cells, turbid reddish background
    - ±   microscopic aggregates.

11. If macroscopic agglutination is not observed, transfer a small amount of the tube contents to a labelled glass slide and examine for microscopic agglutination (take care not to confuse with rouleaux formation).

12. Recipient control:
    - If there is no haemolysis or agglutination noted in the recipient control tube, the results are valid and incompatibilities can be interpreted
    - If there is haemolysis or agglutination present in equal scoring to the donor test samples, the compatibility and suitability of the donor cannot be accurately assessed.

Feline crossmatch abbreviated slide procedure

An alternative procedure for crossmatch analysis in a cat involves visualizing the presence of agglutination on a slide rather than in a test tube.

1. Follow crossmatch procedure steps 1–2 above.

2. For each donor prepare three slides labelled as major, minor and recipient control.

3. Place 1 drop red blood cells and 2 drops plasma on to each slide according to the following:
   - Major crossmatch = donor red blood cells + recipient plasma
   - Minor crossmatch = recipient red blood cells + donor plasma
   - Recipient control = recipient red blood cells + recipient plasma.

4. Gently rock the slides to mix the plasma and red cells and examine for haemagglutination after 1–5 minutes (presence of agglutination indicative of incompatibility); recipient agglutination will invalidate results.

14.2 Crossmatch procedure.

Collection, processing and storage of blood

Blood collection systems

All whole blood collection should take place in an aseptic manner and should use an appropriate anticoagulant. The anticoagulant solutions most often used are ACD (acid–citrate–dextrose), CPD (citrate–phosphate–dextrose) or CPDA-1 (citrate–phosphate–dextrose–adenine). Most of the commercially available blood collection systems contain either CPD or CPDA-1. ACD is more often used in open systems when collecting smaller volumes of blood. The volume of anticoagulant used and the duration of time for which the blood product can be stored varies depending on the composition of the anticoagulant and the collection method. ACD is used at a ratio of 1 ml of anticoagulant to 7–9 ml of blood and CPD and CPDA-1 are typically used in a ratio of 1 ml anticoagulant to 7 ml of blood. Use of other anticoagulants (e.g. sodium citrate, heparin) is not recommended.

Whole blood may be collected using a closed or open collection system. A closed system is one in which the only exposure of the collection bag or its contents to air prior to administration is when the needle is uncapped to perform venipuncture during collection. Examples of a closed system are commercially available 450 ml blood collection bags containing 63 ml of CPD or CPDA-1 anticoagulant with an attached 16 gauge needle. These are most commonly used to collect blood from donor dogs weighing >25 kg. Multi-bag systems with empty transfer satellite bags and red cell preservative may be used for component processing (Figure 14.3). Packed red blood cells prepared from CPDA-1 closed-collection system processing have a storage life of 20 days when maintained at 1–6°C. Whole blood collected into CPD or CPDA-1 in a similar manner has a storage life of 28 days or 35 days respectively.

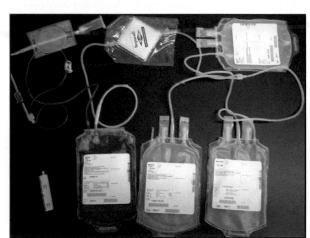

14.3 Example of a commercially available closed collection system with multiple connecting bags allowing processing of whole blood and storage as packed red cells and plasma.

Any system in which there is one or more additional site of potential bacterial contamination during blood collection or processing is by definition an open system. All blood products collected in an open system must be administered within 4 hours, or if stored in a refrigerator (1–6°C) they must be used within 24 hours. Blood collection using syringes or empty bags with added anticoagulant, as used in cats and for other small-volume collections, is classified as an open system (Figure 14.4).

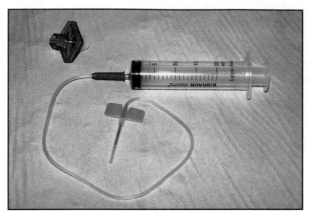

14.4 Example of an open collection system. A syringe and butterfly catheter may be used for small volume blood collections. The paediatric 18 μm filter (Hemo-Nate®, Utah Medical Products Inc.) in the top left corner may be used as an in-line filter during blood administration.

The volume of blood that may be collected safely from canine and feline donors is approximately 20% of their blood volume, every 3–4 weeks. A recommended volume limit is 18 ml/kg for dogs and 10–12 ml/kg for cats. Most volunteer donor schemes using client-owned pets as donors extend the donation interval to every 8 weeks.

Donor health check

Prior to every donation, information on the donor animal is reviewed and a brief questionnaire is completed by the owner. The age and general good health of the donor and the date of the last donation are confirmed. Many aspects will have been covered during the donor selection procedure; however, it is important to assess any changes in status of those that are repeat donors. A full physical examination is performed and noted in the donor file. A small sample of blood for measurement of PCV or Hb level is obtained prior to every donation to ensure the donor has a normal red cell mass. The result is recorded in the donor file. This also allows the recognition of trends in the donor animal's PCV over time.

Blood collection

The jugular vein is the recommended venipuncture site in both dogs and cats, because of its size and accessibility. Collection should be initiated with a rapid, uninterrupted single stick to avoid cell damage or excessive activation of coagulation factors. Strict aseptic technique and the use of sterile equipment minimizes the possibility of bacterial contamination. All donors must be closely monitored during blood collection by assessing their mucous membrane colour, pulse rate and quality, and respiratory rate and effort. If any concerns develop, the donation should be discontinued.

Most dogs are able to donate blood without the use of sedation, and it is preferable to train a donor to the procedure. Placing the dog in lateral recumbency, on a soft blanket on a table, facilitates comfortable restraint (for donor and veterinary personnel) for the period of approximately 10 minutes required for blood collection (Figure 14.5). This position also allows adequate digital pressure to be applied to the venipuncture site for haemostasis whilst the animal maintains a recumbent position following donation. Other positions in decreasing order of author preference include sitting, standing and sternal recumbency.

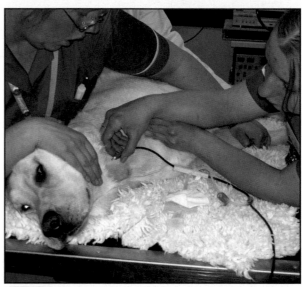

14.5 Blood donation with the donor dog in lateral recumbency using a closed collection system.

Collection of whole blood from dogs using a commercial blood bag may be accomplished via gravity alone (Figure 14.6); however, use of a specialized vacuum chamber may decrease the donation time and therefore the amount of time the donor must be restrained (Figure 14.7). A cylindrical acrylic plastic chamber houses the collection bag during the donation, with the tubing to the donor passing out through a notch at the top of the chamber. A vacuum source that can be regulated at low vacuum pressures (<33.8 kPa (254 mmHg)) is attached to the chamber, and the entire chamber, with collection bag inserted, is placed on a gram scale (Figure 14.8). The gram scale is used to monitor the weight of the bag during collection, to ensure that an adequate but not excessive amount of blood is collected, in order to preserve the appropriate anticoagulant to blood ratio. When collecting blood via gravity alone (Figure 14.6), the bag should be placed on a gram scale and the weight of the bag and anticoagulant measured prior to venipuncture. Again, the bag should be weighed during donation to confirm collection of the correct blood volume. The volume of blood that should be collected into a commercial blood bag is 450 ml, with an allowable 10% variance (405–495 ml). The weight of 1 ml of canine blood is approximately 1.053 g; therefore, the weight of an acceptable unit using one of these bags is approximately 426–521 g.

1. Clip hair over the jugular groove and apply local anaesthetic (e.g. EMLA) cream. This is usually performed at the time of the health check, prior to the donor being placed on the donation table.
2. Restrain the animal securely and comfortably (lateral recumbency on a table is recommended).
3. Prepare the area aseptically.
4. Apply pressure at the thoracic inlet to raise the jugular vein and facilitate palpation and visualization of the vessel. Avoid contamination of the venipuncture site.
5. Use a guarded haemostat or the clamp provided with the blood collection bag on the donor tubing to prevent air from entering the bag when the needle is exposed.
6. Remove the needle cap and perform venipuncture using the 16 gauge needle attached to the collection bag. Remove the clamp or the haemostat. If no flashback of blood is seen in the tubing check the needle placement and check for any occlusion in the donor tubing. The needle may be repositioned, however it should not be fully withdrawn from the patient. If the needle is withdrawn, the line must once again be clamped to prevent entry of air into the bag.
7. The bag should be positioned lower than the donor to aid in gravitational flow. Suction may assist in collection by use of an appropriately designed vacuum chamber (see Figure 14.7).
8. Periodically invert the bag gently to mix blood and anticoagulant.
9. When the bag is full (405–495 ml blood = 426–521 g weight), clamp the donor tubing, remove the needle from the jugular vein and apply pressure to the venipuncture site to prevent haematoma formation.
10. Allow the tubing to refill with anticoagulated blood and clamp the distal (needle) end with a hand sealer clip or heat sealer. If these are not available a tight knot may be tied in the line.
11. Clamp the entire length of tubing in 10 cm segments to be used for subsequent crossmatches.
12. Label the bag with product type, donor identification, date of collection, date of expiration, donor blood type, donor PCV (or Hct or Hb) and phlebotomist identification prior to use and storage.

If using a multiple bag system for blood component preparation, steps 10–12 may be replaced by the processing procedure (centrifugation, plasma extraction).

14.6 Procedure for canine whole blood collection.

1. Place the vacuum chamber on the gram scale.
2. Place the collection bag in the chamber, hanging the bag from the clip on the chamber lid.
3. Exit the donor tubing by placing it in the notch on the top of the chamber. Ensure that enough tubing length remains within the cylinder to prevent occlusion (tight kinking of the line) during collection.
4. Place the lid on the chamber and turn the suction on to a low level (7 kPa (50 mmHg)). Try to gently lift the chamber by the lid to ensure an adequate vacuum seal. If the seal is not tight, or if a whistling noise is heard, place a small piece of moistened cotton at the notch where the tubing exits the chamber.
5. The suction machine must be turned off before venipuncture is performed on the donor. Follow steps 1–6 listed in canine whole blood collection procedure (Figure 14.6).
6. Once a flashback is obtained in the donor tubing line, turn on the suction machine. The recommended vacuum pressure is 6.5–24 kPa (50–180 mmHg). Gentle mixing of the blood and anticoagulant during collection is less necessary during vacuum-assisted collection than gravity flow collection. However, if the chamber must be entered during the collection (slowing or cessation of blood flow, checking tube for occlusion) suction must be discontinued while adjustments are being made.
7. When the bag is full (405–495 ml blood = 426–521 g weight), turn off the suction, clamp the donor tubing, remove the needle from the jugular vein and apply pressure to the venipuncture site to prevent haematoma formation.
8. Allow the tubing to refill with anticoagulated blood and clamp the distal (needle) end with a hand sealer clip or heat sealer. If these are not available a tight knot may be tied in the line.
9. Clamp the entire length of tubing in 10 cm segments to be used for subsequent crossmatches.
10. Label the bag with product type, donor identification, date of collection, date of expiration, donor blood type, donor PCV (or Hct or Hb) and phlebotomist identification prior to use and storage.

If using a multiple bag system for blood component preparation, steps 8–10 may be replaced by the processing procedure (centrifugation, plasma extraction).

14.7 Procedure for vacuum-assisted collection.

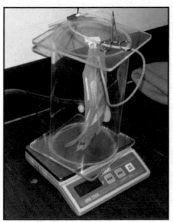

14.8

Vacuum chamber with empty collection bag in place. Suction is applied to the chamber facilitating rapid blood collection. The entire apparatus is placed on a set of scales during donation so that the volume of blood collected can be monitored.

Cats typically require sedation. It is suggested that each practice develop a safe protocol with which they are comfortable, and that works with their donor animals. Examples include combinations of ketamine and midazolam intravenously or isoflurane/oxygen anaesthesia by mask (Figure 14.9). A suggested procedure for collection of feline blood using an open collection system is shown in Figure 14.10. As a safety precaution, cats should have an intravenous catheter placed as part of the donation procedure.

Following donation, food and water are offered to canine donors. Activity should be restricted to lead walks only for the next 24 hours, and it is advised that a harness or lead passed under the chest is used instead of a neck collar and lead, to avoid pressure on

Butorphanol 0.1–0.2 mg/kg ± diazepam 0.5 mg/kg i.v. (same syringe)

Ketamine 2 mg/kg and midazolam 0.1 mg/kg i.v. (same syringe), additional boluses of one quarter to half the original dose as needed

Ketamine 5–10 mg/kg and midazolam 0.2 mg/kg **i.m.** (same syringe) with additional boluses of ketamine 1.0 mg/kg i.v. as needed

Mask isoflurane/oxygen anaesthesia

14.9 Examples of feline donor sedation protocols.

An 18 gauge needle, 19 gauge butterfly catheter, or 18 gauge over-the-needle intravenous catheter is required for dogs; typically a 19 or 21 gauge butterfly catheter is used for cats. Syringes for collection should be prefilled with an appropriate anticoagulant (1 ml CPDA-1 per 7 ml blood).

1. Cats typically require sedation. An intravenous catheter is placed in the cephalic vein of the feline donor, either before (preferable) or after sedation for the purpose of administering intravenous fluids after the blood donation.

2. Steps 1–4 are performed as in the canine whole blood collection method (Figure 14.6). The feline donor is restrained in sternal recumbency, with the forelimbs over the edge of a table and the head raised.

3. Perform venipuncture. Without removing the needle, fill each syringe in turn. The syringe can be gently rocked to ensure mixing of blood and anticoagulant during collection. If an over-the-needle catheter is used, remove the stylet following the venipuncture and advance the catheter into the vein. Attach an extension set, and fill each syringe in turn.

4. Invert the syringes gently several times after collection to mix blood and anticoagulant.

5. After collection remove the needle from the jugular vein and apply pressure to the venipuncture site to prevent haematoma formation.

14.10 Procedure for syringe method of collection. This is most commonly used for collection of feline blood or small volumes of canine blood or when closed collection systems are not available.

the jugular venipuncture site. Donor cats, after completion of the donation, should receive intravenous fluid replacement in the form of 30 ml/kg of intravenous crystalloid solution over approximately 3 hours. The feline donor must be closely observed during recovery from sedation/anaesthesia and may be offered food and water once fully awake.

Blood component processing

Initial blood collection yields fresh whole blood. Whole blood can either be stored or separated into packed red blood cells, fresh plasma, stored plasma or platelet-rich plasma concentrates (Figure 14.11). In large veterinary centres with a high emergency and critical care caseload, preparation of blood components becomes essential to extend resources. The use of blood components permits specific replacement therapy and reduces the number of transfusion reactions.

Blood component processing requires variable-speed, temperature-controlled centrifuges to produce most of the products described. The precise centrifugation protocol used depends on the centrifuge but separation of whole blood into packed cells and plasma typically requires centrifugation at 5000 x g for 5 minutes (not including deceleration time) at 4°C. To prevent microbial contamination a closed collection system must be used, and the transfer of components to satellite bags must be contained within the system by integral tubing. The tubing should be sealed prior to unit storage using either a handheld clip sealer or heat sealer. If blood is collected into an open system it should be refrigerated and administered within 24 hours, therefore use of blood component therapy is less applicable.

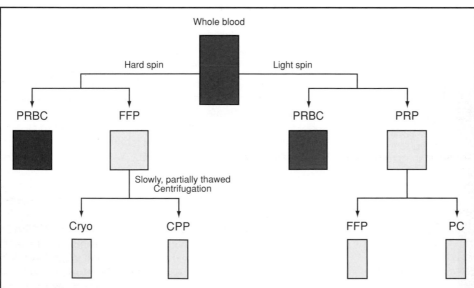

14.11 Component processing (FFP, fresh frozen plasma; PRBC, packed red blood cells; PRP, platelet rich plasma; CPP, cryoprecipitate poor plasma; Cryo, cryoprecipitate; PC, platelet concentrate).

Storage

Red cell products should be stored in a refrigerator maintained at 1–6°C, with the bag in an upright position. Positioning the bag in this manner maximizes gas exchange with the red cell solution to help preserve the viability of the red blood cells during storage and following transfusion. The shelf life of the product is based on the anticoagulant–preservative solution used in collection. Specialized blood storage refrigerators with built-in temperature alarms are available, or a dedicated regular household refrigerator with low in-and-out traffic may be used. The refrigerator thermometer should be checked daily to ensure appropriate storage conditions.

Almost all of the plasma products are stored frozen at −20°C or below. Regular household freezers may suffice, but the temperature may vary depending on the section of the freezer used. The temperature should be checked daily using a thermometer, and opening and closing of the freezer should be minimized. When initially freezing the plasma an elastic band should be placed around the bag, which is removed once it has frozen. This creates a 'waist' in the bag (Figure 14.12). Disappearance of this 'waist' during storage would suggest that the unit has thawed and refrozen, signifying compromise of storage conditions and plasma quality. The entire plasma bag should be enclosed in a sealed plastic bag, in which it should remain during plasma thawing, to protect the injection ports from contamination. The frozen plasma unit is vulnerable to cracking if dropped, and should be handled with care.

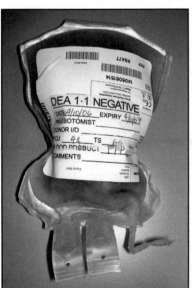

14.12

A unit of fresh frozen plasma showing the 'waist' created by freezing with a rubber band in place.

All blood products should be labelled with product type, donor identification, donor blood type, date of collection and date of expiration.

Use of blood products

Red cell products

Fresh whole blood (FWB) is collected following strict aseptic technique as described above, not refrigerated, and used within 8 hours of collection. All blood components (red blood cells (RBCs), platelets, labile and stable coagulation factors, plasma proteins) are present and functional. FWB is the product most commonly used in private veterinary practices; however, if components are available, the administration of FWB is restricted to those anaemic patients with concurrent haemostatic defects. FWB not used within 8 hours of collection may be stored in a refrigerator at 1–6°C for approximately 28 or 35 days when collected in CPD or CPDA-1, respectively. The unit is then classified as stored whole blood (SWB), which differs from FWB only by the absence of functional labile clotting factors and platelets. When available, SWB may be useful in anaemic animals with concurrent hypoproteinaemia.

Packed red blood cells (PRBCs) are separated from the plasma prior to storage by centrifugation or sedimentation. The unit must be collected in a bag that has attached satellite bags, to allow extraction and transfer of plasma within a closed system. The remaining packed red blood cell unit provides the same red cell properties as a unit of whole blood. PRBC transfusion is indicated in severely anaemic animals that need additional oxygen-carrying support. The packed cell volume of the unit is greater than that of whole blood and is usually in the range of 70–80%, with the volume yield dependent on the donor haematocrit. PRBCs may be stored at 4°C for 20 days, with an extension to 35 days if preservative solution is added.

Plasma products

Fresh frozen plasma (FFP) is separated from PRBCs and frozen within 8 hours of collection. FFP provides the labile coagulation factors V and VIII, as well as all other coagulation factors and plasma proteins. Plasma that is refrozen after thawing or plasma prepared and frozen more than 8 hours post collection loses its labile coagulation factors. Typically, plasma must be placed in the freezer within 6 hours of collection to ensure adequate hard freezing within the 8-hour interval. FFP is indicated in animals with acquired or inherited coagulopathies (inherited factor deficiencies, vitamin K deficiency, disseminated intravascular coagulation (DIC), severe liver disease), and may be used prophylactically in surgical patients with known coagulopathies or at the time of active bleeding. As FFP contains other plasma proteins, it may be used in animals with hypoproteinaemia; however large volumes and repeated transfusions are required to produce a clinically significant and sustained improvement in plasma protein. FFP may be stored for up to 1 year when frozen below −20°C.

Stored frozen plasma (SFP) is FFP that is more than 1 year of age, plasma that was not frozen quickly enough to protect labile factors, or FFP that was thawed and refrozen without opening the bag. Many useful clotting factors and anti-inflammatory proteins will have been lost, but SFP can be used for colloidal support (hypoproteinaemia) and may still provide some vitamin K-dependent factors. SFP may be stored frozen at −20°C for 5 years from the date of collection.

Platelet-rich plasma (PRP) and platelet concentrate (PC) may be prepared from FWB; however, these products are some of the most challenging to prepare due to the delicate nature of platelets. To enhance survival and function of the platelets in the resulting product, extreme care and attention must be given to the unit during all phases of handling. Leucocyte reduction filters (present in many commercially available blood bags) will also remove platelets, thus blood collected for production of platelet products must use a collection bag without an in-line pre-storage leucocyte reduction filter. Fresh whole blood is centrifuged on a 'light' spin, the actual rate and time of which depends on the particular centrifuge, with a goal of producing a platelet unit containing at least 5×10^{10} platelets. An example of a protocol is 2000 x g for 2.5 minutes at 20–24°C (i.e. a lower centrifugation speed and time compared with preparation of PRBCs and FFP), and the product is not refrigerated. PRP is separated from the PRBCs, and may either be administered to the recipient, stored (see below) or further processed into PC and FFP. To make PC, PRP, with an attached empty satellite bag, is centrifuged at 5000 x g for 5 minutes. All but approximately 35–70 ml of the supernatant plasma is transferred into the empty bag and frozen (producing FFP), leaving the platelet concentrate in a small volume of liquid plasma in the second bag. PRP and PC may be stored at 20–24°C, with gentle agitation, for 5 days when collected using a closed system. As they are stored at a higher temperature than other blood products, platelet products are more susceptible to bacterial contamination, and if collected in an open system, they should be used within 4 hours of collection. These products are used when there is uncontrollable, severe or life-threatening bleeding (e.g. intracranial haemorrhage), although the difficulties associated with their production often result instead in the use of more readily available fresh whole blood.

Cryoprecipitate (Cryo) is a plasma component that is prepared by freeze–thaw precipitation of proteins. Preparation of Cryo provides a source of concentrated von Willebrand factor, factor VIII, factor XIII, fibrinogen and fibronectin from a unit of FFP; these precipitated proteins are then resuspended in a small volume of the liquid plasma. Cryo can be prepared from FFP within 12 months of collection. A unit of FFP is slowly thawed until of a slushy consistency or until only approximately 10% of the plasma remains frozen, and then centrifuged at 5000 x g at 4°C for 5 minutes. The cryo-poor plasma (CPP, the cryosupernatant) is expressed, leaving behind the Cryo in a small volume of plasma (10–15 ml). CPP contains many clotting factors (including vitamin K-dependent factors II, VII, IX and X), as well as other anticoagulant and fibrinolytic factors, albumin and globulin, which had been present in the unit of FFP. The Cryo and remaining CPP are immediately refrozen and should be used within 1 year of original collection. The administration of desmopressin (DDAVP) 30–120 minutes prior to donation will increase the amount of von Willebrand factor in the donor's fresh frozen plasma, and increase Cryo yield. Cryo is used in the management of patients with bleeding due to deficiency or dysfunction of factor VIII (haemophilia A), von Willebrand factor or fibrinogen. CPP may be used for treatment of hypoproteinaemia or coagulopathies that do not require supplementation of the Cryo components.

Haemoglobin-based oxygen carriers

Oxyglobin is a sterile solution of purified, polymerized bovine haemoglobin that increases plasma haemoglobin concentration, shifting the majority of the oxygen content of the blood to the plasma and increasing the oxygen-carrying capacity of the blood. It has been approved for use in dogs for the treatment of anaemia, regardless of cause. Although Oxyglobin has been used in cats to provide oxygen-carrying support in cases of anaemia, it is not licensed for use in this species. Oxyglobin should be administered with care. It is a very effective colloid and produces a great deal of intravascular volume expansion, therefore patients receiving it should be monitored for evidence of circulatory overload and possible development of pulmonary oedema and/or pleural effusion. Plasma Hb concentrations of patients who have received haemoglobin-based oxygen-carrying solutions should be monitored using a haemoglobinometer.

Blood product selection

Blood products are used to treat a variety of conditions, including those associated with anaemia (haemorrhage, haemolysis or reduced erythropoiesis), coagulopathies, sepsis, DIC and specific factor deficiencies.

RBC products provide the recipient with additional red cell mass to increase the oxygen-carrying capacity of the blood, and thus improve oxygen delivery to peripheral tissues. There is not a precise packed cell volume (PCV) below which a transfusion is required, although any patient with a PCV <20% should be considered a potential candidate, and almost all patients would benefit once the PCV is ≤12%. In some animals with peracute blood loss and hypovolaemia, red cell transfusions may be used even though their PCV may still be normal. These patients will predictably develop a low PCV following fluid resuscitation with asanguineous fluids. The decision to transfuse red cells is therefore based on several factors, including the haemoglobin concentration (or PCV), onset of anaemia (acute versus chronic), presence of ongoing losses and, most importantly, the clinical signs of the patient. Tachypnoea, tachycardia, bounding peripheral pulses, collapse, lethargy and weakness are all signs that should prompt consideration of a red cell transfusion. If RBCs are not available, Oxyglobin infusion may also be considered.

Plasma products are a source of coagulation factors and various plasma proteins, and deficiencies of these factors or selected proteins are indications for their use. The benefit of plasma transfusion to a hypoproteinaemic patient is limited; the half-life of albumin is very short and in animals with protein-losing diseases many units of plasma would be required to correct the albumin deficit (see Chapter 4). Other modes of therapy (nutritional support, use of colloids) are suggested for this condition.

Blood product administration

Blood products are usually administered intravenously, but may also be given via the intraosseous route if venous access cannot be obtained (e.g. kittens, puppies). They should *not* be given intraperitoneally. An in-line blood filter (170–260 µm) is required for all blood products (including plasma) and is incorporated in standard blood infusion sets. A paediatric filter with reduced dead space, or microaggregate filters of 18–40 µm, can be useful for infusing smaller volumes of products or blood collected in syringes. Stored red cell products do not need to be warmed prior to use, unless they are being given to neonates or very small animals. Plasma products are gently thawed in a warm water bath prior to administration. Packed red cells stored without preservative may be resuspended in or co-administered with 100 ml of physiological saline to decrease their viscosity.

The amount of blood product to be administered depends on the specific product, desired effect and patient's response. A general rule of thumb is that 2 ml of transfused whole blood/kg recipient weight will raise the PCV by 1%. However, it is important to bear in mind that the degree to which the PCV is elevated depends on the extent of ongoing blood loss, and also whether other fluids or colloids are being concurrently administered. Most patients will receive between 10 and 22 ml/kg, and a suggested formula to calculate the amount of whole blood required for transfusion is:

$$\text{Volume (ml)} = 85 \text{ (dog) or } 60 \text{ (cat)} \times \text{BW (kg)} \times [(\text{Desired PCV} - \text{Actual PCV})/\text{Donor PCV}]$$

For PRBC or FFP the average volume for infusion is 6–12 ml/kg.

The rate of blood product administration depends on the cardiovascular status of the recipient. In general, the rate should only be 0.25–1.0 ml/kg/h for the first 20 minutes. If the transfusion is well tolerated, the rate may then be increased to deliver the remaining product within 4–6 hours. In an animal with an increased risk of volume overload (cardiovascular disease, impaired renal function) the rate of administration should not exceed 3–4 ml/kg/h. If it is likely to take more than 4 hours to deliver the desired volume, the product may be divided so that a portion remains refrigerated for later use.

Animals should not receive food or medications during a transfusion, and the only fluid that may be administered through the same catheter is 0.9% saline.

Visual inspection of the product is necessary, especially when using stored red cells or plasma. Discoloration of the red cells (brown, purple) or the suspension fluid, or the presence of clots, may indicate bacterial contamination, haemolysis or other storage lesions. Plasma bags must be examined for evidence of thawing and refreezing, or cracking and tearing of the bag.

The dose listed for Oxyglobin in a normovolaemic dog is 10–30 ml/kg at a rate ≤10 ml/kg/h, although many dogs will require much lower administration rates. It must be remembered that haemoglobin-based oxygen-carrying solutions act as powerful colloids, therefore there is a significant risk of volume overload if they are given at high rates. Off-label use in cats is based on reported clinical experience, with a suggested total daily dose of 10–15 ml/kg administered at rate of 1–2 ml/kg/h. Even lower rates (2–3 ml/h) may be needed in euvolaemic feline patients as cats are more susceptible to volume overload. The administration rate should be chosen based on assessment of the patient and whether the product is being used for oxygen-carrying support in a euvolaemic animal (in which case slow infusion rates are chosen) or whether the product is being used in a hypovolaemic patient, in which case larger bolus doses can be used similar to those of other colloid fluids (see Chapter 4). An in-line filter is not required with use of this solution.

Monitoring transfusions

The following parameters should be measured prior to (baseline), every 15–30 minutes during, and 1, 12 and 24 hours after transfusion:

- Attitude
- Rectal temperature
- Pulse rate and quality
- Respiratory rate and character
- Mucous membrane colour and CRT
- Plasma and urine colour.

The PCV/TP should also be monitored prior to, upon completion and at 12 and 24 hours after transfusion.

It is helpful to design a transfusion monitoring sheet, with time points and monitoring parameters noted, to encourage diligent recording during and after the transfusion. Careful monitoring will allow for prompt recognition and treatment of transfusion reactions as well as evaluation of transfusion efficacy.

Adverse reactions

Any undesired side effect noted as a consequence of a blood product transfusion is considered a transfusion reaction. The reported frequency of transfusion reactions is variable, as is their severity. Transfusion reactions may be classified as immunological (haemolytic or non-haemolytic) and non-immunological, as well as acute or delayed.

Preventative measures necessary to minimize the risk of transfusion reactions include appropriate donor screening, collection, preparation, storage and administration of products. Adherence to standard protocols helps to ensure safety and efficacy of transfusions in practice.

Immunological transfusion reactions

The most concerning type of transfusion reaction is an *acute haemolytic reaction* with intravascular haemolysis. These are antigen–antibody, type II hypersensitivity reactions. This type of reaction is seen in type B cats receiving type A blood as well as DEA 1.1-negative dogs sensitized to DEA 1.1 upon repeated exposure. Clinical signs may include fever, tachycardia, dyspnoea, muscle tremors, vomiting, weakness, collapse, haemoglobinaemia and haemoglobinuria. These reactions may lead to shock, DIC, renal damage and, potentially, death.

Treatment for an acute haemolytic transfusion reaction involves immediate discontinuation of the transfusion, and treatment of the clinical signs of shock, including fluid therapy. Antihistamines and corticosteroids may be administered. Aggressive fluid therapy may be required if the patient becomes hypotensive and patients should be carefully monitored for the development of fluid overload (measurement of central venous pressure (CVP), heart rate, lung auscultation). Blood pressure and urine output should be monitored as hypotension and oliguria may follow (see Chapters 3 and 8).

Febrile non-haemolytic transfusion reactions and reactions to blood that has been contaminated with bacteria may have similar signs, with development of a significant fever during or shortly after the transfusion. The donor and recipient blood type should be confirmed and a crossmatch performed. The product type, date of expiration, volume and rate of administration should be confirmed. A sample of donor and recipient blood should be examined for evidence of haemolysis, and saved for microbial culture and further infectious disease screening if needed. A Gram stain of donor blood may be helpful initially to investigate possible unit contamination, and, if bacterial contamination is suspected, broad-spectrum intravenous antibiotic therapy should be initiated. As DIC and renal failure may occur, monitoring the animals' coagulation profile, urine output, blood urea nitrogen (BUN), creatinine and electrolytes is advisable.

A *delayed haemolytic* reaction with extravascular haemolysis may be recognized 2–21 days post transfusion, with similar although less severe signs to an acute haemolytic reaction (± bilirubinaemia/bilirubinuria). The owner may notice jaundice or anorexia, and on examination the animal may be febrile or have an unexpected decline in PCV. This type of reaction less frequently requires intervention, other than perhaps administration of antipyretics. If the decline in red cells impacts the patient, a crossmatch must be performed prior to any subsequent transfusions.

Non-haemolytic immunological reactions are acute type I hypersensitivity reactions (allergic or anaphylactic), most often mediated by IgE and mast cells. They have a range of clinical signs including urticaria, pruritus, erythema, oedema, vomiting and dyspnoea secondary to pulmonary oedema. If this type of reaction occurs, the transfusion should be discontinued and the patient examined for evidence of haemolysis and shock. Steroid medications (dexamethasone 0.5–1.0 mg/kg i.v.) and antihistamines may be required. Suggested antihistamine dosages are as follows:

- Chlorpheniramine, maximum recommended dose 0.5 mg/kg q12h in both cats and dogs:
  - Dogs: small to medium-sized, 2.5–5 mg i.m. q12h
  - Dogs: medium to large, 5–10 mg i.m. q12h
  - Cats: 2–4 mg/cat orally q12h
- Diphenydramine 1–2 mg/kg i.m. q12h dogs and cats.

If the reaction subsides, the transfusion may be restarted at 25–50% of the previous rate. If there is evidence of an anaphylactic or anaphylactoid reaction/shock, adrenaline, intravenous fluids, antihistamines, H_2 blockers (cimetidine, ranitidine), colloids, dopamine and aminophylline may also be administered in addition to the above treatment measures as needed.

Reactions to leucocytes and platelets may occur, manifested by a febrile non-haemolytic transfusion reaction, which may last up to 20 hours post transfusion. These are recognized as an increase in body temperature of >1°C without an obvious underlying cause.

Other delayed immune-mediated transfusion reactions include post-transfusion purpura (thrombocytopenia noted within the first week after blood transfusion), neonatal isoerythrolysis and immunosuppression of the recipient.

Non-immunological transfusion reactions
Many non-immunological transfusion reactions have been described. Anaphylactoid reactions, which often result from too rapid an infusion rate, may be seen. They tend to subside after discontinuation of the transfusion or reduction of the infusion rate. Circulatory overload may occur in any patient receiving excessive volumes of blood products, or those with cardiac or renal disease. Treatment with diuretics may be required. Hypocalcaemia is identified most commonly following administration of large volumes of plasma or whole blood and is a result of citrate intoxication. Patients with impaired liver function are at greatest risk. Clinical signs of hypocalcaemia may be noted (vomiting, muscle tremors, tetany, electrocardiograph (ECG) changes) and treatment includes supplementation with calcium chloride or calcium gluconate. Other recognized non-immunological reactions include polycythaemia and hyperproteinaemia, hypothermia, coagulopathy, thrombosis, microbial contamination, hyperammonaemia, hypophosphataemia, hyperkalaemia, acidosis, pretransfusion (*in vitro*) haemolysis, haemosiderosis, air embolus and infectious disease transmission.

References and further reading

Blais MC, Oakley DA and Giger U (2005) The canine Dal blood type: a red cell antigen lacking in some Dalmatians. *Proceedings American College of Veterinary Internal Medicine* p. 892

Brooks M (2000) Transfusion of plasma and plasma derivatives. In: *Schalm's Veterinary Hematology, 5th edn*, ed. BF Feldman, JG Zinkl and NC Jain, pp. 838–843. Lippincott Williams and Wilkins, Philadelphia

Bücheler J and Giger U (1993) Alloantibodies against A and B blood types in cats. *Veterinary Immunology and Immunopathology* **38**, 283–295

Callan MB (2000) Red blood cell transfusions in the dog and cat. In: *Schalm's Veterinary Hematology, 5th edn*, ed. BF Feldman, JG Zinkl and NC Jain, pp. 833–837. Lippincott Williams and Wilkins, Philadelphia

Callan MB, Jones LT and Giger U (1995) Hemolytic transfusion reactions in a dog with an alloantibody to a common antigen. *Journal of Veterinary Internal Medicine* **9**, 277–279

Feldman B (2000) Blood transfusion guidelines. In: *Kirk's Current Veterinary Therapy XIII: Small Animal Practice*, ed. JD Bonagura, pp. 400–403. WB Saunders, Philadelphia

Forcada Y and Gibson G (2005) Frequencies of feline blood types in cats at the Royal Veterinary College, London, UK. *Proceedings European College of Veterinary Internal Medicine – Companion Animal* p. 205

Giger U (2000) Blood typing and crossmatching to ensure compatible transfusions. In: *Kirk's Current Veterinary Therapy XIII: Small Animal Practice*, ed. JD Bonagura, pp. 396–399. WB Saunders, Philadelphia

Giger U and Blais MC (2005) Ensuring blood compatibility: update on canine typing and crossmatching. *Proceedings American College of Veterinary Internal Medicine* pp. 721–723

Giger U, Gelens CJ, Callan MB and Oakley DA (1995) An acute hemolytic transfusion reaction caused by dog erythrocyte antigen 1.1 incompatibility in a previously sensitized dog. *Journal of the American Veterinary Medical Association* **206**, 1358–1362

Griot-Wenk ME, Callan MB, Casal ML *et al.* (1996) Blood type AB in the feline AB blood group system. *American Journal of Veterinary Research* **57**, 1438–1442

Griot-Wenk ME and Giger U (1995) Feline transfusion medicine: blood types and their clinical importance. *Veterinary Clinics of North America: Small Animal Practice* **25**, 1305–1322

Hale AS (1995) Canine blood groups and their importance in veterinary transfusion medicine. *Veterinary Clinics of North America: Small Animal Practice* **25**, 1323–1332

Harrell KA and Kristensen AT (1995) Canine transfusion reactions and their management. *Veterinary Clinics of North America: Small Animal Practice* **25**, 1333–1364

Hohenhaus AE (2000) Blood banking and transfusion medicine. In: *Textbook of Veterinary Internal Medicine, Diseases of the Dog and Cat, 5th edn,* ed. SJ Ettinger and EC Feldman, pp. 348–356. WB Saunders, Philadelphia

Hohenhaus A (2000) Transfusion reactions. In: *Schalm's Veterinary Hematology, 5th edn,* ed. BF Feldman, JG Zinkl and NC Jain, pp. 864–868. Lippincott Williams and Wilkins, Philadelphia

Kristensen AT and Feldman BF (1995) General principles of small animal blood component administration. *Veterinary Clinics of North America: Small Animal Practice* **25**, 1277–1290

Niggemeier A, Haberstroh HF, Nelson VE and Giger U (2000) An accidental transfusion of a type A kitten with type B blood causes a transient switch from blood type A to B. *Journal of Veterinary Internal Medicine* **14**, 214–216

Prittie JE (2003) Triggers for use, optimal dosing, and problems associated with red cell transfusions. *Veterinary Clinics of North America: Small Animal Practice* **33**, 1261–1275

Schneider A (1995) Blood components: collection, processing and storage. *Veterinary Clinics of North America: Small Animal Practice* **25**, 1245–1261

Schneider A (2000) Principles of blood collection and processing. In: *Schalm's Veterinary Hematology, 5th edn,* ed. BF Feldman, JG Zinkl and NC Jain, pp. 827–832. Lippincott Williams and Wilkins, Philadelphia

Wardrop KJ, Reine N, Birkenheuer A *et al.* (2005) Canine and feline blood donor screening for infectious disease. *Journal of Veterinary Internal Medicine* **19**, 135–142

Wardrop KJ (1995) Selection of anticoagulant-preservatives for canine and feline blood storage. *Veterinary Clinics of North America: Small Animal Practice* **25**, 1263–1276

Weinstein NM, Blais MC, Greiner K *et al.* (2005) A new blood group antigen in domestic shorthair cats: the feline Mik red cell antigen. *Proceedings American College of Veterinary Internal Medicine* p. 830

15

Reproductive and paediatric emergencies

Gary C.W. England and Marco Russo

Introduction

Numerous reproductive disorders can produce acute onset and potentially fatal clinical disease in dogs and cats. Many of these conditions can be diagnosed and treated relatively easily. Information about the management, diagnosis and treatment of neonatal disease is, however, scant, and for many breeding establishments perinatal losses are a lamentable 20%. This is despite the fact that most neonatal care simply requires an understanding of the normal physiological requirements of this age group. The aim of this chapter is to review the diagnosis and treatment of reproductive tract emergencies as well as the care and management of the neonatal dog and cat.

Reproductive emergencies in the non-pregnant female

Pyometra

Aetiopathology

Pyometra is a disease of the luteal phase of the oestrous cycle, with most bitches and queens showing clinical signs between 5 and 80 days after the end of oestrus. In the queen, a luteal phase only follows ovulation, which is most commonly induced by coitus. Whilst corpora lutea are always present within the ovaries of bitches and queens with pyometra, progesterone concentrations are similar to those in healthy bitches at the same stage of the luteal phase (progesterone concentrations may be low at the time of presentation), and the functioning capacity of the corpora lutea has been shown to be normal. In the spontaneous disease, it appears that anogenital bacteria enter the uterus during oestrus and are able to persist and proliferate during metoestrus (dioestrus). Bacterial contamination of the uterus during oestrus is common, but persistence does not occur unless there is either underlying uterine disease (cystic endometrial hyperplasia) or a particularly pathogenic (adhesive) organism. A further factor that must be considered in the aetiology of pyometra is the use of exogenous progestogens (for the control of oestrus) and oestrogens (for the treatment of unwanted mating). Progestogens have a stimulatory effect upon the uterus whilst oestrogens enhance the effects of progesterone.

Clinical signs

Animals are initially lethargic and inappetent with vomiting, polydipsia and polyuria. Later there may be a vulval discharge, which in some cases is associated with improvement in the clinical signs. In other cases, the animal remains unwell and there is no discharge of pus; if these cases are undiagnosed they generally end fatally, often within 14–21 days from the onset of clinical signs. The cervix remains closed throughout. Death is generally due to septic shock and may or may not be associated with septic peritonitis depending on whether uterine rupture occurs. Occasionally the cervix relaxes and there is an outpouring of pus just before death. In other cases there may be intermittent opening of the cervix, with relatively good health following the discharge of pus, and malaise during the intervening periods. Such cases generally develop signs of sepsis within 6–8 weeks. Some cases of open-cervix pyometra may persist for years with a more or less continuous vulval discharge.

Rectal temperature may be normal in cases of open-cervix pyometra, whilst there is commonly pyrexia in cases of closed-cervix pyometra. In patients with septic shock the temperature may be subnormal.

The character of the vulval discharge may vary considerably; often it is a light chocolate-brown colour and has a characteristic odour. In other cases it is yellow in colour, often blood tinged and varying from watery to a creamy consistency. The vulva is generally enlarged and there may be discoloration or scalding of the perivulval tissues and perineum.

An increased thirst is common and occurs secondary to polyuria caused by reduced water permeability in the collecting duct of the kidney. Renal dysfunction is probably caused by the formation of immune complexes.

Diagnostic features

Most cases can be diagnosed on the basis of the clinical signs. In addition, ultrasonography (Figure 15.1) and radiography are valuable diagnostic tools for the detection of an enlarged or fluid-filled uterus. The total number of leucocytes is frequently increased in cases of pyometra, although the degree of leucocytosis is lower in cases of open-cervix compared with closed-cervix pyometra.

Therapeutic considerations

Renal dysfunction is common and many patients have polydipsia and polyuria. There may also be vomiting

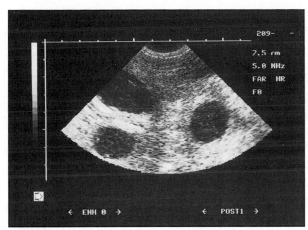

15.1 Ultrasound image of a bitch with pyometra showing three sections of the uterus filled with echogenic fluid (5.0 MHz transducer, scale in cm).

such that fluid, electrolyte and acid–base balance are frequently disturbed. Intravenous fluid therapy is therefore mandatory. Urine output should be maintained at approximately 1–2 ml/kg/h. Balanced electrolytes, for example Hartmann's solution, should be used to restore intravascular volume and allow any acid–base and electrolyte imbalance to be corrected. The rate of fluid administration should be according to individual requirements, but in hypovolaemic animals it may be necessary to give boluses of up to 90 ml/kg (see Chapter 4). Metabolic (lactic) acidosis is a frequent finding which should resolve following restoration of tissue perfusion using fluid therapy; the use of bicarbonate is rarely if ever required. Hypokalaemia may also be present and appropriate addition of potassium to the intravenous fluids may be required. It is often worthwhile monitoring the blood pressure of these patients at presentation and during stabilization and anaesthesia. This can be performed using indirect external methods or by percutaneous direct measurement (see Chapter 3). Mean blood pressure should be maintained above 60–80 mmHg.

Animals with septic shock, including some cases of pyometra, may be hypoglycaemic as a result of depleted glycogen stores or the increased metabolic demand seen with sepsis. If hypoglycaemia is detected, dextrose may be added to the intravenous replacement crystalloid fluid. Dextrose is frequently administered as a 2.5–5.0% solution.

The common bacteria cultured in cases of pyometra are *Escherichia coli*, *Staphylococcus* spp. and *Streptococcus* spp. For these reasons, broad-spectrum bactericidal antimicrobial agents may be administered intravenously, particularly those with actions against both Gram-positive and Gram-negative organisms. Suggested agents include cephalosporins, clavulanic acid-potentiated amoxicillin and trimethoprim-potentiated sulphonamides.

A number of complications may occur in patients with pyometra. Azotaemia may be renal or prerenal in origin. Increased liver enzymes (secondary to sepsis/endotoxaemia or poor hepatic perfusion associated with hypovolaemia) are common but usually return rapidly to normal following removal of the uterus and restoration of fluid and electrolyte balance.

Aspiration pneumonia may occur in debilitated vomiting animals. A non-regenerative normochromic anaemia may also develop subsequent to bone marrow suppression, blood loss at surgery and aggressive fluid replacement. Blood transfusion is rarely indicated, unless the packed cell volume (PCV) decreases to below 20%.

Treatment
Ovariohysterectomy is the treatment of choice for pyometra. Animals that are presented early in the course of the disease are usually a low surgical risk and high success rates should be expected.

The aim of the surgeon is, whenever possible, to stabilize the patient prior to surgery and then to remove the uterus quickly without causing it to rupture. Postoperative management involves continuation of fluid and antimicrobial therapy and ensuring general nursing and analgesic care.

In those cases where it is essential to retain reproductive function, or where surgery is not possible because of intercurrent disease, medical therapy may be considered. There have been several reports of successful medical management using oestrogens (presumably to induce cervical relaxation), as well as drugs to induce uterine contraction, including ergometrine, quinine and etamiphylline. However, since pyometra is a disease of the luteal phase and ovariectomy has been shown to produce resolution of the clinical signs, there has been considerable interest in the use of prostaglandins to cause lysis of the corpora lutea as well as for their uterine spasmogenic action. Prolactin inhibitors such as cabergoline or bromocriptine may also be used for the treatment of pyometra since they remove the support for the corpora lutea and therefore cause a decline in plasma progesterone. A combination of cabergoline (5 µg/kg/day) administered daily for 10 days with cloprostenol (5 µg/kg) administered from day 3 every third day for 10 days (three treatments) has been shown to have a high efficacy. This regime produces a few adverse effects limited to minor restlessness, pacing, hypersalivation, tachypnoea and occasional vomiting and diarrhoea for up to 60 minutes after the administration of the prostaglandin. Careful observation of the patient is necessary immediately after prostaglandin treatment, although it is not uncommon for the adverse effects to be fewer at each administration. The combination regime should naturally be combined with appropriate broad-spectrum antimicrobial agents and intravenous fluid administration.

Whilst prostaglandins alone are not recommended in cases of closed-cervix pyometra because of the risk of uterine rupture, the combined regime appears to have lower risk as long as the prostaglandin is not administered until day 3. This allows time for the cabergoline to cause a decline in progesterone, resulting in softening and opening of the cervix. Following prostaglandin and prolactin inhibitor treatments, up to 80% of bitches have subsequently become pregnant and whelped.

More recently, there has been interest in the use of progesterone receptor antagonists such as aglepristone, which have been shown to be useful for the treatment of pyometra. Whilst these agents appear to produce no adverse effects and a good return to fertility, no uterine contractions are induced to ensure evacuation of pus. Further investigations of combinations of progesterone receptor antagonists with prostaglandins and prolactin inhibitors are warranted.

Prolapse of vaginal hyperplasia

Aetiopathology
Vaginal hyperplasia (commonly termed prolapse) reflects an accentuated response of the caudal vaginal floor to normal circulating oestrogen concentrations. Usually, the vaginal mucosa cranial to the external urethral orifice is involved, becoming oedematous and thickened (Figure 15.2). This rapidly increases in size and a large smooth pink mass protrudes from the vulva. Occasionally, the circumference of the vagina may be involved. In a very small proportion of cases, dysuria may occur due to urethral obstruction by the bulk of the tissue. The condition has not been reported in the queen.

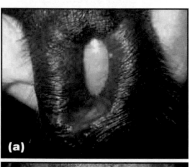
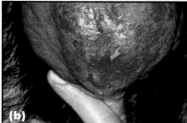

15.2

(a) Vaginal hyperplasia without prolapse. (b) Traumatic bruising and tearing of hyperplastic vaginal wall.

Clinical signs
The features of the condition are easy to identify, since the hyperplastic tissue is evident protruding through the vulval lips. There is often excessive licking, and self-trauma of the site is a common sequel. If self-trauma is severe the tissue may become necrotic.

Diagnostic features
Clinical examination and speculum examination will confirm the nature of the problem.

Therapeutic considerations
In most bitches, the hyperplastic tissue decreases in size at the end of oestrus when oestrogen concentrations decrease and progesterone concentrations increase. The tissue usually completely disappears and is absent even upon careful speculum examination. The greatest problem is often that of reassuring the owner that the mass will regress. The tissue may need to be surgically removed if self-trauma has been severe.

Treatment
Conservative management with local cleansing and lubrication is usually sufficient. Self-trauma should be prevented by the application of an Elizabethan collar. It is possible to speed the termination of oestrus by the administration of progestogens, such as proligestone or megoestrol acetate. Ovariohysterectomy during the subsequent anoestrus will prevent recurrence. Artificial insemination may be necessary in bitches that are required for breeding, or submucosal resection of the tissue may be performed during early oestrus before mating. Submucosal resection may also be required in cases where there has been self-trauma. This surgery involves performing an episiotomy, placing a urinary catheter into the urethra and resecting the hyperplastic tissue. There is often considerable blood loss at the time of surgery. A minority of surgically treated cases will recur and those animals that are not required for breeding should be neutered. The use of surgery in breeding animals has been questioned, since a familial tendency has been reported in certain breeds.

Reproductive emergencies in the pregnant female

Hypocalcaemia

Aetiopathology
Eclampsia or puerperal tetany occurs most commonly during early lactation or late pregnancy in small to medium-sized bitches, and in multiparous queens with a large litter 2–4 weeks postpartum. The aetiology of hypocalcaemia is probably related to calcium loss in the milk, combined with poor dietary availability. In some animals, reduced appetite after parturition contributes to the problem.

Clinical signs
Hypocalcaemia causes loss of cell membrane-bound calcium and subsequent changes in membrane potential. Early clinical signs are restlessness, panting, increased salivation and a stiff gait, which progress to muscle fasciculations and hyperthermia. If untreated, tetany and death result.

Diagnostic features
The condition is most readily diagnosed by the clinical signs and history of late pregnancy or recent parturition. Measurement of plasma calcium concentration is diagnostic; most animals are severely hypocalcaemic with total calcium values less than 1.6 mmol/l or ionized calcium values less than 0.8 mmol/l.

Therapeutic considerations
The principal aim in the short term is to restore plasma calcium concentrations to normal. Factors that increase the protein-bound fraction of plasma calcium may contribute to the development of clinical signs including, for example, systemic alkalosis.

Treatment
The slow intravenous administration of a 10% calcium gluconate solution to effect (50–150 mg Ca/kg) produces a rapid response; the required dose is in the

region of 0.5–1.5 ml/kg of a 10% solution. Cardiac rate and rhythm should be monitored during administration preferably using an electrocardiogram. If bradycardia or premature ventricular complexes are observed, administration should temporarily cease. The response to treatment is usually dramatic; however, the effect is only maintained for between 1 and 12 hours and therefore short-term maintenance therapy is required. In clinical practice this is achieved by giving further supplementation subcutaneously and orally to prevent recurrence (see Chapter 5). Hypocalcaemia may be prevented by oral calcium supplementation in the last few days of pregnancy and during lactation. Excessive oral calcium administration reduces intestinal absorption of calcium and inhibits the secretion of parathyroid hormone; although the inhibition is clinically significant in several species, this does not appear to be the case in the bitch or queen.

In some bitches there is a poor response to treatment, which may be related to either a contributing or primary hypoglycaemia (see below).

Hypoglycaemia

Aetiopathology
It is very rare for a bitch or queen to become hypoglycaemic during pregnancy. Normally, progesterone acts as a potent peripheral insulin antagonist and results in hyperglycaemia (see below). Indeed, metoestrus (dioestrus) and pregnancy diabetes are well recognized, as is the difficulty in stabilizing known diabetics during dioestrus or pregnancy. However, there are reports in bitches of an apparent primary hypoglycaemia of unknown aetiology occurring during pregnancy. In some cases it is thought that hypoglycaemia worsens the clinical signs noted with hypocalcaemia. The condition has not been reported in the queen.

Clinical signs
Bitches with pregnancy hypoglycaemia are weak and may become comatose. The clinical features may be mistaken for those of hypocalcaemia, although tetany is not a usual clinical finding.

Diagnostic features
Diagnosis is based on the measurement of plasma glucose concentration. Blood glucose should be measured as part of the emergency minimum database in any sick animal (see Chapter 1). In whelping bitches investigation may also be stimulated by a lack of effect of intravenous calcium administration given in the initial belief that the bitch was hypocalcaemic.

Therapeutic considerations
The aim of treatment is to restore plasma glucose concentrations and provide frequent intake of glucose until the onset of parturition. The condition disappears following parturition and some authors have suggested that a Caesarean operation may be required in severe cases.

Treatment
Rapid resolution of the clinical signs is achieved following the intravenous administration of glucose to effect (usually 0.5 g/kg i.v. as a 25% solution, followed by addition of glucose to the intravenous fluids as a 2.5–5% solution). Subsequently, increased frequency of feeding can be used to prevent recurrence until the onset of parturition.

Hyperglycaemia
Increased plasma progesterone concentration has a direct antagonistic effect upon insulin and also stimulates the secretion of growth hormone. Progesterone reduces insulin binding and glucose transportation within tissues. Growth hormone also has an antagonistic effect upon insulin, mediated by a decrease in the number of insulin receptors and inhibition of glucose transport. Development of a diabetic state may therefore occur in the bitch during pregnancy; the condition is rare in the queen.

The clinical signs, diagnostic features, therapeutic considerations and treatment of hyperglycaemia associated with diabetes mellitus are discussed in Chapter 16.

Prolonged gestation

Aetiopathology
Prolonged gestation does not normally occur in the queen unless there has been unnoticed uterine inertia or dystocia. However, a common concern of many bitch owners is that parturition is 'overdue' when pregnancy length exceeds 65 or 66 days. In these cases there is a misunderstanding of the normal reproductive physiology, since whilst the 'endocrinological' length of pregnancy is 65 days, there is a large variation in the 'apparent' length of pregnancy. The latter, which is the interval from the day of mating to the day of parturition, can vary from 58–72 days in normal bitches of all breeds (Figure 15.3). Other causes for prolonged gestation include the bitch that has had unnoticed primary uterine inertia or dystocia, or the non-pregnant bitch that is mistakenly thought to be pregnant.

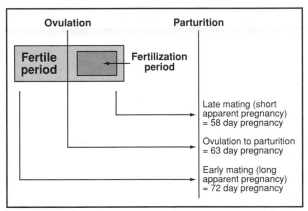

15.3 Schematic representation of the length of pregnancy in the bitch in relation to mating early or late during the fertile period.

Clinical signs
Bitches that are within their physiological pregnancy length and those that are non-pregnant do not have abnormal clinical signs. Those bitches and queens that have had primary uterine inertia may have previously had a small-volume vulval discharge and may have exhibited uterine and possibly abdominal

contractions which were unnoticed by the owner. Subsequently, there is placental separation and the onset of a green-coloured vulval discharge. Dams then become systemically ill as the fetuses die and decompose; a large-volume vulval discharge may be present. Initially, rectal temperature may be normal, but this may subsequently increase and terminally it may become subnormal.

Diagnostic features

Several methods may be used to predict the time of expected parturition in the bitch and may therefore be useful to determine whether this has been exceeded. If the bitch has been monitored during oestrus (using measurement of plasma progesterone concentration to detect the optimal mating time), the time from ovulation to parturition is tightly regulated (63 ± 1 days). Similarly, the use of vaginal cytology during oestrus may be useful since the onset of the metoestrus vaginal smear is related to parturition (58 ± 4 days), although not as precisely as the time of ovulation. A third useful assessment is to measure specific conceptus or fetal components with diagnostic B-mode ultrasound during pregnancy. Some measures (for example head (biparietal) diameter) can predict parturition to within ± 2 days in a large percentage of bitches.

It is also useful to instruct the owner to record the rectal temperature twice daily during the last third of pregnancy, since a decline in rectal temperature precedes parturition by approximately 12–36 hours. In the queen, prediction of the time of expected parturition can be achieved by counting the number of days from mating.

In many bitches, however, none of these procedures has been undertaken and in queens mating is frequently unnoticed. It is important, therefore, to perform a full clinical examination to ensure that the dam is clinically well and that she is pregnant. Measurement of plasma progesterone concentration can then be used to assess whether parturition is imminent. Progesterone concentrations decrease approximately 24–36 hours before parturition in both species (Figure 15.4).

Demonstration of high plasma progesterone concentration therefore indicates that parturition is not imminent, whilst a low progesterone concentration indicates that parturition is imminent or should already

have occurred. Intermediate values are difficult to interpret. Plasma progesterone can be easily measured in the practice laboratory by the use of enzyme-linked immunosorbent assay (ELISA) kits.

From the above, it can be seen that bitches that are still within their normal physiological pregnancy length will have high plasma progesterone concentrations, whilst bitches and queens that have had primary uterine inertia will have low plasma progesterone concentrations. Non-pregnant bitches may have high or low plasma progesterone concentrations, since the luteal phase of pregnancy and non-pregnancy is remarkably similar. Non-pregnant queens will have low plasma progesterone concentrations unless the queen has returned to oestrus and subsequently ovulated.

Treatment

No treatment is required for the bitch that has a normal long apparent pregnancy length or the bitch or queen that is non-pregnant. For the dam that has suffered primary uterine inertia, the best option is to perform a Caesarean operation to remove the retained fetuses, which are likely to be dead. This should be performed as described below, although the requirements for fluid therapy may differ if the bitch is showing signs of septic (distributive) shock.

Dystocia

Aetiopathology

There are many causes of dystocia in the bitch and queen and it is not possible to describe these fully within this review. It is sufficient to classify dystocia as either non-obstructive (primary uterine inertia) or obstructive (dystocia secondary to maternal or fetal causes). Primary uterine inertia occurs most commonly in dams with either a small litter or a very large litter, in obese females or those at their first parturition. Obstructive dystocia may be related to breed, previous injury of the dam or any of several fetal causes. Secondary uterine inertia may develop after the correction of an obstructive dystocia.

Clinical signs

In non-obstructive dystocia, there may be few clinical signs (see prolonged gestation above); however, the observant owner may notice that first-stage parturition has commenced but that this has not progressed.

In cases of obstructive dystocia, the female has entered second-stage parturition and continues to strain unproductively. This may occur during the birth of any of the fetuses depending upon the cause. Unproductive straining for more than 45 minutes should be considered abnormal.

Diagnostic features

Females with non-obstructive dystocia have relaxation of the perineal musculature, dilation of the cervix and already have had a decline in plasma progesterone and, in bitches, a subsequent decline in rectal temperature. Cervical dilation can only be reliably assessed by endoscopic visualization and not digital palpation. If placental separation occurs, a green-coloured vulval discharge will be evident. Early in the

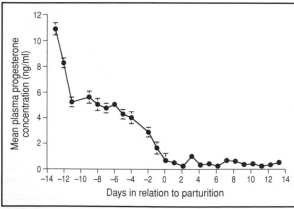

15.4 Changes in mean plasma progesterone concentration (± SEM) in 10 periparturient bitches.

course of the condition the fetuses will be alive, fetal movement may be palpated and fetal movement and heart beats may be detected ultrasonographically. Fetal death can be recognized immediately using ultrasonography by an absence of fetal movement and by a non-moving echogenic appearance to the heart. Fetal death can be detected radiographically by a change in the fetal posture, by the accumulation of gas within the fetus and/or uterus and by overlapping of the bones of the skull, although these changes may not become evident for several days.

Similar diagnostic methods may be used when there is obstructive dystocia, where fetuses can be identified lodged within the birth canal as a result of fetal or maternal abnormalities.

Therapeutic considerations

Females with primary uterine inertia will respond to the administration of exogenous oxytocin. However, the aetiology of the condition is not entirely clear and such therapy should be considered in light of the clinical condition of the dam, as well as the likely number of fetuses to be delivered. For example, it may be preferable to undertake a Caesarean operation in a bitch that has a large number of puppies and is debilitated, rather than to administer oxytocin repeatedly, resulting in an extended parturition with the possibility of dead fetuses.

In females with obstructive dystocia, the primary aim is to remove the obstruction. This can be achieved using retropulsion, realignment and traction techniques if the obstruction is the result of an abnormality of fetal presentation, position or posture. Care should be taken to ensure that parturition continues normally after such correction, since there is a risk of the development of secondary uterine inertia. However, in many cases, the dystocia is the result of a fetal or maternal abnormality that cannot be corrected to allow normal delivery, and in such circumstances it is necessary to perform a Caesarean operation. In such cases it should be remembered that:

- The dam may be 'normal' or she may be debilitated and require careful anaesthetic management
- There is often no time for pre-anaesthetic preparation
- The dam may have been fed recently.

The general aims of the procedure are to ensure adequate oxygenation by intubation and provision of inspired oxygen, to maintain blood volume and prevent hypotension by the administration of intravenous fluid therapy, and to minimize maternal and fetal depression during surgery and after delivery by reducing the dose of anaesthetic agents used. Several factors are important when considering the most appropriate fluid for intravenous administration, for example, there may be loss of acid because of vomiting and there may be loss of blood as a result of the surgery. The best choice is probably an isotonic replacement solution administered at a rate of 10–20 ml/kg/h.

It is not possible to discuss all of the anaesthetic options for Caesarean operation in this text; however, there are a few points worth considering. For premedication, atropine is best not given routinely, since it blocks the normal bradycardic response of the fetus to hypoxia and it relaxes the lower oesophageal sphincter, making aspiration more likely. Phenothiazine tranquillizers are very useful agents, since they smooth anaesthetic induction and reduce the subsequent dose of induction and maintenance agents; they are, however, rapidly transported across the placenta. Alpha-2-adrenoceptor agonists, such as medetomidine and xylazine, are contraindicated because of their severe cardiorespiratory depressant effects. Similarly, the respiratory depressant effect of opioids makes them unpopular. Metoclopramide may be administered intravenously prior to induction to reduce the risk of vomiting during the procedure. For the induction of anaesthesia, dissociative agents such as ketamine are best avoided because they produce profound depression of the fetuses. The ultra short-acting barbiturates and propofol appear to be most useful, since they are either rapidly redistributed or metabolized and therefore have limited effects upon the fetuses after delivery. Some veterinary surgeons successfully use epidural anaesthesia combined with a variety of sedative analgesics.

For maintenance of anaesthesia, the volatile agents are preferable, especially those with low partition coefficients such as isoflurane. This agent has a rapid uptake and elimination by the animal and it may have a better cardiovascular margin of safety than the more soluble inhalants such as halothane.

Whilst nitrous oxide may be used to reduce the dose of other anaesthetic agents, it is rapidly transferred across the placenta and, although it has minimal effects upon the fetus in utero, it may result in significant diffusion hypoxia after delivery. In certain cases, inhalational agents are used for anaesthetic induction, and in this case nitrous oxide is useful for speeding the induction of anaesthesia via the second gas effect.

Treatment

In females with primary uterine inertia, or secondary uterine inertia after the correction of an obstruction, the intramuscular administration of oxytocin (0.25–1.0 IU/kg) may be all that is required to ensure continuation of parturition. In some cases, the effectiveness of uterine contractions can be improved by the slow intravenous administration of 50–150 mg/kg calcium gluconate. When there is a large litter, oxytocin administration may need to be repeated approximately every 30 minutes. In the authors' opinion, no more than three doses of oxytocin should be given if no progression of the delivery has been observed.

In debilitated dams or those with an obstructive dystocia that cannot be resolved, a Caesarean operation should be performed after stabilization and consideration of the anaesthetic requirements discussed above. Operative speed is important since surgical delay is associated with increased fetal depression and asphyxia. Following a conventional Caesarean operation, the uterus should rapidly begin to contract. If this is not the case, oxytocin should be administered to promote uterine involution. This may be required especially if halothane anaesthesia has been used, since this agent is known to delay uterine involution. The administration of oxytocin should, however, not be taken lightly since it may produce peripheral vasodilation and hypotension.

Reproductive emergencies in the postparturient female

Metritis

Aetiopathology
There are several causes of acute metritis in the bitch and queen, some of which are discussed in greater detail below. The common causes include prolonged parturition, poor uterine involution, retained placentae, retained fetuses and obstetrical intervention. The condition is principally a bacterial infection of the uterus, usually with bacteria that are normally considered commensal organisms.

Clinical signs
There is most frequently a purulent or serosanguineous vulval discharge. The dam is often lethargic and anorexic and there may initially be pyrexia, although if untreated the rectal temperature may become subnormal. The dam is often weak, may be dehydrated and may continue to strain.

Diagnostic features
Often the uterus is palpably enlarged, but enlargement can be confirmed radiographically and by the use of ultrasonography. The latter technique usually demonstrates echogenic material present within the uterine lumen, and thickening of the uterine wall.

Therapeutic considerations
Stabilization of the patient by the administration of appropriate fluid therapy is essential, as is the administration of suitable broad-spectrum antimicrobial agents such as ampicillin or trimethoprim-potentiated sulphonamides. In contrast to pyometra, there is no underlying endocrine component of this condition, and the primary aim is to establish drainage of the uterus.

Treatment
Transcervical lavage of the uterus with physiological saline is extremely useful to encourage drainage of the infected material. This can be difficult without endoscopic guidance, although in these cases, the cervix usually remains open. Drainage can also be stimulated by the administration of ecbolic agents such as oxytocin and prostaglandin. Local application of antimicrobial agents into the uterus is valuable; because of the difficulty of intra-uterine administration, however, most agents are given systemically. In severe cases ovariohysterectomy may be necessary.

Haemorrhage

Aetiopathology
Haemorrhage is an uncommon postpartum condition in the bitch and queen that may occur as a result of physical injuries to the uterus or vaginal wall, or as a result of placental necrosis.

Clinical signs
Blood loss is common at the time of parturition, although this is normally limited to the time of delivery of each fetus. A small volume of haemorrhagic fluid may be passed after the termination of parturition in the normal female, but this rapidly decreases in volume and changes in colour due to the release of the pigment uteroverdin from the marginal haematoma. Persistence of a haemorrhagic discharge is abnormal. The dam may initially be unsettled, but later may be depressed and have pale mucous membranes.

Diagnostic features
Inspection of the vaginal wall either digitally or using a speculum or endoscope may demonstrate the site of a physical injury. Uterine bleeding may be detected by the presence of haemorrhagic fluid exiting via the cervix, or by transabdominal ultrasound imaging of the uterus. Although it is not normally necessary to measure the PCV of the fluid, its measurement may occasionally be useful for distinguishing frank haemorrhage from fluid that looks like whole blood but that does not represent pure haemorrhage (PCV in the range 6–10%).

Therapeutic considerations
The principal consideration is to prevent further blood loss and to maintain blood volume as discussed in uterine prolapse (see below).

Treatment
Cases of vaginal trauma can be treated either by direct pressure or the application of a vaginal tampon, or occasionally by clamping of the bleeding tissue using artery forceps followed by ligation. For uterine bleeding in the first instance, it is appropriate to attempt to speed uterine involution by the administration of oxytocin (0.25–1.0 IU/kg) or ergometrine (0.2–0.5 mg/kg). If there is no response, a laparotomy and ovariohysterectomy may be indicated. Presence of a coagulopathy should always be considered and assessments of clotting function should be performed prior to surgery.

Retained fetuses or placentas

Aetiopathology
Retained placentas are very uncommon in bitches and queens, despite the concern expressed by many breeders. Most commonly the condition is wrongly believed to be present, since placentas are not always expelled after each fetus and several are delivered some time later during parturition. Retained fetuses should be investigated as described in primary and secondary uterine inertia (see above).

The aetiology of placental retention is unknown, but it appears to be more common in toy breeds of dog.

Clinical signs
In cases of true placental retention in the bitch, there is usually persistence of a green-coloured vulval discharge, and the bitch may be restless and not allow the puppies to suck. If the condition is not treated, the discharge will become malodorous and the bitch may

become depressed and show signs of sepsis. In general, queens have similar clinical signs, although in some there are no signs of vulval discharge until several weeks after parturition.

Diagnostic features
Diagnosis of the condition soon after parturition can be very difficult without ultrasonographic or endoscopic examination. Transabdominal palpation is often misleading because the involuting uterus may have sections which are dilated, and adjacent regions that are smaller in diameter.

Therapeutic considerations
In many cases placentae have not been retained and the problem is simply the concern of the owner. In true cases the bitch or queen may develop signs of septic shock. In such instances, removal of the infected material is imperative; however, stabilization of the patient with appropriate fluid and antimicrobial therapy is essential. The principles described for pyometra (see above) should be followed.

Treatment
In the early stages, repeated administration of oxytocin may be sufficient to cause expulsion of the retained placentae. This results in resolution of the clinical signs, although the dam should be treated with broad-spectrum antimicrobial agents, such as ampicillin or trimethoprim-potentiated sulphonamides, to prevent the development of a secondary metritis.

In the later stages of the condition, the number of uterine oxytocin receptors has decreased and the administration of exogenous oxytocin has little or no clinical effect. In these instances repeated low-dose prostaglandin treatment may be contemplated; however, it may be difficult to dislodge the placenta, and hysterotomy may be indicated. In animals not required for breeding, ovariohysterectomy is the treatment of choice.

Uterine prolapse

Aetiopathology
Prolapse of one or both uterine horns is rare in the bitch and queen and is only associated with pregnancy. The condition occurs following parturition or abortion. It may occur in females of all ages and, although the aetiology is uncertain, it is claimed to be due to over-relaxation and stretching of the pelvic musculature, uterine atony, trauma of the uterus and prolonged tenesmus during dystocia. Following prolapse, there is commonly rupture of the uterine vessels and the vessels in the broad ligament, resulting in haemoperitoneum and hypovolaemic shock.

Clinical signs
The history is that of a dam that has recently undergone parturition or has aborted, and either one or both uterine horns can be identified at the vulva. Frequently, the patient continues to have abdominal contractions. The prolapsed uterus may be traumatized, in which case there is considerable haemorrhage.

Diagnostic features
The condition can be diagnosed by the history and presenting clinical signs. In the bitch, uterine prolapse can be easily differentiated from vaginal hyperplasia since the latter occurs during oestrus and has an insidious onset.

Therapeutic considerations
The principal consideration is the loss of blood volume. This can be restored by the use of intravenous fluid therapy (crystalloid and/or colloid) at a rate dependent on the degree of hypovolaemic shock (see Chapter 4). Blood transfusion may be considered when the PCV decreases to 20%, or in patients in whom arterial pressure cannot be maintained by infusion of balanced electrolyte solutions. In cases of severe haemorrhage, autotransfusion may be considered by collecting blood aseptically from the peritoneal cavity.

Treatment
Prompt laparotomy with traction of the prolapsed uterus is necessary to allow inspection of the uterine vessels. In cases that are presented early, replacement and pexy of the uterus may be attempted; however, in most cases there is marked pathology of the uterine vasculature, and ovariohysterectomy is the treatment of choice.

Hypocalcaemia
The treatment of postparturient hypocalcaemia should follow the principles described in the section on Hypocalcaemia in Reproductive emergencies in the pregnant female (above), although in some cases it may also be necessary to consider weaning the pups.

Septic mastitis

Aetiopathology
In many cases mastitis is a minor clinical disease. However, acute septic mastitis can occur following the introduction of bacteria during the process of suckling. The condition may occur in a single gland, or occasionally may involve all glands. The common bacteria involved are *Escherichia coli*, *Staphylococcus* spp. and *Streptococcus* spp.

Clinical signs
The affected gland is normally hot, swollen and painful and there may be discoloration of the skin surrounding the teat. The dam is normally pyrexic and lethargic. In certain cases the glands may become gangrenous or abscessated.

Diagnostic features
Examination of strippings from the affected gland or glands often demonstrates a haemorrhagic discoloration of the milk. Microscopic examination may be useful to demonstrate the presence of bacteria, and culture may be undertaken to identify the sensitivity of the organism to antimicrobial agents.

Therapeutic considerations
Topical instillation of antimicrobial agents into the teat canal is not possible. The choice of systemic antimicrobials should be made with care as the aim is to have

high milk concentrations. As this milk may be ingested by the neonates, potential adverse effects should be carefully considered. Antimicrobial drugs contraindicated for neonates include tetracyclines and dihydrostreptomycin. However, in the case of a severe septic mastitis the dam is so unwell that it is often necessary to remove the litter and institute artificial feeding.

Treatment
Stripping of the affected glands and the use of hot compresses are important to encourage drainage of the infected material. The administration of appropriate antimicrobial agents is essential; however, in many cases it is not possible to wait for the results of culture and sensitivity, and therefore broad-spectrum agents are often chosen. Ampicillin is the agent of choice, although chloramphenicol has also been recommended. Agents that are weak bases (e.g. potentiated sulphonamides and lincomycin) tend to achieve high concentrations, since milk from dams with mastitis is slightly more acidic than plasma. Occasionally, severely affected glands become necrotic and surgical drainage is necessary. Chronic persistently infected glands ultimately require mastectomy.

Reproductive emergencies in the male

Paraphimosis

Aetiopathology
Paraphimosis is a failure of the glans penis to be retracted fully into the prepuce. In the dog, this may be the result of a small preputial orifice, inversion of the preputial skin and hair, a short prepuce or neurogenic factors affecting the preputial muscles. In the tom cat, the condition has only been reported associated with an abnormality of the preputial orifice. Paraphimosis may become an emergency because there is swelling of the penis, interference with the circulation within the penis and ultimately ischaemic necrosis. Secondary urethral obstruction may result.

Clinical signs
Initially, the clinical signs are extrusion of the penis, associated with pain and continuous licking. Self-trauma may progress to mutilation. After several hours, the penis becomes cold and the patient may pay less attention to the area.

Diagnostic features
The condition can be diagnosed by inspection, and differentiated from other conditions, since normally the penis is engorged.

Treatment
The application of ice packs and lubricants may be sufficient to allow replacement of the penis, which is the primary goal. In most cases the male resents this manipulation, and sedation is required; this can also be helpful since it reduces systemic blood pressure and causes detumescence of the penis. Surgical enlargement of the preputial orifice may be necessary to allow replacement of the penis, and in some cases amputation of the necrotic organ is required.

Torsion of the spermatic cord (testicular torsion)

Aetiopathology
Rotation of one of the testes around the vertical axis causes occlusion of the pampiniform plexus, followed by swelling and necrosis of the testicle. The aetiology is unknown although it may be related to rupture of the scrotal ligament. Torsion is more common in enlarged neoplastic intra-abdominal testes. The condition has not been reported in the tom.

Clinical signs
Torsion results in severe pain, unilateral swelling of the scrotum and thickening of the spermatic cord (Figure 15.5). Frequently, dogs are unwilling to walk and continually self-traumatize the scrotum. Clinical signs are diagnostic when the condition occurs in a scrotal testis, but may be confusing when the torsion relates to an abdominal testis. In these cases there may be lethargy, inappetence, abdominal pain and vomiting. Later in the course of the condition, the animal may develop ascites and signs of hypovolaemic shock. A firm mass may be palpated within the caudal abdomen.

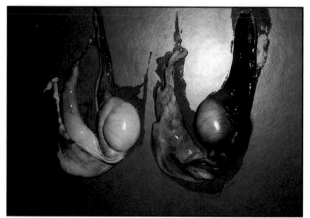

15.5 Normal testicle and testicle with torsion of the spermatic cord demonstrating severe haemorrhage and oedema.

Diagnostic features
Diagnosis can be made based on the clinical signs when the affected testis is scrotal; however, ultrasonography and/or exploratory surgery may be necessary in dogs with torsion of intra-abdominal testes.

Therapeutic considerations
Dogs with this condition require treatment for shock using fluid therapy prior to definitive surgical correction of the problem.

Treatment
Prompt surgical removal of the affected testis is essential.

Acute bacterial prostatitis

Aetiopathology
Adult dogs may develop prostatitis as a result of ascending bacterial infection, commonly *Escherichia coli*, *Staphylococcus* spp. and *Streptococcus* spp.

Prostatitis does not occur in the tom. In dogs, certain conditions increase the likelihood of contamination of the prostate gland, including benign prostatic hyperplasia and squamous metaplasia. It is likely that diseases which increase the number of bacteria within the prostatic urethra, including cystitis, urethral calculi and neoplasia, also increase the risk of development of prostatitis.

Clinical signs
The clinical signs often include systemic illness, with pyrexia, vomiting and caudal abdominal pain. There may be a purulent or haemorrhagic discharge at the prepuce. Urethral obstruction or colonic compression can occur if the prostate becomes large enough.

Diagnostic features
On rectal palpation, the gland is painful and has an irregular contour. There is commonly a neutrophilia on haematological evaluation. Urine culture, urethral washings and ultrasound-guided fine needle aspiration may help with the diagnosis. A technique that is often overlooked is collection of a semen sample with cytological examination of the third fraction of the ejaculate.

Therapeutic considerations
The blood–prostatic fluid barrier is thought to be lost when there is severe inflammation, and therefore many antimicrobial agents can be used for the treatment of prostatitis. Inadequately treated lesions may become chronic and pockets of purulent exudate may form (prostatic abscessation), producing signs of recurrent cystitis. Treatment of these cases is difficult.

Reduction of the size of the gland may be helpful in speeding the resolution of the disease.

Treatment
Prompt antimicrobial treatment should be undertaken, preferably on the basis of microbial culture and identification of sensitivity; potentiated sulphonamides and enrofloxacin are particularly useful if treatment is required before this can be established. Penicillins and cephalosporins have limited penetration into prostatic fluid. Treatment should be continued until no bacteria are found within the prostatic fluid; this may require three or more weeks of therapy, but is necessary to prevent the development of chronic disease. If chronic infection and abscessation are diagnosed, surgical investigation and drainage are required.

Recovery in many cases can be enhanced by reducing prostatic size, either by castration or by the administration of exogenous progestogens or oestrogens. Exogenous drugs produce only a temporary response, and it should be remembered that prolonged oestrogen therapy may produce prostatic metaplasia which predisposes to prostatitis. Most recently, attention has been paid to finasteride, which is a specific 5-alpha reductase inhibitor that prevents the conversion of testosterone into dihydrotestosterone. Finasteride may be useful for managing the underlying prostatic hyperplasia.

Emergencies in the neonate

Resuscitation of neonates
Neonates may require resuscitation following a Caesarean operation, or following a normal delivery. In both cases, the primary cause of mortality is hypoxia, which can be reduced by the rapid removal of fetuses from the amniotic sac. The umbilicus should be cut approximately 3 cm from the fetal abdomen; excessive bleeding can be prevented by the application of a ligature or haemostatic clip. The nostrils and oropharynx should be cleared of fluid using a plastic pipette or cotton swabs. Fluid can also be removed by supporting the head and neck and swinging the neonate slowly downwards in a large arc. Great care must be paid to ensure that a whiplash or concussive injury does not occur. The neonate should be vigorously dried, since this stimulates respiratory drive. Gentle compression of the chest usually results in the establishment of respiratory effort. If this is not the case and the heart is beating, respiratory stimulation should be continued by rubbing the thorax, and flow-by oxygen should be administered. The administration of respiratory stimulant agents such as doxapram hydrochloride (1–2 drops sublingually) may be efficacious although it is less likely to be effective if the brain is hypoxic. If respiration does not commence, then artificial respiration should be performed by endotracheal intubation using a 20 gauge plastic catheter, or by blowing gently into the nose and mouth. Insufflation of air should be performed carefully to induce only slight lung expansion without over-inflation. If the heart is not beating, external cardiac massage combined with artificial respiration may be attempted.

Once regular respiratory efforts are maintained, the neonate may be placed into a prewarmed box or incubator until it is active, when it should be returned to the dam and encouraged to suck. Sucking normally occurs immediately after birth and at intervals of 2–3 hours for the first few days.

Nursing care of neonates
Once born, the puppies and kittens should be carefully examined and their body weight should be recorded. Normal neonates increase in body weight by 5–10% per day; a failure to achieve this rate may indicate ill-health. Examination should ensure that the umbilicus is clean and there should be no evidence of herniation. Respiration should be regular and without excessive noise; the normal respiratory rate is 15–40 breaths per minute. There should be no discharge from the eyes or ears. The neonate should be examined for the presence of congenital diseases. The normal rectal temperature is 32–34°C in the first week after birth.

The environmental temperature is critical; hypothermia is a major cause of neonatal mortality. Recommended temperatures of 25–30°C are only necessary for the first few days; these are often unbearable for the dam and can be safely reduced (22°C) as long as draughts are avoided. One method to reduce heat exposure of the dam is to heat only half of the whelping box. Underfloor heating is the ideal; however, warm hot water bottles or circulating water blankets provide a good alternative. Heat lamps that are suspended above the nest should be used with caution, since the environment may become too hot.

Neonatal puppies and kittens are unable to stand at birth. They should, however, be quite mobile, using their limbs to crawl. Neonates should be assessed for their general strength and the weakest should be carefully observed, since these often do not feed adequately and may fail to thrive. Standing may be seen from 10 days after birth, and most neonates should be able to walk at 3 weeks of age.

Puppies and kittens are born with their eyes closed; separation of the upper and lower lids and opening of the eyes occurs approximately 10–14 days after birth. The cornea at this stage may appear slightly cloudy, although this will resolve over the first 4 weeks. In the first few weeks of life, the dam will provide all the care for her offspring provided that the environment is clean and dry. Many types of bedding material may be used, including shredded paper, newspaper and blankets or newspaper and synthetic rugs. Materials should be washable or easily disposed of. The dam normally licks the perineal region of each neonate for the first 2–3 weeks after birth to stimulate urination and defecation. Puppies and kittens defecate and urinate voluntarily at 3 weeks of age and at this time soiling of the bedding increases; regular changing of the bedding is therefore necessary.

When considering pharmacological therapy for neonates, it should be remembered that drug distribution differs considerably from that of adults because of differences in body composition (lower body fat stores and plasma albumin concentrations, higher percentage of total body water and a poorly developed blood–brain barrier). For these reasons, drug dosages may need to be reduced by up to 50% and the frequency of administration may need to be reduced.

Fading puppies and kittens
Perinatal losses are generally thought to be higher in dogs and cats than in other species; approximately 15% of puppies/kittens are reported to be dead at birth and a further 8% to die shortly afterwards.

Known causes of neonatal loss
Examination of dead puppies shows that asphyxia is the most common cause of neonatal loss and this probably relates to the fact that oxygenation is threatened at birth because:

- There is reduced blood flow to the uterus during contractions
- The umbilicus is stretched (it is very short anyway)
- The placenta separates some time prior to delivery.

Immediately after birth, the neonate experiences marked physiological changes; the arterial oxygen concentrations decrease and the arterial carbon dioxide concentrations increase. Neonates are therefore born with a moderate to severe acidosis. Recovery of normal blood values should occur over a period of 3–6 hours. This is mediated by normal respiration and can

therefore be inhibited by poor respiratory function (i.e. carbon dioxide is not reduced if breathing is poor). It is clear that suitable supervision at the time of parturition can reduce the loss rates considerably; indeed, in high-quality breeding establishments the total losses are in the order of 5%.

In other cases neonatal death occurs because of congenital abnormalities, nutritional disease (including inadequate feeding), abnormally low birth weight, trauma during or immediately after birth, neonatal isoerythrolysis (kittens) and various infectious diseases.

True fading puppy syndrome
In addition to the perinatal losses described above, many puppies and kittens (approximately 55% of total losses) are lost without an apparent cause being found. These neonatal losses are often attributed to 'fading puppy/kitten syndrome'. The first signs of this syndrome can often be detected within a few hours of life, and it is possible that these neonates are not fully viable at birth. Interestingly, it has been shown that true fading puppies (those with no other known cause of death) had significantly lower phosphatidylcholine components of lung surfactant than puppies that died from known causes. Lung surfactant is required for normal respiratory adaptation and maintenance following birth. A significant reduction of surfactant is observed in sudden infant death syndrome in humans, and low values in fading puppies suggest that the production of surfactant may similarly be involved in the aetiology of this disease.

Whatever the cause, there appears to be an early failure to suck and subsequent establishment of a fatal cycle of dehydration and further failure to feed.

Management of sick neonates
Early supplementary feeding may improve survival rates, as may the administration of antimicrobial agents in cases of neonatal sepsis. However, many cases are not related to a primary bacterial infection and such treatment alone is often unrewarding. Intensive therapy, including the administration of intravenous fluids, antimicrobial agents, and intravenous nutrition may be valuable; however, the prognosis for most cases is extremely guarded as their small size limits effective application of these therapies.

Maintaining the puppy or kitten in an oxygen-enriched environment or providing oxygen via a tracheal catheter may help overcome hypoxia. The use of a tracheal catheter may allow artificial ventilation which may be useful to reverse acidosis and encourage lung surfactant production.

Fluid therapy is essential and puppies with pale mucous membranes and a slow capillary refill time are usually at least 10% dehydrated. Rarely fluid may be replaced by oral administration of electrolytes; because of poor gastrointestinal perfusion and absorption, in most cases it is necessary to provide fluids by either intravenous, intraperitoneal or intraosseus administration. The safest fluid to use is a replacement isotonic crystalloid solution at a dose determined by assessment of the patient's hydration and perfusion status (see Chapter 4). If using lactated Ringer's, consider that the neonate has reduced hepatic function and it may be unable to metabolize lactate into bicarbonate. Maintenance potassium (20 mmol/l) can be added once fluid administration rates are at or just above maintenance requirements. Ideally acid–base and electrolyte status should be monitored and corrected, although this may be difficult due to the small size of the patients.

Intravenous catheter placement may be difficult in the dehydrated neonate; human neonatal scalp catheters may be technically easier to place in small vessels. It is always worthwhile spending some time to ensure adequate venous access, and whilst a surgical cut-down may initially seem to lengthen the procedure, in the long term it is often the most sensible option.

Intraperitoneal administration of fluids is a route chosen in some cases where venous access is difficult, or if there is likely to be inadequate ongoing monitoring to ensure successful intravenous administration. The most appropriate intraperitoneal dosing scheme is to provide fluids in three boluses (approximately 10 ml/kg) at approximately 8-hour intervals. Unfortunately intraperitoneal fluids are relatively slowly absorbed, especially in the hypovolaemic neonate.

Intraosseous catheter placement provides a suitable alternative for fluid administration. Rates and doses of fluids administered are the same as for intravenous use. Normally access is via the trochanteric fossa of the proximal femur, or the medial aspect of the proximal tibia. An 18 or 20 gauge needle is pushed longitudinally into the medullary cavity after strict aseptic preparation. In some cases the cortical bone is sufficiently soft to allow the use of an intravenous over-the-needle catheter. Repeated puncture is not advised as holes within the cortical bone can allow fluid leakage; the catheter may be left in position, however, for up to 72 hours.

Hypovolaemia may be complicated by sepsis. Septic shock may result in further depletion of glycogen reserves, an increased peripheral use of glucose and a decrease in gluconeogenesis resulting in hypoglycaemia. In such animals, additional bolus glucose therapy can be provided using a 50% dextrose solution mixed 50:50 with lactated Ringers solution, or by giving 1–2 ml of 10% glucose intravenously.

Broad-spectrum antimicrobial therapy is frequently administered and often it is not appropriate to wait for culture and sensitivity results. It is sensible however to collect bacteriological samples prior to drug administration to allow the potential for changing the antimicrobial preparation once the results are obtained. Culture of whole blood can be useful in many cases.

Prevention of perinatal losses is aimed at:

- The early recognition of weak neonates or dams that have inadequate milk or poor mothering behaviour
- The institution of rapid and aggressive supplementary feeding.

Accurate postmortem examination is essential to establish the causative factors so that these can be eliminated prior to the next breeding.

Artificial nutrition of neonates

Maternal illness, death of the dam, poor nursing, inadequate lactation and a large litter are all factors that contribute to malnutrition of the neonate. In these cases, partial hand-rearing (with rotation of the offspring between the dam and artificial feeding), complete hand-rearing, or a foster dam (a bitch in pseudopregnancy or a bitch/queen which has lost her litter) are required.

When contemplating artificial feeding, a well formulated milk replacer is essential and, whilst home-prepared replacers using cows' milk have been advocated, it is the authors' opinion that a commercially available replacer should be used. It has been suggested that some neonates should be reared entirely artificially rather than alternating the whole litter. However, all neonates should remain with the dam to ensure a normal social development.

It is essential that all neonates receive colostrum from the dam during the first few hours after birth to ensure an adequate uptake of maternal immunoglobulins. Should the dam have died, it may still be possible to milk some colostrum from the mammary glands as long as it is not contaminated with high concentrations of drugs or toxins. If colostrum is unavailable it may be possible to confer some protective immunity by the oral administration of serum or plasma prepared from adult animals (Levy et al., 2001). Orogastric intubation is relatively simple and may be useful in the first few days of life for the rapid feeding of especially sick neonates. A soft polythene tube (2 mm diameter) measured from the mouth to the level of the 9th rib is optimal.

Artificial feeding is time consuming and demanding, particularly if the litter is being reared without the dam. Milk substitutes may be administered using syringe feeders, eye droppers, sucking devices or stomach tube. In most cases it may be easiest to feed from a small syringe (2 ml) for the first 2–5 days. After this time, a small bottle with a nipple may be used; this encourages normal sucking but takes the greatest time. When these devices are used the aperture should be large enough to prevent wind sucking but small enough to prevent excessive volumes being administered, since this may result in aspiration.

Normally neonates feed every 2–4 hours for the first 5 days of life. It is best to mimic this with artificial feeding. The interval can be reduced to every 4 hours after day 5. The milk replacer should be warmed to body temperature (39°C) before feeding and then fed to the manufacturer's instructions, depending upon body weight. After each feeding, the perineal area of the neonate should be stimulated with a moist towel, to mimic the licking action of the dam and stimulate urination and defecation.

Conclusion

It is clear that there are many reproductive disorders which produce acute onset and potentially fatal clinical disease in dogs and cats. Similarly, there are many management factors responsible for perinatal mortality in puppies and kittens. There have been substantial advances in our knowledge of reproductive and neonatal physiology and these, combined with prompt recognition and intervention, may result in greater survival and significantly decreased loss of reproductive performance.

References and further reading

Blunden AS, Hill CM, Brown BD and Morley CJ (1987) Lung surfactant composition in puppies dying of fading puppy complex. *Research in Veterinary Science* **42**, 113–118

England GCW (1998) *Allen's Fertility and Obstetrics in the Dog*. Blackwell Science, Oxford

Gilbert RO, Nothling JO and Oettle EE (1989) A retrospective study of 40 cases of canine pyometra-metritis treated with prostaglandin F-2alpha and broad spectrum antibacterial drugs. *Journal of Reproduction and Fertility Supplement* **39**, 225–229

Gobello C, Castex G, Klima L, Rodriguez R and Corrada Y (2003) A study of two protocols combining aglepristone and cloprostenol to treat open cervix pyometra in the bitch. *Theriogenology* **60**, 901–908

Hoskins JD (2001) *Veterinary Pediatrics, 3rd edn*. WB Saunders, Philadelphia

Jackson PGG (1995) *Handbook of Veterinary Obstetrics*. WB Saunders, London

Levy JK, Crawford PC, Collante WR and Papich MG (2001) Use of adult cat serum to correct failure of passive transfer in kittens. *Journal of the American Veterinary Medical Association* **219**, 1401–1405

Onclin K and Verstegen JP (1999) Comparisons of different combinations of analogues of PGF2 alpha and dopamine agonists for the termination of pregnancy in dogs. *Veterinary Record* **144**, 416–419

Trasch K, Wehrend A and Bostedt H (2003) Follow-up examinations of bitches after conservative treatment of pyometra with the antigestagen aglepristone. *Journal of Veterinary Medicine: A, Physiology, Pathology, Clinical Medicine* **50**, 375–379

16

Endocrine emergencies

Barbara J. Skelly

Diabetic ketoacidosis

A diabetic ketoacidotic crisis can arise in an animal with previously diagnosed diabetes mellitus (DM) or it can appear to occur suddenly in an animal previously thought to be healthy. In this latter group it may provide the first indication that either insulin production has fallen or that mechanisms of insulin resistance are present. Whereas dogs are usually insulin-dependent for life once a diagnosis of DM is reached, cats may provide the further challenge of having waxing and waning insulin requirements. Figure 16.1 lists the most common reasons for diabetic ketoacidosis (DKA) to develop, either in an animal already being treated for DM or in a previously undiagnosed diabetic.

Bacterial infections

Any significant infected focus but especially:
    Urinary tract infection – upper and lower
    Prostatitis
    Pneumonia
    Pyoderma
    Otitis externa
    Severe gingivitis/oral abscesses from tooth root infections

Inflammatory disease
Pancreatitis
Endocrinopathies or physiological endocrine changes
Hyperadrenocorticism (cats and dogs) Acromegaly (cats and dogs, though different mechanisms) Hyperthyroidism (cats) Hypothyroidism (dogs) Phaeochromocytoma Dioestrus phase of oestrous cycle
Iatrogenic causes
Steroid therapy – including intra-aural or ocular

16.1 Conditions that can trigger DKA through insulin resistance.

How does ketoacidosis develop?

For DKA to develop there is usually a triggering condition such as an infection, inflammatory disease (e.g. pancreatitis) or metabolic disturbance superimposed on a background of a loss of insulin activity. This triggering condition then causes the glucagon:insulin ratio to increase, the hormonal hallmark of DKA. Figure 16.2 shows the role of glucagon versus insulin in the development of ketoacidosis. Glucagon promotes

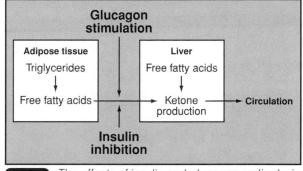

16.2 The effects of insulin and glucagon on lipolysis and ketone production.

glycogenolysis and the formation of ketoacids, while insulin deficiency allows free fatty acids (FFA) from the breakdown of adipocyte triglyceride stores to be released into the circulation and taken up by the liver, again for ketoacid production. Insulin is also required for metabolism of ketones to carbon dioxide and water. While there is a low level of ketone production in uncomplicated DM, the ketones can be metabolized and do not build up to the point at which they might cause clinical signs. The superimposition of further physiological stress, for example in the form of an infection, allows ketone production to accelerate and exceed the rate at which ketones can be metabolized. Ketonuria and a metabolic acidosis then develop.

Clinical signs

The clinical signs of DKA are listed in Figure 16.3. A detailed history may reveal previous signs of DM, if present, for example polyuria and polydipsia, a ravenous appetite and weight loss. Patients in a DKA crisis can also develop acute renal failure so it is useful to know when the animal was last seen to pass urine. Patients are commonly both hypovolaemic and dehydrated on presentation.

Polyuria/polydipsia Anorexia Vomiting and/or diarrhoea Depression Weakness or collapse Poor body condition Hepatomegaly Acetone smell on breath Deeper more rapid respiration reflecting metabolic acidosis

16.3 The clinical signs of diabetic ketoacidosis.

Diagnosis

DKA is an important differential diagnosis for a collapsed, volume-depleted patient. Early recognition of the disease is possible using just a few readily available tests. Firstly, measurement of blood glucose is important in any collapsed animal as both hypo- and hyperglycaemia are possible causes of weakness. Blood glucose measurement is therefore considered part of the emergency minimum database (see Chapter 1). Demonstration of a high blood glucose concentration in an emergency patient prompts the testing of serum or urine ketone levels. This can be done by clinical pathology laboratories, but also by using urine dipsticks with serum or urine as a substrate. One of the predominant ketone bodies (β-hydroxybutyrate) is not measured by standard urine dipsticks. A negative result for ketones in a patient where there is a high clinical index of suspicion for DKA might prompt the addition of hydrogen peroxide to the sample to oxidize β-hydroxybutyrate to acetoacetate. This can then be measured by dipstick, thereby allowing documentation of ketoacidosis.

Initial patient assessment

- Packed cell volume (PCV) and total solids/protein.
- Electrolytes.
- Renal function assessment – urea, creatinine and phosphorus.
- Blood gas analysis.
- Urine analysis:
  - Specific gravity
  - Dipstick analysis – assess for ketones
  - Sediment examination
  - Submit for culture.

Management

Initial management of DKA involves correction of the intravascular volume, hydration and electrolyte abnormalities whilst providing insulin to reduce hyperglycaemia and promote ketone metabolism:

- Place jugular or peripheral vein catheter of the widest bore possible. The benefit of a jugular catheter is that it allows frequent blood sampling without the need for repeated venipuncture
- Begin fluid therapy using an isotonic replacement fluid, e.g. 0.9% NaCl or Hartmann's solution. The latter may be beneficial in cases where the pH is extremely acidic as 0.9% NaCl may, in some circumstances, contribute to acidosis through a dilutional effect
- If the patient is in shock or acute renal failure use fluid boluses to improve pulse quality and initiate urine output. 50–90 ml/kg may be used in the dog and 20–50 ml/kg in cats. Fractions of these volumes (25–30% each time) can be used to effect with careful monitoring between boluses (see Chapter 4)
- Once the patient's cardiovascular status has improved these fluid rates *must be lowered* (see Chapter 4). The aim is to correct the hydration and metabolic abnormalities slowly over 24–48 hours so that complications are avoided. Problems that may be encountered with rapid

correction include:
- Hypokalaemia
- Hypophosphataemia
- Cerebral oedema.

Monitoring potassium

Although many DKA patients have a 'whole body' potassium deficit, the plasma potassium concentration may be disarmingly normal at initial assessment. This occurs because of the effects of solvent drag, whereby high extracellular glucose levels encourage movement of water and potassium out of the cells. When fluid replacement and insulin therapy are given, however, potassium again takes up an intracellular location and hypokalaemia results. Severe hypokalaemia can lead to muscle weakness and can predispose to cardiac dysrhythmias or even respiratory arrest. It is important to monitor potassium levels every 1–2 hours, especially during the first 12 hours of therapy and to supplement the fluids with potassium as appropriate (Figure 16.4).

Serum potassium (mmol/l)	Amount of potassium to add to 1 l fluids (mmol)
>5.5	None – reassess later
4.1–5.4	20
3.1–4.0	30
2.6–3.0	40
<2.5	60–80

16.4 Potassium supplementation of intravenous fluids in patients with DKA.

Monitoring phosphate

Phosphate ions follow the same path as described for potassium above. Severe hypophosphataemia can lead to haemolysis, so again, phosphorus should be monitored during fluid therapy (Willard et al., 1987). Hypophosphataemia often becomes most severe on the second day of therapy. Phosphate supplementation is recommended if the phosphate concentration drops below 0.35 mmol/l. The phosphate supplementation rate suggested in many formularies (0.01–0.03 mmol/kg/h over 4–6 hours) is often insufficient in these patients and doses up to 0.12 mmol/kg/h for 12–48 hours may be required. Regular monitoring of phosphate (every 4–12 hours) is necessary, with the dose adjusted depending on the patient's response. As phosphate is generally supplied as potassium phosphate, the additional potassium supplementation should be taken into account and the dose of potassium chloride reduced accordingly.

Neurological function

During prolonged hyperglycaemia, the central nervous system (CNS) protects itself from dehydration by the generation of idiogenic osmoles that help to conserve water in the intracellular space. If during treatment serum osmolality drops too quickly (e.g. following rapid reduction in blood glucose or rapid rehydration with hypotonic fluid) the osmotic effect of these molecules will tend to pull water into the cells of the CNS and cause oedema. This can lead to worsening neurological function in the early stages of therapy and is an indication that fluid replacement and/or insulin treatment has been too aggressive.

Insulin therapy

Insulin therapy is the cornerstone of treatment, as it allows glucose to be taken up by cells for metabolism and prevents further lipolysis from adding to the ketone burden. It also promotes metabolism of ketones. Hence as serum glucose levels decrease, glucose should be added to the intravenous fluids to allow continued insulin administration until the resolution of ketosis. Neutral (soluble) insulin (termed regular insulin in the USA) should be used, as it facilitates accurate control of glucose levels. Insulin can be given in two ways:

- Method 1 (intramuscular):
  - Begin treatment with a 0.2 IU/kg i.m. bolus of neutral (soluble/regular) insulin
  - Repeat intramuscular injections of 0.1 IU/kg hourly according to blood glucose measurements to keep blood glucose in the 8–15 mmol/l range
  - If blood glucose drops to <8 mmol/l, add 5% dextrose to intravenous fluids, monitor glucose and continue insulin therapy if possible
  - Use neutral/(soluble/regular) insulin for the initial therapy or until the animal begins to eat reliably. At this point, maintenance stabilization using longer-acting insulin can begin
- Method 2 (intravenous constant rate infusion (CRI)):
  - Mix neutral (soluble/regular) insulin with fluids such that it will be delivered at a dose rate of 2.2 IU/kg/day
  - It is easiest to use a separate syringe driver/burette to deliver the insulin dose at a standard fluid administration rate of 1–2 ml/kg/h. This infusion can be run alongside the main fluid source, which can then be adjusted as the patient requires without altering the rate of insulin delivery. Insulin solutions within a burette should be protected from direct light by covering with aluminium foil and should be freshly made up at least once every 24 hours
  - Since insulin binds to plastic tubing in drip lines, before administration to the patient, allow fluids to run through the line until a stable solution has been achieved (30–50 ml expelled)
  - Blood glucose needs to be checked after 1 hour then every 1–2 hours thereafter
  - Again, dextrose can be used as required to maintain the blood glucose between 8 and 15 mmol/l
  - Longer-acting insulin can be introduced when the animal starts to eat.

If a good response is achieved after the first 24 hours, then the intensity of the monitoring can be reduced. The intravenous fluids can be gradually tapered as the patient begins to eat and drink. After the first 24-hour period it may be necessary to change the fluid type depending on the plasma sodium concentration, such that if plasma sodium is >145 mmol/l then a change to Hartmann's solution or 0.45% saline might be advantageous.

Antibiotic therapy

Intravenous antibiotics may be started *after* urine and/or other culture samples have been taken, because there is a strong association between bacterial infection and the precipitation of DKA. Ampicillin 20 mg/kg i.v. q6–8h is a good broad-spectrum choice in an animal that has not previously received antibiotic therapy, until results of cultures or other diagnostic tests allow tailoring of treatment to the specific bacteria involved.

Other therapeutic considerations

It is important to evaluate patients with DKA rigorously for any underlying trigger and treat this as necessary. In patients with profuse vomiting, anti-emetic medication may be required (see Chapter 11) and if voluntary food intake is poor for a prolonged period, alternative methods of supplying nutrition should be considered (see Chapter 23).

Insulinoma

Insulinomas are classically described in middle-aged and older, overweight large-breed dogs and have also been reported rarely in cats (Kraje, 2003). The effect of over-production of insulin is to induce a profound hypoglycaemia, particularly in a fasted animal. Some clinical signs are also attributed to increased activity of the sympathetic nervous system and excessive adrenaline release. Insulinoma-associated polyneuropathy has been reported. The aetiology is not certain but may involve axonal degeneration due to hypoglycaemia and/or immune-mediated mechanisms (Van Ham *et al.*, 1997). The differential diagnosis of hypoglycaemia is shown in Figure 16.5.

Endocrine
Insulinoma Hypoadrenocorticism
Hepatic insufficiency
Neoplasia
Hepatoma Hepatocellular carcinoma Leiomyosarcoma
Sepsis/systemic inflammatory response syndrome
Patient factors
Juvenile (toy breed) hypoglycaemia Hunting dog hypoglycaemia Neonatal hypoglycaemia
Laboratory error
Polycythaemia Aged sample
Iatrogenic
Insulin overdose Oral hypoglycaemic agents
Toxic
Xylitol ingestion (dog)

16.5 Differential diagnosis of hypoglycaemia.

Clinical signs

The history usually involves collapse at exercise or exercise intolerance, weakness, tremors and neurological signs including, more rarely, signs of a polyneuropathy that may present as hindlimb weakness, tetra- or monoparesis. Occasionally animals may present with seizures. The clinical signs are rapidly responsive to feeding and can be controlled by feeding regular small meals.

Diagnosis

The hallmark of insulinoma is the measurement of low serum glucose concentrations with concurrently high serum levels of insulin. Insulin may not be above the normal range (5.0–20 IU/ml) but may still be inappropriately high for the blood glucose; if the pancreatic islet cells are functioning normally, insulin levels should be very low in an animal that has hypoglycaemia. If insulinoma is suspected but the blood glucose is in the normal range, then supervised fasting of the animal can be conducted with glucose measurements every 2–3 hours. In animals with insulinoma, hypoglycaemia will usually result in 6–8 hours. Insulin:glucose and amended insulin:glucose ratios do not contribute to the ease of diagnosis and are not used by this author. The measurement of a low fructosamine (normal range 258–343 μmol/l) can add to the index of suspicion. Glucagon tolerance tests are rarely necessary though they may be used in cases that are difficult to interpret. There are no other consistent abnormalities on clinical pathology measurements.

Radiographs are unlikely to yield diagnostic information. Abdominal ultrasound examination is useful for identification of pancreatic nodules, and also to assess other abdominal organs for abnormalities that suggest the presence of metastatic spread.

Ultimately, a definitive diagnosis is reached if an exploratory laparotomy identifies a pancreatic lesion that is then evaluated by histopathology.

Treatment

Emergency treatment

Patients with neurological signs caused by hypoglycaemia need immediate attention. After collecting blood for glucose and insulin assessment, dextrose should be given as a bolus (10% dextrose solution at 0.2–0.5 g/kg, i.v.). As a rule of thumb, 1 ml/kg of a 50% dextrose solution equates to 0.5 g/kg of dextrose; this should be diluted prior to administration. The clinical response is usually rapid and stability should then be maintained by the addition of 2.5–10% dextrose to the intravenous fluids. If the dextrose concentration is >5% then a central route of administration should be used to avoid problems (thrombophlebitis) caused by administration of a hypertonic solution through a peripheral vein. Alternatively, instead of increasing the dextrose concentration in the fluids, an increase in fluid rate can result in administration of higher doses of dextrose with no change in concentration, as long as the animal tolerates the fluid load.

The use of a glucagon infusion has been reported in a case of insulinoma for a dog that was refractory to dextrose treatment (Fischer *et al.*, 2000). Glucagon was found to induce normal blood glucose for a period of 3 weeks, presumably through the mechanism of insulin resistance.

Longer-term medical management

- Successful medical management involves multiple feeds per day using foods of low glycaemic index.
- Prednisolone (0.2–0.5mg/kg, q12–24h) is also frequently used to induce insulin resistance and is cheap and easily available.
- Diazoxide, a benzothiazide diuretic which inhibits insulin release via stimulation of alpha-adrenergic receptors, can help to maintain euglycaemia in dogs in which prednisolone side effects become dose limiting. Side effects of diazoxide include nausea and sodium retention that may lead to oedema. The latter can be countered by the concurrent use of thiazide diuretics; these also potentiate the effects of diazoxide. The dose rate of diazoxide is 10–30 mg/kg/day which is usually administered in three divided doses.
- Octreotide is a somatostatin analogue that may be of benefit in refractory cases. It also has the potential to worsen clinical signs in that it may lower glucagon and growth hormone concentrations. It is available as an injectable preparation only, so is not suitable for use in every case.

Surgical management

Surgery may be useful in the management of insulinoma in that it may help to confirm a diagnosis and, if removal of a solitary nodule is possible, may allow for a disease-free interval during which no medication is necessary. The argument against surgery is that metastasis is so common that clinical signs will recur, usually within 1 year. In this author's experience there seems to be a clinical spectrum within the diagnosis of insulinoma whereby occasional animals have appropriate clinical signs, low glucose concentrations in the face of elevated insulin and confirmatory histopathology but become completely disease-free after surgical removal of a pancreatic nodule. These insulinomas apparently behave in a benign way and have little metastatic potential. Other animals, however, have extremely aggressive tumours that, even after surgical excision, gain only a short respite from hypoglycaemia and associated clinical signs. Unfortunately it is impossible to predict the biological behaviour of these neoplasms prior to surgery.

Chemotherapy

Streptozotocin is an alkylating agent which has been reported as a treatment for insulinoma. It has been shown to be beneficial in some cases but nephrotoxicity is a limiting factor (Moore *et al.*, 2002).

Hypoadrenocorticism

Hypoadrenocorticism (Addison's disease) is usually caused by immune-mediated destruction of the adrenal cortex leading to a reduction in the output of the steroid hormones, cortisol and aldosterone. This disease occurs in dogs (predominantly young to middle-aged females) and much less frequently in cats. Although a hypoadrenal crisis may occur acutely and deterioration may be rapid, vague, waxing and waning clinical signs have usually been present over a longer period of time. The clinical findings include gastrointestinal signs (anorexia, vomiting and diarrhoea), weight loss, muscle weakness and lethargy. Previous biochemical analysis frequently identifies an intermittent azotaemia and mild electrolyte abnormalities. Some animals are cortisol deficient only at the time of presentation (termed 'atypical' Addisonians), although this group can go on to develop aldosterone deficiency.

Why are adrenal steroid hormones important?

Cortisol and aldosterone have vital roles in the maintenance of many different body systems but particularly in the gastrointestinal tract and in renal function and water homeostasis. The gastrointestinal manifestations of hypoadrenocorticism, caused by cortisol deficiency, are signs of a motility disorder with vomiting and diarrhoea. Aldosterone deficiency allows excessive sodium and therefore water loss through the kidneys and leads to volume depletion. At the same time, the ability to excrete potassium decreases and hyperkalaemia develops.

Clinical signs

An animal presenting in a hypoadrenal crisis is collapsed, hypovolaemic (as evidenced by poor pulse quality, pale mucous membranes, prolonged capillary refill time) and bradycardic. The latter is one of the signs that may alert the clinician to the diagnosis as hypovolaemia is usually accompanied by tachycardia. Vomiting and diarrhoea are also common and may be reported historically. Animals frequently have a history of polyuria and polydipsia.

Diagnosis

Haematology

A complete blood count is often relatively unremarkable although there may be a mild to moderate anaemia, interpreted as anaemia of chronic disease. Less commonly there may be severe anaemia associated with significant gastrointestinal blood loss. An interesting finding is that, because of lack of cortisol up-regulation, there is no stress leucogram (i.e. neutrophilia, lymphopenia, eosinopenia might be expected but are not present), even though disease is severe.

Biochemistry

Hyperkalaemia, hyponatraemia, hypochloraemia and hypercalcaemia may all be present when aldosterone is deficient. Animals may be hypoglycaemic due to the lack of insulin antagonism by cortisol. Azotaemia can be mild to severe and is usually prerenal, but may confuse the diagnosis with one of acute renal failure.

Urine analysis

Urine is usually isosthenuric to mildly concentrated (specific gravity <1.025). This lack of concentrating ability does not reflect renal damage, but merely emphasizes the need for aldosterone in the production of concentrated urine. Hypoadrenocorticism is an important differential diagnosis for young to middle-aged dogs with apparent renal disease defined by azotaemia and isosthenuria, however, the azotaemia of hypoadrenocorticism is prerenal in origin.

Electrocardiography

Electrocardiography may be helpful in determining the nature of the bradycardia noted in most animals with typical hypoadrenocorticism. The rising potassium concentration leads to a blunting of the excitability of conductive tissue in the heart and to a slowing of pacemaker activity. Initially, the P wave becomes depressed and disappears (Figure 16.6) but eventually ventricular activity is also suppressed. Classically, a spiked T wave is described when there is hyperkalaemia but this is a relatively uncommon sign and is less easy to interpret than the disappearance of the P wave.

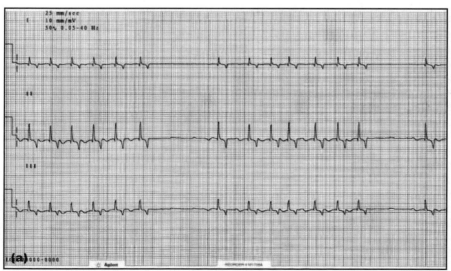

16.6 **(a)** An ECG trace from a dog with hypoadrenocorticism. The potassium was measured as 8.9 mmol/l at the time of the recording. Atrial activity is suppressed, T waves are larger and peaked and there are periods of arrest. (Courtesy of N. Bexfield) (continues) ▶

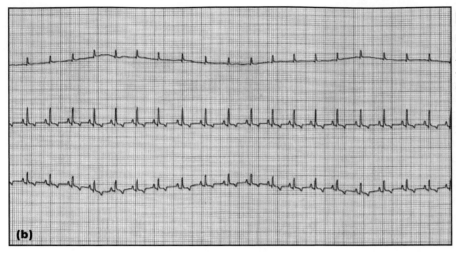

16.6 **(b)** After emergency treatment the potassium had decreased to 6.4 mmol/l. P waves are now visible, the heart rate has increased and the T wave is much smaller. (Courtesy of N. Bexfield)

ACTH stimulation test

An adrenocorticotrophic hormone (ACTH) stimulation test is the definitive test for hypoadrenocorticism. After the measurement of basal cortisol levels, synthetic ACTH is given intravenously at a dose of 125 µg in patients weighing <15 kg and 250 µg in patients weighing >15 kg. A post-ACTH sample is taken 30 minutes to 1 hour later. A classical hypoadrenocorticoid picture would show both a low basal cortisol and no measurable stimulation following ACTH (<20 nmol/l before ACTH and <20 nmol/l following ACTH). The ACTH stimulation test can be performed during the initial stages of volume expansion. The administration of dexamethasone does not interfere with the ability to measure cortisol, although prior administration of either prednisolone or hydrocortisone can cause erroneous results. Frequently the test can be completed before any steroids are given.

Treatment

Emergency treatment

Collapsed, bradycardic and hypovolaemic animals need rapid attention. Urgent volume expansion is required but specific measures may also be necessary to reduce the effects of the hyperkalaemia:

- Begin intravenous fluid therapy using 0.9% sodium chloride at shock doses (90 ml/kg bolus in dogs, 40–50 ml/kg bolus in cats). Administering the total bolus volume in smaller fractions (25–30%) with close monitoring may be preferable and will allow slowing of the fluid rate once adequate volume expansion is achieved, thus reducing the risk of volume overload. Hartmann's solution may also be used; although it does contain some potassium (5 mmol/l) the positive dilutional effects outweigh the impact of the small amount of potassium that is present
- In animals with severe hyponatraemia (<125 mmol/l) rapid increases in serum sodium should be avoided or central nervous system signs can result (see Chapter 5)
- Injectable steroids such as dexamethasone sodium phosphate (0.3–1 mg/kg) or

prednisolone sodium succinate (0.5–1 mg/kg) can be given, although administration of prednisolone should be delayed until after the ACTH stimulation test has been completed. These often improve demeanour and response to shock therapy. Neither of these drugs has a significant mineralocorticoid effect, so they must be followed by administration of fludrocortisone (0.1–0.5mg/kg orally). Alternatively, hydrocortisone sodium succinate or phosphate can be used at a dose rate of 0.5–0.625 mg/kg/h as an intravenous infusion. This drug has the benefit of having both glucocorticoid and mineralocorticoid activity. The rate of sodium retention must be monitored closely when using high fluid rates in combination with mineralocorticoid supplementation, as overzealous correction of hyponatraemia should be avoided.

Treatment of severe hyperkalaemic bradycardia

The level of hyperkalaemia that leads to significant cardiac effects varies between animals, but potassium levels >7.5 mmol/l are usually associated with impairment of cardiac output. In patients with bradycardia <30–40 bpm, which do not respond rapidly to volume replacement, more aggressive treatment to reduce hyperkalaemia, or to protect the heart from its effects, is warranted. Options for treatment include:

- 10% calcium gluconate (0.5–1.5 ml/kg) can be given as a slow infusion with electrocardiograph (ECG) monitoring. This does not reduce serum potassium levels but does raise the cardiac threshold potential so that the difference between the resting and threshold potentials (and thus normal cardiac conduction) is re-established
- Neutral (soluble/regular) insulin (0.2–0.5 IU/kg i.v.) in combination with 2 g of dextrose for every IU of insulin *or* dextrose by itself. This will encourage the redistribution of potassium into an intracellular location and thus rapidly lower the potassium level

- Sodium bicarbonate (1–2 mmol/kg i.v.) will also prompt potassium to move into cells. Treatment with sodium bicarbonate is rarely indicated and should only be used if monitoring of acid–base parameters is possible.

Other treatment considerations

In animals with gastrointestinal haemorrhage or severe hypoproteinaemia, blood products, whole blood or synthetic colloid solutions may be required for volume replacement (see Chapters 4 and 14). Some hypoproteinaemic animals cannot tolerate large volumes of crystalloids because of their tendency to leak fluid out of the vasculature into body cavities and interstitial spaces. These patients may respond better to infusions of colloids such as pentastarch or hetastarch (10–20 ml/kg/day, given as a CRI).

Chronic therapy

Once an acute crisis has been managed, chronic therapy depends on fludrocortisone with or without prednisolone at physiological replacement rates (0.2–0.3 mg/kg/day).

Hyperadrenocorticism

Hyperadrenocorticism (HAC, Cushing's disease) is a chronic disease that is mainly diagnosed after the routine investigation of polyuria/polydipsia in an older dog. HAC may be of pituitary or adrenal origin, although pituitary tumours are the cause in the majority of patients. Uncomplicated HAC is not typically a cause for emergency presentation, and is beyond the scope of this chapter. Occasional animals manifest more critical clinical signs, however, and these are discussed here.

Pulmonary thromboembolism

Pulmonary thromboembolic disease can cause acute dyspnoea and death in animals with HAC. A prothrombotic state is created through the dysregulation of coagulation and anticoagulation mechanisms; for example, excess cortisol has numerous effects on the coagulation system, including the development of hypertension which can lead to proteinuria and loss of antithrombin through the kidney. Obesity, systemic hypertension and an elevated haematocrit are also predisposing factors.

Diagnosis

Radiographs may be unremarkable, may show areas of increased radiolucency representing lung fields with markedly decreased pulmonary perfusion, or have regional or generalized pulmonary infiltrates (alveolar or mixed alveolar/interstitial patterns). Infiltrates may delineate a wedge shape, representing an area of haemorrhage, atelectasis or infarction. When radiographs are unremarkable, ultrasonography may help to identify thrombi in vessels (Figure 16.7). If available, angiography using computed tomography is proving to be helpful in diagnosis of pulmonary thromboembolism.

Arterial blood gas analysis usually shows hypoxaemia and often hypocapnia secondary to hyperventilation. The alveolar–arterial oxygen gradient is increased. A coagulation profile is usually not of great help, although D-dimers may be elevated indicating increased clot turnover (see Chapter 13).

Treatment

Oxygen therapy is used to correct hypoxaemia and to improve cardiopulmonary function. Most thrombi will retract and be broken down spontaneously by the patient's own fibrinolytic system, and many patients will improve over a few hours to days if they can be supported adequately during this time. Anticoagulant drugs may be given to reduce the chance of further thrombi being formed. The management of pulmonary thromboembolism is discussed in Chapters 7 and 13.

Diabetes mellitus

There is an increased risk of diabetes mellitus in animals with HAC, particularly cats. HAC may contribute to insulin resistance in dogs and cats and may increase the risk of DKA. The treatment of both

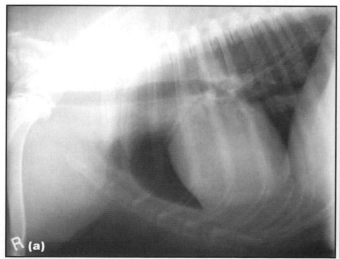
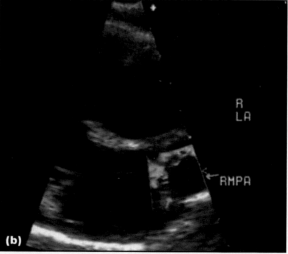

16.7 (a) Lateral thoracic radiograph from a dog showing acute onset dyspnoea. The radiograph is largely unremarkable but shows hyperlucency of the lung fields. (b) Echocardiogram showing right long-axis view from the same dog. A thrombus (arrows) may be seen in the right main pulmonary artery (RMPA) causing turbulent blood flow in this vessel. (Courtesy of A. Holloway)

diseases together is challenging, and if possible diabetic stability should be established before adding a drug to address HAC.

Neurological manifestations

In a proportion of dogs with pituitary tumours (10–15%), the tumour is a macroadenoma rather than a microadenoma, and is therefore more likely to cause neurological signs, principally mental dullness. For some of these dogs, treatment of HAC using either trilostane or mitotane allows a sudden increase in tumour growth or an increase in peritumour inflammation, due to decreased negative feedback as a result of the reduction in circulating steroids. Whilst decreasing the dose of trilostane or mitotane may cause an improvement in these cases, the only other method that has been used to reduce the mass effect of the tumour is radiotherapy (Theon and Feldman, 1998).

Pancreatitis

HAC predisposes to acute pancreatitis through a variety of mechanisms (Hess *et al.*, 1999). HAC patients are often lipaemic and hypercholesterolaemic as well as being polyphagic. Pancreatic duct hyperplasia and inspissated pancreatic secretions have also been reported. Management of acute pancreatitis is addressed in Chapter 11.

Hypertension

HAC frequently leads to hypertension due to the induction of renin secretion by cortisol. Hypertension can cause ocular signs (intraocular haemorrhage, retinal detachment), neurological signs (depression, signs of headache, specific localizable signs reflecting areas of haemorrhage), glomerular disease and thromboembolic disease as discussed above. Hypertension is controlled by addressing the primary underlying disease, HAC, and rarely requires specific treatment other than supportive therapy of associated clinical signs.

Adrenal tumour haemorrhage

A rare consequence of the presence of an adrenal tumour, haemorrhage can occur due to tumour rupture (Figure 16.8). This is a particular risk in animals with malignant adrenal tumours which often invade the caudal vena cava. These animals can present with acute onset of shock due to haemoperitoneum.

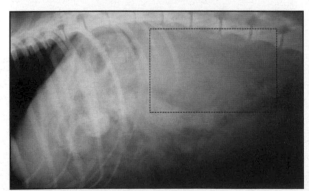

16.8 Lateral abdominal radiograph of a dog showing retroperitoneal haemorrhage due to rupture of an adrenal mass. Image shows dramatic enlargement and streaking of the retroperitoneal space (boxed) with effacement of the kidneys. (Courtesy of A Holloway)

Hyperparathyroidism

Primary hyperparathyroidism can lead to dramatic elevations in blood calcium concentrations as a result of over-secretion of parathyroid hormone (PTH). This disease occurs in dogs of any breed, though Keeshonds have a familial form of the disease and form a significant proportion of total hospital admissions for this endocrinopathy (Refsal *et al.*, 2001) (Figure 16.9). Hyperparathyroidism is rare in cats (Kallet *et al.*, 1991) but may be recognized more easily now that an assay for feline PTH is available.

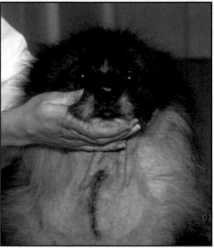

16.9 A Keeshond recovering from surgery to remove a parathyroid nodule.

Clinical signs

The clinical signs of hyperparathyroidism include polyuria, polydipsia, muscle tremors, vomiting, dental pain and bone pain. Serum calcium usually increases slowly over months, so the onset of clinical signs can be insidious and may not be noticed by the owner. Hypercalcaemia causes polyuria through its action on anti-diuretic hormone (ADH) receptors in the renal tubule and the development of nephrogenic diabetes insipidus. The kidneys are also vulnerable to damage by mineralization of renal tubular cells that occurs when there is prolonged hypercalcaemia. A proportion of dogs with primary hyperparathyroidism will present in renal failure, posing a diagnostic dilemma in deciding whether hyperparathyroidism is secondary to renal failure or primary parathyroid disease. These dogs may have vomiting, diarrhoea, anorexia, depression and halitosis alongside the signs of hypercalcaemia (Gear *et al.*, 2005).

Diagnosis

Diagnosis depends on demonstrating hypercalcaemia (both total and ionized) with elevated or inappropriately high PTH, and no other cause for the hypercalcaemia. Usually, renal failure causes an increase in total rather than ionized calcium, but this is not an infallible rule. In addition, comparison of the degree of azotaemia and the degree of hypercalcaemia can give an indication as to which is the primary problem. More reliable is the phosphate level, which will be elevated in cases of renal failure but tends to be suppressed in patients with primary hyperparathyroidism.

Imaging

It is usually possible to image the abnormal parathyroid gland in the neck using ultrasonography or computed tomography (Figure 16.10). Some dogs may have enlargement of more than one gland.

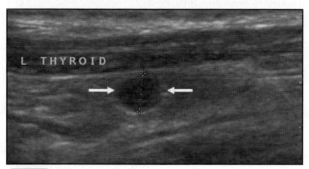

16.10 Ultrasound examination of the ventral neck of animals suffering from hyperparathyroidism usually reveals a parathyroid nodule, appearing as an echolucent mass within thyroid tissue. (Courtesy of A. Holloway)

Treatment

Hypercalcaemia should be dealt with rapidly to avoid precipitating renal failure. Although some dogs survive years without treatment and with no impairment of renal function in the face of severe hypercalcaemia (total calcium >3.8 mmol/l), the degree of renal damage already sustained and the likelihood of developing renal failure is impossible to gauge. Any dog whose treatment is delayed is at risk of developing renal insufficiency. For this reason, severe hypercalcaemia should be treated as a medical emergency.

Fluid therapy

Isotonic (0.9%) sodium chloride is the fluid of choice to induce diuresis and promote calciuresis. Once volume losses have been replaced this can be used in conjunction with furosemide (2–4 mg/kg q12h) to increase further the excretion of calcium.

Surgical management

The treatment of choice for a parathyroid adenoma or parathyroid tissue hypertrophy is surgical removal. This is made easier if a mass has already been identified ultrasonographically, but surgical exploration of the neck is warranted in any dog with a diagnosis of primary hyperparathyroidism whether or not a parathyroid nodule has been identified.

Other methods

Chemical ablation using an ultrasound-directed injection of ethanol has been described (Long et al., 1999). The success of this technique is user dependent and, of course, depends on the reliable identification of abnormal parathyroid tissue.

Hypoparathyroidism

Primary hypoparathyroidism is a rare condition in dogs and there are few reports in cats (Barber, 2004). The disease occurs secondary to destruction of the parathyroid tissue, probably through immune-mediated attack, and the consequent decline in PTH production. This leads to a fall in plasma calcium levels to the point where clinical signs of hypocalcaemia are seen.

Clinical signs

The main signs are those of neuromuscular excitability. Affected animals may have facial twitching progressing to generalized muscle tremors, tetanic spasms and seizures.

Diagnosis

Diagnosis relies on identifying hypocalcaemia and hyperphosphataemia in the face of low serum PTH concentrations. Biopsy of parathyroid tissue can confirm the diagnosis but is not usually necessary.

Treatment

Emergency treatment

Initial emergency treatment involves the immediate use of intravenous calcium gluconate (0.5–1.5 ml/kg of a 10% solution of calcium gluconate). This must be given slowly over 20–30 minutes with ECG monitoring if possible, so that any dysrhythmias can be noted and the infusion slowed or stopped if necessary. If clinical signs recur in the short term, before oral drugs have had a chance to take effect, a CRI of calcium gluconate can be used at a dose of 10 mg/kg/h.

Chronic treatment

Lifelong replacement therapy is required. This is usually given in the form of vitamin D supplementation with or without oral calcium gluconate; the latter can usually be withdrawn once the animal has been stabilized.

Phaeochromocytoma

Phaeochromocytoma is an uncommon adrenal tumour in dogs and is even rarer in cats (Maher and McNiel, 1997). This type of endocrine tumour originates from the chromaffin cells of the adrenal gland; these cells synthesize catecholamines such as adrenaline and noradrenaline. The clinical signs of a phaeochromocytoma may be non-specific and may occur alongside other diseases in older animals, therefore the diagnosis of this condition is particularly challenging.

Clinical signs

Clinical signs include episodic collapse, generalized weakness, weight loss, anorexia, intermittent panting, anxiety, depression and ataxia (Gilson et al., 1994, Bartez et al., 1997). The clinical signs usually reflect the pulsatile nature of the release of large amounts of catecholamines, with their associated influence on blood pressure, cardiac output and heart rate. Animals may also have signs suggestive of systemic hypertension, including retinal haemorrhages, retinal detachment, neurological signs or epistaxis. Cardiac abnormalities may include ventricular premature complexes, supraventricular tachycardia and atrioventricular block (Gilson et al., 1994).

Diagnosis

The antemortem diagnosis of phaeochromocytoma is difficult because of the variable nature of the clinical signs and the lack of a sensitive and specific test with which to confirm the diagnosis. There are no specific clinical pathology abnormalities, but the finding of intermittent or sustained hypertension with an adrenal mass that is not secreting other hormone products (e.g. cortisol and its intermediates) is suggestive. However, phaeochromocytoma may co-exist with adrenal or pituitary-based hyperadrenocorticism which may also cause hypertension.

Measurement of serum levels of specific catecholamines is not readily available in dogs and cats, nor do any veterinary laboratories in the UK offer the facility of measuring urinary metabolites of catecholamines. Perhaps more useful might be the phentolamine suppression test which, when positive in humans, shows a systolic blood pressure decrease of at least 35 mmHg (Maher and McNiel, 1997). This test has not, however, been evaluated in dogs.

Treatment

Management relies on reducing the systemic blood pressure and stabilizing the patient prior to surgical removal of the adrenal mass. Preoperative alpha-adrenergic blockade using phenoxybenzamine (0.2–1.5 mg/kg q12h orally) is useful as this drug is a non-competitive receptor antagonist. When there are significant cardiac dysrhythmias concurrent beta-adrenergic blockade is indicated, although this should never be introduced without prior phenoxybenzamine treatment, otherwise severe hypertension can result.

References and further reading

Barber PJ (2004) Disorders of the parathyroid glands. *Journal of Feline Medicine and Surgery* **6(4)**, 259–269

Bartez PY, Marks SL, Woo J *et al.* (1997) Pheochromocytoma in dogs: 61 cases (1984–1995). *Journal of Veterinary Internal Medicine* **11(5)**, 272–278

Dibartola SP (2005) *Fluid, Electrolyte and Acid-base Disorders in Small Animal Practice, 3rd edn.* WB Saunders, Philadelphia

Feldman EC and Nelson RW (2004) *Canine and Feline Endocrinology and Reproduction, 3rd edn.* WB Saunders, Philadelphia

Fischer JR, Smith SA and Harkin KR (2000) Glucagon constant-rate infusion: a novel strategy for the management of hyperinsulinemic-hypoglycemic crisis in the dog. *Journal of the American Animal Hospital Association* **36(1)**, 27–32

Gear RN, Neiger R, Skelly BJ, Herrtage ME (2005) Primary hyperparathyroidism in 29 dogs: diagnosis, treatment, outcome and associated renal failure. *Journal of Small Animal Practice* **46(1)**, 10–16

Gilson SD, Withrow SF, Wheeler SL *et al.* (1994) Pheochromocytoma in 50 dogs. *Journal of Veterinary Internal Medicine* **8(3)**, 228–232

Gunn-Moore D (2005) Feline endocrinopathies. In: *Veterinary Clinics of North America: Small Animal Practice* **35**, 171–210

Hess RS, Kass PH, Shofer FS, Van Winkle TJ and Washabau RJ (1999) Evaluation of risk factors for fatal acute pancreatitis in dogs. *Journal of the American Veterinary Medical Association* **214(1)**, 46–51

Kallet AJ, Richter KP, Feldman EC *et al.* (1991) Primary hyperparathyroidism in cats: seven cases (1984–1989). *Journal of the American Veterinary Medical Association* **199**, 1767–1771

Kerl ME (2001) Diabetic ketoacidosis: pathophysiology and clinical and laboratory presentation. *Compendium on Continuing Education for the Practicing Veterinarian* **23(3)**, 220–228

Kraje AC (2003) Hypoglycemia and irreversible neurologic complications in a cat with insulinoma. *Journal of the American Veterinary Medical Association* **223(6)**, 812–814

Locke-Bohannon LG and Mauldin GE (2001) Canine phaeochromocytoma: diagnosis and management. *Compendium on Continuing Education for the Practicing Veterinarian* **23(9)**, 807–814

Long CD, Goldstein RE, Hornof WJ, Feldman EC and Nyland TG (1999) Percutaneous ultrasound-guided chemical parathyroid ablation for treatment of primary hyperparathyroidism in dogs. *Journal of the American Veterinary Medical Association* **215(2)**, 217–221

Maher ER and McNiel EA (1997) Pheochromocytoma in dogs and cats. *Veterinary Clinics of North America: Small Animal Practice* **27(2)**, 359–380

Moore AS, Nelson RW, Henry CJ *et al.* (2002) Streptozocin for treatment of pancreatic islet cell tumors in dogs: 17 cases (1989–1999). *Journal of the American Veterinary Medical Association* **221(6)**, 811–818

Refsal KR, Provencher-Bolloger AL, Graham PA and Nachreiner RF (2001) Update on the diagnosis and treatment of disorders of calcium regulation. *Veterinary Clinics of North America: Small Animal Practice* **31**, 1043–1062

Theon AP and Feldman EC (1998) Megavoltage irradiation of pituitary macrotumors in dogs with neurologic signs. *Journal of the American Veterinary Medical Association* **213(2)**, 225–231

Van Ham L, Braund KG, Roels S and Putcuyps I (1997) Treatment of a dog with an insulinoma-related peripheral polyneuropathy with corticosteroids. *Veterinary Record* **141(4)**, 98–100

Willard MD, Zerbe CA, Schall WD *et al.* (1987) Severe hypophosphataemia associated with diabetes mellitus in six dogs and one cat. *Journal of the American Veterinary Medical Association* **190(8)**, 1007–1010

17

Acute management of orthopaedic and external soft tissue injuries

Matthew J. Pead and Sorrel J. Langley-Hobbs

Introduction

Many animals with orthopaedic injuries or wounds also have injuries to vital organ systems. Fractures and wounds are often obvious and may be spectacular but must initially be assigned a low priority in emergency treatment, as they are rarely life threatening. Concurrent injuries, especially those involving the thoracic and abdominal cavities, commonly occur during the trauma. The thoracic problems most frequently encountered include pulmonary contusions (46–66%), pneumothorax (12–50%) and rib fractures (10–25%) (Spackman *et al.*, 1984; Tamas *et al.*, 1985; Houlton and Dyce, 1992; Griffon *et al.*, 1994) (Figure 17.1). If the animal is in shock, the cardiovascular instability should be addressed prior to any investigations or even a full physical examination. Shock can result from internal injury or from the wound or fracture alone. Fluid loss in burns, or osseofascial haemorrhage in fractures, can be sufficient to lead to irreversible shock and death. The initial investigative plan for a trauma case following a complete physical examination should include: conscious thoracic and abdominal radiographs; an electrocardiogram (ECG); and evaluation of blood packed cell volume (PCV) and total solids. If abnormalities are detected, further investigations may be deemed appropriate.

While potentially life-threatening problems are a priority, temporary and emergency management of wounds and fractures should not be ignored. Such treatment should be directed towards prevention of any additional injury or deterioration at the site of trauma, minimizing contamination and improving patient comfort. Emergency management of wounds and fractures should control any systemic implications for the traumatized tissues and prepare them for the start of definitive treatment.

Wounds

Wounds are tissue injuries caused by chemical, thermal or physical trauma. In most cases the skin is damaged and there will be variable involvement of underlying tissues. Particular consideration should be given to the major structures adjacent to the site (Figure 17.2).

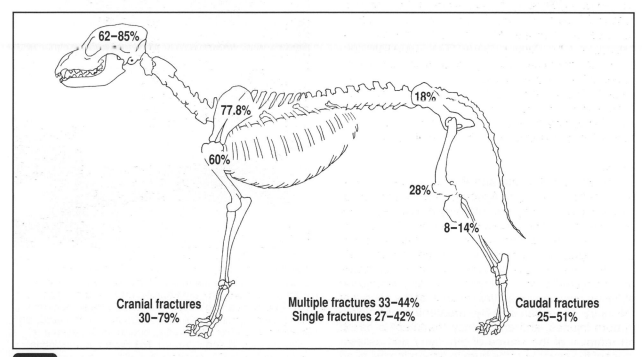

17.1 Schematic diagram illustrating the incidence of thoracic injuries associated with fractures in specific areas.

Area	Examples	Considerations
Head	Cranial fractures	Impacted cranial fractures or jaw fractures need removal of fragments or repair. Risk of meningitis
	Brain damage – swelling, oedema and haemorrhage	Continual monitoring of neurological status required to detect deterioration that may require surgical decompression. Medical management (see Chapter 9)
Neck	Tracheal rupture	Pneumomediastinum and subcutaneous emphysema
	Recurrent laryngeal nerve damage	Assess laryngeal function by observation under a light plane of anaesthesia
	Cervical spinal cord injury	Assess neurological function, evidence of fracture/dislocation of cervical vertebrae
	Carotid artery severance	Emergency haemostasis
	Oesophageal injuries	Exploration for foreign body, consider gastrostomy tube
Thorax	Fractured ribs, pneumothorax, pulmonary contusions	Often treat conservatively. Large wounds must be covered to allow lung expansion. Air may need drainage if severe or a tension pneumothorax. Supplement oxygen. Flail chest – bandage and delay treatment
	Ruptured diaphragm	Usually delay repair until systemically stable, unless there is respiratory distress or the stomach is in the thorax
Appendicular	Bone, ligament, tendon, nerve, artery and vein	Check integrity of tendons, nerves (including spinal cord) and vasculature prior to surgical intervention and anaesthesia
Abdomen	Damage to any abdominal viscera. Abdominal wall or diaphragm rupture with herniation	Monitor for damage by regular physical examination, auscultation, ultrasonography and abdominocentesis. Biochemical and cytological analysis of blood and peritoneal fluid

17.2 Approach to management of wounds affecting specific areas.

Wound types

Wounds related to physical trauma

These wounds result from the breakdown of tissue by physical force and are the most common type seen in veterinary practice. Punctures, lacerations, shearing or degloving of the skin and the impact of projectiles may all cause wounds. They may be complicated by the presence of a foreign body. Recognition of the type of wound can give an early indication of the treatment required (Figures 17.3 and 17.4). In general, the physical breakdown of the skin layer allows damage and exposure of the deeper tissues. The immediate concern is to control haemorrhage and minimize contamination. All wounds should be covered immediately with a sterile dressing to prevent further contamination from the patient and the hospital environment, as nosocomial infection can be more serious and difficult to eliminate than infection resulting from the original injury.

Burns

Burns cause cell death and the subsequent breakdown of tissue integrity. Although common in the human population, they are relatively rare in veterinary practice. In thermal and electrical burns, the build-up of thermal energy cannot be dissipated before the cells are disrupted. In chemical and radiation burns, cellular integrity is directly disrupted by toxic substances or ionizing radiation. In all types of burns, destruction of tissue may continue after removal of the source of the injury. There can be a life-threatening loss of fluid in burn injuries, and emergency treatment is based on removal of the source of the injury and assessment of the severity of the burn to determine the need for fluid therapy. Partial-thickness burns involve the

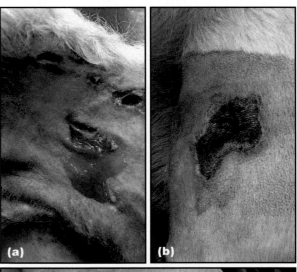

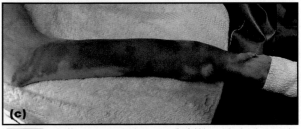

17.3 Different wound types. **(a)** Wounds in the groin of a dog. There is a combination of abrasion, avulsion, burn and contusion injury. The white/grey skin edges to the wounds are necrotic and need debridement. **(b)** A burn on a dog's stifle after a road traffic accident. The pale clipped normal skin contrasts with the hard, dry blackened eschar. The area surrounding the eschar is mildly contused and abraded. **(c)** Severe contusion is apparent in this thin-skinned dog with a simple radius and ulnar fracture that occurred whilst running.

Wound type	Description	Treatment considerations
Abrasion	Superficial wound involving destruction of varying depths of skin by friction or shearing forces. Usually bleeds minimally	When associated with a fracture, normal skin barrier is incompetent – treat fracture as grade I open
Avulsion	Characterized by tearing of tissues from attachments and creation of skin flaps. Limb avulsion injuries with extensive skin loss are called 'degloving'	Blood supply to skin may be compromised leading to skin necrosis 2–5 days after injury. Repeat examinations and consider secondary debridement
Chemical burns	Direct exposure to noxious chemicals	Copious lavage to remove chemical. Ensure animal cannot lick area and ingest harmful substances
Contusion	Blunt trauma may cause blood to pool in the subcutaneous tissue	Application of cold and analgesics. Beware of compartment syndrome
Crushing injuries	Combination of other injuries with extensive damage and contusion to the skin and deeper tissues	Assess neurological and vascular supply prior to treatment
Gunshots	These are contaminated. The heat generated in firing a bullet does not render it sterile. Open fractures may be present	Remove metal if encountered but not usually necessary to remove all fragments unless intra-articular or impinging on major structures such as nerves and arteries. Antibiosis for severe or intra-articular injuries. Treat the wound not the weapon
Laceration	Created by tearing, which damages the skin and underlying tissues and may be superficial or deep and have irregular edges	Debridement and primary closure may be used if treatment is early
Penetrating or puncture wound	Related to the impact of a missile or sharp object such as a knife or tooth. Tissue damage is directly proportional to the velocity of the impact	Excise a 2–3 mm wide full-thickness rim of skin around the puncture site. Check vital signs as there may be significant internal haemorrhage. Penetrating abdominal wounds require exploratory laparotomy
Penetrating foreign bodies	Foreign bodies such as sticks and glass can fragment causing widespread contamination	May need extensive exploration to remove all fragments (90% of glass shards show on radiographs). Protruding foreign bodies should be left in place for transport but can be cut 2–3 cm from the body wall to minimize further internal damage by preventing the protruding shaft acting as a fulcrum
Thermal burns	May see reddened, crusted or blackened skin. Burn injuries around the head and neck may compromise respiration	Beware of systemic complications of the burn. Attend to analgesia and cooling the area

17.4 Recognition and treatment of specific wounds.

epidermis and a variable degree of the dermis. Full-thickness burns involve the entire skin layer. Partial-thickness burns eventually progress to separation between viable and non-viable tissue, but this can take up to 10 days to happen naturally. Full-thickness burns progress to a brown or black eschar, which may become hard to the touch (Figure 17.3b).

In general, any deep partial- or full-thickness burn involving more than 15–20% of the animal's surface will lead to major systemic complications requiring emergency supportive therapy (Pavletic, 1993). Burns are vulnerable to infection, and the same care must be taken to prevent contamination as would be exercised for an open wound.

Treatment of wounds

Although it is advisable to progress to definitive treatment of wounds as soon as possible, other more serious complications of trauma may take priority. Treatment of wounds can be divided into emergency procedures (which can and should be done as soon as possible) and the initiation of definitive treatment. In many cases it is possible to combine these procedures without compromising the animal. It should not be forgotten that wounds themselves might pose a considerable systemic threat to the patient, especially in terms of fluid loss. All animals with wounds should be evaluated for analgesic therapy.

Owners should be made aware as soon as is practical of the implications of treatment in terms of their time and finance. Continued effective communication is important throughout the period of treatment.

Emergency treatment

Emergency treatment of wounds often takes place at the time of initial presentation, while involvement of other body systems is being assessed and stabilization of urgent problems is occurring. Analgesia should be considered as soon as possible. The animal should be muzzled or restrained as necessary to prevent further self-trauma or contamination of the wound, and to ensure that veterinary staff can treat the animal effectively without being bitten.

Haemostasis: Bleeding should be addressed first. Direct pressure can be achieved using a wad of sterile gauze swabs or a bandage, and will be sufficient in most cases to stop minor bleeding. The addition of adrenaline 1:1000 solution (1 ml adrenaline solution with 4–5 ml of sterile saline) to swabs may facilitate haemostasis. Use of adrenaline is contraindicated at extremities, where prolonged vasoconstriction may lead to ischaemia and necrosis, and in the presence of cardiac dysrhythmias. Wounds can also be packed with haemostatic agents such as calcium alginate fibre. With more profuse arterial haemorrhage, it may be necessary to use 'pressure point' haemostasis. At sites where major arteries run superficially, such as the brachial and femoral arteries in the axilla and femoral triangle, respectively, digital pressure is applied over the pressure point proximal to the area of haemorrhage. Head, nose and oral cavity arterial bleeding can be controlled by applying direct digital pressure to the deep area ventral and directly adjacent to the angle of the mandible where the common carotid arteries give rise to the maxillary artery tributaries. Superficial pressure will occlude the jugular, linguofacial or maxillary veins, which can increase venous bleeding, so it is important to apply pressure accurately.

Pressure cuffs and tourniquets: Blood pressure cuffs may be placed proximal to appendicular wounds and inflated 20–30 mmHg higher than measured arterial pressure. These should not be left in place for more than 6 hours, or irreversible neurovascular compromise will occur. Tourniquets made from narrow bands of elastic material, such as Penrose drains, will place excessive pressure on neurovascular structures and may cause permanent deficits. They are not recommended unless the limb is to be amputated, or unless they can be applied distal to the tarsus or carpus where major motor nerves are not present. However even in these sites, narrow tourniquet bands can still only safely be used for 3–5 minutes; in contrast, bands 5–10 cm wide can be used for up to 30 minutes. Ligation, surgical stapling and electrosurgery may then be used for definitive haemostasis. Profuse haemorrhage will require clamping and ligation of major vessels; lesser haemorrhage can usually be controlled by the application of a pressure bandage (Feliciano, 1992).

Initial control of contamination: A 'golden period' of 6 hours exists in which a contaminated wound may be cleaned and primarily closed or covered without development of infection. The procedure for cleaning wounds is summarized in Figure 17.5. Sterile apparel (especially gloves) and instruments should be used to minimize further contamination. A large volume of lavage fluid (minimum 500 ml) is used to remove contaminants, debris and bacteria, and to rehydrate the tissues. The pressure at which the fluid is applied should be sufficient to dislodge contaminants, but applying fluid under too high a pressure and inserting the needle deep into the wound will force contaminated or foreign material deeper, and open up uncontaminated tissue planes. Fluid applied through a 20–50 ml syringe with a 19 gauge needle will produce a satisfactory pressure of 7–9 psi, and will significantly decrease the number of bacteria and thus the incidence of infection. The ideal flushing solution should enhance bacterial removal without being toxic to the tissues. In one *in vitro* study neither phosphate-buffered saline (PBS) nor lactated Ringer's caused any significant fibroblast damage

compared to normal saline and sterile tap water. Lactated Ringer's may be the lavage solution of choice in the clinical situation (Buffa *et al.*, 1997). Detergents and soaps are cytotoxic, as are some antiseptics, however, chlorhexidine 0.05% and povidone–iodine 0.01–1% are safe to use. In wounds with gross contamination, tap water can be used, followed by a sterile lavage solution. However, topical agents such as wound powders, intramammary preparations, hydrogen peroxide and alcohol should be avoided. These substances cause cell death, provoke a foreign body reaction and interfere with the healing process. Finally, the wound is again covered with a sterile dressing. Time spent minimizing contamination (and thus preventing the establishment of infection at the earliest possible stage) can significantly shorten the recovery time of wounds.

Haemostasis

Cover wound with sterile dressing whilst preparing for lavage

Wear sterile gloves (and hat, mask, gown)

Apply gel or sterile saline-soaked swabs to the wound

Clip away hair, working from wound outwards if possible

Flush wound with sterile saline, remove all contaminants from chemical burns

Take a bacterial swab for culture

Apply a sterile dressing and bandage

17.5 Summary of emergency wound care.

Emergency treatment of burns: Evaluation of the area of a burn is critical, and thorough and wide clipping of the area is essential. The damage related to a burn and the surface appearance may change in the first 48–72 hours, therefore the clipped area should be monitored. Burns may appear as reddened areas of inflamed skin with a crust or scab over the surface. The hair may fall out or be easily plucked from full-thickness burns. Partial-thickness burns may be painful when touched; conversely full-thickness burns are typically non-painful as peripheral nerve endings are destroyed. Once the area is assessed, aggressive fluid therapy should be started if the burnt area exceeds 15% of the body surface. Patients should be assessed for evidence of dehydration, anaemia and hypoalbuminaemia. Cardiovascular, pulmonary and renal function should be evaluated and monitored for several days following the injury.

The area of the burn can be cooled by lavage, and in chemical burns all residues should be washed away with copious volumes of water. Large burns should be cooled with care in order to prevent severe heat loss in a debilitated patient. Application of soaked dressings or bags of fluid at 3–10°C for at least 30 minutes is recommended. The necrotic skin in the eschar has great potential for infection and will not be penetrated by systemic antibiotics. Until this tissue can be removed, it should be protected with topical antibiotics, particularly silver sulphadiazine in a water-soluble cream, and covered with a sterile non-adherent dressing. Definitive treatment is initiated using principles and techniques common to the management of other wounds. These are dealt with below.

Starting definitive wound treatment

Once the animal is stable and other injuries have been addressed, more definitive treatment can be initiated (Figures 17.6 and 17.7). Thorough treatment normally requires analgesia and general anaesthesia. The nature and extent of the wound should be evaluated and a plan for subsequent preparation and treatment devised. Such a plan will depend on the nature of the wound (see Figure 17.4). Wounds should be treated in an aseptic fashion using sterile technique and sterile apparel. A large area of normal skin around the wound should be clipped to allow a thorough inspection and to prepare for definitive surgical treatments, such as the use of skin flaps (Fowler, 1999). The skin is scrubbed thoroughly using a proprietary scrub solution. Any exposed areas of the wound can be protected during this initial phase by covering them with a water-soluble gel or swabs soaked in sterile saline. Water-soluble gel can be lavaged away together with any debris from the clipping and preparation.

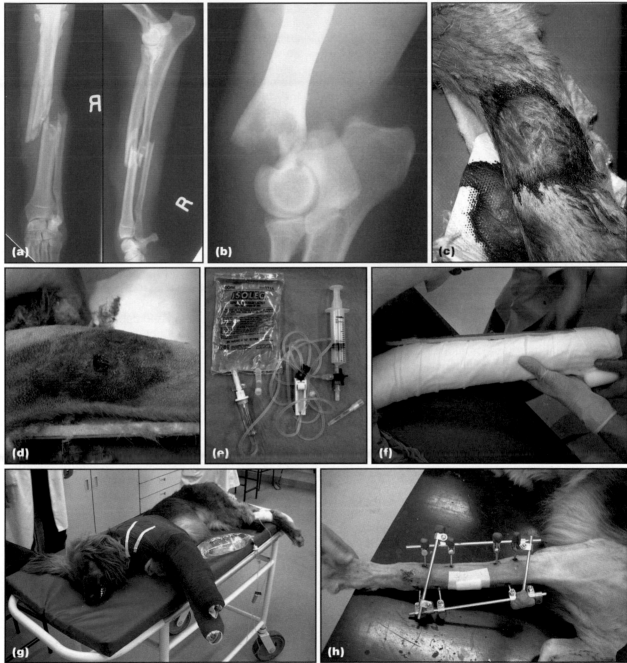

17.6 Early management of a dog with bilateral fractures, prior to surgical stabilization. **(a)** Craniocaudal and mediolateral views of a grade I open radius and ulna fracture; air is visible under the skin shadow adjacent to the fracture on the medial aspect. **(b)** There is a closed distal humeral supracondylar fracture in the left forelimb.
(c) Small wound associated with the open fracture prior to treatment. **(d)** Using aseptic technique, whenever possible, water-soluble jelly is applied to the wound prior to clipping to prevent hair entering the wound. **(e)** The wound is flushed with a 19 gauge needle, 20 ml syringe and lactated Ringer's solution. **(f)** A splinted bandage is applied to support the grade I open radius and ulna fracture. **(g)** A spica splint is applied to support the supracondylar humeral fracture.
(h) Definitive stabilization of the radius and ulna fracture is achieved with a type Ib external skeletal fixator once the patient is stable for anaesthesia. A non-adherent dressing (e.g. Primapore) is applied to the small wound.

Aseptic technique

Evaluation and treatment plan

Preparation of skin and surrounding area

Debridement

Lavage

Bacterial culture and evaluation of contamination

Evaluation and execution of closure if appropriate

Administration of appropriate antibiotics

Application of a sterile dressing and bandage

17.7 Summary of initial definitive wound care.

Debridement:

1. Remove all foreign debris such as gravel and superficial gun shot (the tissue should not be aggressively explored to retrieve all shot).
2. Dissect out and remove obviously necrotic tissue, especially muscle, fat and skin. Nerves, blood vessels, tendons, ligaments and bone with soft tissue attachments should be preserved.
3. Leave tissue that has a good chance of viability, especially when major structures are involved or the wound involves the distal extremities. If viability is questionable, a delayed debridement can be performed several days later if necessary.
4. Remove partial-thickness burn eschar by 'tangential section', sharply cutting back the tissue parallel to the surface until healthy bleeding dermis is encountered.
5. Debride full-thickness burn eschar vigorously, as early as possible, to define its extent.
6. Control haemorrhage carefully, as blood provides the ideal conditions for bacterial proliferation. Use pressure and diathermy where possible, with ligation for larger vessels.
7. Lavage the wound with sterile saline as described above.
8. Take a swab for culture at the end of cleaning and debridement as this timing has been found to produce the most significant results.

Decisions on the amount of tissue to remove can be difficult. The most common cause for delayed wound healing and infection is inadequate debridement, therefore aggressive debridement, especially with expendable structures, is often the best policy. There is some variation in recommendations for different types of tissue, and the following general guidelines are useful:

- Assess skin viability based on colour, temperature, bleeding and pain sensation. Non-viable skin will appear black, blue–black or white, feel cool, lack pain sensation and not bleed. Skin of questionable viability may appear blue or purple
- Debride muscle until it bleeds and contracts following appropriate stimuli
- Remove small bone fragments from open fractures, as they may prevent complete granulation
- Excise contaminated fat aggressively as it is easily devascularized, harbours bacteria and is expendable.

Other techniques that have been used to assess tissue viability include dye injection, the use of radiographic contrast media, transcutaneous oxygen and carbon dioxide measurements, and laser and Doppler velocimetry (Bellah and Krahwinkel, 1985; Rochat *et al.*, 1993). However, visual examination is feasible in most situations and was found to be as accurate as dye infusion in one study (Bellah and Krahwinkel, 1985).

Assessment of bacterial contamination: Wound closure and antibiotic therapy are influenced by the degree of bacterial contamination. Swabbing for culture and sensitivity at the end of debridement and lavage is sufficient for most wounds healing by second intention, as antibiotic therapy can be targeted accurately. However, infection is a significant source of morbidity in prematurely closed wounds, and further precautions may be needed if closure is contemplated. Gross inspection will not determine whether a wound is infected or not, but quantitative bacterial counts and culture can provide insights into the advisability of wound closure. If there are $>10^5$ organisms/g or β-haemolytic streptococci present, then the wound should not be closed (Gfeller and Crowe, 1994). The rapid slide test (RST) can be performed prior to attempting wound closure. The method involves swabbing 1 cm^2 of the deepest surface of the prepared wound with a sterile cotton-tipped swab. The swab is rubbed over 1 cm^2 of a clean microscope slide. The slide is examined under microscopy and if even one bacterium is seen, the wound should not be closed (Gfeller and Crowe, 1994).

Closure: After cleaning and debridement, the wound may either be closed immediately (primary), left for 3–5 days and then closed (delayed primary), closed after the granulating bed has matured (10 days; secondary closure), or left to heal by granulation and re-epithelialization (second-intention healing). The wound should only be closed if one is confident that all necrotic tissue and debris have been removed and if closure can be achieved without excessive tension. Tension-relieving techniques, such as undermining, walking sutures, subdermal suture patterns (inverted vertical mattress pattern), vertical mattress sutures, far–near–near–far and far–far–near–near suture patterns, stented sutures, relaxing incisions, bipedicle flaps, V–Y plasties or Z plasties, may be useful in closing selected wounds (Pavletic, 1993).

For wound repair, a small-diameter monofilament non-absorbable suture material should be selected, although, if available, stapling is faster than suturing and is associated with a lower infection rate. Wounds treated by primary closure should initially be covered, as it takes 24–48 hours for a fibrin seal to form that will resist bacterial invasion. Unpublished studies suggest a 50% higher infection rate in uncovered wounds. For selected wounds, drainage should be provided because wound fluids and exudates interfere with normal healing. A drain can be used for dead space obliteration, to eliminate established fluid, and for prophylactic prevention of fluid or air accumulation within a wound. Active suction drains are particularly useful under these circumstances (Bellah and Krahwinkel, 1985; Rochat *et al.*, 1993). In-depth discussions of protracted wound management and surgical reconstruction of wounds can be found in the *BSAVA Manual of Canine and Feline Wound Management and Reconstruction* as well as other specialized texts (e.g. Pavletic, 1993).

Selection of antibiotics: Clean wounds primarily closed within 6–8 hours of the injury, and more extensive wounds correctly treated with debridement and lavage, do not need antibiotic therapy provided tissue damage is minimal. Antibiotic therapy is indicated in the management of deep wounds involving muscle, wounds with severe tissue damage or where tissue of doubtful viability is left after debridement and in patients with systemic infection or which are immunocompromised. If antibiotics are given in the first 3 hours after injury, they will contact bacteria via the fluid in the wound, before debris and fibrin surround them. To exploit this opportunity, intravenous therapy should be started as soon as possible to maximize antibiotic levels in tissue and wound fluid. As results from culture will not be available at this stage, simple guidelines are used to select a broad-spectrum antibiotic. Most wounds are exposed to contamination from *Staphylococcus* and *Streptococcus* species. Bite wounds may contain *Pasteurella* and Gram-negative species such as *Escherichia coli*. Gram-negative species may also be found in puncture wounds and in potentially contaminated areas such as the perineum. Cephalosporins, trimethoprim–sulphonamides, amoxicillin–clavulanate and enrofloxacin all have activity against these organisms and can be given intravenously. When there is a possibility of extensive Gram-negative contamination, an aminoglycoside should be considered. Ampicillin and penicillin should only be used after culture results confirm susceptibility, as in more than two thirds of cases the bacteria isolated are resistant to these agents (Hirsch and Smith, 1978).

During definitive treatment, antibiotic therapy can be modified on the basis of culture and RST results. Unless there is an indication to change or extend the course, the most effective, narrowest-spectrum, cheapest and safest antibiotic available should be continued by injection or orally for 5–7 days. If the appearance of the wound does not improve or the patient's systemic condition deteriorates, a change in antibiotics coupled with re-swabbing the wound is indicated. Antimicrobial medication can usually be discontinued once a good granulation bed has become established (Figure 17.8).

Systemic antibiotics alone will be adequate in most situations, but heavily contaminated wounds and burns are best treated with a combination of topical and systemic therapy (Figure 17.9). Gentamicin, nitrofurazone, bacitracin/polymixin and neomycin may all be delivered to the wound via the primary dressing layer. Topical antibiotics are particularly useful when the contaminants are resistant or difficult to treat systemically, such as *Pseudomonas* spp. Soaking the primary dressing in tris–EDTA (ethylene diamine tetra-acetic acid – tromethamine) also aids the control of *Pseudomonas* (Farca *et al.*, 1997). Tris–EDTA is made by combining 1.2 g of EDTA with 6.05 g tris (a buffer),

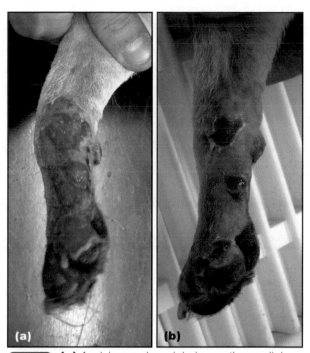

17.8 **(a)** Avulsion or shear injuries on the medial aspect of a dog's antebrachium and carpus. **(b)** 10 days later, after the use of wet to dry dressings, and then non-adherent dressings, healthy granulating tissue is present with evidence of early epithelialization and wound contraction. At this stage antimicrobial therapy should no longer be necessary.

For simple wounds, which are treated correctly, do not use antibiotics

For serious wounds start broad-spectrum intravenous therapy immediately

Re-assess therapy on the basis of culture, rapid slide test results, wound progress and patient's condition

Once therapy is started, continue for 5–7 days

Consider combinations of multiple systemic and topical drugs in heavy contaminated wounds with resistant bacterial species

---

17.9 Summary of antibiotic selection.

added to 1 l of sterile water for injection. The pH is adjusted to 8.0 using dilute NaOH solution and the resulting tris–EDTA solution autoclaved for 15 minutes. Topical water-soluble silver sulphadiazine cream can be applied to the eschar in burn cases, to prevent the necrotic tissue becoming infected.

Dressings and bandages
Dressings are required as a primary contact layer with the wound. Maintaining the apposition of the wound, provision for the storage of exudates and mechanical stability can be achieved using various combinations of bandages, adhesives, sutures and external skeletal fixation (ESF). Individual bandages are addressed in the section on musculoskeletal trauma. The principal decision relates to the choice of dressing; selection of appropriate dressings depends on evaluation of the state of the exposed tissue, the degree of contamination and the anticipated production of fluid from the wound surface (Figure 17.10). Ideally a dressing should:

Description (and proprietary examples)	Properties	Uses	Contraindications
Thin perforated polyester film, backed with absorbent cotton and acrylic fibre pad (Melonin, Smith & Nephew; Primapore, Smith & Nephew; Figure 17.6h)	Semi-occlusive Non-adherent May have adherent surround, e.g. Primapore	Clean sutured wounds, abrasions, lacerations and minor burns	Necrotic wounds or those requiring debridement
Open-weave gauze impregnated with paraffin jelly (Jelonet, Smith & Nephew)	Non-adherent Free draining into absorbent secondary dressing May be antibiotic impregnated	Low viscosity exudative wounds	Avoid on granulating wounds as interdigitates with expanding granulating tissue which causes damage at removal
Outer polyurethane film, hydrophilic core, polyurethane wound contact layer (Allevyn, Smith & Nephew; Figure 17.15a)	Non-adherent Controlled exudate absorption Absorbs ten times its own weight Keeps wound moist	Granulating wounds with some exudation Can be left in position for up to 5 days	Necrotic debris
Hydrocolloid gel (Intrasite, Smith & Nephew; Granuflex, ConvaTec Ltd)	Moist environment Non-adherent Interactive, conformable Waterproof (Granuflex) Absorbs exudate	Granulating wounds including those with some necrotic debris Can assist in microdebridement Vehicle for antimicrobial agents, e.g. metronidazole	Highly exudative wounds
Calcium alginate fibre (Kaltostat, ConvaTec Ltd)	Interactive ion exchange Haemostatic Absorbs 20 times weight	Bleeding and exudative wounds	Dry wounds or wounds with necrotic slough
Open-weave gauze saturated with sterile saline Wet to dry or wet to wet (Figure 17.11b)	Adherent Saline dilutes exudate and facilitates absorption Debriding – necrotic material entrapped as gauze dries, and removed at dressing change	Open degloving wounds, especially if contaminated or necrotic. Use in early stages to aid debridement, soak with tris-EDTA and antibiotics or perfuse solutions to moisten dressing continuously	Healthy granulating and epithelializing wounds

17.10 Characteristics of a variety of dressing materials.

- Prevent further contamination
- Assist the process of debridement
- Conduct fluid away from the surface preventing pooling, maceration and the formation of an environment conducive to bacterial proliferation
- Prevent desiccation and maintain a moist, well oxygenated environment to promote repair.

The primary consideration for initial management of wounds is whether to use an adherent or non-adherent dressing. Adherent dressings, such as dry swabs or sterile saline-soaked swabs that are allowed to dry in contact with the wound (wet to dry), aid debridement (Figure 17.11). Such dressings are useful in wounds that have a considerable amount of necrotic debris and where surgical debridement is delayed. However, they can be painful to remove and removal may disrupt granulation tissue. The wound surface may become desiccated if the dressing is too dry, and macerated if it is too wet. Non-adherent dressings prevent disruption and damage to epithelializing or granulating tissue at removal. They vary in their

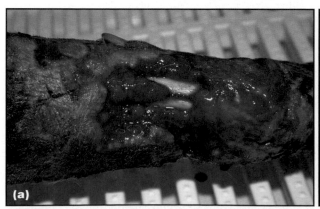
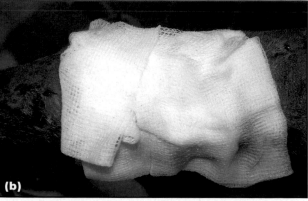

17.11 **(a)** This wound over a dog's carpus occurred as a result of a dogfight. There is some granulation tissue present but further superficial debridement of the necrotic mucoid layer would be beneficial. **(b)** 'Wet to dry' dressings with sterile swabs soaked in sterile lactated Ringer's solution are applied to the wounds.

degree of absorbency, and conduct fluid away from the surface to a greater or lesser extent (see Figure 17.15a). In addition, some of them have interactive properties that promote the removal of necrotic debris and bacteria from the wound surface, but they are not as valuable in the process of debridement as the adherent dressings. Non-adherent dressings are easier to manage, less painful to change and maintain a more constant wound environment.

Ideally, initial treatment of most wounds should be with an adherent dressing to assist microdebridement, followed by non-adherent dressings once granulation commences. However, to ease the management of dressing changes, in many cases non-adherent dressings can be used throughout the healing process. Recent improvement in the properties and variety of these dressings, particularly the ability of some of them to participate in microdebridement, allow selection of a dressing with properties appropriate to the stage of wound healing. Whatever dressing materials are used, a schedule for dressing changes should be devised based on the severity of the wound. Frequent dressing changes allow more accurate monitoring, but may retard healing and distress the patient. Dressings on contaminated wounds and those with severe skin loss should be changed within the first 24 hours. Dressings over simple lacerations should be changed after 48–72 hours. Removal of adherent dressings can be painful; pain can be ameliorated by soaking the primary layer with sterile saline or 2% lidocaine. The protocol described for initial wound management, particularly the need to maintain asepsis, should be followed as far as possible at dressing changes.

Musculoskeletal trauma

Although they are often the most obvious and impressive part of a case, musculoskeletal injuries have a low priority in the initial handling of the trauma patient, and emergency care must be directed primarily towards systemic injuries. Even after evaluation of the major organ systems, musculoskeletal injuries cannot be considered in isolation. The haemorrhage and local disruption of the surrounding soft tissue may pose more problems than the injury itself, therefore the integrity of all tissue involved and its systemic implications must be considered before definitive fixation (Figures 17.12 and 17.13).

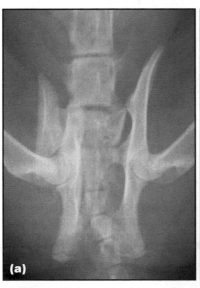
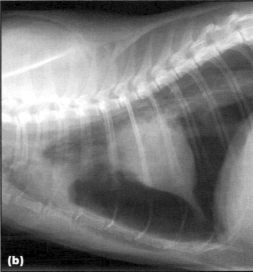

17.12 Prioritization of therapy: radiographs of a cat which had recently been involved in a road traffic accident. **(a)** The cat has a displaced ilial fracture and a sacroiliac luxation; it was unable to ambulate and had neurological deficits.
(b) However the cat was also in respiratory distress with a tension pneumothorax, which required emergency thoracocentesis.

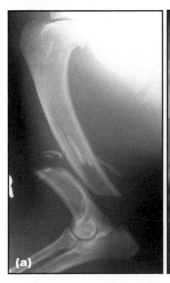
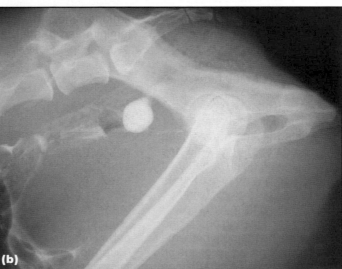

17.13 Soft tissue complications of fractures. **(a)** This dog presented with a severe comminuted humeral fracture.
(b) In addition the bladder was ruptured. Leakage of positive contrast from the cystogram into the abdomen clearly demonstrates the problem.

Definitive treatment frequently requires a prolonged period of anaesthesia to allow accurate evaluation and corrective surgery. Most definitive treatment should thus be outside the remit of emergency care. However, the emergency management of a specific injury can be important in improving the systemic condition of the animal, and can have as much impact in achieving complication-free healing as definitive fixation.

Fractures and luxations

Most fracture or luxation presentations are simple, acute and have a clear history related to external trauma. Clinical signs include pain, deformity, swelling, crepitus and instability. The systemic consequences can be severe. The osseofascial haemorrhage that occurs in closed femoral and humeral fractures can result in up to 30% of circulating blood being sequestered at the fracture site. Fractures and luxations in which direct trauma is clearly not involved require less consideration of systemic problems in the early phase of treatment. These include isolated luxations (both traumatic and congenital or developmental) and simple fractures, such as condylar fractures in puppies which can occur when a shear force is transferred indirectly to the bone by an axial compression force along the antebrachium. In these less common cases, investigation can progress more rapidly to a definitive evaluation of the fracture or luxation and the underlying cause, once simple support and analgesia have been implemented.

Evaluation

There are numerous systems by which to evaluate and classify fractures. These sytems are mostly used in decisions related to definitive treatment, rely on accurate imaging and are unnecessary for initial treatment. A basic evaluation should therefore be made of the position of the injury, its relationship to critical structures and whether it is open or closed. The accompanying systematic examination should include a general evaluation of the extremities, assessing pulses, neurological status and the presence of wounds or devitalized skin. Oedema indicates impaired venous and/or lymphatic return caused by haematoma or mechanical impingement. On the basis of this information, the problem can be categorized in the following manner:

- Fractures and luxations that require prompt treatment due to life-threatening complications (impacted cranial fractures, spinal fractures/luxations and open fractures involving major structures)
- Fractures that will benefit from being treated immediately, provided the animal is not at increased risk from anaesthesia (open fractures and luxations)
- Fractures that should be treated within 24–48 hours for optimal results (articular and epiphyseal fractures and all other luxations)
- Fractures that need to be treated within 5 days of occurrence (all other fractures).

Evaluation of position: Although evaluation of abnormal range of movement, swelling and crepitus is useful, manipulation and palpation of fractures or luxations should be minimized to prevent discomfort and further damage to adjacent tissue. If the animal will lie quietly, it is often possible to take a survey radiograph to give information on the position and extent of the injury. Even though such radiographs may not be accurate enough for use in the definitive fixation, they are often the best and least distressing method of evaluating the position of the fracture.

Evaluation of open fractures: The main feature of open fractures is that there is direct exposure of the bone to the outside environment. Evaluation of the grade of open fracture allows straightforward selection of therapy and an early indication of prognosis. The guidelines for evaluation are:

Grade I   Penetration of the skin by a bony fragment from the fracture. The fragment frequently retracts back beneath the skin. Prognosis is as good as a closed fracture, providing that there is aseptic wound handling and early fixation

Grade II   The fracture is created by an external force, which also creates a wound. The bone is not directly exposed but communicates with the wound and there is variable damage and/or loss of skin and underlying tissue. Prognosis depends on the degree of soft tissue loss and contamination

Grade III   Severe injuries which are commonly associated with high-energy trauma. The fractures are often comminuted and there is a high degree of tissue loss, contamination and devitalization. Bony union is normally delayed and there are often complications during the healing period.

The prognosis in grade III fractures is variable. In some cases it may not be possible to treat the fracture successfully and initial treatment should be aimed towards an amputation. In humans, the grade III group has been further subdivided to help in this decision (Caudle and Stern, 1987):

Grade IIIA Despite extensive soft tissue loss and/or high-energy trauma, there is still adequate soft tissue covering bone. There is a fair prognosis despite extended healing time

Grade IIIB Soft tissue loss is more severe with exposure of bone and periosteal stripping present; often highly contaminated. The prognosis is guarded and in some cases will force amputation

Grade IIIC There is severe tissue damage with major arterial damage. The prognosis is poor and amputation should be considered.

Principles of emergency treatment of fractures and luxations

The principles of emergency management of fractures and luxations consist of:

- Limiting swelling
- Prevention of further compromise of blood supply
- Limiting further soft tissue damage resulting from instability
- Increasing patient comfort and minimizing movement (Figure 17.14)
- Provision of analgesia
- Treating wounds over open fractures in the same way as described previously for other wounds.

Bone affected	Method of stabilization
Mandible	None, or tape muzzle
Maxilla and cranium	None
Cervical spine	Neck splint
Scapula or humerus	None or full spica splint (see Figures 17.21c and 17.22a)
Radius and ulna or tibia	Support bandage or splinted bandage
Carpus or tarsus and all bones distal	Support bandage
Thoracolumbar spine	Back splint (see Figure 17.24)
Caudal lumbar spine	None
Pelvis	None
Femur	None or a full spica splint

17.14 Emergency stabilization of fractures.

Application of these principles is primarily dependent on the position of the injury. Some techniques for fracture management are valid for one area and wholly inappropriate for another.

Open injuries should be considered as wounds involving a fracture or luxation. The same considerations of emergency treatment, debridement, contamination, antibiotics and dressings should be applied as outlined earlier. The depth of tissue involved in grade II and III injuries dictates the application of maximal care to these injuries. Early stabilization, where possible, reduces discomfort and can speed recovery. Temporary stabilization should always be considered concurrent with early treatment of the wound, as stability promotes wound-healing processes, decreases pain and reduces complications. External coaptation can be used if it is appropriate to the site. External skeletal fixation (ESF) is often the optimal definitive fixation for open fractures. However, ESF should also be considered during initial management, as an alternative to external coaptation. ESF can be placed rapidly in a closed fashion, and is therefore applicable during anaesthesia for wound debridement. Unlike external coaptation, ESF allows the stability of the site to be maintained during dressing changes, thus reducing pain, the need for sedation for dressing changes and the amount of bandaging material required. Transarticular ESF (TESF) (Figure 17.15) can be used to control the stability of a wound over a joint, even when no fracture is present, for example after a traumatic luxation with shear injury.

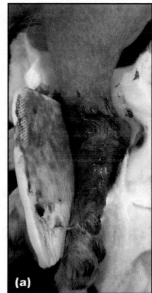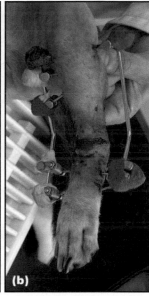

17.15 **(a)** The hock of the dog shown in Figure 17.8 with a dislocation and an avulsion or shear wound on the cranial flexor aspect of the hock. A non-adherent absorbent dressing (Allevyn, Smith and Nephew) and hydrocolloid gel (Intrasite gel, Smith and Nephew) have been used. **(b)** 10 days later, after stabilization of the hock with a transarticular external skeletal fixator and appropriate wound management consisting of daily wound flushing and application of 'wet to dry' or non-adherent dressings as dictated by the appearance of the wound.

Selection and use of bandages

Bandages can be used to stabilize traumatized areas and to hold dressings in place. However, it can be difficult to place bandages correctly on a distressed patient and the benefit of a bandage, particularly complex ones such as slings and spica splints (Figures 17.16 and 17.21), must be weighed against the problems of possible incorrect placement. Simple bandages also have limitations. The Robert Jones bandage, when applied above the elbow or stifle, tends to slip down and form a 'pendulum' of extra weight at or below the joint. Thus, when considering emergency stabilization there are several situations in which it is better not to apply an extensive bandage, but to use cage rest, analgesia and sedation to restrict further damage at the fracture site (see Figure 17.14).

Specific situations in which certain bandage configurations are appropriate are outlined in Figures 17.16 and 17.19 and in the text below. Dressings can be held in place over the body with wraps, particularly using the newer elasticated and conformable materials. The most useful general configuration is the support bandage.

Support bandage: Support bandages minimize swelling and oedema, aid haemostasis, provide stabilization and increase patient comfort. True pressure bandages are rarely necessary. The Robert Jones bandage is known as a pressure bandage but, with the deformable materials used, pressure is generally not maintained for a significant length of time. Pressure gauges placed on the skin under such bandages soon return to normal. The bandage should be applied with

Type of bandage	Description	Uses	Comments and specific contraindications
Support (modified Robert Jones dressing)	Use deformable secondary layer applied under compression. Leave pads of middle two digits protruding to allow checking for swelling	Stable fractures distal to the elbow or stifle. Positioning of a dressing, especially over an exudative wound	Do not use in proximal limb fractures, rarely of use in elbow or stifle injuries. In these cases the bandage may slip down and become a pendulum weight
Splinted bandage	Augment a support bandage with a splint to increase rigidity without extra bulk	Unstable fractures distal to elbow or stifle	Do not use in proximal limb fractures, rarely of use in elbow or stifle injuries
Velpeau sling	Bandage placed around leg and over body to flex carpus, elbow and shoulder	Holds entire forelimb in flexion to prevent weightbearing and movement of distal limb	Provide sufficient padding to prevent sores
Carpal flexion	Figure-of-eight bandage applied over padding from distal radius to metacarpals	Flexion of carpus and prevention of forelimb weightbearing, although limb can still be moved	Do not use for antebrachial or distal injuries
Ehmer sling	Figure-of-eight bandage from metatarsals to distal femur with the bandage all medial to the tibia	Internal rotation of hip and stifle reduces the chance of re-luxation after reduction of ventral hip luxations	Difficult to apply, especially on cats or short-legged dogs
Hobble	Bandage connection between both distal tibias	Prevents abduction and reduces the chance of re-luxation after reduction of ventral hip luxations	
Spica splint	Flat splint strapped from toe to dorsum. Held in place with support bandage distally and body bandage	Fractures proximal to the elbow (use in hindlimb is also reported)	Not usually recommended for injuries distal to the elbow or stifle

17.16 Bandages (see also Figures 17.17, 17.18, 17.21 and 17.22).

a primary layer covering any wound, a secondary layer of a conformable material such as cotton wool, a tertiary layer using a tightly wound bandage and an outer protective bandage. The bandage should be placed to follow the normal aspect of the limb (Figure 17.17) and can be reinforced by a splint placed after the secondary layer has been pressurized. Splints can be made from strips of cast material and therefore conformed and customized to the patient, but commercial off-the-shelf products are particularly useful for temporary and emergency usage (Figure 17.18).

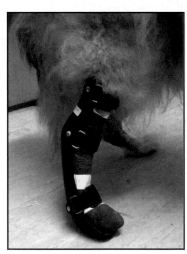

17.18
A commercial splint with Velcro tapes can be applied rapidly to provide temporary support during healing or while awaiting definitive repair.

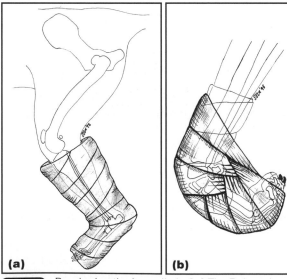

17.17 Bandaging the lower limb. **(a)** The Robert Jones bandaging provides a column of support following the conformation of the limb. **(b)** Carpal flexion bandage prevents weightbearing but allows movement of the upper limb joints (elbow and shoulder).

Ischaemic injury
Ischaemic injury can occur after incorrect application of a bandage (Anderson and White, 2000). This is attributed to direct pressure necrosis related to inadequate or uneven application of padding, or to a tourniquet effect resulting in secondary ischaemic oedema. All owners of cases discharged with bandages in place should be given written instructions on home care and inspection of bandages. If possible the nails/pads of the third and fourth distal phalanges should be left visible at the bottom of the bandage for monitoring. Owners can be asked to assess the apposition of the nails – when swelling occurs the nails will part or splay. If an animal shows signs of pain or excessive licking or chewing at the bandage, it should be removed as soon as possible. All bandages should be reassessed within 24 hours to minimize the risks

inherent in inadvertent misapplication of the bandage. Bandages placed on limbs with vascular injury or deep lacerations should be rechecked and changed frequently to monitor for increased tissue pressure due to oedema.

Luxations

Traumatic luxations require definitive treatment as early as the systemic condition of the animal allows, in order to minimize cartilage destruction, muscle contracture and periarticular fibrosis. Examination under general anaesthesia and the use of two orthogonal radiographic views are essential to confirm the presence and direction of the luxation, concurrent periarticular injuries and pre-existing disease, such as hip dysplasia, which may influence management. There is likely to be damage to some part of the bone, muscle, tendon and ligament complex that confers stability on the normal joint. In some joints, surgical repair of this damage, coupled with postoperative support,

is indicated to maintain reduction (Figure 17.19). The hip, elbow, temporomandibular joint and occasionally the shoulder have enough inherent stability to remain reduced despite some damage, and closed reduction of these joints is indicated as a primary treatment (Figure 17.20). The Ehmer sling can be used to assist stability of the hip joint after reduction, and the Velpeau sling may be applied to support the shoulder (Figure 17.21). In general, surgical reduction and repair of any joint should be considered if:

- Closed reduction is impossible
- The joint is still unstable or luxates easily after closed reduction
- Periarticular or articular fractures prevent reduction or require fixation
- Exploratory surgery is required to evaluate periarticular structures such as nerves
- Developmental or congenital abnormalities are present which can cause instability.

Affected joint	Direction of luxation	Technique for reduction (under general anaesthetic)	Postoperative support	Comments
Temporomandibular	Rostrodorsal	Lever in mouth and close mouth	Tape muzzle 7–10 days	Associated fractures may require surgery
	Coronoid displacement	Open mouth further and move mandible towards midline	None	Partial zygomatic arch resection if recurrent
Scapulohumeral	Medial	Manipulate proximal humerus/acromion	Velpeau 2–3 weeks	Small dogs, often congenital
	Lateral	Manipulate proximal humerus/acromion	Spica	Large dogs, often traumatic
Elbow	Lateral	See Figure 17.20	Maintain extension	Very rarely medial. May need surgical reduction
Carpus	Variable	Surgical	Support bandage	Arthrodesis may be required if function is unsatisfactory
Phalangeal	Lateral or abaxial	Closed for pet animals, surgical treatment in working dogs	Support bandage	Require surgical imbrication of collaterals, or arthrodesis
Hip	Craniodorsal	See Figure 17.20	Ehmer sling or cage rest	Surgical stabilization ultimately required in many cases (15–71%)
	Ventral	Externally rotate and abduct hip (and adduct stifles) whilst gently pushing dorsally. If reduction is unsuccessful and hip displaces craniodorsally, treat as in Figure 17.20	Hobble	Closed reduction usually successful
Stifle	Cranial	Surgical	Spica or ESF	Repair combination injuries of collaterals and cruciates
Tibiotarsal	Variable	Surgical	Bandage, splint or ESF	Repair fractured malleoli and collateral ligaments if possible

17.19 Management of luxations.

Technique for elbow reduction
1. Fully flex elbow and abduct and pronate antebrachium whilst applying medial pressure to caudal ulna to engage anconeus.
2. Extend elbow slightly and then slowly extend elbow further and pronate and adduct antebrachium whilst applying medial pressure to radial head.
3. Use high support bandage or spica, to maintain extension, or carpal flexion bandage to avoid weightbearing.

Technique for reduction of craniodorsal hip luxation
1. Externally rotate femur; distract limb against countertraction.
2. Adduct then internally rotate, extend and abduct limb.
3. Manipulate through full range of movement to dispel clots.

17.20 Technique for reduction of elbow and hip luxations.

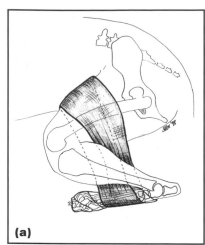
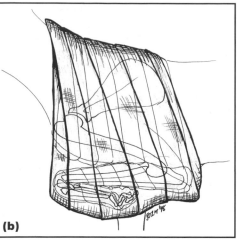
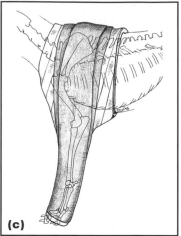

17.21 Bandaging the upper limb. **(a)** The Ehmer sling is a figure-of-eight bandage, which internally rotates the hip and prevents re-luxation. **(b)** The Velpeau sling provides stability for the shoulder area and prevents weightbearing by limiting movement of the limb. **(c)** The spica splint stabilizes the elbow and humerus and can also be used on the hindlimb. The antebrachium is padded with a Robert Jones bandage and there is some padding over the scapula. A flat lateral splint is placed over the midline at the tip of the scapula and all the way down to the foot. The splint can be made from a sheet of thermosetting cast material and pleated for resistance to bending. It is held in place with adhesive tape over the Robert Jones dressing and a body bandage around the thorax.

Articular fractures

Articular fractures should be treated definitively within 24–48 hours, provided the animal can be safely anaesthetized. Accurate reconstruction of articular surfaces, compression and rigid internal fixation are essential. Early return to function minimizes periarticular fibrosis and joint stiffness. Bandages or splints applied prior to treatment will be beneficial in decreasing swelling and increasing comfort, but are contraindicated in some situations. Cats in particular do not tolerate bandages well and, with closed injuries, cage rest may be preferable to bandaging. In general, the joints below the elbow and stifle can be supported with a bandage or splint. The elbow and stifle can be supported if necessary using a spica splint (Figures 17.6g, 17.21c and 17.22a). Support of either the shoulder or hip joint

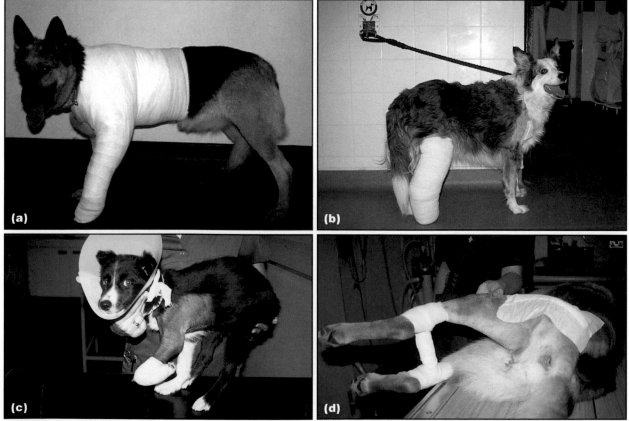

17.22 Bandages in use on dogs. **(a)** Spica splint on a German Shepherd Dog after closed reduction of a lateral shoulder luxation. **(b)** Robert Jones dressing. **(c)** Carpal flexion bandage. **(d)** Hobbles placed on a dog while still anaesthetized after surgery.

prior to definitive treatment is generally not necessary, as the large muscle mass surrounding these joints provides sufficient support.

Diaphyseal fractures

Fractures involving the pelvis, scapula, femur and humerus should generally be left unbandaged. The muscle mass surrounding these bones provides some support, and bandages for these areas are cumbersome and restricting. Tubular bandages are ineffective in supporting these fractures and tend to form a pendulum of extra weight swinging at the level of the fracture. Femoral and humeral fractures may be supported with spica splints for transport or if repair must be delayed. Cage rest with suitable analgesia may be preferable. Fractures of the bones below the elbow and stifle should be supported with a bandage or splint. The combination of a splint and bandage (Figure 17.6f) usually provides better stability to a fractured part than a bandage in isolation, even a well padded bandage.

Spinal fractures

Spinal fractures are candidates for immediate treatment, despite the high (40–50%) incidence of concurrent problems (Selcer *et al.*, 1991). The potential for injury to the spinal cord itself is high and early intervention is essential to allow the maximum chance of conserving spinal cord function. There is a risk of further injury to the spinal cord during transport and examination of the patient. Animals should be transported on a flat board, a firm stretcher or slung in a strong blanket.

Examination: Early neurological examination is important, but extensive testing involving movement of the animal may cause further problems. Particular attention should be paid to whether deep pain sensation is present, and the testing of local reflexes, where all the muscle groups should be observed acting coherently. Repeated monitoring is important to assess any change in status. Survey radiographs of the conscious patient are indicated, as sedation, muscle relaxation and positioning for radiographs may cause further damage at the site of instability. Lateral views of the entire spine are advisable as multiple fractures can occur. Oblique views assist evaluation of the articular processes and can be taken with the animal in lateral recumbency. Positioning for dorsoventral views can be hazardous, and a horizontal beam view is the preferred option (Wheeler and Sharp, 1994). Orthogonal views should be taken if the site of injury is not obvious on one view (Figure 17.23).

It is important to assess the stability of the fracture. Bending, shear, rotational and axial loading forces all act on the spine. Radiographic evaluation of the damaged areas can indicate the residual capacity of the spine to resist these forces, and indicate the optimum fixation technique. The key areas of evaluation are the ventral spinal component (i.e. the vertebral body and the intervertebral discs) which resists load and bending, and the articular processes, which resist a combination of forces. If one or both of

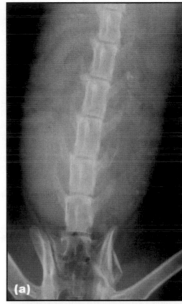

17.23

This cat presented with sudden onset hindlimb paraparesis. Patellar reflexes were exaggerated and sciatic myotatic reflexes reduced. **(a)** Ventrodorsal radiograph of the cat's lumbar spine. There is a left ilial fracture. The unusual sacroiliac joint was considered to be an incidental finding. **(b)** Lateral radiograph shows a compression fracture of the body of the sixth lumbar vertebra.

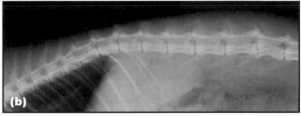

these areas are severely compromised, the fracture will be unstable and a candidate for surgical fixation. More complex systems for staging the damage in relation to stability can be consulted, but the information is often difficult to apply to commonly occurring fracture patterns (Smith and Walter, 1985; Patterson and Smith, 1992; Shores, 1992). Stress radiography under fluoroscopy to evaluate instability should only be undertaken with extreme caution (Wheeler and Sharp, 1994). If available, other imaging techniques such as computed tomography may also be beneficial, providing information about the spinal cord as well as the bony injury.

Treatment: Owners of animals that are being treated for spinal fractures need to commit themselves to a 4–6-week recovery period to allow an opportunity for return to function. Animals without deep pain sensation have a poor prognosis for any return to function. Although conservative and medical therapy coupled with continual reassessment, or exploratory surgery to identify a malacic cord, are possible in these patients, euthanasia should be considered.

The treatment of spinal fractures has three components: medical therapy; stabilization; and decompression (Figure 17.24). Selection of appropriate therapy is initially based on the clinical presentation. Indications for conservative treatment are:

- Animals that can walk or are paraparetic
- Animals that exhibit strong voluntary movement and have peripheral pain perception
- Animals that have minimal pain or pain that can be controlled by drugs.

Treatment	Indications	Advantages	Disadvantages
Cage rest. Confine in very small space until radiographic evidence of healing	Ambulatory or paraparetic animals with stable thoracolumbar injuries	Economical. No exposure to lengthy surgery and anaesthesia	Difficult to restrict some animals. Animals may suffer prolonged discomfort, and neurological deficits may worsen or even become irreversible
Back splinting (Patterson and Smith, 1992)	Caudal cervical, thoracic and lumbar injuries	Economical. Provides better stability than cage rest. Can combine with internal fixation	Intensive nursing required especially for large dogs. Not ideal if ventral component involved
Vertebral body pinning	Lumbar fractures	Economical. Implants often readily available	Weakest form of internal fixation
Dorsal spinous process plating. Apply a metal or plastic plate to dorsal spinous processes either side of lesion	Thoracic and lumbar fractures	Effective combined with vertebral body plating in resisting bending forces	Difficult to apply to small dorsal spinous processes. Processes may fracture
Modified segmental fixation. Secure a pin or pins to two dorsal spinous processes cranial and caudal to the lesion	Thoracic and lumbar injuries in small dogs and cats	Economical. Equipment usually readily available	Articular processes may fracture. Immobilizes a long segment of spine. Ideally require intact ventral component
Vertebral body plating. Plate applied to dorsolateral vertebral bodies above transverse processes	Thoracic and cranial lumbar vertebrae (application caudal to L3 requires sacrificing nerves to the lumbosacral plexus)	Effective versus bending forces, enhanced when combined with dorsal spinous plating. Can combine with hemilaminectomy	Difficult to apply plate in thoracic region as need to disarticulate ribs. Little resistance to rotational forces
Pins or screws and polymethylmethacrylate	Any location	Very versatile technique. Provides rotational stability	Occasionally see wound infection and pin migration
Trans-ilial pinning. Pin through wings of ilium dorsocaudal to the bone of the dorsal spinous process of L7	Lumbosacral injuries	Can combine with dorsal spinous body plating or stapling	Pins may migrate and may provide inadequate stability if used in isolation

17.24 Treatment options for spinal fractures and luxations.

Major indications for surgery are:

- Non-ambulatory animals
- Palpably unstable or significantly displaced injuries
- Animals that deteriorate with conservative treatment
- Animals with peripheral pain perception but no voluntary movement
- When decompression is required for displaced spinal segments, bone fragments or extruded disc material
- Non-ambulatory animals with no deep pain
- Animals with significant pain associated with the fracture.

Medical management: Acute injury to the spinal cord initiates a sequence of vascular, biochemical and inflammatory events that result in secondary tissue damage. Medical management includes appropriate analgesia once the neurological evaluation is complete. Patients presented within 8 hours of acute cord trauma may benefit from methylprednisolone sodium succinate (MPSS) treatment (see Chapter 9), although this is controversial. Some would argue that it has no benefit and the possible complications, including an increased risk of pneumonia, gastrointestinal haemorrhage and perforation, may outweigh the possible benefits. Analgesics, including opioids and non-steroidal drugs, together with confinement and immobilization are probably the mainstay of non-surgical management.

Stabilization: Stabilization can be carried out conservatively (Figure 17.25) or surgically depending on the clinical signs, radiographic indications of stability and anatomical position (Figure 17.24). If surgery is indicated, a myelogram or CT can be used to determine if there is a significant lesion that requires decompression; however, evaluation of the survey radiographs alone may be sufficient to deduce this information. Hemilaminectomy should be used for decompression as it has minimal effect on spinal stability. Decompression should always be accompanied by appropriate internal fixation.

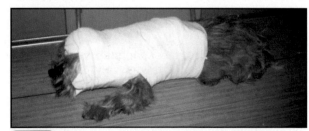

17.25 Temporary neck splinting for atlantoaxial subluxation fracture. The splint should extend from the mandible to the thorax. Careful monitoring is required; upper airway obstruction and inability to move the chest wall are common concerns.

Compartment syndrome

Acute compartment syndrome following trauma has been reported in the dog (De Haan and Beale, 1993). Bleeding or tissue swelling within a fascial compartment can cause a rapid rise in pressure in that compartment, which is responsible for the problem. The condition is common in humans, especially associated with tibial fractures. Due to the non-specific nature of the signs and the difficulty of making a definitive diagnosis, the condition may be underdiagnosed in the dog.

Pathogenesis

Physiological compartments are enclosed by skin, epimysium, fascia or bone. The term osseofascial is used to describe a compartment where bone and fascia are the barriers to swelling (Basinger *et al.*, 1987). Extraneous material, such as a dressing or a cast, can also define a compartment. In dogs, osseofascial compartments have been reported in:

* Craniolateral crus
* Caudal crus
* Caudal antebrachium
* Femoral compartment (complex multifascial envelope).

If the pressure in one of these compartments rises, the veins will collapse and local venous pressure will rise. This reduces the arteriovenous gradient, blood flow and tissue perfusion, leading to ischaemia and necrosis. Peripheral nerves and muscles have limited resistance to hypoxia and are damaged first by the rise in pressure, leading to impaired neuromuscular function (Rorabeck and McGee, 1990). As there is an inverse linear relationship between pressure and the time taken for the tissue damage to become irreversible, early treatment is essential. Reperfusion injury, for example after cast removal, may also play a part in the pathophysiology of the condition. Pressure can increase for several reasons:

* Bleeding into the compartment after trauma
* Increased capillary permeability and swelling following ischaemia (reperfusion injury may occur here too)
* External pressure constricting a compartment, for example a bandage.

Normal pressures in muscle average 4 mmHg, with a range of 0–8 mmHg. Measurements of muscle pressure in dogs with compartment syndrome reported in the literature were 26–30 mmHg (De Haan and Beale, 1993).

Diagnosis and treatment

Compartment syndrome should be considered in trauma patients with swollen and tense limbs, where there is little compliance to surface finger pressure and which are especially uncomfortable and resistant to analgesia (Figure 17.26). Arterial pulses are still palpable, as the pressure does not generally rise enough to stop arterial blood flow. There is decreased sensation due to nerve compression. It can be difficult to differentiate compartment syndrome from arterial occlusion and neuropraxia.

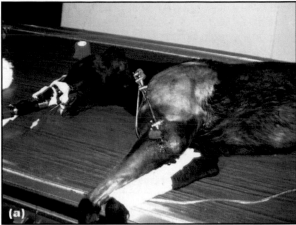
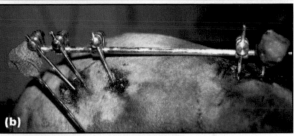
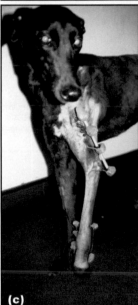

17.26 A dog with suspected compartment syndrome. **(a)** A 2-year-old Greyhound presented with a comminuted humeral fracture with severe brachial swelling and intense pain associated with the area. The dog had intact deep pain sensation and weak pulses distal to the fracture. **(b)** Close-up view of the brachial area showing the swollen tense brachium. **(c)** The dog developed severe muscle atrophy and carpal contracture, similar to Volkmann contracture which is seen in humans as a sequela to compartment syndrome. A transarticular external skeletal fixator was placed across the carpus to prevent further contracture.

The only reliable method of diagnosis is to measure tissue pressures. Slit catheters, wick catheters, needle manometers and continuous infusion systems have been used to measure pressure. However, the simplest practical system is to use a standard CVP manometer linked to an ordinary needle and zeroed to atmospheric pressure; the tip of the needle is then placed into the compartment and the pressure measured.

Compartment syndrome should be treated as an emergency. Rapid relief of the pressure is necessary to prevent irreversible damage resulting from the hypoxia and ischaemia. For cases of confirmed or suspected compartment syndrome, the treatment is to remove the barrier to swelling by cutting the skin, fascia and epimysial layer. In humans, after fasciotomy the incision is left open for delayed closure or split skin grafting 7–8 days later, but postoperative management in animals is facilitated by closure of the skin (De Haan and Beale, 1993). Fractures concurrent to compartment syndrome should be rigidly fixated to promote soft tissue healing, but this can be delayed if necessary. Removal of dressings or bivalving casts can reduce compartment pressures by 50–85% and should be considered if there is a potential for compartment syndrome to occur. Untreated compartment syndrome causing prolonged muscle ischaemia can lead to Volkmann contracture.

References and further reading

Anderson DM and White RA (2000) Ischemic bandage injuries: a case series and review of the literature. *Veterinary Surgery* **29(6)**, 488–498

Basinger RR, Aron DN, Crowe DT and Purinton PT (1987) Osteofascial compartment syndrome in the dog. *Veterinary Surgery* **16**, 427–434

Bellah JR and Krahwinkel DJ (1985) Xylenol orange as a vital stain to determine the viability of skin flaps in dogs. *Veterinary Surgery* **14**, 124–126

Buffa EA, Lubba AM, Verstraete FA and Swaim SF (1997) The effects of wound lavage solutions on canine fibroblasts: an in vitro study. *Veterinary Surgery* **26**, 460–466

Caudle RJ and Stern PJ (1987) Severe open fractures of the tibia. *Journal of Bone and Joint Surgery* **69A**, 801–807

DeHaan JJ and Beale BS (1993) Compartment syndrome in the dog: case report and literature review. *Journal of the American Animal Hospital Association* **29**, 134–140

Farca AM, Piromalli G, Maffei F and Re G (1997) Potentiating effect of EDTA-Tris on the activity of antibiotics against resistant bacteria associated with otitis, dermatitis and cystitis. *Journal of Small Animal Practice* **38(6)**, 243–245

Feliciano DV (1992) Trauma to the peripheral vascular system. In: *Principles and Practice of Emergency Medicine,* ed. CR Schwartz, CG Cayten and MA Magelson, p. 1098. Lea and Febiger, Philadelphia

Fowler D (1999) Tension relieving techniques and local skin flaps In: *Manual of Canine and Feline Wound Management and Reconstruction,* ed. D Fowler and JM Williams, pp. 57–68. BSAVA Publications, Gloucester

Gfeller RW and Crowe DT (1994) The emergency care of traumatic wounds: current recommendations. *Veterinary Clinics of North America: Small Animal Practice* **24**, 1249–1274

Griffon DJ, Walter PA and Wallace L-J (1994) Thoracic injuries in cats with traumatic fractures. *Veterinary Comparative Orthopaedics and Traumatology* **7**, 98–100

Hirsch DC and Smith TM (1978) Osteomyelitis in the dog. Microorganisms isolated and susceptibility to antimicrobial agents. *Journal of Small Animal Practice* **19**, 679–687

Houlton JEF and Dyce J (1992) Does fracture pattern influence thoracic trauma? *Veterinary Comparative Orthopaedics and Traumatology* **5**, 90–92

Patterson RH and Smith G (1992) Back splinting for treatment of thoracic and lumbar fracture luxation in the dog: principles of application and case series. *Veterinary Comparative Orthopaedics and Traumatology* **5**, 179–187

Pavletic MM (1993) *Atlas of Small Animal Reconstructive Surgery.* JB Lippincott, Philadelphia

Rochat MC, Payne JT, Pope ER, Wagner-Mann CC and Pace LW (1993) Evaluation of skin viability in dogs, using transcutaneous carbon dioxide and sensor current monitoring. *American Journal of Veterinary Research* **54**, 476–480

Rorabeck CH and McGee HMJ (1990) Acute compartment syndromes. *Veterinary Comparative Orthopaedics and Traumatology* **3**, 117–122

Selcer RR, Bubb WJ and Walker TL (1991) Management of vertebral column fractures in dogs and cats: 211 cases (1977–1985). *Journal of the American Veterinary Medical Association* **198,** 1965–1968

Shores A (1992) Fractures and luxations of the vertebral column. *Veterinary Clinics of North America: Small Animal Practice* **22**, 171–175

Smith GK and Walter MC (1985) Fractures and luxations of the spine. In: *Textbook of Small Animal Orthopaedics,* ed. CD Newton and DM Nunamaker, pp. 307–332. JB Lippincott, Philadelphia

Spackman EJA, Caywood DD, Feeney DA and Johnston GR (1984) Thoracic wall and pulmonary trauma in dogs sustaining fractures as a result of motor vehicle accidents. *Journal of the American Veterinary Medical Association* **185**, 975–977

Swaim SF and Henderson RA (1997) *Small Animal Wound Management.* Williams and Wilkins, Philadelphia

Tamas PM, Paddleford RR and Krahwinkel DJ (1985) Thoracic trauma in dogs and cats presented for limb fractures. *Journal of the American Animal Hospital Association* **21**, 161–166

Wheeler SJ and Sharp NJH (1994) *Small Animal Spinal Disorders.* Mosby-Wolfe, London

Whitney WO and Mehlhaff CJ (1987) High-rise syndrome in cats. *Journal of the American Animal Hospital Association* **191**, 1399–1403

18

Dermatological emergencies

Petra J. Roosje

Introduction

Dermatological conditions in small animals are most often chronic problems that do not require emergency care. Some acute problems, although not life threatening, may be alarming to the owner, for example hot spots. Other rare conditions, which may not appear severe initially, can eventually prove to be fatal to the animal, e.g. toxic epidermal necrolysis (TEN).

As some of the more serious skin diseases can be difficult to differentiate from each other on the basis of history, physical examination and basic clinico-pathological testing, it is important to perform multiple skin biopsies of early lesions and submit these specimens to a pathologist with a special interest in dermatology. It is imperative to obtain a precise history, description of lesions, possible previous treatments and response to treatment. This chapter describes a selection of acute dermatological conditions, emphasizing those that may have serious consequences for the animal's health.

Juvenile cellulitis

Juvenile cellulitis (puppy strangles or juvenile pyoderma) is an uncommon disease that affects puppies between the ages of 3 weeks and 4 months. The condition has also been described rarely in adult dogs (Jeffers *et al.*, 1995; Neuber *et al.*, 2004). It can occur in numerous breeds, although Gordon Setters, Golden Retrievers and Dachshunds appear to be predisposed (Mason and Jones, 1989; Scott *et al.*, 2001a). The cause of the disease is unknown. Secondary infection with *Staphylococcus* spp. may occur.

Clinical signs

Initially, affected puppies have a painful and swollen face. The eyelids, muzzle and lips are especially affected (Figure 18.1). Papules and pustules develop within a few days. The pinnae are also often involved and, occasionally, the preputial and perianal areas may be affected. Other findings commonly include enlarged mandibular and prescapular lymph nodes, which may become abscessed, rupture and drain in some cases. Lethargy, anorexia and fever occur in around 50% of the puppies. Small numbers of affected animals show joint pain. Occasional puppies may have a concurrent sterile pyogranulomatous panniculitis.

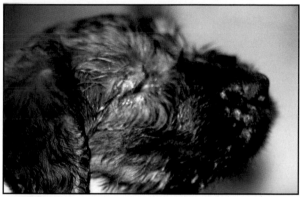

18.1 Briard puppy with swollen eyelids, nose and pinnae due to juvenile cellulitis.

Diagnosis

Differential diagnoses should include staphylococcal pyoderma, demodicosis, drug reaction and angioedema. Multiple deep skin scrapings should be taken to exclude demodicosis. A thorough history will provide information about previous drug administration. Aspirates of intact lymph nodes and pustules should be taken for cytology and bacterial culture. Cytology of intact pustules will reveal pyogranulomatous inflammation without microorganisms. Bacterial cultures of intact pustules should be negative unless there is secondary staphylococcal infection. Skin biopsy specimens of early lesions show multiple discrete or confluent periadnexal granulomas and pyogranulomas consisting of macrophages and neutrophils.

Clinical management

Oral prednisolone (1–2 mg/kg/day) should be given until the clinical signs improve, usually within 1–2 weeks. Corticosteroid administration should then be tapered and stopped over 4–6 weeks. Concomitant administration of antibiotics is often indicated as secondary bacterial infection is common. Affected puppies generally do not recover with antibiotic therapy alone (White *et al.*, 1989). Cefalexin (40–60 mg/kg/day divided into two doses) is the drug of choice. Antiseptic washes or shampoos containing 2–3% chlorhexidine have been recommended, but may cause struggling and stress in the puppy. If anorexia or fever is present, more intensive therapy is required, including the use of intravenous fluid and electrolyte administration. Euthanasia may be indicated in severe cases (Mason and Jones, 1989). The prognosis is generally good, although permanent facial scarring can occur.

Pyotraumatic dermatitis

Pyotraumatic dermatitis ('hot spots' or acute moist dermatitis) is a condition frequently seen in dogs and less often in cats. Hot spots are especially observed in young dogs. The condition is most commonly reported in heavily coated breeds such as St Bernards, Golden Retrievers and German Shepherd Dogs but can be seen in any breed (Holm *et al.*, 2004). In breeds with a dense coat, increased temperature and slow drying of the coat make the skin surface favourable to bacterial colonization and overgrowth. Many 'hot spots' occur as complications of one or more of the factors listed in Figure 18.2. These factors can induce the itch–lick or scratch cycle that varies in intensity with individuals. Lesions may be induced within a few hours.

Flea-bite hypersensitivity
Otitis externa
Atopic dermatitis
Foreign bodies in the coat
Food hypersensitivity
Dirty, matted, unkempt coat
Ectoparasite infestations
Painful musculoskeletal disorders
Anal sac problems

18.2 Causes of pyotraumatic lesions.

Clinical signs

These animals are presented with a history of acute onset of disease. The self-induced painful lesion consists of a well circumscribed area of moist matted hair, glued together with exudate (Figure 18.3). Predilection sites are the cheek, neck, lumbar region and flank.

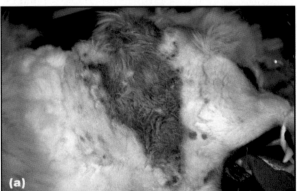

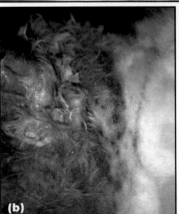

18.3 (a) A Pyrenean Mountain Dog with severe pyotraumatic dermatitis involving the neck. (b) This dog presented with fever and was treated with cefalexin.

Diagnosis

The diagnosis is based on the clinical appearance and a history of acute onset. The lesion usually occurs in an area where the dog can cause self-trauma. The primary cause may not always be apparent. Clinically it is hard to differentiate true pyotraumatic dermatitis from a pyotraumatic folliculitis. Moreover, pyotraumatic dermatitis lesions often have histological evidence of folliculitis (Holm *et al.*, 2004). It may be, however, that folliculitis is a time-related effect. True pyotraumatic dermatitis is a superficial process consisting of a flat erosive or ulcerated lesion. The hair is lost from the lesion but a clear margin is present between the lesion and the normal surrounding skin. In pyotraumatic folliculitis, the lesion is thickened, plaque-like and surrounded by satellite papules and pustules. In most patients, hairs epilate easily from the inflamed area.

Clinical management

The hair on and around the lesion should be clipped to allow a better examination of the lesion and thorough cleaning of the area. As this can be very painful for the dog, sedation or anaesthesia may be needed. Initial cleaning with a chlorhexidine solution is recommended. In dogs with severe lesions, the owner should continue with daily rinsing or washing of the affected area followed by light towel drying of the area. A combination product containing antibiotics and corticosteroids should be applied twice daily. In subacute cases or in the presence of folliculitis and furunculosis, oral cefalexin (40–60 mg/kg/day divided into two doses for 3 weeks) should be given. Initially, an Elizabethan collar, T-shirt or socks may be used to prevent further trauma to the lesion. Topical treatment should be continued until the lesion has dried, usually 7–10 days. Many dogs do not need oral corticosteroids but if pruritus is persistent these patients may benefit from a short course of prednisolone (1 mg/kg/day for 3–5 days, then tapered).

Flea-bite hypersensitivity is often an underlying cause, and therefore it is advisable to recommend stringent flea control measures. To prevent relapses in dogs with a dense coat and without an underlying cause (see Figure 18.2), clipping the whole body during summer can be helpful.

Urticaria and angioedema

Immunologically mediated urticaria, angioedema and anaphylaxis can be thought of as the same disease, with variations in severity and target organ. Urticaria (hives) consists of focal superficial anaphylactic reactions visible as erythematous wheals. Possible causes are listed in Figure 18.4. Dogs are more commonly affected than cats. Urticaria lesions often disappear within a day but may persist longer, with the development of new lesions. A chronic form also exists. In angioedema, deep blood vessels are affected and the resulting oedema causes diffuse swelling. Both diseases result from mast cell or basophil degranulation, which may have an immunological (type I hypersensitivity) or non-immunological origin. The

| Foods |
| Drugs |
| Antisera, bacterins and vaccines |
| Stinging and biting insects |
| Blood transfusions |
| Plants |
| Intestinal parasites |
| Infections (staphylococcal pyoderma, canine distemper)[a] |
| Sunlight[a] |
| Excessive heat or cold[a] |
| Oestrus[a] |
| Atopy[a] |
| Psychogenic factors |

18.4 Factors reported to have caused urticaria in dogs and cats. [a] Reported in dogs only (Scott *et al.*, 2001)

cause of the wheal formation is often hard to identify. Wheals can be irritating to the animal and there is a risk that associated swelling of the mucous membranes may obstruct the airway.

Clinical signs
Urticaria can develop within a few hours. Lesions may be single or multiple and may occur all over the body (Figure 18.5). Animals are variably pruritic. Signs of angioedema consist typically of facial swelling and sometimes swelling of the extremities. Angioedema usually does not cause pruritus.

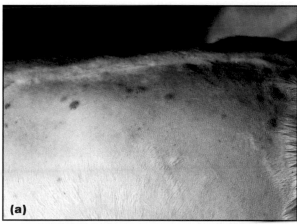
(a)

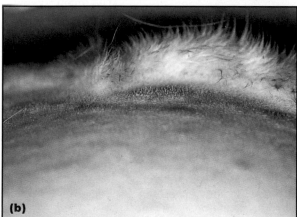
(b)

18.5 **(a)** Multiple urticaria that developed within 2 hours. **(b)** Close-up showing erythematous wheals.

Diagnosis
The differential diagnosis for urticaria includes folliculitis, erythema multiforme, vasculitis and neoplasia. Definitive diagnosis is based on obtaining an extensive history, and a thorough physical examination. Staphylococcal folliculitis can be mistaken for urticaria, especially in short-coated dogs, where hairs can stand out focally. In staphylococcal folliculitis lesions, hairs can be easily epilated and, compared with urticaria, lesions are more exudative. Clipping of the coat can help to identify the lesions. Skin biopsy can be helpful for differentiation when the lesions persist.

Clinical management
Therapy includes avoidance and elimination of the aetiological factors. In cases of urticaria, the wheals will resolve within a day unless exposure to the initiating factor continues or recurs. In this situation new lesions may continue to develop. If the animal is not distressed by the lesions and pruritus is minimal, therapy is not always necessary. It is important, however, to inform the owner of the risk of development of angioedema. The prognosis for angioedema varies with the severity and location. Angioedema of the larynx may produce potentially fatal airway obstruction.

In cases of pruritic urticaria, oral administration of prednisolone at 1 mg/kg/day for 1–2 days is often sufficient. Antihistamines are not always useful in acute urticaria but may help in preventing chronic urticaria. Identification and avoidance of the causative factor is the most successful long-term treatment. When there is life-threatening angioedema, dexamethasone 0.1–0.2 mg/kg i.v. and diphenhydramine 2 mg/kg s.c. should be given. The animal should be closely monitored for signs of respiratory distress (see Chapter 7). Anaphylaxis with associated hypotension is rarely encountered, but should be managed with intravenous fluids, supportive care, and possibly even additional treatment with adrenaline 0.01–0.02 mg/kg i.v. or i.m., while carefully monitoring the patient (see Chapter 3).

Cutaneous drug reactions

Drugs can induce various cutaneous adverse reactions with a wide range of clinical manifestations, which can mimic many other skin diseases (Figure 18.6). The severity of the lesions ranges from local, benign reactions to extensive skin lesions that may result in death of the animal. Cutaneous drug reactions can occur as the result of immunological and non-immunological mechanisms. The latter may be due to overdosage, cumulative toxicity, genetic predisposition, interaction of drugs or idiosyncratic metabolism. These reactions can be evoked by any type of drug, including topically applied drugs, shampoos and insecticides. Although drug reactions occur in a very small number of patients, the incidence may be higher than is reported in the literature (Affolter and von Tscharner, 1993).

Vaccinations, antisera, bacterins

Blood transfusions

Antibiotics (e.g. sulphonamides, penicillins, cephalosporins, gentamicin, neomycin, tetracyclines, chloramphenicol, lincomycin)

Corticosteroids (e.g. triamcinolone)

L-Thyroxine

Aurothioglucose, ciclosporin, azathioprine, cyclophosphamide, chlorambucil, hydroxyurea

5-Fluorocytosine

Retinoids

Primidone

Griseofulvin, ketoconazole, itraconazole

Shampoos (especially insecticidal)

D-Limonene

Diethylcarbamazine, thiasetarsamide

Levamisole, ivermectin

18.6 Drugs reported as causing drug reactions in dogs and cats. (Scott *et al.*, 2001).

Clinical signs

Lesions can be urticarial, angioedematous, papular, exfoliative, vesiculobullous, erythrodermatous or ulcerative. Draining nodular lesions, focal or diffuse alopecia, fixed drug eruptions (focal to multifocal sharply demarcated erythematous lesions) and pseudolymphomatous changes can also be seen (Affolter and von Tscharner, 1993). Diseases that can be caused by drug reactions include vasculopathies, panniculitis, drug-induced pemphigus foliaceous, bullous pemphigoid, superficial suppurative necrolytic dermatitis of Miniature Schnauzers, erythema multiforme (EM), Stevens–Johnson syndrome (SJS), toxic epidermal necrolysis (TEN) and SJS–TEN overlap syndrome. Signs of systemic illness can accompany the cutaneous signs.

Diagnosis

In addition to an extensive history and complete physical examination, other skin diseases should be excluded by means of multiple skin scrapings, bacterial culture, fungal culture and cytology. Skin biopsies may help to define a specific cause for the animal's lesions, may reduce the list of differential diagnoses and can strongly support the diagnosis of a drug reaction. It is important to perform multiple skin biopsies at different lesion sites or at sites bordering an ulcerated area. Disease-specific histopathological changes are sometimes apparent in a few lesions only. Although a histological pattern is not always pathognomonic for a drug reaction, the knowledge that a drug reaction can be the cause of the cutaneous lesions should lead to a careful review of the patient's history. The following list may help in making a tentative diagnosis of a drug reaction:

- When a skin condition worsens suddenly and unexpectedly after initiating drug therapy, or when there is a sudden deterioration after an initial improvement
- When skin lesions occur during drug treatment for a non-dermatological condition
- When observed manifestations do not resemble known pharmacological actions of the drugs
- When there is a history of previous exposure to the drug or related drugs, although prior exposure to the drug may have been tolerated without adverse effects
- When biopsy specimen examination results indicate histological features that can be consistent with a drug eruption
- When a physical examination demonstrates clinical signs consistent with a drug eruption
- When resolution of the signs occurs following withdrawal of the drug. This may take 1–2 weeks and is dependent on the severity of the initial skin lesions and the presence of secondary infections
- When there is a negative challenge with other concurrently used drugs and the appropriate elimination of other causes.

The ultimate test of a causative association is to challenge with the suspect drug. This is however not without serious risk and is therefore generally not recommended.

Clinical management

The most important part of the therapy is to discontinue the suspect causative drug and prevent further administration. When animals are receiving several drugs (including topical medication or shampoos) they should all be discontinued at the same time. If this is not possible, the drugs that were added to the regimen last should be stopped first. Most drug reactions improve spontaneously within 7–14 days upon drug withdrawal. Complete healing may take longer and depends on the severity of the skin lesions. Reactions due to repositol or body-stored agents (i.e. gold salts) respond more slowly after the drug has been withdrawn, and can continue for long periods.

Supportive therapy is not necessary unless animals have a more severe form of drug reaction such as SJS–TEN. If lesions have healed but animals are pruritic because of remaining crusts, a mild shampoo can be used. The choice of shampoo should be based on history of previous use. If the suspected causative agent was a sulpha-containing drug it may be safer to avoid use of a shampoo containing salicylic acid (Noli *et al.*, 1995).

To prevent future drug reactions it is important to inform the owner about the causative agent if known. Patients allergic to penicillins should not be treated with any other drug from the penicillin group. Cephalosporins should be used with care in these patients as they have a β-lactam ring in common with penicillins.

Erythema multiforme, Stevens–Johnson syndrome and toxic epidermal necrolysis

EM, SJS and TEN are rare diseases. Clinically, severe cases of erythema multiforme (EM major), SJS, SJS–TEN overlap syndrome and TEN can be hard to differentiate in dogs and cats.

The pathogenesis of these diseases is a matter of debate, but lesions are a manifestation of a polyaetiological reaction pattern of the skin, caused by cytotoxic attack on keratinocytes (Fritsch and Ruiz-Maldonado, 2003). In humans, SJS, SJS–TEN overlap syndrome and TEN are more often associated with drug administration, whereas EM is usually associated with herpesvirus infections (Roujeau and Revuz, 1994). A retrospective study demonstrated an absence of drug history in dogs with EM, and indications of a drug reaction in SJS, SJS–TEN overlap syndrome and TEN (Hinn *et al.*, 1998). Other reports, however, have suggested an association of EM with a drug history in cats and dogs (Affolter and von Tscharner, 1993; Scott and Miller, 1999). In cats, EM has been reported to occur with herpes infections (Olivry *et al.*, 1999). Infection with parvovirus was demonstrated in one dog with EM (Favrot *et al.*, 2000).

Erythema multiforme

Clinical signs

Lesions are variable but are initially characterized by acute onset of symmetrical erythematous macules or papules that spread peripherally and clear centrally, producing annular lesions (target lesions) or arciform patterns (Figure 18.7). Urticarial plaques, vesicles and bullae or a combination of lesions may be seen. Later in the course of the disease, the epidermis sloughs and erosions and ulcerations appear. Mucosal lesions consist of vesicles, bullae and ulceration. Animals may have cutaneous pain. Some animals may have a positive Nikolsky's sign, which is elicited by applying pressure with a blunt object like a pencil on a vesicle or to the edge of an ulcer, erosion or normal skin. The Nikolsky's sign is positive when the outer layer of the skin (epidermis) is easily rubbed off or pushed away, indicating poor cell cohesion. In dogs the ventrum, mucocutaneous junctions, oral cavity, pinnae and footpads are often affected. In cats, lesions are most commonly seen on the trunk, oral cavity and mucocutaneous junctions. The mild form of erythema multiforme (EM minor) can run a short course with less extensive skin lesions.

Diagnosis

The diagnosis of EM is based upon history, indication of a previous or concurrent viral infection, clinical features, exclusion of other diseases and histopathology of multiple skin biopsy specimens. The list of differential diagnoses includes bacterial folliculitis, dermatophytosis, demodicosis, urticaria, vasculitis, Sweet's syndrome, SJS, SJS–TEN overlap syndrome, TEN and autoimmune diseases. Clinical differentiation between EM, SJS, SJS–TEN overlap syndrome and TEN is currently based on an adapted clinical classification for dogs (Hinn *et al.*, 1998) (Figure 18.8). Of note, if the disease is initially recognized at an early stage, the lesions may still progress. Additionally, it is important to look carefully at the haired skin and mucosae to ensure that the extent of the disease is not underestimated. The most characteristic histological change in EM is apoptosis with lymphocyte satellitosis. An interface dermatitis is invariably present.

Clinical management

The disease may be mild with spontaneous regression of lesions within a few weeks. It is of great importance to try to identify an underlying cause and treat accordingly. The use of glucocorticoids is controversial. In contrast, if extensive vesiculobullous lesions or ulceration are present, the prognosis is guarded. Anecdotal reports suggest that ciclosporin (5 mg/kg/day) and pentoxifylline (25 mg/kg twice daily) are helpful (Scott *et al.*, 2001b). Care should be taken to avoid the use of immunosuppressive drugs in cases of virus-associated EM in both dogs and cats.

When animals suffer from severe forms of EM, they may need more intensive therapy, as discussed below for SJS and TEN.

Stevens–Johnson syndrome, SJS–TEN overlap syndrome and toxic epidermal necrolysis

Clinical signs

Many animals have an acute onset of fever, anorexia and depression with development of extensive vesiculobullous lesions all over the body, as well as

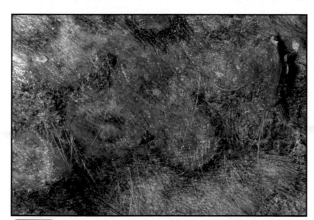

18.7 Target lesions in a dog with erythema multiforme. The causative drug was not identified because the dog had received multiple drug therapy.

Clinical lesions	EM minor	EM major	SJS	SJS–TEN overlap syndrome	TEN
Flat or raised, focal to multifocal, target or polycyclic lesions	Yes	Yes	No	No	No
Number of mucosal surfaces involved	None or >1	>1	>1	>1	>1
Erythematous or purpuric, macular or patchy eruption (% total body surface area (TBSA))	<50	<50	>50	>50	>50
Epidermal detachment (% TBSA)	<10	<10	<10	10–30	>30

18.8 Proposed criteria for the clinical classification of erythema multiforme (EM), Stevens–Johnson syndrome (SJS) and toxic epidermal necrolysis (TEN). (Hinn *et al.*, 1998)

mucous membranes (including the conjunctiva), mucocutaneous junctions and footpads. Vesiculobullous lesions have a very short lifespan, and may progress to epidermal sloughing and ulceration within hours (Figure 18.9). These patients often have cutaneous pain and show a positive Nikolsky's sign.

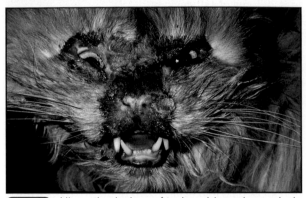

18.9 Ulcerative lesions of toxic epidermal necrolysis due to a trimethoprim–sulfadiazine reaction.

Diagnosis
The differential diagnoses include burns, autoimmune diseases, erythema multiforme, vasculitis and epitheliotropic lymphoma. Clinical differentiation between EM and SJS–TEN is based on the adapted clinical classification for dogs (Hinn *et al.*, 1998) (Figure 18.8). For histopathology, it is important to perform biopsies of intact epidermis. Areas of erythema without ulceration should be chosen.

Histopathology will show hydropic degeneration of basal epidermal cells, full-thickness coagulation of the epidermis and typically minimal dermal inflammation ('silent dermis'). Dermoepidermal separation results in subepidermal vesicles.

Unfortunately there is often an overlap between the histological changes in EM, SJS and TEN. The clinical diagnosis supported by compatible histopathological findings should be used to examine whether causative drug exposure is likely (SJS, SJS–TEN overlap syndrome, TEN) or not (EM).

Clinical management
The treatment of SJS–TEN includes elimination of the underlying cause and symptomatic and supportive measures. These animals may lose a considerable part of the epidermis. Fluids, electrolytes and proteins are lost and secondary bacterial infections occur. It is therefore imperative to handle these patients with the utmost care and keep their surroundings as clean as possible. The success of management of patients with TEN may increase when they are not bathed or clipped (Reedy *et al.*, 1997).

In addition to the skin, other organ systems may become involved during the course of the disease. It is helpful to collect blood and urine samples to establish baseline values. Oedema may develop and many animals succumb to the development of secondary factors such as shock, sepsis or disseminated intravascular coagulation (DIC).

As well as supportive intravenous fluid administration and pain management, antibiotics are indicated to address secondary bacterial infection, the choice

being based upon earlier drug administration. The benefit of corticosteroid administration in these cases is controversial and the response may be poor. SJS, SJS–TEN overlap and TEN in humans are often treated with intravenous administration of purified human immunoglobulins (IVIG) (Prins *et al.*, 2003). Successful treatment with IVIG was reported in a dog with SJS, a dog with TEN and a cat with EM major (Byrne and Giger, 2002; Nuttall and Malham, 2004). IVIG should be administered slowly over 6–8 hours at a recommended dosage of 0.5–1 mg/kg (Hohenhaus, 2005). The same dose can be repeated on the following day. In humans several reports describe the successful use of ciclosporin, and use of this drug could be considered in veterinary patients.

The prognosis is generally guarded or poor. In humans, the extent of the skin lesions gives an indication of the prognosis. Whether this is true for animals is not clear.

Primary irritant contact dermatitis

Irritant material coming into contact with animal skin can cause irritant dermatitis (Figure 18.10). The mechanism by which the epidermal cells are affected varies with the substance. Irritant dermatitis is therefore a heterogeneous disease with variable clinical manifestations.

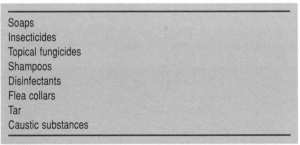

Soaps
Insecticides
Topical fungicides
Shampoos
Disinfectants
Flea collars
Tar
Caustic substances

18.10 Substances that may cause irritant contact dermatitis.

A thorough history may give an insight as to whether any irritant substances were used on the animal or whether there are possible agents in the environment that could cause irritant dermatitis. The location of the lesion should fit with possible contact with the agent.

Clinical signs
Environmental irritants typically produce lesions where the hair coat is thin or missing and where the body parts have contact with the irritant. Susceptible areas are the abdomen, thorax, interdigital spaces, legs, axillae, scrotum and flank (Figure 18.11). Oral lesions can occur when the animal has licked the primary skin lesion. When the offending agent is a liquid or a collar, the skin lesions occur where the substance touched the skin. Erythema or papules are primary lesions. In more chronic cases erosions, crusts, lichenification or ulcerations may occur. Pruritus may occur and can influence the appearance of the primary lesions.

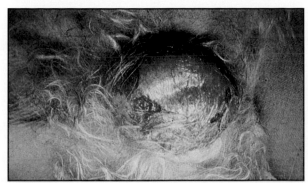

18.11 Erythema and crusts due to an irritant contact dermatitis.

Diagnosis

A careful history and physical examination may lead to a tentative diagnosis. When the irritants are less toxic, obtaining a definitive diagnosis is more difficult. The differential diagnoses should include atopic dermatitis, adverse food reaction, allergic contact dermatitis, *Malassezia* dermatitis, drug hypersensitivity and ectoparasite infestations.

Clinical management

The causative agent should be removed and further contact avoided. Washing of the animal may help to dilute or eliminate the agent. If the dog or cat tries to lick or bite at the lesion, an Elizabethan collar or bandaging of the affected area may help. With removal of the agent the lesions should heal spontaneously. When animals are very pruritic, oral prednisolone 1 mg/kg/day for 1 week may be indicated.

Canine uveodermatological syndrome

This syndrome occurs in many breeds but is most often seen in Arctic breeds such as Huskies, Samoyeds, Malamutes or Akita Inus. Acute clinical signs consist of uveitis with depigmentation primarily of the nasal planum, eyelids and lips. The skin changes usually occur simultaneously with or shortly after the ocular signs. Leucoderma (nonpigmented skin) and leucotrichia (white hairs) develop in the more chronic phase and can become widespread. Although the exact pathogenesis is unknown, it is considered to be an immune-mediated disease in which melanocytes are the immunological target.

Clinical signs

In dogs, the syndrome is characterized by acute onset of uveitis and/or depigmentation of the iris. Dermatological signs may occur concurrently with, or subsequent to, the ophthalmological problems and include depigmentation of the nasal planum, eyelids or mouth and erosive, crusting lesions around the eyes, muzzle and ears (Figure 18.12a).

Diagnosis

After a thorough history and physical examination, multiple skin biopsies should be performed. Differential diagnoses include pemphigus foliaceous, discoid

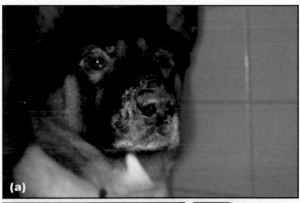

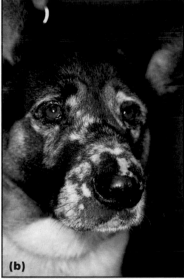

18.12
(a) Depigmentation of the nasal planum, perinasal and periocular erosions and erythema. **(b)** Repigmentation of the nasal planum and leucotrichia after 4 months of therapy with azathioprine and prednisolone.

lupus erythematosus, leishmaniasis, vitiligo and thallium toxicosis. Histopathology will reveal an interface dermatitis with melanin drop-off and macrophages loaded with melanin.

Clinical management

Dogs with this disease can be considered dermatological emergency patients. Treatment of ocular pathology is required to prevent the development of a panuveitis and possible blindness (see Chapter 10). Ophthalmic examinations should be periodically performed even when the cutaneous changes are in remission. The skin lesions are treated with a combination of azathioprine 1–2 mg/kg/day and prednisolone 2 mg/kg/day. Initial haematology is indicated to facilitate monitoring for azathioprine-induced bone marrow depression. Generally, azathioprine should be given at the above dosage for at least a month or until lesions have resolved, whereas prednisolone may be tapered to an alternate day regimen after 1–2 weeks, depending on effect. Monthly rechecks and repeat haematology should be scheduled. Unfortunately, many of these animals require lifelong treatment and it is therefore important to try to taper the medication to the lowest effective dose. Where animals respond to lower doses of treatment drugs, the prognosis for the dermatological changes is usually good, with repigmentation often occurring, although leucotrichia may remain (Figure 18.12b).

Burns

Burns may result from radiation therapy, microwave radiation and thermal or chemical insult to the skin. Thermal burns may result from the use of fires, heating pads/lamps (Figure 18.13), hair dryers, improperly grounded electrosurgical units, boiling water or oil. Chemical burns may result from contact with caustic or acid materials. Burns are classified according to their depth.

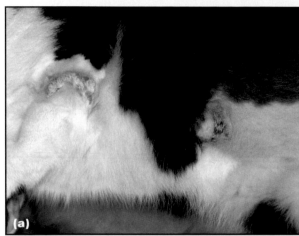

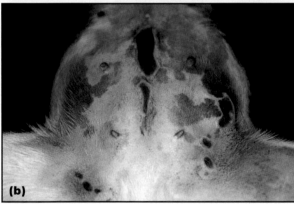

18.13 **(a)** A cat with burn wounds caused by electric current. Note the dry crusts. (Courtesy of Dr Peter Kronen, Vetsuisse Faculty-University of Berne) **(b)** Burn wounds caused by heating lamps.

Superficial partial-thickness burns affect only the epidermis, which becomes thickened and erythematous and ultimately desquamates. The burn usually heals by re-epithelialization in 3–6 days, and hair regrowth is likely.

Deep partial-thickness burns involve the epidermis and part of the dermis. In these cases a marked subcutaneous oedema and inflammatory response occur. These burns heal by re-epithelialization from the remnants of hair follicles and sebaceous glands and from the wound edge. Healing rate and quantity of hair regrowth depend on the depth of the burn.

In full-thickness burns, destruction of all cutaneous structures occurs and a dark brown insensitive leathery covering (eschar) is formed. After removal or sloughing of the eschar these wounds heal slowly by contraction and re-epithelialization. Hair regrowth will not occur and full-thickness burns often need surgical intervention.

Burn wounds may not only cause local tissue damage but can also cause severe systemic pathology. The respiratory system should be carefully evaluated in case of concurrent smoke inhalation (Chapter 7). Burn patients exhibiting clinical signs of shock require intensive aggressive therapy, including management of fluid and electrolyte balance and body temperature; due to increases in metabolic demand, a nutritious, high-calorie, high-protein diet should be fed if liver and kidney function are adequate. Monitoring of vital signs, mental status, body weight and urine output should occur throughout treatment. The minimum database should include a complete blood count, chemistry screen, urinalysis and blood gases (where available). Depending on the total body surface area involved, secondary bacterial infection is common due to tissue necrosis and loss of barrier function. This can lead to life-threatening sepsis.

Clinical signs

Burns in haired areas caused by microwave radiation, electric currents, chemicals, heating pads, or cage dryers may not be obvious to the owner for a few days after the injury. Well demarcated erythema occurs initially, and the lesions often feel hard and dry. This stage is followed by development of adherent crusts, erosions or the odour of necrosis. The shape of the lesion (angular borders, 'drip-pattern' or symmetry) may suggest the origin of the burn.

Burns caused by hot metals or fire are usually immediately obvious but it may take 24–48 hours before the full extent of the lesion is visible. Chemical burns are erosive and necrotic in nature and it can take 24–48 hours before their maximum extent is seen.

Diagnosis

The diagnosis is clear when the burn incident was observed, but may be less so if it was not witnessed, especially when the burn is superficial. A complete history and physical examination, including eyes, ears, oral cavity, respiratory tract, urogenital tract, anus and footpads should be performed. The presence of circulatory shock and/or respiratory thermal injury should be assessed. Biopsy specimens of different points of the lesion (especially the margins) can be helpful to discern between chemical or thermal burns and electrical burns.

Clinical management of thermal wounds

If an owner calls immediately after a burn due to hot water or a chemical substance the best immediate therapy is to rinse the site with cold tap water for at least 10 minutes. Identification of the chemical substance is useful for choosing a neutralizing agent that can be applied after lavage. The depth and the extent of the burn (percentage of total body surface area, TBSA) should be assessed. A decision should be made whether:

- The thermal injury is minor, requiring only local therapy
- Local wound care and systemic therapy are indicated

- The animal is burnt to such an extent that euthanasia is indicated. Euthanasia should be considered when full-thickness burns cover more than 30–50% of the TBSA or when there are severe burns of the face or genitalia with a chance of permanent deformity (Swaim and Henderson, 1997).

Extensive burns generate extensive costs and this should be communicated to the owner at an early stage.

Evaluation of the depth of a burn may be difficult in the early stages following injury. If hair is still present and epilates easily, it generally indicates a deep burn. Analgesia should be provided, and the patient may be sedated to facilitate treatment. Care should be taken if ventilatory or cardiovascular function is compromised. Hair should be clipped carefully from the burned surface. If the burn has just occurred, application of saline or water (3–17°C) for at least 30 minutes may relieve pain and arrest the progression of the burn. When large burns are present, care should be taken to avoid hypothermia.

The following procedures should be considered:

- Topical antibacterial prophylaxis is the basis for bacterial control. Wounds should always be handled with gloves to minimize the risk of further infection
- To help soften and separate viable from non-viable tissue in superficial and deep partial-thickness burns, the wound can be gently spray lavaged with warm water. Alternatively a wet bandage impregnated with an antimicrobial agent such as povidone–iodine and used as a wet to wet bandage can be applied. Necrotic tissue can be debrided from the wound after the lavage or in between the wet to wet bandages, which should be kept in place for several hours at a time. It must be kept in mind that moist applications can accelerate bacterial proliferation. Between lavages, bandages with a water-soluble medication should be applied. A silver sulfadiazine medication is used most commonly
- Superficial partial-thickness burns can be allowed to heal as an open wound
- In deep partial-thickness burns, the resulting wound can be allowed to heal by contraction and re-epithelialization with regular bandage changes and systemic medication. Wound healing is supported by a moist environment. Alternatively, a combination of reconstructive techniques and healing as an open wound may be used
- In full-thickness burns with areas of demarcated devitalized tissue, the tissue can be debrided by wound excision and eschar removal. An eschar may protect the underlying tissue from electrolyte, fluid and protein loss, but it can also harbour bacteria and influence wound contraction. Total removal of the eschar is indicated when the animal is stable enough for anaesthesia

- When all of the devitalized tissue has been removed from a full-thickness burn, it should be decided if the wound can be closed by relocation of local tissue using a skin flap. Consultation with a surgical specialist is advised for animals with extensive lesions or systemic signs.

References and further reading

Affolter VK and Von Tscharner C (1993) Cutaneous drug reactions: a retrospective study of the histopathological changes and their correlation with clinical disease. *Veterinary Dermatology* **4**, 79–86

Byrne KP and Giger U (2002) Use of human immunoglobulin for treatment of severe erythema multiforme in a cat. *Journal of the American Veterinary Medical Association* **220(2)**, 197–201

Favrot C, Olivry T, Dunston SM, Degorce-Rubiales F and Guy JS (2000) Parvovirus infection of keratinocytes as a cause of canine erythema multiforme. *Veterinary Pathology* **37**, 647–649

Fritsch PO and Ruiz-Maldonado R (2003) Erythema multiforme, Stevens–Johnsons syndrome, and toxic epidermal necrolysis, In: *Fitzpatrick's Dermatology in General Medicine, 6th edn*, ed. IM Freedberg, AZ Eisen *et al.*, pp. 543–557. McGraw-Hill, New York

Hinn AC, Olivry T, Luther PB, Cannon A and Yager J (1998) Erythema multiforme, Stevens–Johnson syndrome, and toxic epidermal necrolysis in the dog. *Veterinary Allergy and Clinical Immunology* **6**, 13–20

Hohenhaus AE (2005) Blood transfusions, component therapy, and oxygen-carrying solutions. In: *Textbook of Veterinary Internal Medicine, 6th edn*, ed. SJ Ettinger and EC Feldman, pp. 464–468. Elsevier Saunders, St. Louis

Holm BR, Rest JR and Seewald W (2004) A prospective study of the clinical findings, treatment and histopathology of 44 cases of pyotraumatic dermatitis. *Veterinary Dermatology* **15**, 369–376

Jeffers JG, Duclos DD and Goldschmidt MH (1995) A dermatosis resembling juvenile cellulitis in an adult dog. *Journal of the American Animal Hospital Association* **31**, 204–208

Mason IS and Jones J (1989) Juvenile cellulitis in Gordon Setters. *Veterinary Record* **124**, 642

Neuber AE, van den Broek AH, Brownstein D, Thoday KL and Hill PB (2004) Dermatitis and lymphadenitis resembling juvenile cellulitis in a four-year-old dog. *Journal of Small Animal Practice* **45**, 254–258

Noli C, Koeman JP and Willemse T (1995) A retrospective evaluation of adverse reactions to trimethoprim-sulfonamide combinations in dogs and cats. *Veterinary Quarterly* **17**, 123–128

Nuttall TJ and Malham T (2004) Successful intravenous human immunoglobulin treatment of drug-induced Stevens–Johnson syndrome in a dog. *Journal of Small Animal Practice* **45**, 357–361

Olivry T, Guaguère E, Atlee BA and Héripret D (1999) Generalized erythema multiforme with systemic involvement in two cats. *Proceedings of the Annual Meeting of the European Society of Veterinary Dermatology*. Stockholm, Sweden: pp. 20–22

Prins C, Kerdel FA, Padilla RS *et al.* (2003) Treatment of toxic epidermal necrolysis with high-dose intravenous immunoglobulins: multicenter retrospective analysis of 48 consecutive cases. *Archives of Dermatology* **139**, 26–32

Reedy LM, Miller WH and Willemse T (1997) *Allergic Skin Diseases of Dogs and Cats, 2nd edn*, pp. 239–245. WB Saunders, Philadelphia

Roujeau JC and Revuz J (1994) Toxic epidermal necrolysis: an expanding field of knowledge. *Journal of the American Academy of Dermatology* **31**, 301–302

Scott DW and Miller WH (1999) Erythema multiforme in dogs and cats: literature review and case material from the Cornell University College of Veterinary Medicine (1988–96) *Veterinary Dermatology* **10**, 297–09

Scott DW, Miller WH, and Griffin CE (2001a) Miscellaneous Diseases. In: *Small Animal Dermatology, 6th edn*, ed. DW Scott, WH Miller and CE Griffin, pp. 1125–1183. WB Saunders, Philadelphia

Scott DW, Miller WH, and Griffin CE (2001b) Immune-mediated disorders. In: *Small Animal Dermatology, 6th edn*, ed. DW Scott, WH Miller and CE Griffin, pp. 667–779. WB Saunders, Philadelphia

Swaim ST and Henderson RA (1997) *Small Animal Wound Management, 2nd edn*, pp. 87–101. Williams & Wilkins, Baltimore

White SD, Rosychuk RAW, Stewart LJ, Cape L and Hughes BJ (1989) Juvenile cellulitis in dogs: 15 cases (1979–1988). *Journal of the American Veterinary Medical Association* **195**, 1609–1611

19

Toxicological emergencies

Robert H. Poppenga

Recognition of the intoxicated patient

Given the wide range of effects caused by the ingestion of poisons, recognition of an intoxicated patient can be difficult, particularly in the absence of a history of exposure. Alternatively, animal owners are often convinced that the illness of a pet is due to malicious poisoning or exposure to an industrial or environmental poison. The clinician should not be misled by allegations of intoxication, but rather the objective historical and clinical findings should guide the case work up.

Historical clues to possible poison exposure include recent changes in routine, such as dietary change or access to a new environment, acute illness after a period of being unsupervised, acute onset of neurological or gastrointestinal signs, and liver and/ or kidney failure. Correlation of the onset of illness with recent use of pesticides or household products may be important. Illness from poisons such as lead can be associated with renovation of older buildings. Access to human medications and herbal remedies should be included in initial questioning.

Identification of affected organ systems from the initial physical examination and laboratory work up of a patient is extremely useful in formulating a list of differentials. The occurrence of several clinical signs characteristic of a particular toxic syndrome can be helpful. For example, muscarinic receptor overstimulation manifested clinically by DUMBELS (diarrhoea, urination, miosis, bronchospasm, emesis, lacrimation and salivation) is strongly suggestive of intoxication by a cholinesterase-inhibiting insecticide. Visual examination of vomitus may reveal coloured baits or fragments of medications. Detection of specific odours may provide useful clues, e.g. organophosphorus has a garlic-like odour that might be detected in vomitus or on the skin.

Management of the intoxicated patient

Each situation is unique and the approach must be tailored ultimately to the individual patient. In some circumstances, certain steps may be unnecessary. For example, there may not be an antidote for a given poison or a way to enhance its elimination once it has been absorbed systemically. A general approach to management of the intoxicated patient should adhere to the following principles (Shannon and Haddad, 1998):

- Stabilize vital signs
- Obtain a history and clinically evaluate the patient
- Prevent continued systemic absorption of the poison
- Enhance elimination of absorbed poison
- Provide symptomatic and supportive care
- Administer an antidote if indicated and available
- Closely monitor the patient.

In recently exposed animals, the severity of poison exposure must be determined in order to choose the appropriate sequence of management steps (Figure 19.1). Several factors must be considered, including the inherent toxicity of the chemical, the dose, the species and age of the animal and the presence of underlying disease conditions. For example, close monitoring at home for several days may be sufficient for management of recent ingestion of an anticoagulant rodenticide at well below reported toxic doses (less than or equal to one tenth of an LD_{50}). Ingestion of higher doses of a toxicant may warrant administration of an adsorbent, a cathartic and/or a specific antidote, followed by close monitoring in the clinic.

If a known or suspected poison has been ingested, specific veterinary advice and information may be sought from a central database of veterinary toxicities. In the UK registered practices can contact the Veterinary Poisons Information Service (VPIS) on 0207 635 9195 or 0113 245 0530. In the USA, the ASPCA Animal Poison Control Center can be contacted on 888-426-4435. If there is no information available about toxicity to the particular animal species exposed, toxicity may be extrapolated from other species. Ultimately, the advice to "treat the patient and not the poison" is sound.

Specific approaches to stabilization of vital signs are discussed in other sections of this manual. Attention should be paid to maintaining a patent airway and providing adequate ventilation, maintaining cardiovascular function with attention to appropriate fluid and electrolyte administration, maintaining acid–base balance, controlling central nervous system (CNS) signs, such as seizures, and maintaining body temperature.

Once vital signs are stable, a thorough history should be obtained while the animal is being further evaluated. If blood or urine samples are obtained, specimens should be set aside for possible toxicological testing (Figure 19.2).

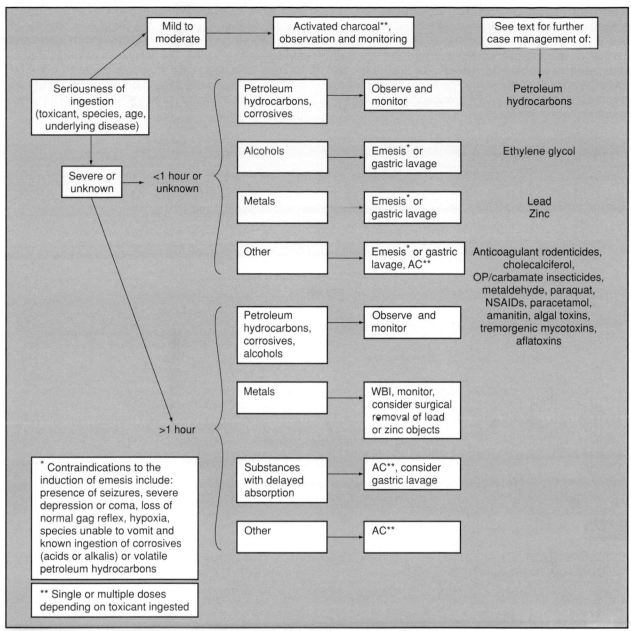

19.1 Treatment algorithm for initial management of small animal intoxications (AC, activated charcoal; WBI, whole bowel irrigation).

Sample*	Amount
Whole blood	5 ml, EDTA/heparin tube, refrigerate
Serum/plasma	5–10 ml, serum clot tube or plastic vial, frozen
Vomitus, stomach contents, lavage fluid	100 g, plastic bag or vial, frozen
Liver	100 g, plastic bag, frozen
Kidney	100 g, plastic bag, frozen
Brain	Right or left half, plastic bag, frozen
Urine	5–20 ml, plastic container, frozen
Feed	1 kg, plastic container, frozen if wet food otherwise refrigerated (dry or semi-moist food)
Water	1 litre, plastic or clean glass container, refrigerated or frozen
Environmental samples (bedding, soil, paint)	Check with laboratory

19.2 Routine samples and amounts to submit for toxicological investigations. * The best sample for some intoxicants may be other than those listed. For example, lung tissue is one of the best samples to submit for the postmortem detection of paraquat.

Administration of specific antidotes

Antidotes should be administered if indicated and available. In some situations, it may be critical to administer an antidote quickly. For example, in suspected cholinesterase-inhibiting insecticide intoxications, administration of atropine may be essential to control life-threatening signs before proceeding with subsequent management steps.

Figure 19.3 lists antidotes that should be immediately available, based on the frequency with which intoxications occur as reported by animal poison control statistics. Figure 19.4 lists antidotes that may be needed less frequently. A source such as a human hospital or pharmacy should be identified for obtaining the latter antidotes, prior to their need in an emergency situation.

Indication	Antidote	Dosage
Paracetamol	N-Acetylcysteine	Loading dose of 140–280 mg/kg orally or 140 mg/kg in 5% dextrose/water i.v. followed by maintenance dose of 70 mg/kg orally q6h for 2–3 days
Anticoagulant rodenticides	Vitamin K1	1st generation anticoagulants: 1 mg/kg orally in divided doses q8–12h for 4–6 days For 2nd generation anticoagulants: 2.5–5.0 mg/kg orally for 2–6 weeks in divided doses q8–12h
OP/carbamate insecticides	Atropine sulphate	0.1–0.2 mg/kg (given until muscarinic signs controlled), $^1/_4$ initial dose given i.v. with the remainder given i.m. or s.c. Given as needed
	Pralidoxime chloride (2-PAM)	20 mg/kg i.m. or slow i.v. q8–12h
Cholecalciferol	Calcitonin	4–6 IU/kg s.c. q6–12h
Ethylene glycol	Ethanol (20%)	Dogs: 5.5 ml/kg by slow i.v. infusion every 4 hours for five treatments then every 6 hours for four treatments Cats: 5 ml/kg by slow i.v. infusion q6h for five treatments then q8h for four treatments
	Fomepizole	Dogs: initial dose of 15 mg/kg slow i.v. in 5% dextrose or 0.9% saline solution. This is followed by 10 mg/kg q12h for four doses and then 5 mg/kg q12h (ideally until ethylene glycol serum levels fall below 3222 µmol/l) Cats: 125 mg/kg i.v. at 1, 2, and 3 hours after ethylene glycol ingestion followed by 31.25 mg/kg i.v. at 12, 24 and 36 hours post-ingestion (Thrall *et al.*, 2006)
Lead, arsenic	Succimer	10 mg/kg orally q8h for 5 days followed by 10 mg/kg orally q12h for 2 weeks
Lead, zinc	CaNa$_2$ EDTA	25 mg/kg q6h as a 1% solution (in 5% dextrose/water) for 5 days. Provide 5-day rest period between courses of treatment

19.3 Antidotes for some common intoxications.

Indication	Antidote	Dosage
Arsenic, cyanide	Sodium thiosulphate	30–40 mg/kg of a 20% solution i.v., may be repeated
Copper, lead	D-Penicillamine	Copper: 10–15 mg/kg/day orally Lead: 110 mg/kg/divided q6h orally for 1–2 weeks, re-evaluate animal 1 week after cessation of initial course
Cyanide	Sodium nitrite	16 mg/kg of a 1% solution i.v., given only once
Iron	Deferoxamine mesylate	Not determined; for children the dose is 20 mg/kg i.m. or slow i.v. followed by 10 mg/kg at 4-hour intervals depending on clinical response. Subsequent doses of 10 mg/kg may be given every 4–12 hours
Cholecalciferol	Pamidronate	Not determined. In dogs, 1.3 mg/kg i.v. in 150 ml normal saline 1 and 8 days after ingestion of a toxic dose of cholecalciferol was effective in decreasing hypercalcaemia
Nitrites, chlorates	Methylene blue	Dogs: 8.8 mg/kg of a 1% solution given by slow i.v. drip Cats: not recommended
Opioids	Naloxone	Not determined. In children a dose of 2 mg is given i.v. If there is no response, a second dose of 2 mg is given. This dose is repeated every 2 minutes until there is a clinical response or 10–20 mg has been given (if no response to this dose, opioid overdose can be ruled out)
Venomous spiders, snakes, fish and marine invertebrates	Antivenins	Follow specific antivenin recommendations
Arsenic and mercury	Dimercaprol (BAL)	2.5–5.0 mg/kg of a 10% solution in oil i.m. q4h for 2 days then q12h for the next 10 days or until recovery

19.4 Less commonly used antidotes.

Gastrointestinal decontamination
Gastrointestinal decontamination (GID) is a critical component of case management, which may prevent the onset of clinical signs, significantly decrease their severity or shorten the course of intoxication. GID consists of (Shannon and Haddad, 1998):

- Gastric evacuation
- Administration of an adsorbent
- Catharsis.

Gastric evacuation
Approaches to gastric evacuation include induction of emesis with emetics such as syrup of ipecacuanha, 3% hydrogen peroxide, washing soda (sodium carbonate) crystals, apomorphine or xylazine (Figure 19.5), and gastric lavage. Induction of emesis is contraindicated in the presence of seizures, severe depression or coma, loss of normal gag reflex, hypoxia, species unable to vomit (e.g. rat) and known ingestion of corrosives or volatile petroleum products. Syrup of ipecacuanha and 3% hydrogen peroxide may be available in the home and their administration can be considered prior to transport to the hospital. Hydrogen peroxide can be administered relatively easily and if emesis does not occur within 10 minutes, the dose can be repeated once. Emesis is often more effectively induced when the stomach is full; feeding a small amount of food prior to induction can improve efficacy. Owners may have difficulty administering syrup of ipecacuanha to cats due to its objectionable taste. Other disadvantages of ipecacuanha include prolonged emesis, and the possibility of its adsorption by activated charcoal (AC). Administration of AC may have to be delayed to allow the emetic action of syrup of ipecacuanha to occur. Apomorphine is the emetic of choice for dogs, but it is not recommended for cats. Xylazine has been used instead as an emetic for cats (also suitable for dogs). While apomorphine and xylazine induce emesis quickly, they may also cause

undesirable CNS depression. Fortunately, specific reversal drugs are available for both apomorphine and xylazine to minimize undesirable side effects.

Gastric lavage
Gastric lavage can be employed when administration of an emetic is contraindicated. Patients should be anaesthetized and the airway should be protected with a cuffed endotracheal tube. Once the patient is anaesthetized, the largest possible gastric tube, with terminal fenestrations, is introduced into the stomach. Tube placement is confirmed by aspiration of gastric contents or air insufflation with a stethoscope placed over the stomach. After gastric intubation, the mouth should be kept lower than the chest. Tepid tap water or normal saline (5–10 ml/kg) is introduced into the stomach under minimal pressure and is withdrawn by aspiration or gravity flow. The procedure is repeated until several lavages are clear, often requiring numerous cycles. AC (with or without a cathartic) can be administered just before tube removal. The initial lavage sample should be retained for possible toxicological analysis.

Activated charcoal and cathartics
AC is the only adsorbent routinely used in companion animal medicine, although others such as Fuller's earth may be indicated rarely for specific poisons (see paraquat). AC is an effective adsorbent for most poisons, with several notable exceptions, including alcohols, corrosives and metals, such as iron and lithium (Howland, 1994). It is available as a powder, an aqueous slurry or combined with cathartics such as sorbitol. Repeated doses of AC are effective in interrupting enterohepatic recycling of several poisons, and continued presence of AC in the gastrointestinal tract may create a sink for trapping poison passing from the circulation into the intestines (gut dialysis). Repeated administration of AC is usually safe.

Agent	Indication	Dosage
Syrup of ipecacuanha	Emesis	Dogs: 1–2 ml/kg orally Cats: 3.3 ml/kg orally diluted 50:50 with water
3% Hydrogen peroxide	Emesis	1–2 ml/kg orally; if no emesis, repeat once
Apomorphine	Emesis	Dogs: 0.03 mg/kg i.v. or 0.04 mg/kg i.m. or s.c. Do not use in cats
Activated charcoal (AC)	Adsorption	All animals: 1–4 g/kg orally as an aqueous slurry (~1 g per 5 ml water); may be repeated at 4–6 hour intervals
Sodium or magnesium sulphate	Catharsis	Dogs: 5–25 g mixed in AC slurry Cats: 2–5 g mixed in AC slurry Give only once
Sorbitol	Catharsis	Often included in AC formulations. If not, give 3 ml/kg orally of 70% sorbitol. Give only once
Polyethylene glycol	Whole bowel irrigation	Not established for animals; however, young children are given 20–40 ml/kg per hour until clear rectal effluent noted
Sodium bicarbonate	Urine alkalinization	Generally, 1–2 mEq/kg administered every 3–4 hours; goal is to achieve urine pH of 7 or above. For selected weak acids
Xylazine	Emesis	Cats: 0.44 mg/kg i.m.

19.5 Common gastrointestinal and systemic decontamination agents.

Both saline (sodium sulphate or magnesium sulphate or citrate) and saccharide (sorbitol) cathartics are available (Figure 19.5). Cathartics hasten the elimination of unabsorbed poison via the stools and are safe, particularly if used only once. Repeated administration of magnesium-containing cathartics can lead to hypermagnesaemia manifested as hypotonia, altered mental status and respiratory failure, while repeated administration of sorbitol can cause fluid pooling in the gastrointestinal tract, excessive fluid losses and severe dehydration.

Recent innovations in human medicine

Recently in human medicine there has been a movement away from combining gastric evacuation with an adsorbent, toward the administration of only the adsorbent, especially in mild to moderate intoxications (Perry and Shannon, 1996). Early administration of AC alone has been shown to be as efficacious as gastric evacuation followed by AC. The case for or against inclusion of a cathartic with AC is less clear-cut, but a single dose of a cathartic along with the initial dose of AC is currently recommended. AC formulations that include a cathartic should be administered once, followed by AC alone if repeated doses are indicated. Unless emesis can be immediately and safely induced, it may be better to administer AC as soon as possible after exposure to poisons amenable to adsorption, rather than to waste valuable time attempting to evacuate the stomach.

One newer approach to human GID is whole bowel irrigation (WBI), the oral administration of large volumes of an electrolyte-balanced solution until a clear rectal effluent is produced. A polyethylene glycol solution, routinely employed to cleanse the gastrointestinal tract for surgical or radiographic procedures, is used (Perry and Shannon, 1996). WBI may be efficacious when an ingested poison is poorly adsorbed to AC, or when sustained-release medications, small metal objects or lead-based paint have been ingested. WBI is well tolerated by human paediatric patients, but its utility in veterinary medicine has not been determined.

Enhancing elimination via the urinary tract

Removal of absorbed poisons via urinary excretion may be indicated in several specific situations. For example, alkalinization of the urine to a pH above 7.0 with sodium bicarbonate enhances the urinary elimination of weak acids such as ethylene glycol, salicylates, phenobarbital and the herbicide 2,4-D. Administration of ammonium chloride to acidify the urine (pH 5.5–6.5) may enhance the elimination of weak bases such as amphetamines and strychnine. Urinary alkalinization or acidification requires close patient monitoring to avoid acid–base disturbances. In human medicine, urinary acidification is currently not recommended due to complications associated with metabolic and urinary acidosis.

Extracorporeal methods of poison elimination

Extracorporeal methods for removal of poisons are occasionally utilized in human medicine, and the increasing availability of such methods in veterinary medicine makes their use in poisoned small animal patients more likely. The two most commonly used methods are haemodialysis and charcoal haemoperfusion (Orlowski et al., 2001). Physical characteristics of poisons amenable to removal by haemodialysis include a short tissue distribution time, low endogenous clearance (≤ 4 ml/min/kg), small volume of distribution (≤ 1 l/kg), low protein binding, water solubility and low molecular weight (≤ 500 daltons). Physical characteristics of poisons effectively removed by haemoperfusion are similar, but additionally poisons that have high protein binding, are lipid soluble and are large (up to 40,000 daltons) can be eliminated. The use of haemoperfusion also requires that the poison can be effectively adsorbed to AC.

General guidelines and indications for the use of extracorporeal methods include the following (Orlowski et al., 2001):

- An expectation that clearance of the poison may be increased by 30% or more
- Severe or potentially lethal exposure
- Impairment of natural removal mechanism(s)
- Deteriorating clinical condition in spite of supportive care
- Clinical signs consistent with severe poisoning (i.e. hypotension, coma, metabolic acidosis, respiratory depression, dysrhythmias or cardiac decompensation)
- Known ingestion of a poison with serious delayed effects.

Intoxications routinely treated by extracorporeal methods in human medicine include those caused by lithium, ethylene glycol, methanol, salicylates, barbiturates and theophylline.

Supportive care and monitoring

Fortunately, many intoxicated patients will recover if attention is paid to appropriate symptomatic and supportive care. For example, even if GID is not possible following the ingestion of strychnine, effective control of muscle rigidity with pentobarbital may result in complete recovery from intoxication. Other sections of this manual should be consulted for appropriate symptomatic care protocols.

Use of a toxicology laboratory

Effective use of a toxicology laboratory requires submission of appropriate antemortem and postmortem samples for analysis. Appropriate samples vary depending on the poison. For example, whole blood is required for diagnosis of lead intoxication, whereas plasma, serum or urine is required for diagnosis of chocolate intoxication. Often, several samples are necessary to detect a poison; urine may contain detectable concentrations whereas plasma or serum may not. Figure 19.2 lists samples commonly used for toxicological diagnoses. Most samples can be kept frozen for extended periods of time without interfering with the analysis. Thus, postmortem histopathological examination of tissues can be performed first, perhaps suggesting an alternative diagnosis or identifying a need for specific toxicological analyses.

It is a common misconception that the clinician needs to have some idea which poisons to look for before toxicological testing will be useful. In fact, many toxicology laboratories offer relatively inexpensive organic and inorganic screens that may detect an otherwise unanticipated poison. Despite the availability of screens, it remains necessary to develop appropriate differential lists based on historical or clinical findings.

In most cases, toxicological testing does not change initial clinical management, due to delays in obtaining laboratory results and the fact that relatively few poisons have specific antidotes. However, detection of a specific poison may confirm a tentative diagnosis, have prognostic value and identify human health hazards. In addition, toxicological testing may produce negative results, which may allay client fears of environmental contamination or malicious poisoning.

Specific poisons

Anticoagulant rodenticides

The anticoagulant rodenticides are among the most common poisons of small animals, particularly dogs. Anticoagulant rodenticides derived from coumarin include warfarin, brodifacoum, bromodiolone and difenacoum. Indandione derivatives include pindone, chlorophacinone and diphacinone. New compounds, such as difethialone, are routinely added to those already in commercial use. Most modern 'second-generation' anticoagulants are potent, single-feeding rodenticides; these have largely replaced older 'first-generation' rodenticides such as warfarin, pindone, chlorophacinone, dicoumarol and valone.

Anticoagulant rodenticides competitively inhibit vitamin K epoxide reductase, which converts vitamin K epoxide to its active reduced form. Final activation of clotting factors II, VII, IX and X depends on the availability of reduced vitamin K epoxide. Coagulopathies ensue once the supply of active clotting factors is consumed, generally 1–3 days following ingestion of a toxic dose. Second-generation anticoagulants such as brodifacoum are more effective at inhibiting vitamin K epoxide reductase and have longer half-lives than first-generation anticoagulants. The indandione derivatives are considered to be long-acting.

Clinical signs are due to a coagulopathy. Haemorrhage can be acute and massive or slow and sustained. The most common site of haemorrhage is within the respiratory tract with development of haemothorax, parenchymal haemorrhage or submucosal tracheal bleeding. Subcutaneous haematomas, epistaxis, melaena and haematemesis may also be apparent. Presenting signs depend on the location of haemorrhage and may not include external signs of bleeding. For example, haemorrhage into the CNS may cause ataxia, convulsions or sudden death, whereas pulmonary haemorrhage may cause respiratory distress.

Diagnosis relies on demonstrating prolonged coagulation and detection of a specific anticoagulant. Tests of coagulation such as prothrombin time (PT), partial thromboplastin time (PTT) and activated coagulation time (ACT) are affected at different times following ingestion, due to differences in the half-lives of the affected clotting factors. Since factor VII has the shortest half-life, the extrinsic coagulation pathway is affected first and PT is prolonged before and more severely than the PTT. PT should be used to monitor coagulation times in asymptomatic animals after exposure to an unknown amount of anticoagulant, when vitamin K1 is not given prophylactically, or following cessation of vitamin K1 therapy. All coagulation tests are likely to be prolonged in animals presenting with clinical signs.

Many veterinary diagnostic laboratories offer anticoagulant screens of whole blood or serum antemortem, or liver postmortem. Generally, the most commonly used anticoagulants are included in the screen, but some less commonly used compounds may not be included. Analysis of stomach contents is inappropriate since exposure of a symptomatic animal was 1–3 days prior to presentation.

Vitamin K1 is used as an antidote and the dose and duration of therapy depends on the specific compound ingested; the longer the half-life of the anticoagulant, the longer the duration of vitamin K1 therapy. A recommended dose for treatment of warfarin intoxication is 1 mg/kg for 4–6 days. For other anticoagulants, doses of 2.5–5.0 mg/kg for a minimum of 2–6 weeks are suggested. When the specific compound is unknown, it should be assumed that exposure was to one of the more potent compounds. The oral bioavailability of vitamin K1 is greatly improved if it is fed with a small fatty meal such as canned dog food. PT should be checked 1, 3 and 5 days after cessation of therapy to detect recurrence of a coagulopathy. During emergency management, vitamin K1 can be given subcutaneously at several sites with a small-gauge needle. Intramuscular administration should be avoided due to the possibility of haemorrhage at the injection site, and intravenous administration is not advisable because of the possibility of an anaphylactic reaction. A delay of 6–12 hours occurs before synthesis of sufficient new clotting factors. More rapid resolution requires preformed clotting factors in blood products. In severely symptomatic animals, plasma or blood transfusions may be necessary.

If pregnant or lactating animals are exposed to anticoagulant rodenticides, haemorrhage may occur during delivery and the toxins can be eliminated in milk. Nursing puppies or kittens should be removed from the exposed dam and supplemented with vitamin K1 orally for 2–3 weeks. Alternatively, nursing animals can be placed on vitamin K1 while the coagulation status of the dam is monitored. If the dam remains normal, vitamin K1 can then be discontinued. Anticoagulant-exposed pregnant animals should be maintained on vitamin K1 until birth, and newborns should be maintained on vitamin K1 for at least 1 additional week or until their coagulation status can be monitored.

Cholecalciferol (vitamin D3)

Cholecalciferol is a newer rodenticide, which kills rodents within 1–3 days of ingestion. After absorption, it is metabolized to 25-monohydroxyvitamin D in the liver, then metabolized to the active 1,25-dihydroxyvitamin D by the kidney. Active vitamin D increases calcium absorption from the intestine, osteoclastic resorption of bone and calcium reabsorption from the renal distal tubules. Toxic doses result in hypercalcaemia, which causes cardiac conduction disturbances and metastatic tissue mineralization. Clinical signs develop 12–36 hours after ingestion of a toxic dose and include depression, anorexia, emesis, polydipsia and polyuria. Azotaemia and renal failure may develop.

A presumptive diagnosis relies on detecting high serum calcium concentrations. Cholecalciferol toxicosis must then be differentiated from hypercalcaemia of malignancy, primary hyperparathyroidism and primary renal failure. Measurement of parathyroid hormone (PTH), PTHrP, 25-monohydroxyvitamin D and total and ionized calcium can be used to differentiate the causes of hypercalcaemia. With cholecalciferol toxicity, hyperphosphataemia is a consistent finding that may precede hypercalcaemia.

Case management is challenging, with several approaches to lowering serum calcium available. Normal saline, with furosemide at 1–2 mg/kg i.v. followed by 1 mg/kg i.v. q8h, should be given to promote calciuresis. Furosemide should not be administered if the animal is dehydrated. Prednisolone (2 mg/kg orally q8–12h) inhibits the release of osteoclast-activating factors, reduces intestinal calcium absorption and promotes calciuresis. Salmon calcitonin has been used when hypercalcaemia is severe or refractory, but is ineffective when used alone. Pamidronate disodium, a bisphosphonate drug used to treat hypercalcaemia of malignancy in humans, shows promise for reversing cholecalciferol-induced hypercalcaemia in dogs at 1.3 mg/kg i.v. in 150 ml normal saline, 1 and 8 days after cholecalciferol ingestion (Rumbeiha et al., 1997).

Cholinesterase-inhibiting insecticides: organophosphorus and carbamates

While the use of organophosphorus (OP) and carbamate insecticides for flea and tick control has declined in recent years, environmental exposure remains common. OPs and carbamates inhibit cholinesterase enzymes, particularly acetylcholinesterase, which breaks down acetylcholine. Acetylcholine propagates nervous impulses at a number of sites within the central and peripheral nervous systems. Overstimulation of muscarinic and nicotinic receptors causes most of the clinical manifestations of intoxication.

Clinical signs related to overstimulation of parasympathetic muscarinic receptors include diarrhoea, increased urination, miosis, bradycardia, bronchospasm and dyspnoea, emesis, excessive lacrimation and salivation. Excessive stimulation of nicotinic receptors initially results in muscle stimulation, followed by a depolarizing blockade. Death usually results from respiratory failure.

Diagnosis depends on a history of exposure, detection of a specific chemical in gastric contents and demonstration of low cholinesterase enzyme activity in whole blood antemortem or in the brain postmortem. Enzyme activities below 50% of normal indicate exposure to a cholinesterase-inhibiting insecticide. Often, enzyme activity is depressed by more than 80%.

In the period following exposure before clinical signs occur, the management priority is decontamination. If the animal is symptomatic, atropine should be given before decontamination. Atropine specifically blocks muscarinic receptors and at high doses it can provide immediate but short-lived relief. It must be re-administered when signs begin to recur. Atropine is administered to effect and precise dosages may vary. Once signs of muscarinic overstimulation are controlled, decontamination can begin.

Pralidoxime hydrochloride (2-PAM) reverses enzyme inhibition and prevents 'ageing' (i.e. the irreversible binding of cholinesterase) following OP exposure (20 mg/kg q8–12h i.m. or slowly i.v.). Once 'ageing' has occurred, 2-PAM is ineffective; therefore, the efficacy of 2-PAM is greatest soon after intoxication. Nevertheless, if treatment is delayed, 2-PAM therapy may still be helpful and it is continued until the patient is asymptomatic or shows no improvement of nicotinic signs after 24–36 hours of therapy. Pralidoxime is not effective for treating carbamate intoxication, since the mechanism of enzyme inhibition is slightly different and ageing does not occur. When it is uncertain whether intoxication is due to OP or a carbamate, 2-PAM should be administered. Diphenhydramine (1–4 mg/kg orally q6–8h) has been suggested to reverse signs due to nicotinic receptor stimulation, but its clinical efficacy has not been established.

Pyrethrins and pyrethroids

OP and carbamate insecticides for use on animals and in their environment have largely been replaced by other insecticides, especially the pyrethrins and pyrethroids (PP). Pyrethrins are naturally occurring chemicals from Chrysanthemum cinerariaefolium. Pyrethroids are synthetic derivatives of pyrethrins that exhibit enhanced potency and stability. Most PPs, when used as directed, are safe and present little poisoning risk to animals. However, cats are more sensitive to PPs than are other species, probably due to differences in their metabolism. The most common poisoning scenario is the misuse on cats of concentrated PP canine formulations (primarily products containing the pyrethroid, permethrin). Reports of intoxication of cats by permethrin have occurred following the dermal application of concentrated products on dogs followed by cat contact with treated areas. Products intended for use on cats containing the pyrethroid phenothrin were recently withdrawn from the market in the US due to numerous reports of intoxication.

The insecticidal and toxic properties of PP insecticides are due to their ability to alter the activity of neuronal sodium ion channels. PPs prolong the period of sodium conductance, which increases the duration of depolarization and causes repetitive nerve firing (Hansen, 2006). Clinical signs associated with intoxication include emesis, diarrhoea, depression, ataxia, hyperaesthesia, muscle tremors, seizures, hyperthermia and death. Signs can develop within hours of exposure or be delayed for up to 72 hours (Richardson, 2000). Topical allergic reactions have also been reported and can be manifested as generalized dermal urticaria, hyperaemia, pruritis and alopecia (Hansen, 2006).

GID is generally not warranted when PPs have been applied dermally. In rarer intoxications following oral exposure, standard GID procedures should be considered. Bathing of dermally-exposed animals using a mild dishwashing detergent is recommended. In mild cases of intoxication, diazepam alone may control muscle tremors. However, if animals are experiencing seizures, seizure control can be difficult. A combination of diazepam and methocarbamol may be the most efficacious intervention. Methocarbamol is administered intravenously at 50–150 mg/kg with one third to half the dose given as a slow bolus and the remaining dose given as needed to control tremors. A maximum dose of 330 mg/kg/day should not be exceeded (Hansen, 2006). If diazepam is not effective for seizure control, other options include barbiturates, propofol and isoflurane. Control of muscle tremors and seizures will often result in relatively rapid resolution of hyperthermia. Intravenous crystalloids should be given to minimize renal damage secondary to rhabdomyolysis. The response to therapy and therefore the prognosis is worse for animals presenting with seizures. Allergic reactions generally resolve following bathing; diphenhydramine may also be useful.

Paraquat

In general, herbicides are not a significant hazard to pets. Serious intoxications of dogs most commonly involve exposure to paraquat and the related herbicide diquat. Reported LD_{50} values for dogs are 25–50 mg/kg. Both the herbicidal action and the toxicity are believed to be due to production of free radicals resulting in lipid membrane damage. Paraquat is concentrated in alveolar cells where it causes oxidant damage. Initial clinical signs following ingestion include mucosal irritation, emesis, hyperexcitability and ataxia. In dogs, proximal tubular necrosis and renal failure often occur. The hallmark of paraquat intoxication is pulmonary oedema and congestion, occurring several days after exposure and resulting in dyspnoea. Necrosis of alveolar cells occurs, resulting in scarring and fibrosis, and death due to respiratory failure. Diquat does not cause lung damage.

Management includes decontamination with bentonite or Fuller's earth, which are clays that bind paraquat and diquat. However, if clays are not immediately available, AC should be given. Supportive and symptomatic care are important. Superoxide dismutase and N-acetylcysteine have been recommended and both have theoretical benefits, but their clinical efficacy for preventing oxidant damage due to paraquat has not been proven. Prognosis is grave if damage to the pulmonary parenchyma is severe.

Metaldehyde

Metaldehyde is the active ingredient in many slug and snail baits (at 3.5–4.0%). Reported lethal doses are 100–1000 mg/kg for dogs and approximately 200 mg/kg for cats. Metaldehyde decreases brain concentrations of γ-aminobutyric acid (GABA), resulting in loss of its CNS inhibitory action. Early clinical signs include anxiety and restlessness followed by salivation, mydriasis, tremors and ataxia. Advanced signs include tachypnoea, tachycardia, muscle tremors, opisthotonos,

continuous seizures, cyanosis and hyperthermia. The diagnosis can be confirmed by detection of metaldehyde in gastric contents. Treatment involves GID if ingestion was recent, and control of seizures with diazepam or barbiturates. Methocarbamol may be useful for controlling muscle tremors.

Particular care should be taken to monitor and maintain appropriate acid–base status. Prognosis is good if aggressive seizure management is instituted at an early stage but poor if seizures are uncontrolled.

Non-steroidal anti-inflammatory drugs

Non-steroidal anti-inflammatory drugs (NSAIDs) are a large group of drugs that share pharmacological actions and side effects. They are classified chemically as carboxylic acids and enolic acids. Carboxylic acids are further divided into: salicylic acid derivatives, including aspirin and diflusinal; acetic acid derivatives, including diclofenac, indomethacin, tolmetin and sulindac; proprionic acid derivatives, such as carprofen, fenoprofen, flurbiprofen, ibuprofen, ketoprofen and naproxen; and fenamic acids, including meclofenamic acid, meclofenamate sodium, flunixin meglumide and mefenamic acid. The enolic group is divided into: pyrazolone derivatives, which include phenylbutazone, dipyrone and apazone; and oxicam derivatives, such as piroxicam.

NSAIDs act by inhibiting prostaglandin synthesis, which reduces inflammatory mediators such as prostaglandins E_2 and $F_{2\alpha}$ and endoperoxides, and also causes the adverse effects noted following their ingestion. The toxicity of NSAIDs varies considerably and cats tend to be more sensitive than dogs. The most common adverse effects of NSAIDs are mild epigastric pain, erosive gastritis, peptic ulcers and haemorrhage. Anaemia and hypoproteinaemia may occur secondary to gastric and intestinal ulceration. Nephrotoxicity is manifested as acute interstitial nephritis, acute papillary necrosis, nephrotic syndrome and acute and chronic renal failure.

Single ingestions of ibuprofen of 300 mg/kg can cause acute renal failure, while repeated dosages of 8 mg/kg/day can produce gastrointestinal irritation and haemorrhage. Doses of 15 mg/kg naproxen are considered toxic to dogs and repeated dosages of 5 mg/kg cause significant gastrointestinal damage. Aspirin doses of 50 mg/kg q12h cause emesis in dogs and higher dosages cause depression and metabolic acidosis.

Diagnosis of NSAID intoxication relies on the history, detection of a specific NSAID in gastric contents, plasma or urine and compatible clinical signs. Management of acute ingestion involves GID and supportive care. Repeated doses of AC should be administered every 4–6 hours for NSAIDs with long half-lives and significant enterohepatic recirculation (carprofen, indomethacin, piroxicam, sulindac, meclofenamic acid, meclofenamate and diclofenac). Gastrointestinal ulcers can be treated with cimetidine or ranitidine, omeprazole and sucralfate. Acute renal failure may be reversible but severe papillary necrosis is most likely to be irreversible. Fluid therapy is the most important component in treating acute renal failure. If oliguria persists after fluid therapy, medical therapy (furosemide, mannitol) should be initiated with the aim of inducing diuresis (see Chapter 8). Hyperkalaemia and acid–base disturbances should be corrected.

Paracetamol (acetaminophen)

Paracetamol (acetaminophen) is a non-opiate derivative of p-aminophenol, which produces analgesia and antipyresis by a mechanism similar to that of salicylates. Paracetamol is detoxified by the liver via conjugation with glucuronide, sulphate or glutathione. Cats lack the glucuronide conjugation pathway and are quite sensitive to paracetamol toxicity. If the conjugating ability of the liver is surpassed, N-acetyl-p-benzoquinone (NAPQI), a toxic metabolite, causes severe oxidative stress to hepatocytes and red blood cells. Oxidative damage to erythrocytes causes oxidation of haemoglobin to methaemoglobin and the formation of Heinz bodies with subsequent anaemia. Cats may also experience swelling of the face and paws. Potentially toxic doses of paracetamol for cats are 50–100 mg/kg, while a reported toxic dose for dogs is 600 mg/kg.

Clinical signs of intoxication include depression, weakness, anorexia, emesis, tachypnoea, tachycardia, hypersalivation and facial oedema in cats. Methaemoglobinaemia imparts a muddy colour to the mucous membranes and there may be haematuria and haemoglobinaemia. Acute hepatic necrosis is the most important toxic effect in dogs.

Routine decontamination should be attempted early after a known or suspected ingestion. N-Acetylcysteine (NAC) is a specific antidote that provides one of the limiting precursors (cysteine) for glutathione synthesis. A loading dose of 140–280 mg/kg orally or 140 mg/kg i.v. in 5% dextrose/water is followed by a maintenance dosage of 70 mg/kg orally q6h for 2–3 days. Although AC binds orally administered NAC, both should be administered as soon as possible after ingestion, as the recommended oral dosage of NAC provides sufficient cysteine despite reduced systemic absorption (Howland *et al.*, 1994). Ascorbic acid can be administered (30 mg/kg orally or s.c. q6h) to help reduce methaemoglobin to haemoglobin. Oxygen support may be necessary.

Chemotherapeutic emergencies

Antineoplastic drugs, including cyclophosphamide, methotrexate, 5-fluorouracil and cisplatin, may occasionally cause serious adverse effects. Antineoplastic drugs kill the actively dividing cells in malignant tumours. Unfortunately, cells such as intestinal epithelial cells, bone marrow cells, hair follicles, lymphoid cells and gonadal cells also undergo rapid division and are susceptible to their effects. Most serious intoxications are related to haematological and gastrointestinal effects.

Leucocyte, platelet and red blood cell precursors can be damaged by antineoplastic drugs, with resulting effects on peripheral blood counts depending on the circulating half-life of each cell type. Since the half-life of circulating neutrophils is the shortest (4–8 hours), neutropenia occurs first, followed by thrombocytopenia (platelet circulating half-life of 5–7 days).

The most serious potential consequence is sepsis, which positively correlates with the severity and duration of neutropenia. Broad-spectrum, bactericidal antibiotics and appropriate fluid therapy should be instituted. Thrombocytopenia can result in petechiae, ecchymoses and mucosal haemorrhage. If needed, platelet replacement therapy consists of either whole blood or platelet-rich plasma.

Gastrointestinal toxicity is manifested by nausea, emesis and gastroenterocolitis. Anti-emetics, such as metoclopramide, ondansetron or butorphanol, may reduce the incidence of emesis, but animals with persistent emesis may require hospitalization for fluid therapy. Gastroenterocolitis is treated symptomatically with demulcents, and fluid and electrolyte therapy. Broad-spectrum antibiotics may be required in severe cases to reduce the risk of sepsis secondary to bacterial translocation across the damaged gastrointestinal mucosa.

Herbal remedies

A complete discussion of intoxication risks from herbal remedies is available elsewhere (Tyler, 1993; Lewin *et al.*, 1994; Poppenga, 2006). Since there are many herbs with a wide range of biologically active constituents, it is important to ask about their use when presented with an ill animal. Haematological, gastrointestinal, cardiac, neurological, hepatic and renal signs may occur. The source of the herbal remedy is important, as many imported Chinese patent medicines are adulterated with metals, pesticides and drugs such as NSAIDs and sedatives. Chinese patent medicine formulations may also contain cinnabar (mercuric sulphide), realgar (arsenic sulphide) or litharge (lead oxide). The risk of intoxication depends on the dose administered, the duration of use and the presence of pre-existing diseases. The potential for adverse drug reactions increases when herbal medicines are given concurrently with traditional pharmaceuticals.

A human poison control centre may be consulted regarding the active constituents of herbal remedies, particularly if the label is incomplete or in a foreign language. Toxicological testing of fluid or tissue samples may identify some active ingredients, although many potentially toxic constituents are not detected by routine screens. Testing for contaminants such as metals and drugs may be indicated when an imported patent remedy has been used. In general, acute ingestion of potentially toxic herbal products should be managed by following standard decontamination protocols and symptomatic treatment. Decontamination may not be helpful when a herbal remedy has been given chronically.

Ethylene glycol

Ingestion of ethylene glycol (EG) remains one of the most common toxicoses of dogs and cats. It is readily consumed by animals and the incidence of toxicoses is highest in late autumn and early spring when antifreeze use increases. EG has been replaced in some formulations by relatively non-toxic propylene glycol. EG itself is not particularly lethal, but its metabolites cause serious toxicity. One metabolite, glycolic acid, causes severe metabolic acidosis within several hours of ingestion. In addition, another metabolite, oxalic acid, combines with calcium to form calcium oxalate crystals in blood vessels and renal tubules. Renal tubular damage with subsequent renal failure occurs 1–3 days after ingestion.

EG toxicosis can be divided into three clinical phases. Phase 1 occurs 1–4 hours after ingestion, and is manifested by ataxia, tachycardia, tachypnoea, diuresis, polydipsia and dehydration. Phase 2 occurs 4–6 hours after ingestion and coincides with the onset of metabolic acidosis due to EG metabolites. Clinical signs include anorexia, depression, emesis, miosis and hypothermia. Following large ingestions, severe depression, tachypnoea, coma and death ensue unless treatment is initiated. With smaller doses these clinical signs may resolve only to be followed by phase 3, characterized by oliguric renal failure 2–7 days after ingestion.

Diagnosis of EG toxicosis can be difficult. Increased serum osmolality, metabolic acidosis and an anion gap greater than 40–50 mmol/l are often observed, but isopropanol, salicylates, methanol, paraldehyde, toluene, formaldehyde and ibuprofen toxicoses can cause similar changes. Birefringent rosette-shaped calcium oxalate crystals may be seen in urine sediment, particularly under polarized light. Laboratory detection of EG or glycolic acid in serum or urine confirms exposure. Colorimetric kits allow detection of EG in serum within 24 hours of exposure, when serum EG concentrations are high. Unfortunately, animals may recover from phases 1 and 2, only to be presented in renal failure, which is associated with a guarded prognosis.

Management depends on the time of presentation following ingestion. Unless an animal is presented immediately following ingestion, GID is not useful, since EG is rapidly absorbed from the gastrointestinal tract. Specific antidotes include ethanol and fomepizole, which prevent metabolism of EG to toxic metabolites by inhibiting alcohol dehydrogenase. In dogs, a 20% ethanol solution is given at 5.5 ml/kg by slow intravenous infusion every 4 hours for five treatments, then every 6 hours for four additional sessions. In cats the recommended dose is 5.0 ml/kg i.v. every 6 hours for five treatments then every 8 hours for four treatments. The dose should be titrated to maintain severe depression for up to 72 hours during which time the patient will require intensive supportive care. In dogs, fomepizole is administered by slow intravenous infusion of 15 mg/kg as a 5% solution, then 10 mg/kg every 12 hours for four doses followed by 5 mg/kg every 12 hours until plasma EG concentrations fall below 3222 µmol/l. If EG concentrations cannot be monitored, the 5 mg/kg dose should be continued for at least 24 hours. Fomepizole has fewer side effects than ethanol and is the antidote of choice for dogs. Early work in EG-exposed cats did not show efficacy using doses of fomepizole that were effective in dogs. However, more recent work has shown fomepizole to be effective in cats if given at 125 mg/kg i.v. at 1, 2 and 3 hours after EG ingestion followed by 31.25 mg/kg i.v. at 12, 24 and 36 hours post-ingestion (Thrall *et al.*, 2006). Mild CNS depression was the only adverse effect associated with high-dose fomepizole administration. Since metabolism of EG occurs quickly, the antidotes need to be given as soon as possible after ingestion. Supportive care should be provided; correction of metabolic acidosis and maintenance of urine flow are critical to successful case management. For patients with acute oliguric renal failure an antidote is unlikely to be helpful and prognosis is poor.

Household agents
There are hundreds of chemicals in the household to which animals may be exposed and some of these are listed in Figure 19.6. Many household products are, however, generally considered to be non-toxic (Figure 19.7). The majority of toxic exposures are managed using standard GID protocols and supportive treatment.

Product	Toxicity rating	Ingredients	Clinical presentation
De-icer	4	~75% ethylene glycol and isopropyl alcohol	Disorientation, ataxia, weakness, depression, irritation of mucous membranes and eyes
Fertilizer	2	Mainly nitrogen (e.g. potassium nitrate, urea), phosphorous, potassium; may contain small amounts of metals or pesticides	Gastrointestinal irritation, emesis, diarrhoea, methaemoglobinaemia
Fuels (cooking fuels, lighter fluid)	3	Petroleum hydrocarbons, kerosene, or methanol	Depression, coma, seizures, emesis
Glues	3–4	Carriers include aliphatic hydrocarbon solvents (e.g. petroleum solvents, acetone, toluol, toluene, methyl acetate, naphtha)	Direct irritation, depression
Paint and varnish removers	4	Benzene, acetone, toluene, methylene chloride, methanol	Direct irritation, depression
Radiator cleaners	4	Oxalic acid	Direct irritation of mucous membranes and gastrointestinal tract, muscle twitching, tetany, seizures, depression, paralysis, renal failure

19.6 Toxicity of common household products. Toxicity is based on a scale of 1–6, where 1 is relatively harmless (probable oral lethal dose of >15 g/kg) and 6 is extremely toxic (probable oral lethal dose <1 mg/kg). Reproduced from Osweiler (1996) with permission of the publisher. (continues) ▶

Product	Toxicity rating	Ingredients	Clinical presentation
Rust removers	4	Hydrochloric acid, phosphoric acid, hydrofluoric acid, naphtha and mineral oil	Necrosis
Thawing salt	2–3	Calcium chloride, sodium chloride, or potassium chloride	Erythema, exfoliation, ulceration, general irritation of the gastrointestinal tract, emesis, anorexia, diarrhoea, direct irritation of footpads, mouth, or pharynx from contaminated water
Fire extinguisher chemicals	2–4	Chlorobromomethane, methylbromide, or halogenated hydrocarbons consisting of brominated or chlorinated fluoromethanes	Irritation of the skin and eyes, emesis, CNS signs, hypotension, coma, pulmonary failure
Fireplace colours	3–4	Coke dust, sawdust, heavy metal salts (e.g. copper, rubidium and caesium compounds, lead, arsenic, selenium, tellurium, barium, molybdenum, antimony, zinc), chloride, borate and phosphate	Severe gastroenteritis, emesis, diarrhoea, followed by depression, shock and renal failure
Fireworks	3–4	Oxidizing agents (e.g. potassium nitrate, chlorates), heavy metal salts (e.g. mercury, antimony, copper, strontium, barium, phosphorus)	Emesis, severe abdominal pain, bloody faeces, rapid shallow breathing, methaemoglobinaemia and death from respiratory or cardiac failure; other signs relate to specific effects of toxic heavy metals
Fluxes	3–4	Zinc chloride, hydrochloric acid, salts of aniline, glutamic and salicylic acid, aliphatic alcohols, terpenes, hydrocarbons, boric acid and fluorides (silver solder)	Irritation of the mouth, gastrointestinal tract or skin; nausea, emesis, diarrhoea, ataxia, delirium and excitement progressing to stupor or coma
Matches	2	Potassium chlorate	Methaemoglobinaemia with cyanosis and haemolysis
Photographic developer	4–5	Boric acid, *p*-methyl aminophenol sulphite, ammonium thiosulphate, potassium thiocyanate, sodium hydroxide	*p*-Methyl aminophenol sulphite causes methaemoglobinaemia; corrosive effects may result from acids and alkalis
Bleach	3	~5% sodium hypochlorite	Acid solutions combined with hypochlorite bleaches can cause release of chlorine gas and hypochlorous acid, presenting an acute inhalation hazard characterized by pain and inflammation of the mouth, pharynx, oesophagus and stomach; oral ingestion results in irritation with oedema of the pharynx, glottis, larynx and lungs
Drain cleaners	No rating	Sodium hydroxide, sodium hypochlorite	Necrosis and ulceration of the oral mucosa and, possibly, the oesophagus; sequelae include strictures, laryngeal or glottal oedema, asphyxiation and pneumonia
Furniture polish	3	Petroleum distillates, mineral spirits, petroleum hydrocarbons	Depression, coma, seizures, emesis
Metal cleaners, oven cleaners	3–4	Caustic soda or potash (alkaline cleaners), kerosene, high concentrations of chlorinated ethylenes or 1,1,1-trichoroethane (solvent cleaners), hydrochloric, sulphuric, chromic or phosphoric acids	Necrosis, emesis
Pine oil disinfectants	3	Pine oils (terpenes), phenols, synthetic phenol derivatives (e.g. o-phenyl phenol)	Gastritis, emesis, diarrhoea are followed by depression, unconsciousness, or mild seizures followed by depression and renal failure
Shoe polish	2	Animal, petroleum or vegetable waxes, mineral spirits, turpentine, aniline dyes; nitrobenzenes or terpenes may also be present	Large amounts could produce methaemoglobinaemia
Deodorant/ antiperspirants	3	Cream base and an antibacterial agent, antiperspirants also contain 15–20% aluminium salts (e.g. aluminium chlorohydrate, aluminium chloride); less commonly used agents include titanium dioxide, oxyquinoline sulphate and zirconium salts	Gingival necrosis and haemorrhagic gastroenteritis, sometimes accompanied by ataxia and nephrosis; severe effects are rare unless large amounts of active ingredient are ingested

19.6 (continued) Toxicity of common household products. Toxicity is based on a scale of 1–6, where 1 is relatively harmless (probable oral lethal dose of >15 g/kg) and 6 is extremely toxic (probable oral lethal dose <1 mg/kg). Reproduced from Osweiler (1996) with permission of the publisher. (continues) ▶

Product	Toxicity rating	Ingredients	Clinical presentation
Denture cleaners	4	Perborates decompose to hydrogen peroxide and sodium borate, which are strongly alkaline and very irritating	Salivation, emesis, early stimulation of the CNS followed by depression, non-specific liver and kidney damage
Perfumes	3–4	Alcohols, essential oils (e.g. savin, rue, tansy, apiol, juniper, cedar leaf, cajupute)	Essential oils are often hepato- or nephrotoxic and may irritate the skin, mucous membranes and lungs resulting in aspiration, pulmonary oedema and pneumonitis; albuminuria, haematuria and glycosuria result from renal damage; CNS effects include excitement, ataxia, disorientation and coma
Rubbing alcohol	2–3	Ethanol or isopropyl alcohol	Disorientation, ataxia, weakness, depression, irritation of mucous membranes
Shampoos	3	Surfactants, fragrance, sodium lauryl sulphate or triethanolamine dodecyl sulphate; antidandruff shampoos contain one or more metals (e.g. zinc pyridinethione, selenium sulphide) coal tar derivatives or salicylic acid	Only mild toxicosis is expected in most cases; progressive blindness has been reported in dogs and cats ingesting zinc pyridinethione (lesions include retinal detachment and severe exudative chorioretinitis)
Suntan lotion	2	Alcohol	See Rubbing alcohol
Styptic pencil	2	Potassium alum sulphate	Corrosive lesions from sulphuric acid formed during hydrolysis of the salt
Paintballs	No rating. Clinical signs reported in a 41 kg Labrador that ingested 15 paintballs	Ingredients vary depending on manufacturer but may include: polyethylene glycol, glycerol, gelatin, sorbitol, dipropylene glycol, mineral oil, dye, ground pig skin and water	Emesis, ataxia, diarrhoea and tremors are the most common clinical signs reported. Hypernatraemia is the most common laboratory abnormality (hyperchloraemia and hypokalemia can also occur)
Play dough (homemade)	No rating. Estimated toxic dose is 1.9 g/kg	Recipes vary in amounts of each ingredient but consist of flour, sodium chloride and water	Emesis, polydipsia, seizures, polyuria, tremors, hyperthermia. Hypernatraemia is the most significant laboratory abnormality
Gorilla glue	No rating	Urethane polymer and polymeric isocyanate liquid compound	Physical obstruction of the gastrointestinal tract

19.6 (continued) Toxicity of common household products. Toxicity is based on a scale of 1–6, where 1 is relatively harmless (probable oral lethal dose of >15 g/kg) and 6 is extremely toxic (probable oral lethal dose <1 mg/kg). Reproduced from Osweiler (1996) with permission of the publisher.

Abrasives
Adhesives
Air fresheners
Aluminium foil
Antacids
Antibiotics
Ashes (from non-treated wood/ fireplace)
Baby product cosmetics
Baby wipes (without alcohol)
Ballpoint pen inks
Bath oil beads
Bath oils
Birth control pills
Bleach with <5% sodium hypochlorite
Body conditioners
Bubble bath soaps
Calamine lotion
Candles (beeswax or paraffin wax)
Carboxymethyl cellulose
Chalk
Charcoal and charcoal briquettes
Chewing gum
Cigarette ash

Clay
Clotrimazole cream
Colognes (low alcohol)
Corticosteroids
Cosmetics
Crayons marked AC, CP
Cyanoacrylate
Deodorizers
Elmer's glue
Erasers
Eye make-up
Fabric softeners
Felt tip pens
Fish bowl additives
Glow stick/jewellery
Glycerol
Grease, motor oil
Gypsum
Hair products (dyes, sprays, tonics)
Hand lotions/creams
3% Hydrogen peroxide
Incense
Indelible markers
Ink (blue and black)

Iodophil disinfectant
Lactaid
Lanolin
Latex paints
Laxatives
Lip balm
Lipstick
Lubricants
Magic markers
Mascara
Mineral oil
Modelling clay
Newspaper
Oral contraceptives
Pencil (graphite lead and colouring)
Petroleum jelly
Photographs
Plant foods and fertilizers
Plaster
Play-Doh
Polaroid picture coating fluid
Porous tip marking pens
Putty
Rouge
Rubber cement

Sachets
Shaving creams and lotions
Silica gel
Silly-Putty
Soaps and soap products
Spackle
Starch
Stick-em glue traps
Styrofoam
Sunscreen products
Sweetening agents [a]
Tallow
Thermometers (mercury)
Titanium oxide
Toothpaste (without fluoride)
Vitamins (without iron)
Wallboard
Wallpaper paste
Washing powder (except those for dishwashers)
Watercolours
Wax
White glue/paste
Zirconium oxide

19.7 Household items generally considered to be non-toxic to children. [a] The artificial sweetener xylitol is toxic to dogs, causing hypoglycaemia and occasionally hepatic failure.

Petroleum-based products

With the exception of petroleum distillates serving as vehicles for more toxic chemicals, ingestion of petroleum-based products is not considered to be life threatening. Aspiration pneumonia is the most serious sequel of ingestion of volatile petroleum products such as paraffin (kerosene), naphtha or petroleum distillates. Aspiration risks increase with spontaneous or induced emesis and GID should be avoided. When co-ingestion of another toxic chemical has occurred, GID should be considered.

Thoracic radiographs should be considered for all patients who have ingested petroleum-based products. Those who remain asymptomatic with normal thoracic radiographs 4 or more hours after ingestion can be discharged after a 1-day observation period, with no further treatment. However, patients with radiographic and/or clinical evidence of pneumonitis require close monitoring, symptomatic oxygen supplementation and serial arterial blood gas determinations. Indications for antibiotic therapy include documented bacterial pneumonia, or worsening of radiographic infiltrates, leucocytosis and fever after the first 40 hours. There appears to be no benefit from the administration of corticosteroids.

Illicit drugs

While the documented incidence is unknown, the widespread availability of drugs such as cocaine, narcotics and amphetamines makes exposure of pets likely. Drug sniffer dogs may be at particular risk. Most illicit drugs are rapidly absorbed and target the CNS. Therefore, illicit drug exposure should be considered in any animal with acute neurological signs.

Cocaine intoxication is manifested by CNS excitation, peripheral vasoconstriction, hyperthermia and increased muscular activity. Death results from respiratory or cardiac arrest, or hyperthermia. Narcotics such as heroin exert their effects on the gastrointestinal, cardiovascular and central nervous systems. Early clinical signs may include drowsiness, ataxia, decreased sensory pain perception, transient excitation, emesis, defecation and tachypnoea. Late clinical signs include delirium, seizures, miosis, coma, respiratory depression and hypotension. Pulmonary oedema often occurs in fatal cases and death is often attributed to respiratory arrest. Amphetamine overdoses cause restlessness, behavioural changes, hyperactivity, mydriasis, polypnoea, hyperthermia, tachycardia, tremors, respiratory depression, cardiac dysrhythmias, heart block and circulatory shock.

Treatment is largely symptomatic. Early after ingestion GID should be considered. Treatment of seizures, hyperthermia, respiratory depression and cardiac dysrhythmias is of primary concern. The toxic effects of most narcotic agents can be reversed by naloxone (0.01–0.02 mg/kg i.v., i.m. or s.c.) to effect; repeated doses may be needed. Chlorpromazine (0.1–0.5 mg/kg i.v.) may antagonize many of the effects of cocaine and amphetamines. Haloperidol (1 mg/kg i.v.) may be protective against the lethal effects of amphetamines.

Plants

While scores of potentially toxic plants may be ingested, relatively few plants (Figure 19.8) account for the majority of exposures (Buck, 1995; Hornfeldt and Murphy, 1995). In cases of plant exposure, plants should be positively identified in order to determine their potential toxicity. Whole plant samples are preferred for identification, but it may be possible to identify a plant based upon examination of plant parts either from the environment of the animal or from vomitus. With few exceptions, treatment of toxic plant ingestions involves symptomatic and supportive care.

Common name	Scientific name	Poison	System(s) affected	Clinical signs	Treatment
Philodendron	*Philodendron* spp.	Insoluble calcium oxalate	GI, respiratory	Painful burning of lips, oral mucosa, throat; if severe, oedema, dyspnoea	Pain and oedema resolve slowly without treatment, symptomatic
Dumbcane	*Dieffenbachia* spp.				
Rhododendron Azalea	*Rhododendron* spp.	Andromedotoxins	GI, cardiovascular	Transitory burning in mouth followed by salivation, emesis and diarrhoea; muscular weakness; bradycardia; hypotension; coma and convulsions terminally	GID, monitor ECG, fluids, atropine for bradycardia
Easter and tiger lilies	*Lilium loniflorum* and *L. tigrinum*	Unknown	Renal	Consistent with acute renal failure: anorexia, depression, emesis	GID, treatment for acute renal failure
Marijuana	*Cannabis sativa*	Tetrahydrocannabinol (THC)	CNS	Ataxia, depression, hallucinations evidenced by barking and agitation, emesis, dry mucous membranes	GID (antiemetic properties of THC may negate emetics), place in warm quiet environment
Poinsettia	*Euphorbia pulcherrima*	Unknown	GI	Not generally toxic; emesis most severe sign	Not generally needed, symptomatic

19.8 Most commonly implicated poisonous plants. (continues) ▶

Common name	Scientific name	Poison	System(s) affected	Clinical signs	Treatment
Onion, wild onion, leek, garlic (onion powder, dehydrated onions, cooked onions)	*Allium* spp.	Sulphides such as *n*-dipropyl sulphide, dimethyl, di-1-propenyl and di-2-pronenyl disulphides Cats are more sensitive; some Japanese dogs are more sensitive	Haemopoietic system – specifically the red blood cells (toxins cause oxidant damage to haemoglobin and red blood cell membrane)	Lethargy, weakness, pale mucous membranes, tachycardia, tachypnoea, haematuria or dark-coloured urine, haemoglobinuria, Heinz body anaemia, haemoglobinaemia, altered red blood cell morphology, emesis, diarrhoea	GID, lactated Ringer's solution to promote diuresis, symptomatic and supportive. Monitor PCV and renal function

19.8 (continued) Most commonly implicated poisonous plants.

Grapes and raisins

Recently, ingestion of grapes or raisins by dogs has been associated with acute renal failure (Mazzaferro *et al.*, 2004). The proximate toxin has not been identified and not all dogs that ingest grapes or raisins are affected. In addition, there is no apparent relationship between the number of grapes or raisins ingested and the occurrence of acute renal failure. Clinical signs of intoxication are those of acute renal failure, including anorexia, emesis, diarrhoea, lethargy, abdominal pain and oliguria followed by anuria. Histopathological lesions include proximal renal tubule degeneration and necrosis. Diagnosis of intoxication relies on a history of recent ingestion of grapes or raisins. Treatment includes early GID and symptomatic and supportive care. Haemodialysis or peritoneal dialysis should be considered if available. The prognosis is poor based upon reported cases to date.

Methylxanthines (caffeine, theobromine)

Caffeine and theobromine are alkaloids of plant origin found in a variety of foods, beverages, dietary supplements and over-the-counter (OTC) products. Intoxication of animals most often occurs following the ingestion of chocolate (containing primarily theobromine, but also caffeine), caffeine-containing dietary supplements or OTC stimulant tablets. Less frequently, dogs have reportedly been intoxicated following the ingestion of cocoa bean shells used as mulch for plants. The theobromine content of chocolate varies, with unsweetened baking chocolate containing 1360–1600 mg/100 g and milk chocolate containing 155–212 mg/100 g (Carson, 2006). The lethal doses of caffeine and theobromine for dogs vary from 110–200 mg/kg and 100–250 mg/kg, respectively. Most cases of intoxication occur in dogs. Dogs may be predisposed to intoxication from theobromine due to slower metabolism. The half-life of theobromine in dogs is approximately 17.5 hours compared to 6–10 hours in humans.

Methylxanthines inhibit cyclic nucleotide phosphodiesterases and are adenosine receptor antagonists. These actions result in cerebral cortical stimulation, seizures, increased myocardial contractility, smooth muscle relaxation and diuresis (Carson, 2006). Additionally, caffeine stimulates catecholamine release. The onset of clinical signs following ingestion of methylxanthines at toxic doses is rapid. Initially, restlessness, hyperactivity, behavioural abnormalities and emesis are commonly noted. Signs progress rapidly to panting, tachycardia, weakness, ataxia, diuresis, diarrhoea, hyperexcitability, severe hyperactivity, muscle tremors, hyperthermia and clonic seizures. Death is most often due to cardiac dysrhythmias, especially ventricular fibrillation (Holmgren, 2004; Carson, 2006). Caffeine and theobromine can be detected in a variety of samples (stomach contents, plasma, serum, urine and liver) to confirm exposure when needed.

Early treatment of the intoxicated animal involves stabilization of respiratory and cardiac function. Once stable, appropriate GID should be undertaken. Administration of multiple doses of AC is useful to increase caffeine or theobromine clearance; 0.5 g/kg every 3 hours for 72 hours has been recommended (Carson, 2006). Hyperactivity, hyperexcitability and seizures can be controlled with diazepam at 0.5–2 mg/kg i.v.; if unresponsive to diazepam, barbiturates can be used. Hyperthermia can resolve rapidly once hyperactivity or seizures are controlled, although persistent hyperthermia should be treated aggressively. Cardiac function should be monitored closely and cardiac dysrhythmias treated appropriately. Tachycardia can be treated with a beta blocker such as metoprolol (0.5–1.0 mg/kg orally q8h for dogs and 2–15 mg orally q8h for cats). Premature ventricular contractions should be treated with lidocaine (initially a slow intravenous bolus of 2–6 mg/kg in dogs or 0.5–1.0 mg/kg in cats is followed by a constant rate infusion of 20–70 µg/kg/min in dogs or 10–20 µg/kg/min in cats). Intravenous crystalloids should be given to minimize renal damage secondary to rhabdomyolysis. Urinary catheterization may be useful to increase methylxanthine clearance, since reabsorption can occur across the bladder wall. Haemoperfusion or haemodialysis can also increase methylxanthine clearance.

Mushrooms

A variety of mushrooms are toxic (Spoerke, 2006), with the most poisonous mushrooms containing cyclopeptide toxins, especially amanitin. Several genera of mushrooms contain amanitin, but ingestion of *Amanita* spp. and *Galerina* spp. are most often involved in intoxication. Ingestion of amanitin-containing mushrooms results in fulminant liver failure. Renal failure and coagulopathy can also occur. Amanitin toxins inhibit protein synthesis by ribosomes within hepatocytes. Following mushroom ingestion, there can be a latent period before the onset of clinical signs. Clinical signs include hyperglycaemia followed by hypoglycaemia, coagulation abnormalities, ataxia, listlessness, bradycardia and shock. Antemortem diagnosis of *Amanita* intoxication relies on a history of recent mushroom ingestion and, if testing is available, detection of amanitin in serum, urine or gastrointestinal contents. Whether amatoxin testing is available or not, an attempt should be made to identify the genus and species of mushroom ingested. Unfortunately, mushroom identification often requires specialized expertise that may or may not be readily available and fresh samples are necessary.

Once liver damage has occurred, treatment is often unrewarding. GID is warranted if the animal is presented early after ingestion. Multiple doses of activated charcoal are indicated because enterohepatic recirculation of the toxins occurs. Apart from standard supportive care, penicillin G and silymarin (derived from *Silybum marianum*, or milk thistle) have been used, but their efficacy is uncertain. Silymarin at a total dose of 1.4–4.2 g per day can be given orally for 4–5 days. Alternatively, *N*-acetylcysteine at doses similar to those for treating paracetamol intoxication can be administered. Silymarin and *N*-acetylcysteine are thought to be hepatoprotective. Vitamin K1 and blood transfusions are indicated in cases with coagulopathy.

Mycotoxins

Mycotoxins are secondary fungal metabolites that can intoxicate humans and animals (Puschner, 2002). Several mycotoxins have been characterized and shown to cause animal disease. However, two major classes of mycotoxins are responsible for the majority of small animal intoxications: aflatoxins and tremorgenic mycotoxins.

Aflatoxins

Aflatoxins are produced by certain fungal species in the genus *Aspergillus*, which grow on corn, peanuts and other agricultural products during warm and humid conditions. Under natural conditions, four major aflatoxins are produced (aflatoxins B_1, B_2, G_1 and G_2), with aflatoxin B_1 being both the most prevalent and most toxic. Aflatoxins are metabolized by the liver to reactive epoxides which bind covalently with cellular macromolecules such as DNA, RNA and proteins. Such binding results in damage to hepatocytes leading to impaired liver function, bile duct proliferation, bile stasis and liver fibrosis. Cases of toxicity have occurred in dogs but have not been reported in cats.

In dogs, most reported cases have resulted in acute liver failure. Signs can include weakness, depression, anorexia, emesis, diarrhoea, icterus and signs associated with coagulopathy. Haemorrhage, secondary to clotting factor deficiency as a result of inhibition of protein synthesis, is often the immediate cause of death. Liver enzymes, ammonia and bilirubin concentrations are increased in serum and coagulation times can be prolonged. Testing of biological specimens for aflatoxins is not widely available. An antemortem diagnosis relies on occurrence of characteristic signs, ruling out other causes of acute liver failure and detection of aflatoxins in representative food items. Recognition of aflatoxicosis often does not happen sufficiently early for GID procedures to be useful. Treatment is symptomatic and supportive. The prognosis is related to the severity of the liver damage. If liver damage is extensive, the prognosis is poor.

Tremorgenic mycotoxins

Penitrem A and roquefortine are two mycotoxins produced by *Penicillium* spp. Toxigenic *Penicillium* spp. have been found on mouldy dairy products, bread, walnuts and compost. Penitrem A and roquefortine affect the CNS. Penitrem A may cause presynaptic changes in acetylcholine release, decreased production of glycine or GABA receptor agonism; the mechanism of action of roquefortine is unknown.

Most reported cases of intoxication involve dogs. Signs of intoxication in dogs include emesis, increased irritability, weakness, muscle tremors, rigidity, hyperactivity, sensitivity to noise, panting and hyperthermia (Puschner, 2002). Tremors can become severe, and opisthotonus, seizures, nystagmus, recumbency and paddling can occur. Rhabdomyolysis, dehydration and metabolic acidosis are potential complicating factors. Signs can occur within 30 minutes of ingestion of contaminated materials or be delayed for several hours. A diagnosis of intoxication relies on a history of ingestion of mouldy materials, occurrence of characteristic signs and detection of penitrem A or roquefortine in samples such as food items, gastrointestinal contents, serum or urine. A number of other poisons such as metaldehyde, organophosphate and carbamate insecticides, pyrethrin/pyrethroid insecticides, bromethalin and illicit drugs cause similar clinical signs, so obtaining a detailed history and performing analyses on appropriate samples are keys to confirming mycotoxin exposure. Treatment involves GID if instituted early after a suspected exposure. Additional therapy involves controlling seizures and hyperthermia, correcting metabolic acidosis and maintaining hydration and urine flow.

Cyanobacterial toxins

Cyanobacteria or blue-green algae are commonly found in fresh or salt water in temperate regions of the world. Under favourable environmental conditions, algae can undergo rapid proliferation resulting in algal 'blooms', and elaborate extremely toxic compounds. Blooms can become concentrated along shorelines as a result of wind or wave action. Pets are exposed to the toxins when they ingest bloom material secondary to water ingestion. *Microcystis* and *Nodularia* spp. can produce hepatotoxins and *Anabaena*, *Aphanizomenon*, *Lyngbya* and *Oscillatoria* spp. can produce neurotoxins (Hooser and Talcott, 2006). The hepatotoxicants include microcystins or nodularin while the neurotoxicants include anatoxin-a or anatoxin-a$_s$.

Microcystins and nodularin inhibit protein phosphatases within hepatocytes which leads to rapid and massive hepatic necrosis, intrahepatic haemorrhage and shock. Anatoxin-a is a postsynaptic depolarizing blocking agent and anatoxin-a$_s$ is an acetylcholinesterase inhibitor. Clinical signs associated with hepatotoxicant ingestion include emesis, diarrhoea, lethargy, weakness, pallor and circulatory shock. Anatoxin-a causes acute onset of muscle rigidity, tremors, seizures, paralysis and respiratory paralysis. Anatoxin-a$_s$ causes rapid onset of signs of muscarinic receptor stimulation (DUMBELS), seizures and respiratory paralysis. Confirmation of exposure relies on a history of access to contaminated water, observation of bloom material on the haircoat or around the mouth, detection of an odour suggestive of exposure to stagnant water, occurrence of compatible clinical signs, identification of toxigenic algal species in water samples or gastrointestinal contents and identification of specific toxins in water samples or gastrointestinal contents.

Treatment includes standard GID procedures if initiated soon after exposure to bloom material, and symptomatic and supportive care. Circulatory shock is of immediate concern in animals exposed to hepatotoxicants, while seizure control and respiratory support are critical for animals exposed to the neurotoxicants. Atropine will reverse the muscarinic signs associated with anatoxin-a$_s$ intoxication. The prognosis is poor for symptomatic animals and the rapidity of onset of clinical signs often precludes effective therapeutic intervention.

Lead

Lead intoxication is still common, despite efforts to decrease environmental sources of exposure. The incidence is highest in young dogs and in pets kept in older houses. Sources of exposure include paint and paint residue or dust from sanding, lead objects such as curtain and fishing weights, improperly glazed ceramic food or water bowls, plumbing materials, solder, putty and linoleum.

Lead interacts with sulphydryl groups and interferes with numerous enzymes, including those involved in haem synthesis, resulting in increased fragility and reduced survival of red blood cells. Damage to CNS capillaries may account for acute CNS effects. Clinical signs are related to the gastrointestinal and nervous systems. Gastrointestinal signs are prominent in animals with chronic low-level exposure to lead, and include emesis, diarrhoea, anorexia and abdominal pain. Neurological signs are more common in animals with acute exposure, and include lethargy, hysteria, seizures and blindness. Diagnosis relies on detection of clinically significant lead concentrations in whole blood. A large number of nucleated red blood cells and basophilic stippling suggest lead exposure, but their absence does not rule out lead toxicosis. Radio-opaque material in the gastrointestinal tract may be an important clue to ingestion of lead objects or paint chips.

Case management should be tailored to the individual situation. AC is not effective in binding lead. Sodium sulphate may hasten the elimination of lead from the gastrointestinal tract by forming lead sulphate, which is not well absorbed. Whole bowel irrigation to remove small metallic objects or paint chips seems reasonable, although such a decontamination approach has not been evaluated for efficacy. Alternatively, metal objects may be removed via endoscopy or surgery. Calcium disodium edetate (CaNa$_2$EDTA)

and succimer (dimercaptosuccinic acid or DMSA) are effective lead chelators. The use of succimer is relatively new; it has several major advantages over CaNa$_2$EDTA, including oral efficacy and fewer side effects (Graziano, 1994). CaNa$_2$EDTA should be diluted to a 1% solution with 5% dextrose in water and administered subcutaneously at 25 mg/kg q6h for 5 days (Poppenga, 1997). Animals with blood lead concentrations greater than 1 ppm often need multiple treatments separated by 5-day rest periods. Blood lead concentrations should be monitored several days after cessation of treatment to determine whether additional chelation will be necessary. Succimer is administered orally at 10 mg/kg q8h for 5 days, followed by 10 mg/kg q12h for 2 weeks. Extended treatment should be separated by 2-week rest periods. Seizures should be controlled with diazepam.

Zinc

Zinc intoxication may occur following the ingestion of zinc-containing objects such as coins, galvanized hardware materials or ointments containing zinc oxide. It is most frequently reported in dogs and pet birds. Zinc causes severe gastrointestinal irritation and intravascular haemolysis. Multiple organ failure, disseminated intravascular coagulation and cardiopulmonary arrest have been reported. Diagnosis relies on the measurement of elevated serum zinc concentrations. Metallic objects may be detected on abdominal radiographs and may be an important clue to zinc intoxication in patients with a haemolytic crisis.

Specific treatments for zinc toxicosis include removal of metallic objects from the gastrointestinal tract and the administration of CaNa$_2$EDTA, which chelates zinc (succimer does not chelate zinc effectively). Symptomatic and supportive care should be instituted and liver, renal, coagulation and cardiac function monitored. Removal of the source of zinc often results in gradual improvement over 48–72 hours.

References and further reading

Buck WB (1995) Top 25 generic agents involving dogs and cats managed by the national animal poison control centre in 1992. In: *Current Veterinary Therapy XII: Small Animal Practice*, ed. JD Bonagura, p. 210. WB Saunders, Philadelphia

Carson TL (2006) Methylxanthines. In: *Small Animal Toxicology*, ed. ME Peterson, PA Talcott, pp. 845–852. Elsevier Saunders, St. Louis

Dumonceaux GA (1995) Illicit drug intoxications in dogs. In: *Current Veterinary Therapy XII: Small Animal Practice*, ed. JD Bonagura, pp. 250–251. WB Saunders, Philadelphia

Graziano JH (1994) Antidotes in depth: 2,3-dimercaptosuccinic acid (DMSA, succimer). In: *Toxicologic Emergencies*, ed. LR Goldfrank *et al.*, pp. 1045–1047. Appleton and Lange, Norwalk

Hansen SR (2006) Pyrethrins and pyrethroids. In: *Small Animal Toxicology*, eds. ME Peterson and PA Talcott, pp. 1002–1009, Elsevier Saunders, St. Louis

Holmgren P, Norden-Petterson L and Ahlner J (2004) Caffeine fatalities: four case reports. *Forensic Science International* **139**, 71–73

Hooser SB and Talcott PA (2006) Cyanobacteria. In: *Small Animal Toxicology*, eds. ME Peterson and PA Talcott, pp. 685–689, Elsevier Saunders, St. Louis

Hornfeldt CS and Murphy MJ (1995) Incidence of small animal poison exposures in a major metropolitan area. In: *Current Veterinary Therapy XII: Small Animal Practice*, ed. JD Bonagura, pp. 209–210. WB Saunders, Philadelphia

Howland MA (1994) Antidotes in-depth: activated charcoal. In: *Toxicologic Emergencies*, ed. LR Goldfrank *et al.*, pp. 66–71. Appleton and Lange, Norwalk

Howland MA, Smilkstein J and Weisman RS (1994) Antidotes in depth:

N-acetylcysteine. In: *Toxicologic Emergencies,* ed. LR Goldfrank *et al.,* pp. 498–500. Appleton and Lange, Norwalk

Lewin NA, Howland MA and Goldfrank LR (1994) Herbal preparations. In: *Toxicologic Emergencies,* ed. LR Goldfrank *et al.,* pp. 963–979. Appleton and Lange, Norwalk

Mazzaferro EF, Eubig PA, Hackett TB *et al.* (2004) Acute renal failure associated with raisin or grape ingestion in 4 dogs. *Journal of Veterinary Emergency and Critical Care* **14**, 203–212

Orlowski JM, Hou S and Leikin JB (2001) Extracorporeal removal of drugs and toxins. In: *Clinical Toxicology,* eds. Ford MD *et al.,* pp. 43–50. WB Saunders, Philadelphia

Osweiler GD (1996) Clinical toxicology of common household chemicals. In: *The National Veterinary Medical Series: Toxicology.* Williams and Wilkins, Baltimore

Perry H and Shannon M (1996) Emergency department gastrointestinal decontamination. *Pediatric Annals* **25**, 19–29

Poppenga RH (2006) Hazards associated with the use of herbal and other natural products. In: *Small Animal Toxicology,* eds. ME Peterson and PA Talcott, pp. 312–344, Elsevier Saunders, St. Louis

Poppenga RH (1997) Lead poisoning. In: *The 5 Minute Veterinary Consult: Canine and Feline,* ed. LP Tilley and FWK Smith, Jr, pp. 760–761. Williams and Wilkins, Baltimore

Puschner, B (2002) Mycotoxins. *Veterinary Clinics of North America* **32**, 409–419

Richardson, JA (2000) Permethrin spot-on toxicosis in cats. *Journal of Veterinary Emergency and Critical Care* **10**, 103–105

Roberston J, Christopher M and Rogers Q (1998) Heinz body formation in cats fed baby food containing onion powder. *Journal of the American Veterinary Medical Association* **212**, 1260–1266

Rumbeiha WK, Kruger J, Fitzgerald S *et al.* (1997) The use of pamidronate disodium for treatment of vitamin D3 toxicosis in dogs. Proceedings, American Association of Veterinary Laboratory Diagnosticians, 40th Annual Meeting, p. 71. Louisville, KY

Shannon MW and Haddad LM (1998) The emergency management of poisoning. In: *Clinical Management of Poisoning and Drug Overdose,* ed. LM Haddad *et al.,* pp. 2–31. WB Saunders, Philadelphia

Solter P and Scott R (1987) Onion ingestion and subsequent Heinz body anemia in a dog: a case report. *Journal of the American Animal Hospital Association* **23**, 544–546

Spoerke D (2006) Mushrooms. In: *Small Animal Toxicology,* eds. ME Peterson and PA Talcott, pp. 860–887. Elsevier Saunders, St. Louis

Thrall MA, Connally HE, Grauer GF and Hamar D (2006) Ethylene glycol. In: *Small Animal Toxicology,* eds. ME Peterson and PA Talcott, pp. 860–887. Elsevier Saunders, St. Louis

Tyler VE (1993) *The Honest Herbal: A Sensible Guide to the Use of Herbs and Related Remedies.* Pharmaceutical Products Press, New York

20

Cardiopulmonary–cerebral resuscitation

Edward Cooper and William W. Muir

Introduction

Cardiopulmonary–cerebral resuscitation (CPCR) continues to command a great deal of interest and occupy a large number of written pages in both research and clinical journals because of its catastrophic nature, the development of new treatment modalities, the clinical use of sophisticated monitoring techniques and the natural aversion to death. Cardiopulmonary arrest is defined as an abrupt cessation of spontaneous and effective ventilation and systemic perfusion (circulation), which leads to inadequate oxygen delivery to tissues, shock and death. Common causes include anaesthetic overdose, trauma (multiple fractures, head injury, coma) with or without exsanguination, acute cardiac failure from cardiac dysrhythmias or myocardial disease (cardiomyopathy, valvular insufficiency) and debilitating diseases.

CPCR is an organized pre-planned approach for providing artificial support of ventilation and circulation (basic life support) until spontaneous breathing and circulation can be restored and sustained (advanced life support). Regardless of the progress made in our understanding of pathophysiological processes and therapies, little or no improvement in long-term survival (patient leaves the hospital) following CPCR has been reported. Indeed, although several studies suggest initial survival rates ranging from 20–75%, most critical reviews of long-term survival following cardiopulmonary resuscitation in dogs and cats note that less than 5% of the patients resuscitated ever leave the hospital (Kass and Haskins, 1992; Wingfield and Van Pelt, 1992). There are many reasons for the discrepancies in the survival rate percentages reported, including the criteria used to determine when resuscitation should be initiated, which patients were selected for resuscitation, definitions of successful resuscitation and a host of patient-related (e.g. age, disease status), personnel (training, preparedness) and environmental (monitoring capabilities) considerations. Unfortunately no recent studies have been published to account for these variables, or to aid in determining whether there has been any increase in CPCR success rates. Certainly the best methods for improving patient survival are to maximize patient monitoring, have immediate access to drugs and equipment and to be familiar with the techniques and therapies necessary to perform CPCR. Stated in different terms, 'an ounce of prevention is worth a pound of cure' and 'practice makes perfect'.

When to resuscitate

The decision to begin CPCR is based upon clinical signs, consideration of the potential outcome and a previous agreement (if possible) with the animal owner (Figure 20.1). It is important to establish a code and technical approach for any critical patient or one that is to undergo general anaesthesia. That way, all personnel will be able to respond to the arrest appropriately. Resuscitation should be attempted in patients that have a treatable disease. CPCR should not be performed: in animals in the terminal stages of an incurable disease (hepatic, renal, cardiac failure, etc.); in those that have suffered severe head trauma with brain damage, where there is no reasonable chance of restoring near-normal mentation; or when the owner of the animal has instructed the veterinary surgeon not to resuscitate.

Changes in the effort, rate or rhythm of breathing
Dyspnoea (abdominal breathing)
Gasps (gurgling sounds)
Tachypnoea
Bradypnoea
Apnoea
Altered patterns of breathing:
   Periodic breathing
   Agonal breathing

Absence of pulse
The peripheral arterial pulse becomes difficult, if not impossible, to palpate at mean arterial blood pressures <30–40 mmHg

Irregular or inaudible heart sounds
Heart sounds of varying intensity suggest a cardiac dysrhythmia (atrial fibrillation, ventricular tachycardia)
Heart sounds become difficult to hear at mean arterial blood pressures <40 mmHg

Changes in heart rate or rhythm
Tachycardia
Bradycardia
Irregular rhythm

Absence of bleeding

Altered peripheral perfusion
Change in mucous membrane colour:
   Pale or white
   Blue or cyanotic: 50 g/l of reduced haemoglobin produces a
   bluish discoloration of the mucous membranes regardless of the
   haemoglobin concentration. Anaemic animals (<50 g/l
   haemoglobin; PCV ~ 15%) do not demonstrate cyanosis

Pupillary dilation
The pupils dilate within 1–2 minutes of cardiac arrest

Depression or coma

20.1 Signs and symptoms of impending cardiopulmonary arrest.

Phases of basic life support

Once the decision to perform CPCR has been made, basic and advanced life support should be initiated as rapidly as possible in a sequential, orderly and predetermined manner (Figure 20.2). All pertinent personnel should be prepared for and have practised appropriate CPCR techniques. Basic life support includes establishing and maintaining an airway (A), controlling breathing (B) and circulatory (C) support via the initiation of manual chest compression. There has been some suggestion that priority should be given to establishing circulation first, the CAB approach (Shapiro, 1998). This is based largely on the fact that primary cardiac disease often plays a role in human cardiac arrest. Additionally, thoracic compression alone has been shown to produce adequate ventilation, at least for a short period of time (Evans, 1999). However, since most cardiopulmonary arrests in veterinary medicine are respiratory or vagally induced, it seems that A–B–C is still the most appropriate sequence in our species. Advanced life support includes measures that lead to the establishment and maintenance of spontaneous breathing and circulation at or above normal values, via the administration of drugs (D), evaluation of the electrocardiogram (E) and treatment of cardiac dysrhythmias, including ventricular fibrillation (F). Figure 20.3 lists emergency cart supplies.

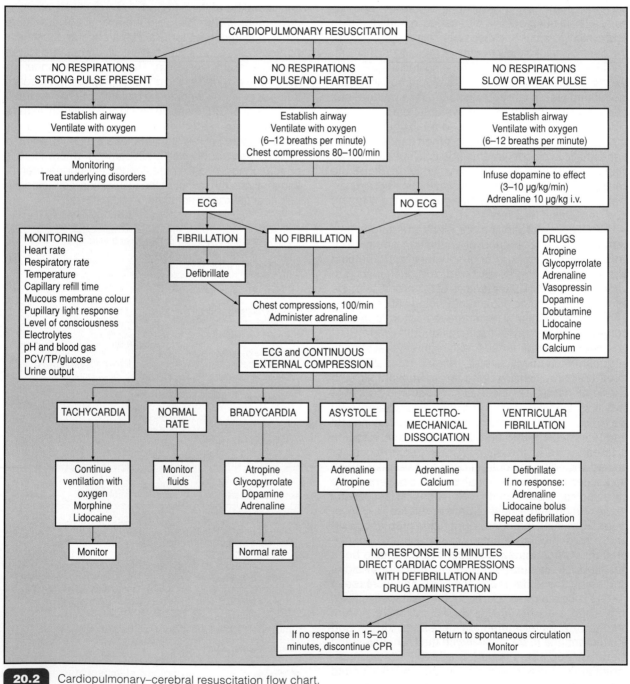

20.2 Cardiopulmonary–cerebral resuscitation flow chart.

Drugs
Atropine/glycopyrrolate
Calcium gluconate
Adrenaline
Dopamine
Dobutamine
Vasopressin
Lidocaine
Furosemide
Mannitol
Sodium bicarbonate
Diazepam
50% dextrose
Lactated Ringer's solution

Supplies
Pressure bag for rapid fluid infusion
Ambu bag
Various sizes of endotracheal tubes
Laryngoscope
Isopropyl alcohol
Antiseptic scrub
Hypodermic needles, various sizes
Assorted intravenous catheters
2 x 50 mm, 4 x 100 mm gauze sponges/swabs
12 mm, 25 mm, 50 mm tape
50 mm roll of gauze
Polyethylene urinary catheters
Suture material
Three-way stopcocks
Thoracostomy tray with loaded scalpel
Clippers
Electrocardiogram monitor
Doppler blood pressure monitor
Defibrillator
External and sterile internal defibrillator paddles

20.3 Emergency cart supplies.

Airway

An essential step in performing CPCR is the establishment of a secure and patent airway. The most effective way to achieve this goal is by endotracheal intubation with a cuffed endotracheal tube. The head should be extended and pulled forward prior to endotracheal intubation. Occasionally, animals become cyanotic and subsequently unconscious because mucus, soft tissue structures (soft palate, tongue) or foreign material such as food obstructs the upper airway. Brachycephalic breeds are particularly susceptible to upper airway obstruction during recovery from anaesthesia. Placement of an endotracheal tube ensures access to an unobstructed airway, and allows mucus or foreign material to be removed manually or by suction.

When airway obstruction is severe or cannot be removed, an emergency tracheostomy should be performed (see Chapter 7). A 3–5 cm incision is made on the ventral midline parallel to the trachea, 2–4 cm caudal to the larynx (Figure 20.4). The tissue over the trachea is bluntly dissected and an incision is made between the tracheal rings, through which an endotracheal tube is placed. In animals with incomplete upper airway obstruction, transtracheal catheter

ventilation, an alternative to tracheostomy, is less traumatic (Reich and Mingus, 1990). Ventilation is achieved by transcutaneously puncturing the trachea with a 14 gauge plastic intravenous over-the-needle catheter assembly. The catheter is attached to venous extension tubing and a hand-operated oxygen release valve (Figure 20.5). Oxygen flow rates are adjusted initially to 50 ml/kg. This technique has the advantage of providing 100% oxygen directly into the trachea and is relatively atraumatic. Tracheostomy generally remains the technique of choice, however, because it may allow spontaneous breathing of room air until the obstruction can be resolved. Tracheostomy can also

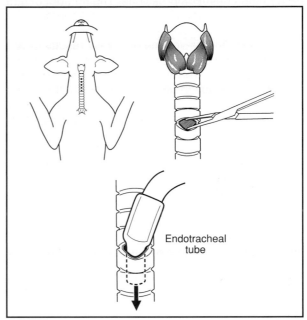

Endotracheal tube

20.4 A tracheostomy is performed as illustrated after creating a ventral midline incision.

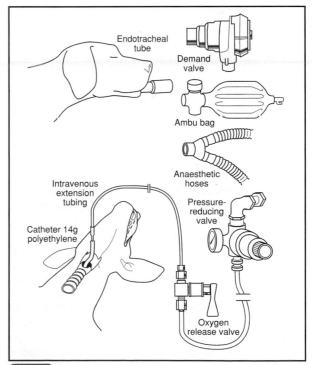

Endotracheal tube
Demand valve
Ambu bag
Anaesthetic hoses
Pressure-reducing valve
Intravenous extension tubing
Catheter 14g polyethylene
Oxygen release valve

20.5 Methods of providing oxygen.

be useful in conscious animals that require ventilatory assistance, because of the difficulty in maintaining orotracheal intubation without general anaesthesia.

Breathing

Controlled or assisted ventilation can be accomplished by connecting a properly placed endotracheal tube to a self-inflating Ambu bag, demand valve or anaesthetic machine (see Figure 20.5). Respiratory rate should be between 6 and 12 breaths per minute in animals with normal lungs. Ratios of one breath to five chest compressions or two breaths per 10–15 chest compressions are used when simultaneously performing chest compressions. The amount of gas volume delivered (tidal volume) should approximate 15 ml/kg at a maximum peak inspiratory pressure of 20–25 cmH$_2$O. This volume generally results in visible but minimal expansion of the chest or movement of the abdomen. The lungs of cats and neonates, and normal alveoli in patients with restrictive types of lung disease (e.g. pneumonia, adult respiratory distress syndrome (ARDS), pulmonary fibrosis, diaphragmatic hernia) are easily overinflated. Lung overexpansion can lead to pulmonary barotrauma, inflammation, haemorrhage and pneumothorax. Smaller tidal volumes (6–10 ml/kg) at higher respiratory rates (15–20 breaths per minute) should be used in these patients.

Poor training and the excitement associated with CPCR can often lead to overly aggressive ventilation. This should be avoided as it can be harmful for a number of reasons. Hypocapnia associated with hyperventilation can lead to decreased cerebral perfusion from reflex vasoconstriction, thereby worsening neuronal injury. In addition, studies in experimental swine have demonstrated that hyperventilation during CPCR is associated with lower coronary perfusion pressures and reduced survival (Aufderheide and Lurie, 2004). Furthermore, excessively long inspiratory times (>3 seconds) or the maintenance of positive end expiratory pressure (PEEP) greater than 10 cmH$_2$O increase intrathoracic pressure, thereby decreasing venous return, cardiac output and arterial blood pressure. Small amounts (3–5 cmH$_2$O) of PEEP, however, are not harmful, are inconsequential when the thoracic cavity is open to the atmosphere during internal cardiac massage and may improve arterial oxygenation. Mechanical artificial respiratory assist devices, particularly pressure-cycled ventilators, perform poorly during CPCR. The intrathoracic pressure fluctuations produced by chest compression cause mechanical respirators to initiate or terminate the inspiratory cycle prematurely, resulting in inadequate ventilation.

Mouth-to-nose ventilation is performed if endotracheal tubes and ventilatory assist devices are not available. It is accomplished by cupping both hands around the animal's muzzle, placing the operator's mouth against the thumbs (attempting to produce an airtight seal) and blowing air into the animal's mouth. Inflation of the stomach with air may occur, but can be avoided by pushing the larynx dorsally in order to occlude the oesophagus. This technique is inefficient, but easily performed and can be life saving in puppies and kittens or in larger dogs and cats in acute respiratory distress situations after removal of foreign material from the upper airway.

Kinking or mucus obstruction of the endotracheal tube, oesophageal intubation and accidental intubation of a mainstem bronchus make it difficult to inflate the lungs (high inspiratory pressure) and frequently produce dyspnoea and cyanosis. Other conditions that restrict breathing include pleural effusions, diaphragmatic hernia and pneumothorax. Auscultation and percussion of the chest are helpful diagnostic techniques which may differentiate between these problems. Muffled heart sounds and a damped response to percussion may indicate fluid or tissue in the thoracic cavity. Normal heart sounds and a hyper-resonant chest may indicate pneumothorax or tension pneumothorax. Thoracocentesis, a chest drain or an open-chest approach should be used to remove excessive fluid or air, particularly when tension pneumothorax is suspected.

Ventilatory support should not be stopped once signs of spontaneous ventilation begin. Intermittent positive pressure ventilation is usually necessary until the patient regains consciousness. Listening to the end of the endotracheal tube, watching for normal ventilatory movement of the chest wall and continued monitoring of mucous membrane colour and capillary refill time will help to assess the adequacy of ventilation. Measurement of arterial pH and blood gases on a point-of-care analyser, or non-invasive assessment of oxygen saturation using pulse oximetry (S_pO_2 >90%) and ventilation using end-tidal (ET) capnography (ETCO$_2$ 30–40 mmHg) are also important techniques. Following extubation, nasal oxygen and oxygen cages help to maintain arterial oxygenation in conscious animals (Fitzpatrick and Crowe, 1986).

Acupuncture stimulation of governor vessel 26 (GV 26; Jen Chung) has been used successfully to restore respiratory and cardiac function in cats, dogs, kittens and puppies. Acupuncture therapy consists of vigorous pricking and twirling of a 25 gauge needle 2–4 mm deep in GV 26, a point located in the 'T' formed in the philtrum below the nose or in the midline of the nasolabial cleft at the level of the lower canthi with the nostrils (Janssens et al., 1979; Altman, 1997).

Circulation

Closed-chest CPCR

The restoration of normal cardiac electrical and pumping activity depends upon the early restoration of myocardial oxygenation and blood flow. Blood flow is initiated and supported by compressing the chest wall. Blood moves through the heart and vessels during chest compression due to direct cardiac compression in cats and narrow-chested dogs (cardiac pump mechanism), and phasic increases in intrathoracic pressure, which collapses intrathoracic veins, in larger animals (thoracic pump mechanism; Peters and Ihle, 1990). The ideal chest compression rate in dogs and cats is approximately 100 compressions per minute, devoting equal time to compression and relaxation.

Effective chest compression in small animals is accomplished by compressing the chest wall from side to side with the animal in lateral recumbency (Figure 20.6). The heel of one hand compresses one side of the chest wall while the palm of the other hand or a sand-filled pillow is placed under the opposing chest wall for support. The thumb and forefinger can be used to accomplish the same manoeuvre in cats and very small dogs. Attention should be focused upon how fast the heel of the hand compresses the thorax, not the force necessary to compress the chest, although enough force must be generated to produce an obvious indentation of the chest wall of approximately 1–3 cm depending on patient size. Alternatively, mechanical chest compression devices have been investigated in dogs and, while there was some improvement in haemodynamic parameters, there was no impact on survival or neurological outcome when compared to manual compressions (Wik *et al.*, 1996).

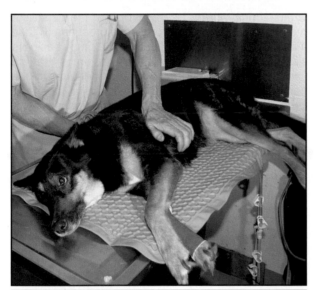

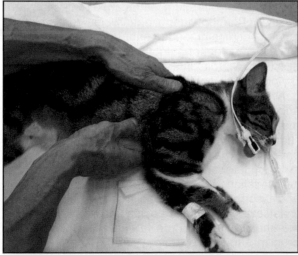

20.6 Correct hand positioning for performing chest compressions in the dog and cat.

A breath should be given once every fifth or sixth chest compression, or 2–3 times for every 10–15 chest compressions. Blood flow to the brain and heart was more effectively maintained by administering chest compressions simultaneously with ventilation at relatively high airway pressures (30–40 cmH$_2$O), combined with abdominal binding (Koehler *et al.*, 1983). Intermittent slow abdominal compression (counterpressure) appears to be another effective means of improving blood flow during resuscitative efforts. A recent meta-analysis of studies involving humans, dogs and pigs concluded that this method was effective and safe at improving organ perfusion and overall survival (Babbs, 2003). Abdominal counterpressure is accomplished by having a second person use the palms of both hands to compress the abdominal cavity slowly at approximately 20-second intervals. Alternatively, the abdomen may be temporarily bound during CPCR with an elastic bandage or towel if extra help is not available.

Signs of restoration of effective peripheral blood flow include improvement in mucous membrane colour, decrease in capillary refill time, reduction in pupil size and restoration of a peripheral arterial pulse. The peripheral arterial pulse should be evaluated during a short pause in chest compression because pulse waves carried into the femoral veins during chest compression may be mistaken for an arterial pulse.

Open-chest CPCR
Attempts to maintain peripheral blood flow by chest compression should be evaluated within 3–4 minutes of initiating CPCR. If signs of successful resuscitation are not evident or if the patient continues to deteriorate (bradycardia or cardiac arrest), the chest should be opened and internal (direct) cardiac massage initiated. Severe chest trauma, fractured ribs, pneumothorax, haemothorax, pericardial effusion, diaphragmatic hernia and other primary thoracic diseases (neoplasms, foreign bodies) are reasons for immediately initiating direct cardiac compression in patients that require CPCR. The chest is opened by making an incision from the top of the scapula to approximately 4 cm from the sternum on the left thoracic wall, at the cranial aspect of the fifth rib (fourth intercostal space) avoiding the intercostal vessels and nerves. To limit contamination, the hair should be clipped and antiseptic solution applied to the skin prior to making the approach. Care must be taken not to damage the lung when entering the thoracic cavity. Once the chest is entered, the fourth and fifth ribs are spread apart and the lungs are reflected dorsally and caudally. The pericardium is grasped and opened near the apex of the heart, and reflected dorsally exposing the ventricles. In smaller patients the heart is grasped between the thumb and forefinger and direct cardiac massage initiated at a rate of approximately 100 compressions per minute. In larger patients the heart is held between the palm and fingers using a reverse-milking motion to compress the heart. Excessive force during direct cardiac compression should be avoided as it can result in severe cardiac trauma, cardiac dysrhythmias and ventricular fibrillation.

The colour, tone and rhythm of the heart can be evaluated once the chest is open. The presence of adequate ventricular filling can be assessed, and a decision made whether additional fluid resuscitation is required. Cardiac colour can be improved by appropriate ventilation and cardiac compression. Cardiac contractile function and rhythm can be improved by normalizing acid–base and electrolyte balance and the administration of cardiotonic or anti-dysrhythmic drugs. In larger dogs, the aorta can be compressed dorsally against the spine with the thumb of the opposite hand, which promotes blood flow to the heart and brain. Direct cardiac compression always produces better blood flow than closed-chest compression and has been associated with improved survival and neurological outcome (Benson *et al.*, 2005). However, this technique does require surgical intervention and predisposes to infection.

Fluid therapy

Fluid therapy is another important consideration when trying to re-establish effective circulation during a cardiopulmonary arrest. If cardiac arrest is thought to be secondary to hypovolaemia, aggressive fluid resuscitation may be warranted, especially once a spontaneous heart beat has occurred. However, in the euvolaemic patient large amounts of intravenous fluids may be detrimental, especially if lung disease is also present. Furthermore, coronary perfusion is dictated by the difference between ventricular pressures. Excessive fluid therapy could lead to right-sided pressure loading and significant impairment of myocardial blood flow in animals with poor cardiac function (Voorhees *et al.*, 1987). Therefore only small amounts of intravenous fluid (1–2 ml/kg/h), if any, should be administered until cardiac function is restored.

Monitoring circulation during CPCR

Whether cardiac compressions are performed with an open or a closed chest, it is important to determine whether adequate blood flow is being achieved. Invasive monitoring of direct arterial pressures or cardiac output is ideal, but is rarely possible or practical. Palpation of femoral pulses can be helpful but is not a very sensitive indicator of perfusion, especially regarding more vital structures (heart, lungs, brain). Monitoring end-tidal carbon dioxide can be a useful and non-invasive marker of pulmonary perfusion. If there is inadequate venous return and delivery of blood to the lungs, carbon dioxide cannot be exchanged and expired and thus end-tidal carbon dioxide is low. Attaining higher end-tidal carbon dioxide levels during resuscitation is associated with improved survival, and is potentially a better marker of adequate perfusion than cardiac output or cerebral blood flow (Blumenthal *et al.*, 1997). Another way of determining if cerebral blood flow is being established is the assessment of transcorneal Doppler blood flow. The same Doppler crystal used to measure blood pressure can be placed directly on the cornea and pulsatile blood flow can be heard with each compression (Figure 20.7). While this technique does not provide quantitative information it can help determine whether cardiac compressions are producing blood flow to the head.

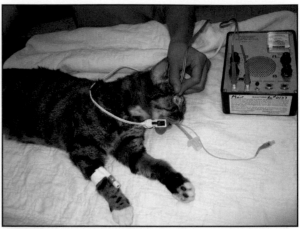

20.7 Use of transcorneal Doppler for detection of cerebral blood flow.

Drugs

Drugs should not be used to replace the establishment of an airway (A), restoration of breathing (B) and manual support of the circulation (C). Once basic life support has been initiated, however, drugs may be used to promote restoration of spontaneous circulation or to address the underlying cause of the arrest. Drugs should always be administered by bolus injection and followed by 1–3 ml of crystalloid flush through a peripheral vein (Figure 20.8). Drug administration should occur simultaneously with chest compression, if possible, since the chest compressions are responsible for blood flow and the delivery of the drug to the heart and brain. Intravenous drug administration is preferred, although intracardiac and intratracheal (endobronchial) routes can be used when venous access is not readily available (Mazkereth *et al.*, 1992). Using the intracardiac route, drugs are deliberately injected into the lumen of the left ventricle in order to hasten their delivery to the coronary arteries and ventricular myocardium. Intracardiac injections are easily performed during open-chest resuscitation, but are not recommended prior to opening the chest, since inadvertent pneumothorax, haemopericardium or intramyocardial injections leading to cardiac dysrhythmias can occur. The intracardiac drug dose is generally one half the intravenous dose, while the endobronchial dose is two to three times the recommended intravenous dose. Adrenaline, atropine and lidocaine can all be administered by the endobronchial route. The drugs are diluted in saline to administer 1 ml/5 kg, and followed by two or three manual lung inflations in order to promote drug distribution and absorption from the lung. It can be helpful to pass a sterile red rubber or male dog urinary catheter down the endotracheal tube to facilitate instillation of the drug into the lower airways. Sodium bicarbonate should never be administered by the endobronchial route as it causes severe airway irritation.

Adrenaline, a catecholamine, is the first drug selected for the treatment of severe bradycardia that is non-responsive to atropine, severe hypotension and cardiac arrest. The administration of adrenaline during CPCR significantly improves myocardial and

Drug	Indications	Dosage	Action
Adrenaline	Severe bradycardia Ventricular fibrillation Ventricular asystole Pulseless electrical activity	0.01–0.2 mg/kg i.v. bolus q3–5min 0.04–0.4 mg/kg intratracheal 0.1–1 µg/kg/min i.v. CRI	α- and β-adrenergic agonist
Atropine sulphate	Sinus bradycardia Atrioventricular block Ventricular asystole	0.04 mg/kg i.v 0.4 mg/kg intratracheal	Parasympatholytic
Calcium gluconate (10%)	Hyperkalaemia Hypocalcaemia Calcium channel-blocker toxicity Hypermagnesaemia	0.5–1.0 ml/kg i.v. to effect; closely observe the ECG	Positive inotrope Affects cardiac threshold potential to normalize cardiac conduction
Diltiazem	Supraventricular tachycardia Ventricular fibrillation Hypertrophic cardiomyopathy	Dogs: 0.5–1.5 mg/kg q8h orally Cats: 1.75–2.4 mg/kg q8–12h orally Dogs, cats: 0.25 mg/kg i.v. bolus, to cumulative dose of 0.75 mg/kg 5–10 µg/kg/min CRI	Calcium channel blocker
Dobutamine	Myocardial failure Low cardiac output	5–20 µg/kg/min CRI	Positive inotrope β-adrenergic agonist
Dopamine	Bradycardia Low cardiac output Hypotension	5–10 µg/kg/min CRI for increased contractility and cardiac output 10–20 µg/kg/min CRI for vasoconstriction	Noradrenaline precursor Dose-dependent α- and/or β-adrenergic agonist
Flumazenil	Benzodiazapine overdose	0.02 mg/kg i.v.	Benzodiazapine antagonist
Glycopyrrolate	Sinus bradycardia Atrioventricular block Ventricular asystole	0.004–0.010 mg/kg i.v.	Parasympatholytic
Furosemide	Cerebral/pulmonary oedema Congestive heart failure Hypertension Oliguria/anuria	Dogs: 2–4 mg/kg i.v., i.m. Cats: 1–2 mg/kg i.v., i.m.	Loop diuretic
Lidocaine	Ventricular tachycardia Ventricular fibrillation	Dogs: 2–8 mg/kg i.v. bolus followed by 30–80 µg/kg/min CRI Cats: 0.25–0.5 mg/kg i.v. bolus followed by 10–20 µg/kg/min CRI	Class 1B ventricular anti-dysrhythmic
Magnesium chloride	Unresponsive ventricular dysrhythmias (torsade) Chemical defibrillator Severe hypotension	10–15 mg/kg i.v. given slowly over 5 min	Electrolyte chemical defibrillator
Mannitol	Cerebral oedema Free radical scavenger Oliguria	0.5–1.0 mg/kg i.v. given slowly over 10 min	Osmotic diuretic
Morphine sulphate	Analgesia/sedation Vasodilator Pulmonary oedema	0.04–0.08 mg/kg i.v., i.m., s.c.	Narcotic analgesia
Naloxone	Electromechanical dissociation Narcotic overdose	0.03 mg/kg i.v. or intrathecal	Opiate antagonist
Sodium bicarbonate	Severe metabolic acidosis	0.5–1.0 mEq/kg i.v.	Alkalinizing agent
Vasopressin	Ventricular fibrillation Asystole Pulseless electrical activity	0.8 IU/kg once	Vasoconstriction

20.8 Drugs commonly employed during and following cardiopulmonary resuscitation.

cerebral blood flow by causing intense vasoconstriction of peripheral vascular beds, thereby centralizing blood volume. Adrenaline increases heart rate, arterial blood pressure and blood flow. Although large doses of adrenaline (0.2 mg/kg i.v.) are recommended when cardiopulmonary arrest is unwitnessed and resuscitation is delayed, smaller doses (0.01–0.02 mg/kg i.v.) should be used to treat the acute development of bradycardia or ventricular asystole (Figure 20.9) (Brown *et al.*, 1992). Adrenaline overdose can produce ventricular dysrhythmias, ventricular fibrillation and cardiac contracture ('stone heart').

Route	Dose (mg/kg)	Comments

Intravenous:
  Arrest/fibrillation
  Severe hypotension
  Bradycardia
	0.01–0.05
	0.01–0.02
	0.01–0.02
		Used to treat unwitnessed cardiac arrest [a]
		Used to treat witnessed cardiac arrest and bradycardia

Intracardiac	0.005–0.01	For bradycardia
Intratracheal	0.05–0.2	Dilute with 0.9% saline to deliver total volume of 1 ml/5 kg and provide three to four positive pressure breaths following administration

20.9 Emergency doses of adrenaline. [a] Note that larger doses of adrenaline (0.1–0.2 mg/kg i.v.) are used if arrest is unwitnessed *and* suspected to have been present for more than 2–3 minutes.

Atropine and glycopyrrolate are anticholinergics that are particularly effective in treating bradydysrhythmias caused by increases in vagal tone. Opioids (morphine, oxymorphone, fentanyl), α-2 agonists (xylazine, medetomidine, romifidine) and occasionally inhalant anaesthetics (halothane, isoflurane, sevoflurane) can produce bradydysrhythmias that are responsive to anticholinergic therapy. Profound bradycardia, asystole and bradydysrhythmias that are unresponsive to initial doses of either atropine or glycopyrrolate should be treated with adrenaline. Excessive doses of anticholinergics can produce sinus tachycardia and predispose to ventricular dysrhythmias. If the cause of bradycardia is unknown, or due to anaesthetic overdose, low doses (0.01 mg/kg i.v.) of adrenaline should be administered.

Once heart rate, rhythm and a palpable pulse have been restored, either dopamine (3–10 μg/kg/min i.v.) or dobutamine (5–20 μg/kg/min i.v.) can be used to maintain arterial blood pressure and blood flow. Dopamine is the preferred drug if the heart rate continues to be slow, while dobutamine is preferred when the heart rate is within normal limits or elevated. Dopamine is more likely to increase heart rate than dobutamine, but both drugs increase arterial blood pressure and systemic blood flow. As with all catecholamines, excessive doses can cause sinus tachycardia, ventricular dysrhythmias and ventricular fibrillation.

Lidocaine, a local anaesthetic, possesses potent anti-dysrhythmic, antishock and analgesic effects. Lidocaine is particularly effective in treating ventricular dysrhythmias if the patient is not hypokalaemic (potassium <3.0 mmol/l). Neurological side effects (muscle twitching, seizures) may occur if excessive doses are administered, particularly to cats. Initial bolus doses should not exceed 4 mg/kg in dogs and 1 mg/kg in cats. A lidocaine infusion (30–80 μg/kg/min) is used to produce sustained effects for periods of up to 24–48 hours when necessary.

Sodium bicarbonate is used to treat non-respiratory (metabolic) acidosis. Severe lactic acidosis is common following cardiopulmonary arrest and results from anaerobic metabolism due to tissue hypoxia. Severe acidosis leads to central nervous system (CNS) depression, myocardial depression, decreased catecholamine responsiveness and the production and release of tissue destructive metabolites. Sodium bicarbonate may be administered either during prolonged resuscitation attempts or in the immediate post-arrest period to try and reduce some of these effects. Excessive sodium bicarbonate administration, however, produces alkalaemia, decreases serum ionized calcium and impairs the release of oxygen from haemoglobin. The required dose of sodium bicarbonate can be calculated from blood gas results, using the base excess (BE), according to the following equation:

Total bicarbonate deficit = 0.3 x BW (kg) x BE

Although this equation gives the total deficit of bicarbonate, the initial dose administered should be approximately one third to one half the calculated total. The acid–base status should then be re-assessed and the remainder given only if necessary. In the absence of blood gas analysis, the initial dose of sodium bicarbonate should not exceed 1 mEq/kg unless there is evidence of severe non-respiratory acidosis (dehydration, diarrhoea, lactic acidosis). Subsequent doses (0.5 mmol/kg i.v.) of sodium bicarbonate may be administered every 10 minutes until the circulation is restored or resuscitative efforts are terminated.

Vasopressin was added to the 2000 Guidelines for Advanced Life Support, as an alternative or an addition to adrenaline. Vasopressin causes vasoconstriction and, unlike catecholamines, is not affected by acidosis. Therefore, it may be effective when adrenaline is not. A number of experimental studies, primarily conducted in pigs, have shown increased cerebral and coronary perfusion using vasopressin, when adrenaline has failed to produce a response. One study showed improved neurological recovery when vasopressin and adrenaline were administered together after prolonged CPCR (Stadlbauer *et al.*, 2003). Human patients with higher vasopressin levels are more likely to survive CPCR (Lindner *et al.*, 1996), suggesting that vasopressin supplementation during arrest could be of benefit. Preliminary trials in people suggested that administration of 40 IU of vasopressin improved resuscitation and 24-hour survival following ventricular fibrillation (Lindner *et al.*, 1997). Despite these encouraging results, a recent meta-analysis of several human studies (Aung *et al.*, 2005) found no clear advantage for the use of vasopressin in CPCR. Although there have been only rare case reports and no published clinical trials, the use of vasopressin during CPCR in dogs is still a potential consideration (0.8 IU/kg, once i.v.).

Other drugs that have been used for the acute treatment of cardiac arrest include calcium gluconate, diltiazem and magnesium chloride (see Figure 20.8) (Capparelli *et al.*, 1992). None of these drugs has been shown to improve long-term outcome, although the administration of calcium-containing solutions is therapeutic in patients with hypocalcaemia, hyperkalaemia, overdose of a calcium channel blocking drug (verapamil, diltiazem) or inhalant anaesthetic arrest. However, calcium has been shown to play a significant role in ischaemia–reperfusion injury and secondary brain injury in the post-resuscitation period. Therefore, calcium-containing solutions are not recommended for routine use in CPCR.

Electrocardiography

An electrocardiogram (ECG) is essential for accurate diagnosis of cardiac rhythm disturbances (Figures 20.10 and 20.11) and provides valuable insights for appropriate drug selection. A normal ECG, however, does not ensure that cardiac contractile function is adequate to maintain arterial blood pressure or peripheral blood flow.

Cause	Peripheral pulse	Auscultation of heart sounds	ECG	Visual observation of heart
Pulseless electrical activity	Very weak or absent	Normal, muffled or none	Normal P-QRS-T, rapid, normal or slow heart rate. P-QRS-T may become increasingly wide and bizarre if treatment is unsuccessful	Weak or absent cardiac contractions, poor filling
Bradycardia	Slow, may be irregular	Normal or muffled, infrequent	Infrequent P-QRS-T or ventricular complexes; junctional or ventricular escape complexes	Infrequent coordinated ventricular contractions
Supraventricular tachycardia	Rapid, may be weak, pulse deficit	Normal or muffled intensity; may be irregular	Normal QRS-T; may have inverted or abnormal P waves, P wave may be buried in previous T wave	Rapid, occasionally irregular heart beat
Ventricular tachycardia	Weak and rapid with pulse deficits; may be irregular	Muffled, may be of variable intensity	Wide QRS complexes, absence of P-QRS relationship; large T waves	Disorganized rapidly beating heart
Ventricular asystole (cardiac arrest)	None	None	Absent QRS-T complexes; straight flat-line ECG	No cardiac movement
Ventricular fibrillation	None	None	Absent QRS-T complexes; fibrillation waves	Fine to coarse rippling of the ventricular myocardium

20.10 Distinguishing characteristics of several types of cardiac rhythm or arrest disorders.

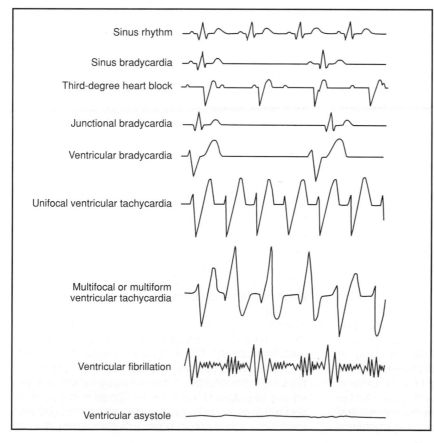

Sinus rhythm

Sinus bradycardia

Third-degree heart block

Junctional bradycardia

Ventricular bradycardia

Unifocal ventricular tachycardia

Multifocal or multiform ventricular tachycardia

Ventricular fibrillation

Ventricular asystole

20.11

Cardiac rhythms observed during CPCR in the dog and cat.

Pulseless electrical activity (PEA) is a catch-all term used to describe patients that have electrocardiographic evidence of a cardiac rhythm, but a very weak or non-palpable peripheral arterial pulse. Patients may or may not have an auscultatable heart beat. Clinically, patients in normal sinus rhythm but with a systolic arterial blood pressure below 40–50 mmHg are considered to be demonstrating PEA. The most extreme form of PEA is electromechanical dissociation (EMD), where there is electrocardiographic evidence of organized electrical activity (sinus or ventricular rhythm), but complete absence of effective myocardial contraction. Anaesthetic overdose, acute hypoxia, severe acidosis, systemic toxicity and cardiogenic shock are potential causes of EMD. The term PEA has largely supplanted the use of the term EMD in clinical practice. Treatment of PEA involves addressing the underlying cause(s), and the administration of adrenaline.

Bradydysrhythmias (sinus bradycardia, third-degree heart block, ventricular escape rhythm) are potential causes of cardiac arrest or fibrillation, and are common occurrences in traumatized, anaesthetized or endotoxaemic patients, or immediately after successful CPCR. Sinus bradycardia and junctional escape rhythms are frequently observed during hypoxia and prior to ventricular asystole or fibrillation, while junctional and ventricular (idioventricular) escape rhythms can develop after defibrillation (Figure 20.11). These rhythm disturbances are impossible to distinguish from one another without an ECG. Their haemodynamic consequences are similar, resulting in hypotension and poor systemic blood flow. Patients that present with slow junctional or idioventricular escape rhythms should be suspected of suffering from severe hypoxia, hyperkalaemia or systemic toxicity. Therapy includes anticholinergics (atropine, glycopyrrolate), adrenaline or specific techniques to lower serum potassium. Normal saline, sodium bicarbonate, dextrose with or without insulin, and hyperventilation may help to lower serum potassium when acute hyperkalaemia is responsible for the bradydysrhythmia. Calcium gluconate can be used to rapidly reverse the bradycardia and improve cardiac contractility until the other measures have diminished the hyperkalaemia. If cardiac arrest secondary to hyperkalaemia is suspected (e.g. urethral obstruction), calcium gluconate should be the first drug used during resuscitation. When the cause for the acute onset of bradycardia is unknown, the first steps should be to administer oxygen, begin chest compression and administer adrenaline and/or atropine. Adrenaline should also be administered intravenously when the heart rate is rapidly slowing and peripheral pulses are not palpable.

Ventricular tachycardia may be difficult to distinguish from sinus tachycardia without the aid of an ECG, since both can produce a weak peripheral pulse. Lidocaine is the drug of choice for the treatment of most ventricular dysrhythmias and is administered intravenously as a bolus or infusion. Intravenous procainamide (5–10 mg/kg i.v.) can be used as an alternative if lidocaine is not effective in restoring normal sinus rhythm. The serum potassium concentration should be determined and normalized (4–5 mmol/l), since most anti-dysrhythmics are ineffective in hypokalaemic patients and toxic in hyperkalaemic patients. If the peripheral pulse remains weak after normal sinus rhythm has been restored, infusions of fluids, dopamine or dobutamine can be administered to improve cardiac contractility, increase arterial blood pressure and enhance peripheral perfusion. Alternatively, low intravenous doses of adrenaline can be administered. In the post-arrest patient, intravenous sodium bicarbonate can assist with restoration of normal sinus rhythm if metabolic acidosis is present.

Ventricular asystole is difficult, if not impossible, to distinguish from ventricular fibrillation without an ECG (see Figure 20.11). This distinction is important, since ventricular asystole may respond to chest compression and the administration of adrenaline, while ventricular fibrillation requires electrical defibrillation. In either case, an airway should be established, and breathing and chest compression should be instituted immediately. All anaesthetic drugs should be discontinued. Adrenaline and sodium bicarbonate should be administered intravenously. Adrenaline can be re-administered at 3–5-minute intervals if asystole persists. External electrical defibrillation is required if asystole converts to ventricular fibrillation. Dopamine or dobutamine are administered by infusion once heart rhythm is restored. Ventricular asystole usually results from severe myocardial depression and is associated with a poor prognosis.

The most common ECG rhythm in humans experiencing cardiopulmonary arrest is ventricular fibrillation, occurring as the initial disturbance in approximately 60–70% of patients (Holmburg et al., 2000). In veterinary patients, however, PEA is the most common rhythm, occurring in 23.3% of all arrests in one study (Rush and Wingfield, 1992). Ventricular asystole is almost as common, occurring in 22.8% of arrests. Other frequently recognized rhythms included ventricular fibrillation (19.8% of arrests) and sinus bradycardia (19.0%). This difference in frequency of arrest rhythms between species is probably attributable to the different circumstances under which CPA occurs. Cardiac arrest in humans most commonly involves myocardial infarction secondary to coronary artery disease, predisposing to ventricular fibrillation. In veterinary patients, cardiac arrests are more frequently associated with systemic illness, with anaesthesia, or preceded by respiratory arrest. Unfortunately, at least in human medicine, the prognosis for survival in patients with ventricular fibrillation is much better than in those with either asystole or PEA (Holmburg et al., 2000).

Fibrillation and defibrillation

Ventricular fibrillation is an irregular quivering motion of the ventricles caused by continuous disorganized electrical activity. The ECG demonstrates fibrillatory waves (no QRS complexes) which are not effective in creating the coordinated myocardial contractions necessary to propel blood forward. Blood is not pumped and patients are pulseless. Lidocaine cannot convert ventricular fibrillation to normal sinus rhythm, but can be used to prevent ventricular dysrhythmias following defibrillation. The inability to convert ventricular fibrillation to sinus rhythm, or the recurrence of ventricular fibrillation after restoration of a cardiac rhythm, is an indication of myocardial hypoxia, acidosis, depression or severe systemic disease. The adequacy of ventilation, chest or cardiac compression and initial therapies should be re-evaluated frequently. Intravenous or intracardiac adrenaline should be administered prior to repeated attempts to defibrillate the heart. Occasionally during open-chest CPCR, drugs are deliberately injected into the left ventricle (intracardiac) in order to hasten their delivery to the coronary arteries and ventricular myocardium. Once a stable cardiac rhythm is produced, dobutamine or dopamine can be used to maintain arterial blood pressure and systemic blood flow.

Electrical defibrillation remains the method of choice for the conversion of severe unresponsive ventricular dysrhythmias or ventricular fibrillation to sinus rhythm (Figure 20.12). Electrical defibrillation should be performed as soon as ventricular fibrillation is diagnosed, because survival decreases linearly with increasing time to defibrillation. In order to achieve the most effective defibrillation, the electrical current should be transmitted directly across the heart. To facilitate this in closed-chest defibrillation, the patient should be placed in dorsal recumbency allowing placement of the paddles on either side of the chest, avoiding contact between the paddles and the table. Ideally, the hair should be clipped on both sides of the chest (although the urgency of the situation may preclude this) and a liberal amount of contact gel applied to

both paddles to ensure adequate contact. Care should be taken to ensure that the two gelled areas on the patient remain separate, and that the paddles do not touch each other, or the electrical discharge will occur along these lower resistance routes rather than through the thoracic cavity. Prior to discharging the defibrillator the operator should announce 'clear' and make sure that no one is in contact with the patient or the table, to avoid inadvertent shock to personnel. Adrenaline (0.01–0.05 mg/kg i.v.) should be administered and defibrillation repeated if initial attempts to restore a perfusing cardiac rhythm are unsuccessful. Few data are available on the clinical efficacy of chemical methods of producing defibrillation.

Monitoring

Proper post-resuscitation monitoring and therapy are as critical as the resuscitation period itself if the patient is to survive. The period of hypoxia and ischaemia, regardless of how brief, results in metabolic acidosis and reperfusion injury to multiple organ systems. These effects can lead to temporary or permanent blindness, neurological deficits, pulmonary oedema, gastrointestinal mucosal sloughing, renal failure, hypothermia and shock. At particular risk is the CNS where ischaemia/reperfusion is characterized by neuronal damage and an increase in capillary and blood–brain barrier permeability, resulting in cerebral oedema and increased intracranial pressure. Careful monitoring of CNS signs (mental status), heart rate and rhythm (ECG), the peripheral pulse (arterial blood pressure), packed cell volume, total protein/solids, arterial blood gas and acid–base parameters (pH, pO_2, pCO_2), electrolytes (Na^+, K^+, Ca^{2+}), and urine production (1–2 ml/kg/h) is essential. Mechanical ventilation may be required for many hours following resuscitation in order to enhance success. Infusions of dopamine or dobutamine are useful in maintaining cardiac contractility and peripheral blood flow during the post-resuscitation period. Judicious use of isotonic replacement solutions, with frequent auscultation of the chest and measurement of central venous pressures and urinary output, helps to prevent pulmonary or cerebral oedema (Fischer and Hossmann, 1996).

Brain ischaemia

The clinical consequences of partial or complete brain ischaemia include sensory deficits, blindness, cerebral oedema, seizures and coma, culminating in respiratory arrest and cardiovascular collapse. These signs can be used to determine the progression of neurological status and emphasize the importance of monitoring the patient's level of consciousness, voluntary and involuntary body movements, extraocular reflexes, pupil position and response to light, respiratory rate and pattern and heart rate and rhythm. Bilateral pupillary constriction is an early response to brain ischaemia and suggests interruption of sympathetic tracts. Altered patterns of breathing, including Cheyne–Stokes respiration (alternating periods of

---

Ventricular tachycardia with severe hypotension or ventricular fibrillation
Direct-current defibrillators
    Internal: 0.5–2.0 Watt-seconds (Ws)/kg
    External: 5–10 Ws/kg
        Small patient (<7 kg)
            Internal: 5–15 Ws
            External: 50–100 Ws
        Large patient (>10 kg)
            Internal: 20–80 Ws
            External: 100–400 Ws
Alternating-current defibrillators
    Small patient
        Internal: 30–50 V
        External: 50–100 V
    Large patient
        Internal: 50–100 V
        External: 150–250 V

Unresponsive ventricular fibrillation
Evaluate ventilation
Evaluate thoracic wall or cardiac compression
Evaluate fluid therapy
Repeat and increase dose of adrenaline
Repeat sodium bicarbonate administration
Administer lidocaine for ventricular dysrhythmias
Repeat electrical defibrillation (direct-current; see above)

20.12 Defibrillation techniques. Modified from Muir and Bonagura (1985).

tachypnoea and apnoea), suggest respiratory centre depression. Loss of corneal reflexes and widely dilated pupils indicate severe cerebral hypoxia or brainstem herniation and are usually followed by respiratory arrest.

Long-term recovery of normal brain function is possible after resuscitation if resuscitative efforts are initiated early (within 1–3 minutes) and optimized. Clinical signs of neurological injury, however, may not become apparent for several hours after successful resuscitation and often do not develop for 4–12 hours following resuscitation (White et al., 1983). The delay in onset of clinical signs is difficult to explain and suggests that the transient restoration of near normal brain function followed by gradual deterioration may be due to the maturation or continuation of mechanisms responsible for poor brain blood flow. Brain ischaemia causes cytotoxic or cellular oedema due to failure of cell membrane pumps (Na^+/K^+, Ca^{2+}). Relatively short periods of hypoxia can cause disruption of the blood–brain barrier; in conjunction with increases in intracranial pressure caused by chest compression, this promotes increased transfer of water and protein, predisposing the patient to cerebral oedema. Cerebral oedema caused by the net gain in brain water may eventually impede cerebral blood flow, causing delayed clinical signs. Capillary vasospasm and abnormal vasoconstrictive activity due to local release of prostaglandins and calcium from damaged cells are responsible for large increases in post-ischaemic vascular resistance. In addition, damaged neurons can release excitatory neurotransmitters, such as glutamate, which stimulate surrounding tissues, increasing oxygen demand and exacerbating injury. Highly tissue-destructive oxygen free radicals are produced following resuscitation and the reintroduction of oxygenated blood. These pathological consequences of brain ischaemia and reperfusion are responsible for the delayed onset of hypoperfusion of the brain and the neurological signs following cardiac arrest and resuscitation in dogs and cats.

Treatment of post-resuscitation brain ischaemia

The prevention of post-resuscitation neurological abnormalities is dependent upon rapid re-establishment of cerebral blood flow, control of intracranial pressure and inhibition of the products and detrimental processes triggered by brain ischaemia and reperfusion (Figure 20.13). The duration of circulatory arrest prior to the initiation of CPCR and the time required to re-establish normal haemodynamics and breathing are paramount in limiting complications and determining outcome. If resuscitation takes longer than 10–15 minutes when conventional closed-chest cardiac massage is used, neurological prognosis is poor because closed-chest compression techniques do not provide adequate brain blood flow. If CNS injury is to be avoided, CPCR should begin promptly at chest compression rates of approximately 100/min. The intravenous administration of adrenaline (0.01–0.02 mg/kg) concurrent with ventilation, abdominal compression or abdominal binding helps to maintain higher levels of blood flow to the brain.

Problem	Therapy/drug	Dose
Hypotension	Lactated Ringer's 6% Dextran 70; Hetastarch 7% NaCl 7% NaCl in 6% dextran 70 Dopamine Dobutamine	35–70 ml/kg i.v. 10 ml/kg i.v. 3–5 ml/kg i.v. 5–7 ml/kg i.v. 3–10 µg/kg/min i.v. 5–20 µg/kg/min i.v.
Seizures	Pentobarbital Thiopental Diazepam Propofol	1–3 mg/kg i.v. 1–3 mg/kg i.v. 0.2–0.5 mg/kg i.v. 1–3 mg/kg i.v.
Cerebral oedema or increased intracranial pressure	Oxygenation Hyperventilation Furosemide Mannitol	P_aO_2 >80 mmHg P_aCO_2 >25–35 mmHg 1.0 mg/kg i.v. 0.5–1.0 g/kg i.v.
Cerebral vasospasm	Diltiazem	0.2 mg/kg i.v. bolus x2, 5–10 µg/kg/min CRI

20.13 Brain-orientated resuscitation. Modified from Muir (1989).

Fluids must be administered judiciously with close patient monitoring during and following CPCR. The administration of crystalloids or colloids during resuscitative efforts improves arterial blood pressure and blood flow, but can also cause dramatic increases in intracranial pressure (ICP) if given at shock doses (20–40 ml/kg i.v.). The increase in interstitial fluid volume and ICP occurs because venous return may be hampered by resuscitative efforts and because the brain lacks a lymphatic drainage system. Hypertonic saline (7% NaCl, 5 ml/kg i.v.) produces rapid, but transient, restoration of haemodynamics, increases cerebral blood flow (CBF) and decreases ICP. The administration of hyperoncotic or hyperosmotic solutions (5 ml/kg of 7% NaCl in 6% dextran 70) also minimizes increases in ICP. Head elevation and neck extension during spontaneous or controlled ventilation may help to alleviate increases in ICP and ensure a patent airway.

Cerebral blood flow is increased by high P_aCO_2 and/or low P_aO_2. Maximal vasodilation occurs when P_aCO_2 is greater than 60 mmHg, while P_aO_2 values less than 50 mmHg are required to increase brain blood flow. Increases in cerebral blood flow increase the vascular to interstitial compartment fluid flux, thereby increasing ICP and predisposing to or causing cerebral oedema. Following successful CPCR and extubation, nasal oxygen or an oxygen cage is helpful in maintaining P_aO_2 above 100 mmHg (Fitzpatrick and Crowe, 1986). In intubated patients, ventilation using an inflatable Ambu bag, anaesthetic machine or respirator helps prevent potentially detrimental increases in cerebral blood flow by normalizing P_aCO_2 (between 35 and 45 mmHg) and maintaining P_aO_2 values above 90 mmHg. Long-term use of high levels of F_iO_2 (>60% for more than 12 hours) should be avoided, to prevent oxygen toxicity and oxygen free radical formation. Determination of pH and blood gases (P_aCO_2, P_aO_2) using a point-of-care blood analyser is the most practical and accurate method of assessing pH and blood gas disorders. Central venous blood samples are superior to arterial blood samples when assessing the severity of acid–base abnormalities, while arterial blood samples provide more information about lung function. Sodium bicarbonate may be administered at 0.5–1.0 mEq/kg if severe metabolic acidosis (pH <7.1) persists despite appropriate fluid therapy and maintenance of blood pressure.

Care must be taken not to overventilate the patient in the post-resuscitation period. Overventilation (P_aCO_2 <20 mmHg) can cause constriction of cerebral vessels, cerebral hypoxia and increases in cerebrospinal fluid (CSF) lactate concentrations. Large tidal volumes during controlled ventilation may also increase intrathoracic pressure, thereby elevating cerebral venous pressure, causing disruption of the blood–brain barrier. High tidal volumes also lead to decreases in venous return to the heart, thereby decreasing cardiac output and systemic blood flow.

Loop diuretics (furosemide, bumetanide) and osmotic diuretics (20% mannitol) are capable of rapidly decreasing ICP. Furosemide inhibits Cl^- and Na^+ reabsorption in the ascending limb of the loop of Henle, producing immediate large-volume diuresis, and redistributes blood to peripheral vascular beds by dilating venules. The net effect of diuresis and redistribution of blood favours the movement of fluid from the brain (or lung) to the intravascular space, decreasing brain water and ICP. Furosemide also inhibits carbonic anhydrase, decreasing Na^+ uptake by the brain, which decreases brain swelling. Furosemide is initially administered at 1 mg/kg i.v. or 2 mg/kg i.m., followed by 0.5 mg/kg i.v. every 2–4 hours, if required. The patient's electrolyte, hydration and intravascular volume status should be carefully monitored during diuretic therapy. Although furosemide has the potential to produce hypokalaemic metabolic alkalosis, this is generally not a concern during acute administration.

Mannitol produces an osmotic diuresis and establishes an osmotic gradient that moves water from the brain to the intravascular space. In addition, mannitol has the ability to promote reperfusion by causing haemodilution and increasing cerebral blood flow. These effects, combined with its properties as a scavenger of oxygen free radicals, make it an excellent choice for the prevention and treatment of increases in ICP and cerebral oedema. Dosages of 0.5–1.0 g/kg i.v. are recommended, and repeat doses of 0.5 g/kg i.v. may be given approximately every 4 hours.

Diazepam and midazolam (0.1–0.2 mg/kg) are centrally acting muscle relaxants that produce mild calming effects and help to prevent seizures following resuscitation. If anaesthesia is required, low dosages of either sodium pentobarbital (1–3 mg/kg i.v.) or sodium thiopental (1–3 mg/kg i.v.) given to effect will help limit CNS damage and control seizures, although care must be taken to avoid barbiturate-induced cardiovascular compromise. Benzodiazepines and barbiturates decrease cerebral metabolic rate (oxygen consumption) by decreasing neuronal activity, protect membranes from free radicals and other excitatory neurotransmitters, decrease intracranial blood volume and ICP and increase tolerance to brief periods of complete brain ischaemia. Isoflurane and propofol have been advocated as alternatives to barbiturates for acute seizure control in dogs and cats; propofol (1–3 mg/kg) may be an excellent option in dogs. Finally, lidocaine administered by infusion (40–60 µg/kg/min) significantly reduces brain metabolic rate and stabilizes cell membranes.

Calcium channel blockers are believed to produce beneficial effects by preventing or reducing large increases in the concentration of intracellular Ca^{2+}, thereby inducing vasodilation and increases in brain blood flow. Diltiazem at 5–10 µg/kg/min produces long-term increases in cerebral blood flow and improves outcome (see Figure 20.8) (Capparelli et al., 1992). Blood pressure should be monitored during infusion, since calcium channel blocking drugs can produce hypotension due to their vasodilatory and negative inotropic effects.

Another emerging technique for post-resuscitation neuroprotection involves the use of induced or permissive hypothermia. The most logical benefit of hypothermia comes from a reduction in cerebral metabolic rate and overall oxygen demand. In addition, hypothermia leads to decreased excitotoxicity, free radical formation, cerebral oedema, ICP, destructive enzyme activity, apoptosis and inflammatory response (Safar et al., 2002; Polderman, 2004). Induction of mild hypothermia (33–36°C) has been found to provide benefit without the deleterious effects of moderate hypothermia (28–32°C). A meta-analysis of human studies demonstrated a significant improvement in short-term neurological recovery and overall survival (Holzer et al., 2005). This benefit has also been demonstrated in a number of canine studies, including one study which showed that induction of mild hypothermia during CPCR resulted in preservation of extracerebral organs as well as neuronal tissue (Nozari et al., 2004). Most evidence suggests that, to maximize this protective effect, the onset of hypothermia should be as close to the cardiopulmonary arrest as possible, if not during CPCR itself. Generally, external cooling is too slow, and hypothermia is most effectively and rapidly achieved by intravenous delivery of chilled crystalloid fluids (approximately 20–30 ml/kg to effect to reach a temperature of 33–36°C). Hypothermia should be maintained for 12–24 hours by further active cooling or warming as needed. Shivering, which can increase metabolic demands, may be prevented by administration of opioids, tranquillizers or neuromuscular blockers (if the patient is ventilated). The patient should be re-warmed gradually to prevent rebound hyperthermia, which could be detrimental. Potential side effects associated with hypothermia can include dysrhythmias, coagulopathies, increased risk of infection and electrolyte and fluid imbalances from 'cold diuresis'. These effects most commonly occur at temperatures below 32°C and should be minimal if mild hypothermia is used.

Conclusion

Clinical experience suggests that when complete brain ischaemia lasts for longer than 5 minutes and the cardiac resuscitative effort lasts in excess of 10–15 minutes, neurological outcome is poor and long-term survival is reduced. Age, concurrent disease and current medical or surgical complications are all important factors in determining outcome. Important prognostic indicators include the level of consciousness, pupil, eyelid and upper airway reflexes, breathing patterns and the ability to maintain a normal body temperature. The presence of the oculocephalic (doll's eye) and oculovestibular (caloric) reflexes are useful indicators of prognosis, but are suppressed by sedatives, anaesthetics and hypothermia. These reflexes are generally absent when body temperature falls below 36°C in the dog and cat. Rapid recovery of eyelid, pupillary and swallowing reflexes, resumption of a normal arterial pulse and breathing pattern, improving level of consciousness and the maintenance of normal body temperature are considered good prognostic signs. Most dogs and cats that show signs of recovery within 5 minutes of restoration of spontaneous circulation will recover with normal brain function. Progressive mental deterioration, seizures or unconsciousness, particularly after initial partial recovery, dilated fixed pupils, loss of eyelid and swallowing reflexes, prolonged respiratory arrest and gradual decreases in body temperature are poor prognostic signs. Inability to maintain a strong arterial pulse and normal heart rate, and failure to resume breathing, regardless of specific therapies, are excellent indicators of impending death. Close monitoring should be continued for at least 24 hours after cardiorespiratory function is restored.

References and further reading

Altman S (1997) Acupuncture as an emergency treatment. *California Veterinarian* 33, 6–8

Aufderheide TP and Lurie KG (2004) Death by hyperventilation: A common and life-threatening problem during cardiopulmonary resuscitation. *Critical Care Medicine* 32(9 Suppl), S345–S351

Aung K, Htay T (2005) Vasopressin for cardiac arrest. *Archives of Internal Medicine* 165, 17–24

Babbs CF (2003) Interposed abdominal compression CPR: a comprehensive evidenced based review. *Resuscitation* 59(1), 71–82

Benson DM, O'Neil B, Kakish E *et al.* (2005) Open-chest CPR improves survival and neurological outcome following cardiac arrest. *Resuscitation* 64(2), 209–217

Blumenthal SR and Voorhees WD (1997) The relationship of carbon dioxide excretion during cardiopulmonary resuscitation to regional blood flow and survival. *Resuscitation* 35(2), 135–143

Brown CG, Martin DR, Pepe PE *et al.* (1992) A comparison of standard-dose and high-dose adrenaline in cardiac arrest outside the hospital. *New England Journal of Medicine* 327, 1051–1055

Capparelli EV, Hanyok JJ, Dipersio DM *et al.* (1992) Diltiazem improves resuscitation from experimental ventricular fibrillation in dogs. *Critical Care Medicine* 20, 1140–1145

Evans AT (1999) New thoughts on cardiopulmonary resuscitation. *Veterinary Clinics of North America: Small Animal Practice* 29, 819–829

Fischer M and Hossmann KA (1996) Volume expansion during cardiopulmonary resuscitation reduces cerebral no-reflow (review). *Resuscitation* 32, 227–240

Fitzpatrick RK and Crowe DT (1986) Nasal oxygen administration in dogs and cats: experimental and clinical investigations. *Journal of the American Animal Hospital Association* 22, 293–300

Holmberg M, Holmberg S and Herlitz J (2000) Incidence, duration and survival of ventricular fibrillation in out-of-hospital cardiac arrest patients in Sweden. *Resuscitation* 44(1), 7–17.

Holzer M, Bernard SA, Hachimi-Idrissi S *et al.* (2005) Hypothermia for neuroprotection after cardiac arrest: systematic review and individual patient data meta-analysis. *Critical Care Medicine* 33(2), 414–418

Janssens L, Altman S and Rogers PAM (1979) Respiratory and cardiac arrest under general anaesthesia: treatment by acupuncture of the nasal philtrum. *Veterinary Record* 105, 273–276

Kass PH and Haskins SC (1992) Survival following cardiopulmonary resuscitation in dogs and cats. *Journal of Veterinary Emergency and Critical Care* 2, 57–65

Koehler RC, Chandra N, Guerci AD *et al.* (1983) Augmentation of cerebral perfusion by simultaneous chest compression and lung inflation with abdominal binding after cardiac arrest in dogs. *Circulation* 67, 266–275

Lindner KH, Haak T, Keller A, Bothner U and Lurie KG (1996) Release of endogenous vasopressors during and after cardiopulmonary resuscitation. *Heart* 75, 145–150

Lindner KH, Dirks B and Strohmenger HU (1997) A randomised comparison of epinephrine and vasopressin in patients with out-of-hospital ventricular fibrillation. *Lancet* 349, 535–537

Mazkereth R, Paret G, Ezra D *et al.* (1992) Adrenaline blood concentrations after peripheral bronchial versus endotracheal administration of adrenaline in dogs. *Critical Care Medicine* 20, 1582–1587

Muir WW (1989) Brain hypoperfusion post-resuscitation. *Veterinary Clinics of North America: Small Animal Practice* 19, 1151–1166

Muir WW and Bonagura JD (1985) Cardiovascular emergencies. In: *Medical Emergencies*, ed. RG Sherding, p. 90. Churchill Livingstone, New York

Nozari A, Safar P, Stezoski SW *et al.* (2004) Mild hypothermia during prolonged cardiopulmonary cerebral resuscitation increases conscious survival in dogs. *Critical Care Medicine* 32(10), 2110–2116

Peters J and Ihle P (1990) Mechanics of the circulation during cardiopulmonary resuscitation – pathophysiology and techniques (part I). *Intensive Care Medicine* 16, 11–19

Polderman KH (2004) Application of therapeutic hypothermia in the ICU: Opportunities and pitfalls of a promising treatment modality. Part 1: Indications and evidence. *Intensive Care Medicine* 30, 556–575

Reich DL and Mingus M (1990) Transtracheal oxygenation using simple equipment and a low-pressure oxygen source. *Critical Care Medicine* 18, 664–665

Rush JE and Wingfield WE (1992) Recognition and frequency of dysrhythmias during cardiopulmonary arrest. *Journal of the American Veterinary Medical Association* 200(12), 1932–1937

Safar P, Behringer W, Bottiger BW and Sterz F (2002) Cerebral resuscitation potentials for cardiac arrest. *Critical Care Medicine* 30(4 Suppl), S140–144

Shapiro BA (1998) Should the ABCs of basic CPR become the CBAs? *Critical Care Medicine* 26(2), 214–215

Stadlbauer KH, Wagner-Berger HG, Wenzel V *et al.* (2003) Survival with full neurologic recovery after prolonged cardiopulmonary resuscitation with a combination of vasopressin and epinephrine in pigs. *Anesthesia and Analgesia* 96, 1743–1749

Voorhees WWD, Ralston SH, Kougias C and Schmitz PM (1987) Fluid loading with whole blood or Ringer's lactate solution during CPR in dogs. *Resuscitation* 15, 113–123

White BC, Winegar CD, Jackson RE *et al.* (1983) Cerebral cortical perfusion during and following resuscitation from cardiac arrest in dogs. *American Journal of Emergency Medicine* 1, 128–138

Wik L, Bircher NG and Safar P (1996) A comparison of prolonged manual and mechanical external chest compression after cardiac arrest in dogs. *Resuscitation* 32(3), 241–250

Wingfield WE and Van Pelt DR (1992) Respiratory and cardiopulmonary arrest in dogs and cats: 265 cases (1986–1991). *Journal of the American Veterinary Medical Association* 200, 1993–1996

21

Anaesthesia and sedation of the critical patient

Richard Hammond

Introduction

Many critically ill patients will need sedation or even anaesthesia at one or more points during the hospitalization period.

Sedation

Sedation is used in various ways in intensive care unit (ICU) patients including:

- To allow minor procedures, diagnostic or therapeutic, to be performed without the need for general anaesthesia
- To augment the effects of analgesics, where the level of distress or anxiety requires central behavioural modification. Sedation is never a substitute for the provision of adequate analgesia
- To provide strategic neuroprotection in animals with head injury or those in status epilepticus
- To modify sleep patterns to permit sleep in an otherwise distressed and insomniant patient
- To modify behavioural signs such as vocalization and pacing due to separation/hospitalization anxiety. The additional stress response in an animal that is suffering disease and may be in pain further promotes a catabolic state, prolongs recovery from surgery and increases the potential for infection. When using a sedative to modify behaviour, the patient should be evaluated to ensure that the behavioural signs do not represent an early manifestation of another disease such as cerebral hypoxia. In addition, in an animal displaying these signs, sedation does not replace the provision of basic nursing care, with consideration of both physical comfort (e.g. checking for a full bladder, full litter tray, wet bedding etc.) and the patient's emotional requirements.

Anaesthesia

Anaesthesia is a necessary procedure in many ICU patients:

- To facilitate procedures where sedation alone would be inadequate. Anaesthesia allows the establishment of a protected airway, the provision of increased inspired oxygen concentrations and the potential for ventilatory support where appropriate. In anaesthetized cases, cardiovascular and respiratory monitoring (such as capnometry) may also be easier to perform. Anaesthesia, with the associated increase in patient support, may therefore be associated with a better outcome than a period of heavy sedation alone. Anaesthesia should therefore be considered 'first line' in most cases where a *short* period of 'patient control' is required
- To facilitate intermittent positive pressure ventilation (IPPV). Small animals are poorly tolerant of endotracheal intubation when conscious. Anaesthesia is therefore often necessary to allow long-term assisted or mandatory ventilation.

Assessment prior to sedation or anaesthesia

Assessment of the critical patient is qualitatively no different to that of any patient presumed healthy prior to anaesthesia. Findings form the basis of a structured and prioritized checklist of potential problems that may arise during the peri-anaesthetic period. Awareness of these potential problems allows preparedness and, where required, further pre-induction stabilization and support. It also forms the basis for the choice of anaesthetic protocol. Because of the variable response to a given dose of agent in patients with severe compromise, patients should be examined to assess suitability for anaesthesia, even if sedation only is intended at that stage. An ABC body systems approach is one such method of assessment (Figure 21.1).

Neural and hormonal responses in the critically ill or injured patient will act to preserve circulation to essential organs, including the brain and myocardium. This effectively centralized circulation may make the patient more susceptible to the adverse effects of sedative or anaesthetic agents. This effect may be exacerbated by the concomitant presence of hypothermia, hypoalbuminaemia and acid–base and electrolyte disturbances. Careful preoperative assessment, stabilization of vital parameters and attention to detail are essential if potentially catastrophic effects of additional centrally depressant agents are to be avoided. Few procedures require sedation or general anaesthesia to be performed on an emergency basis and whenever possible patients should undergo a period of stabilization prior to the anaesthetic. Occasionally, due to the nature of the patient's disease, stabilization is not possible; in this scenario the nature of the patient's

Airway	Breathing/gas exchange	Circulatory
Questions:		
Can the patient maintain an airway?	Is the patient dyspnoeic and/or tachypnoeic?	Is heart rate normal at rest?
Is there a potential need for tracheostomy?	Is oxygen supplementation required to maintain normal arterial oxygen saturation at rest?	Is there a dysrhythmia that is likely to result in reduced cardiac output?
Will patency be lost at induction (e.g. brachycephalic airway obstruction syndrome BAOS)?	Can the patient maintain an adequate arterial oxygen content (in the context of the circulating haemoglobin level)?	Does the type or frequency of the patient's dysrhythmia preclude general anaesthesia?
Is there a need or potential need for airway clearance (i.e. suction)?		Does the patient have adequate tissue perfusion to vital organ beds?
		Is urine production adequate (>0.5 ml/kg/h)?
Comments:		
Airway obstruction at, or rostral to, the larynx (e.g. laryngeal trauma/paralysis/BOAS) will be managed by orotracheal intubation. Excessive sedation prior to induction should be avoided	Ventilatory drive, tidal volume, pulmonary gas exchange and blood oxygen-carrying capacity are assessed	Pulse pressure is not a reliable indicator of the status of circulatory volume, although presence of a poor peripheral pulse suggests reduced peripheral perfusion
Patients at risk of airway obstruction should be carefully monitored during sedation	When intrathoracic disease is suspected survey thoracic radiographs should be obtained. Any air or fluid within the pleural space should be removed by needle thoracocentesis or placement of a chest drain	Capillary refill time is a poor indicator of circulating volume
The potential for failed intubation necessitates preparation for alternative techniques for securing the airway (including tracheostomy)	The patient's ability to oxygenate may be evaluated by techniques such as pulse oximetry and arterial blood gas analysis where available	Central venous pressure is considered the most reliable method of assessing both circulating volume and response to the administration of intravenous fluids
Obstruction of the airway between the larynx and carina presents a considerable problem and is unlikely to be resolved by normal endotracheal intubation techniques	As arterial oxygen content also depends on haemoglobin concentration, patients with acute falls in haematocrit to below approximately 20% or Hb <70 g/l will require transfusion if severe tissue hypoxia is to be avoided during anaesthesia	Circulating volume should be optimized prior to sedation or anaesthesia by the use of intravenous crystalloids and colloids as appropriate
Patients at risk of aspiration or obstruction due to the presence of fluid and/or debris in the pharynx may require clearance using suction techniques		When a significant dysrhythmia is found, anaesthesia should be delayed if possible and therapy directed at the underlying cause (e.g. electrolyte disturbances, hypoxia, cardiac disease, hypercapnia and pain)
Prolonged airway suction quickly leads to marked arterial desaturation, and intermittent supplementation of F_iO_2 is mandatory		

21.1 Assessment of the critical patient based on ABC body systems approach.

underlying disease, the effects of the anaesthetic agents and clinician familiarity with the drugs should all be carefully considered when making a rational choice of agent(s) to use. More detailed information on anaesthetic concerns with specific procedures can be found in the *BSAVA Manual of Canine and Feline Anaesthesia and Analgesia*.

Interactions with concurrently administered medications

Animals rarely pass though intensive care without the benefits of polypharmacy. In addition, emergency patients may have been exposed to long-term drug regimens. The direct and indirect effects of these agents on the anaesthetic protocol must be considered.

Drug groups that may have an effect on anaesthesia include:

- Diuretics (hypovolaemia, hypokalaemia, acid–base disturbances)
- Non-steroidal anti-inflammatory drugs (NSAIDs) (gastrointestinal ulceration, renal damage, increased potential for overdose through altered protein binding)
- Anticonvulsants (altered protein binding, liver enzyme induction)
- Steroids (interaction with NSAIDs)

- Antibiotics (potentiation of neuromuscular blockade with aminoglycosides and macrolides)
- Beta blockers (lack of response to inotropes, competition for hepatic elimination with midazolam, propofol altering propranolol distribution in the dog (Perry *et al.*, 1991)).

In most cases of long-term therapy, drugs should not be withdrawn prior to sedation or anaesthesia, as their withdrawal may increase the potential for complications.

Choice of agent

Many drugs used for sedation in ICU may also produce anaesthesia (or more specifically hypnosis) at a higher dose (Figure 21.2). The effects of the drug on the patient (both wanted and 'unwanted') increase predictably, and in most cases linearly, over clinical dose ranges. The point of 'anaesthesia' is usefully defined in this situation by the ability to perform and maintain endotracheal intubation. The clinician may therefore encounter a situation whereby the animal is on the 'cusp' between sedation and anaesthesia at the dose of agent required to produce the desired

Propofol	Diazepam/midazolam	Medetomidine	Etomidate	Ketamine	Acepromazine
Sedation					
25–100 µg/kg/min No maximum duration in dogs. Limited to 12 hours in cats Add 50ml of propofol to a 500ml bag of 0.9% saline: 1.5 ml/kg/h = 25 µg/kg/min 6.0 ml/kg/h = 100 µg/kg/min OR use undiluted propofol with a syringe pump	0.1–0.4 mg/kg bolus Used in combination with propofol: 40–100 µg/kg/h	1–3 µg/kg bolus i.v. Used in combination with propofol: 1 µg/kg/h Analgesia is also provided at this dose		1–2 mg/kg/h in both dogs and cats Analgesia is also provided at this dose. Lower doses of 0.1–0.2 mg/kg/h provide analgesia without sedation	0.005–0.03 mg/kg repeated q3–6h for short-term sedation
Premedication/induction of anaesthesia					
Alone 1–6 mg/kg to effect (lower doses in more unstable patients)	Premedication dose 0.1–0.4 mg/kg in both dog and cat. If followed by propofol may lead to a period of apnoea	1–3 µg/kg i.v. bolus of medetomidine prior to propofol 3–4 mg/kg	0.05–0.2 mg/kg diazepam or midazolam followed by 0.2–2.0 mg/kg etomidate i.v. over 10–15 seconds. Do not repeat dose or top up as *adrenocortical suppression will be prolonged for up to 24 hours*	0.05–0.2 mg/kg diazepam or midazolam followed by 3–10 mg/kg ketamine in both cats and dogs	
Maintenance of anaesthesia					
Cat 0.05–0.22 mg/kg/min Dog 0.05–0.40 mg/kg/min					

21.2 Drugs commonly used for sedation and anaesthesia in veterinary intensive care. For further information on drug effects at different doses, please see text.

effect (e.g. treatment of status epilepticus by propofol infusion). In such cases, the advantages of a protected airway, and ability to perform IPPV where necessary, must be weighed against the potential for airway drying and increased risk of respiratory infection due to compromise of upper airway integrity. In the following text, agents and combinations that might be used for sedation or anaesthesia are discussed together. Opioids are discussed in Chapter 22.

Propofol

Advantages

- Can be used at low doses to produce sedation. Increasing doses result in anaesthesia. Recovery from anaesthesia is smooth and rapid and does not rely on hepatic metabolism for initial plasma clearance.
- Relatively non-cumulative over long-term infusion.
- Rapid response to change in infusion rate, thus easy to titrate dose.
- Potent anticonvulsive.
- Reduces intracranial pressure.
- Can be mixed in intravenous fluid bag to facilitate constant rate infusion (CRI) without loss of potency.
- May be used in the presence of disease including renal and hepatic failure.

Disadvantages

- Lack of preservative and good bacterial medium properties mean asepsis must be scrupulous. When used as a CRI, the intravenous line and connections must be diligently maintained and regularly replaced (every 24 hours).
- High or bolus doses may result in apnoea.
- High doses lead to vasodilation and reduce cardiac output.
- Long-term infusion may lead to hyperlipidosis and may represent a significant proportion of the caloric needs of the patient without providing amino acids. This must be taken into consideration when calculating nutritional support formulas.
- Limited to 12 hours of infusion in cats due to reduced clearance and potential for Heinz body anaemia.
- No analgesia.
- Apparent tolerance is seen after 48 hours of higher dose infusion in some dogs (unpublished observation) requiring gradual increase of infusion.
- Individual animal response is highly variable especially where there is hypoalbuminaemia.
- Expensive.

Properties

Propofol is an intravenous sedative–hyponotic that has become the mainstay of human intensive care sedation and anaesthesia. Propofol decreases intracranial pressure, is a potent anticonvulsive, anti-oxidant and bronchodilator and has some anti-inflammatory properties. Pharmacokinetic properties of propofol that make it suitable for long-term sedation by infusion include rapid tissue redistribution, rapid metabolic clearance in most species (even with reduced hepatic function) and slow return to the circulation. These properties account for the rapid onset of action and short duration, making titration of dose by infusion easier and more effective. The low reliance on hepatic function for plasma clearance makes propofol suitable for sedation in dogs even in the presence of severe hepatic compromise (Heldman *et al.*, 1999). The relative safety of propofol in the human ICU appears to be good. Cardiovascular effects are primarily due to vasodilation without the concomitant baroreceptor mediated increase in heart rate. This makes propofol useful in most ICU patients where increased myocardial work would be detrimental. Blood pressure should however be carefully monitored. Hypotension is less severe if propofol is given slowly to effect or via infusion, and is dose dependent, but may still be of significance in patients with hypovolaemia or haemodynamic instability. Heart rate is normally slightly reduced – again this is dose dependent. Respiratory depression is dose dependent at sedative doses and is not normally of significance; the rapid clearance means that the effects are quickly reversed. At high sedation doses, or when anaesthesia is maintained by continuous infusion, the ability to perform IPPV (Ambu bag or breathing attachment and anaesthetic machine) should be available. Despite early reports of 'propofol syndrome' in infants and, more recently, some adults (cardiac failure, metabolic acidosis and rhabdomyolysis) such complications are rare in human patients and not reported in veterinary species at the time of writing.

Practical use

Sedation is dose dependent and is achieved by infusion with no requirement for a loading dose. Infusion should be initiated at 25 µg/kg/min and increased incrementally by 10 µg/kg/min at 10–15-minute intervals; maintenance of sedation requires a constant infusion of propofol with discontinuation resulting in prompt awakening. At higher doses, anaesthesia may be induced and the airway may not be protected. There is a high inter-patient variability in dose requirement and this may change over time. Thus, equipment to perform endotracheal intubation should be easily accessible before initiating even a low-dose sedation infusion. Vomiting during propofol infusion is an infrequent complication but is potentially catastrophic in an animal with reduced airway protection. Animals on higher-dose sedation should be monitored and observed as if anaesthetized, and even an apparently stable patient should be under 24-hour observation. Propofol is a suitable sedative/anaesthetic for use in cats in ICU but the duration of sedation and the number of anaesthetics in a given time is limited due to the reduced ability of cats to conjugate, and therefore eliminate, phenolic compounds. Repeated use of propofol may result in significant Heinz body anaemia in this species. It is recommended that sedation (via CRI) is limited to 12 hours and a 48-hour wash-out period allowed between anaesthetics.

Benzodiazepines (midazolam and diazepam)

Advantages

* May be used in combination with other agents for more stable sedation in ICU patients.
* Minimal cardiovascular effects at standard doses.
* Relatively inexpensive when used in combination with other agents.
* Potent anticonvulsive and muscle relaxant properties.

Disadvantages

* Sedation is unreliable when used as a sole agent. In some animals, especially cats, profound dysphoria is seen. May produce disinhibition (loss of learned behaviour).
* High doses produce respiratory depression.
* Increasing doses do not result in anaesthesia.

Properties

Benzodiazepines act centrally to produce muscle relaxation and some sedation. These agents possess minimal cardiovascular and respiratory depressant properties and may significantly reduce the dose requirement of anaesthetic induction agents. Sedation is less reliable and of shorter duration than with acepromazine, but is often more profound in debilitated patients. Benzodiazepines are potent anticonvulsants. Diazepam is metabolized to products with pharmacological activity and is available as an emulsion preparation for intravenous use, an injectable form for intramuscular administration (containing benzyl alcohol) as well as a rectal tube preparation more suitable for treatment of status epilepticus. Midazolam is a water-soluble preparation that can be used by any parenteral route. Accumulation of these products may result in a prolonged half-life, and makes them less suitable for longer-term infusion. In combination with other agents such as opioids, synergy of sedative effects is seen. This is the usual mode of use in the veterinary ICU. In cases of overdose, a benzodiazepine antagonist (flumazenil) is available. It has a short shelf life, short half-life and is expensive.

Practical use

These agents are widely used in the human ICU, where the degree of sedation produced is greater and more predictable. Although midazolam is a more potent sedative than diazepam in humans, this is not reflected in veterinary use. There is little practical use of benzodiazepines alone in the veterinary ICU, apart from their first-line use for management of seizures. Diazepam (and probably midazolam) is reduced in potency by addition to an intravenous fluid bag (Kowaluk *et al.*, 1982), limiting its use in the absence of a syringe driver. For intravenous use, Diazemuls™ (distributor: AH Cox & Co Ltd, Barnstaple), the emulsion preparation, should be used, as it does not contain propylene glycol. In combination, benzodiazepines may be infused alongside propofol or fentanyl. The advantages of such combinations are a significant dose reduction of the other sedative/analgesic (and therefore reduction of unwanted effects) as well as a more stable and reliable response. A suggested protocol would be to initiate intravenous infusion of the benzodiazepine at a fixed rate (40–100 µg/kg/**h** of midazolam or diazepam) followed 15–20 minutes later by propofol infusion at a variable rate titrated to effect and starting at 25 µg/kg/**min**. Cumulative effects can be managed by a gradual reduction of the CRI dose over time, depending on the response of the patient. Midazolam is less likely to be cumulative if the infusion is to be prolonged for more than 24 hours.

Medetomidine and dexmedetomidine

Advantages

- Marked sedation with only mild reduction in minute ventilation.
- Analgesic properties.
- Titratability and rapid, complete reversibility with atipamezole.
- Inhibition of stress response improves recovery times.
- Reduction of intracranial pressure with a matching of cerebral oxygen demand and supply.

Disadvantages

- Significant increase in systemic vascular resistance and decreased cardiac output may be extremely risky in unstable animals.
- Prolonged elimination in the presence of hepatic dysfunction.
- Bradycardia.
- Emesis at higher doses.
- Hyperglycaemia.

Properties
Medetomidine provides sedation, analgesia, muscle relaxation and anxiolysis. Medetomidine has replaced xylazine in dogs and cats, due to its greater alpha-2:alpha-1 affinity. This increased selectivity results in more predictable and effective sedation and analgesia and fewer side effects.

The sedative–hypnotic effects of alpha-2 agonists are a result of inhibition of noradrenaline release from noradrenergic receptors (autoreceptors) in the locus coeruleus. Analgesic effects are principally but not exclusively due to spinal anti-nociception via binding to non-noradrenergic receptors (heteroreceptors) located on the dorsal horn neurons of the spinal cord (Shaham *et al.*, 2000). These heteroreceptors are found presynaptically, where they inhibit the release of neurotransmitters and neuropeptides, and postsynaptically, where they decrease ascending spinal nociceptive transmission. There is also some evidence for supraspinal analgesic mechanisms; suppression of noradrenaline release in the locus coeruleus leads, via disinhibition of certain catecholaminergic nuclei in the pons, to increased release of noradrenaline from dorsal horn terminals and consequent activation of presynaptic and postsynaptic heteroreceptors (Ruiz-Ortega *et al.*, 1995).

Dexmedetomidine is one of the optical enantiomers of medetomidine and has twice the potency. Qualitatively its effects are the same as those of medetomidine, and the two will be considered together. Medetomidine is in widespread clinical veterinary use as a sedative and as part of anaesthetic combinations. Its use has traditionally been reserved for the healthy animal due to concerns with regard to unwanted cardiovascular effects. There is an emerging popularity and increased use of dexmedetomidine in human ICU practice. This, coupled with more detailed studies as to the effects of low doses of medetomidine in dogs and cats, has resulted in revived interest in its use as a sedative in the veterinary ICU. Low doses of medetomidine, 5–20 µg/kg, produce qualitatively similar cardiovascular changes which, in the dog, include a biphasic blood pressure response, bradycardia and increased systemic vascular resistance. Coronary blood flow is preserved in conscious dogs (Schmeling *et al.*, 1991). In anaesthetized patients, the effect is less clear, a coronary arterial vasocontrictive effect being balanced by a high degree of local metabolic control. Cardiac output is reduced primarily, but not entirely, due to increased afterload and reduced rate, as contractility is preserved. Perfusion to vital organs is preserved, despite a reduction in cardiac output, due to peripheral vasoconstriction. At micro doses of 1–2 µg/kg the cardiovascular effects of medetomidine are, however, markedly reduced. These doses still result in effective sedation and some analgesia in most animals. In addition, these micro doses are highly effective in improving the quality of concomitantly administered sedatives. Microdose medetomidine has been shown to be as effective as high-dose diazepam (0.4 mg/kg) in the reduction of propofol requirement for sedation in dogs (Ko *et al.*, 2006).

Practical use
Micro-dose medetomidine may be used as an infusion either alone or, more usefully, to reduce the dose of concurrently administered propofol required for sedation in animals without serious cardiovascular instability or hepatic compromise. A bolus of 1–3 µg/kg i.v. is given followed by infusion of propofol, starting 5–10 minutes later at a variable rate titrated to effect and starting at a propofol dose of 10 µg/kg/min. The medetomidine bolus is repeated at approximately 90-minute intervals. Alternatively, where the equipment is available, an infusion of medetomidine at 1 µg/kg/h may be started instead of a bolus, and the propofol infusion started 10–15 minutes later. Opioids have a semi-synergistic effect when combined with alpha-2 agonists. Receptors for both compounds occupy similar sites in the brain and on some neurons, and produce similar actions (membrane-associated G protein activation leading to neuronal hyperpolarization and a reduced response to excitatory input). This combination results in an improved quality and duration of analgesia.

Etomidate

Advantages

- Minimal or no cardiovascular effects when used as a single bolus for induction of anaesthesia.
- Inexpensive.
- Very short duration of activity with rapid smooth recovery.

Disadvantages

- Profound and potentially long-lasting suppression of adrenocortical activity occurs, which could be detrimental in patients with critical disease. The duration of suppression of adrenocortical activity is dose dependent, lasting a few hours at low doses. Recently, there have been calls for the withdrawal of etomidate from use in human ICU patients (Annane, 2005), although some controversy remains (Jackson and Ramos, 2006). It is difficult to recommend the use of etomidate in the ICU setting for all but a very limited group of patients. It may still have some use for the emergency induction of anaesthesia in critical patients.
- Frequently causes pain and phlebitis on intravenous injection, owing to its high osmolarity.
- Clonic seizure-like movements on induction.
- Duration of anaesthesia is too short for most procedures and requires follow up by maintenance with a volatile or other injectable agent. High inspired concentrations or continuous infusions of another injectable drug are then required to maintain anaesthesia in the absence of residual hypnosis from an injectable agent.

Properties and practical use

Etomidate retains an indication for use in the critical patient either with significant ventricular dysrhythmia or primary myocardial failure that cannot be further stabilized prior to necessary anaesthesia. In this situation, a dose of 0.05–0.2 mg/kg midazolam or diazepam (as emulsion) is given by intravenous bolus followed by 0.2–2.0 mg/kg etomidate as an intravenous bolus over 10–15 seconds.

Ketamine

Advantages

- Analgesia and sedation effects.
- Minimal cardiovascular and respiratory depression in normal patients.

Disadvantages

- Indirect sympathomimetic effects include an increase in heart rate, which may be detrimental in hypertrophic cardiomyopathy and ischaemic heart disease.
- Produces increases in cerebral blood flow, causing increased intracranial pressure and should be avoided in patients with head trauma.
- Cumulative and limited to 24 hours' use.
- Renal elimination, therefore may have increased effects in patients with renal insufficiency.

Properties

There is renewed interest in ketamine not only as an analgesic, but also as an adjunct to general anaesthesia and as a sedative and analgesic in the ICU and post-trauma setting. Low doses of ketamine produce minimal cardiovascular depression and there may even be some support of heart rate in healthy animals. In addition, ketamine reduces or limits the potentiation of nociceptive 'wind up' at the level of the spinal cord following injury (see Chapter 22). The benefit of an additional modality of analgesia and sedation in the ICU patient is tempered by the potential for psychomimetic adverse effects, such as dysphoria and vocalization. In veterinary species, dysphoria is a problem when ketamine is administered alone. In the ICU setting, ketamine is used either as a repeated bolus or, ideally, as an infusion alongside either propofol or fentanyl. This ensures more profound and more stable sedation as well as additional analgesia. Ketamine is metabolized to an active metabolite (nor-ketamine) which requires renal elimination. Care should be taken in animals with renal or hepatic dysfunction as this may increase the effects and the rate of accumulation of the drug or its metabolites. Ketamine is cumulative and administration is limited to 24 hours at normal doses.

Practical use

When sedation and analgesia are required, ketamine is administered at a rate equivalent to 1–2 mg/kg/h in both dogs and cats. If ketamine is to be administered concurrently with propofol the rate may be similar, or may be reduced to 0.1–0.2 mg/kg/h, at which dose there is minimal additional sedation but provision of analgesia (Figure 21.3).

Example – low-dose infusion

Loading dose = 1–2 mg of ketamine per kg, intravenously
Desired CRI dose: 0.1 mg/kg/h

CRI: Add 60 mg of ketamine to a 1 l bag (or 30 mg to a 500 ml bag) of 0.9% saline
This produces a solution of 0.06 mg/ml; therefore 0.1 mg = 1.67 ml
To deliver the desired dose of 0.1 mg/kg/h:
- With an infusion pump set rate at body weight (kg) x 1.67 ml/h
- With a 60 drops/ml intravenous drip set, use the animal's body weight (kg) to set the number of drops per minute (e.g. a 5 kg cat will get 5 drops/min, i.e. one drop every 12 seconds). This gives an infusion rate of 1 µg of ketamine/kg/min, equal to 0.06 mg of ketamine/kg/h

21.3 Calculating the dose of ketamine required for a continuous rate infusion.

Acepromazine

Advantages

- Low doses can produce selective arteriolar vasodilation, thereby reducing afterload. This may improve cardiac output in some patients.
- May protect the heart from the dysrhythmogenic effects of adrenaline.
- Inexpensive.

Disadvantages

- Hypotension may be seen in hypovolaemic patients or when higher doses (>0.03 mg/kg) are used. Hypotension may also be associated with an increase in vagal tone in some dog breeds.
- Use of the drug in patients with a predisposition towards seizures (e.g. head trauma) is controversial. It is suggested that it may reduce the threshold at which seizures occur, although clinical evidence for this phenomenon is lacking.
- Poor titratability.

Properties and practical use

Although an 'old' drug, acepromazine (ACP) has a role in sedation and premedication in the critical patient. Relative contraindications remain animals with hypovolaemia or reduced preload and possibly animals with head trauma or a history of epileptiform seizures. Otherwise, renal disease, hepatic disease and even cardiac disease are not contraindications to use of a low dose of ACP (0.005–0.03 mg/kg i.m. or i.v.). The sedative effects at these low levels are less reliable but can be potentiated if necessary by combination with an opioid such as butorphanol (0.1 mg/kg) or pethidine (3–5 mg/kg). In patients with cardiac disease, the selective arteriolar dilation and reduction in afterload may actually increase cardiac output. These low doses of ACP will have an effective duration of action of 1.5–2 hours, which should not be significantly prolonged even in the presence of hepatic disease. ACP is less useful compared to other agents regarding its flexibility of dosing (ceiling effect and increased hypotensive effects) and for long-term sedation where titration and flexibility are important.

Volatile agents

Sub-anaesthetic concentrations of volatile agents, such as isoflurane and more recently desflurane, have been successfully used for sedation in the human ICU (Kong and Willatts, 1995; Meiser et al., 2003). Their advantages are excellent titratability, minimal cardiovascular effects and smooth emergence. This technique is more applicable to patients on long-term ventilation and for practical reasons requires placement of an endotracheal tube. It has minimal application in current veterinary use for non-ventilated ICU patients.

Induction of anaesthesia in the critical patient

The aim of induction is to produce a smooth passage to the unconscious state with minimal compromise of ventilatory or cardiovascular function. Induction allows a secure patent airway to be obtained. Pre-oxygenation is recommended in all patients where possible, and is mandatory in patients with respiratory compromise if it can be achieved without undue patient stress. This helps to reduce the desaturation associated with induction apnoea. To be effective, pre-oxygenation must be performed for a period of at least 5 minutes. High flows are indicated to maximize FiO_2.

Mask induction

Advantages

- Permits provision of a high FiO_2.
- Obviates the need for the use of intravenous agents and their associated unwanted effects.
- Useful where protein binding or total protein is reduced, making estimation of the dose of usually heavily albumin-bound intravenous agents difficult.

Disadvantages

- Often stressful to the patient.
- Does not allow rapid control of the patient's airway.

Practical use

Mask induction of anaesthesia is a practical option for debilitated patients with CNS depression and/or hypoproteinaemia, but who are not at immediate risk of airway collapse. The available volatile agent of choice is currently sevoflurane. Lack of airway irritation, low solubility and hence rapid rate of rise of alveolar concentration (and therefore speed of induction) coupled with a rapid smooth recovery are all properties that favour use of this agent. For further information see the BSAVA Manual of Canine and Feline Anaesthesia and Analgesia. Nitrous oxide has traditionally been a useful adjunct to mask induction, as the second gas effect reduces induction time by hastening the uptake of the volatile agent. Use of nitrous oxide will, however, reduce the F_iO_2. Use of sevoflurane probably negates the need for nitrous oxide in this situation.

Mask induction should be avoided in:

- Patients with upper airway obstruction
- Patients at risk of regurgitation/reflux
- Patients with severe dyspnoea and/or intrinsic pulmonary disease
- Patients with reduced pulmonary blood flow
- Patients with severe cardiovascular instability (a period of hypoxia may be significantly detrimental to already compromised tissue oxygen delivery).

Use of drug combinations

The agents most commonly used for induction of anaesthesia in critical patients are propofol, ketamine and etomidate (see above). When anaesthesia is to be induced using these agents, the concurrent use of potent opioids and/or benzodiazepines allows the administration of lower doses of individual agents, thereby minimizing unwanted side effects. In severely debilitated patients, the combination of a benzodiazepine and a potent opioid such as fentanyl may be sufficient to allow endotracheal intubation. Suggested combinations are given in Figure 21.4.

Combination	Comments
Dogs and cats	
Diazepam or midazolam 0.2 mg/kg i.v. followed 20 seconds later by fentanyl 5–10 µg/kg i.v.	Endotracheal intubation may be possible in many debilitated animals. When anaesthesia is insufficient add propofol to effect (1–2 mg/kg) to allow intubation
Midazolam 0.2 mg/kg i.v. + propofol to effect (1–5 mg/kg)	Wait only 15–20 seconds until animal starts to show signs of midazolam efficacy. If propofol administration is delayed longer than 20 seconds, midazolam-induced dysphoria may occur, necessitating increased propofol dosing
Acepromazine 0.02 mg/kg + pethidine 2 mg/kg i.m. followed 30 minutes later by propofol to effect (1–5 mg/kg)	
Cats	
Midazolam 0.2 mg/kg i.v. + ketamine 5 mg/kg	Produces short-term (5–10-minute) anaesthesia and will need to be followed by maintenance with a volatile agent

21.4 Suggested combinations of agents for effective induction of anaesthesia in the critical veterinary patient.

Maintenance of anaesthesia

Anaesthesia may be maintained by the use of intravenous agents, volatile inhalational agents or a combination of the two.

Intravenous infusions

Anaesthesia may be maintained by intravenous infusion of a sole agent when the agent has suitable pharmacokinetics (e.g. propofol). Practically, production of a stable plane of anaesthesia is difficult in all but prolonged procedures (e.g. positive pressure ventilation). In addition, infusion of propofol at a rate sufficient to maintain anaesthesia may be associated with unwanted effects such as hypotension and vomiting. The use of adjuncts to anaesthesia in critical patients has found favour in both human and veterinary clinical practice. Suitable adjuncts include medetomidine and ketamine (see above) as well as rapid-onset, short-duration, highly potent opioids, such as fentanyl, combined with sedatives, such as midazolam. Such adjuncts reduce induction and maintenance requirements for propofol and result in a more stable anaesthetic plane. These drugs also provide profound analgesia and will usually ablate the patient's response to noxious surgical stimuli. Administration may be in response to signs occurring as a result of surgical stimulus (inferred from changes in cardiovascular parameters) or pre-emptively either by bolus or infusions. For suggested doses, see Figure 21.5. It should be noted that both ketamine and fentanyl at the doses suggested might produce ventilatory depression when used in an anaesthetized patient. Although this does not usually warrant use of IPPV, facilities for assisted ventilation should be available.

Inhalational agents

Volatile inhalational agents still form the mainstay of anaesthesia maintenance in critical patients. As with propofol infusion, combination with an adjunct, enabling reduction of inspired concentration, usually results in significant improvement of cardiovascular parameters, even when sevoflurane or isoflurane are used.

Suggested adjuncts to anaesthesia in the critical patient	Comments
Fentanyl 1–2 µg/kg i.v. bolus repeated every 15–20 minutes	Heart rate will fall initially and then return towards normal as the effect wanes. The dose may be repeated at this point. Some tolerance may be seen (shorter time between doses). Ventilation rate will fall but IPPV is rarely required at these doses
Fentanyl infusion 3–30 µg/kg/h after initial bolus as above	Less tolerance seen than with intermittent boluses. Some reduction in heart and ventilation rate expected. Cumulative effects can occur with long (>90 minutes) duration of infusion, but can be managed by dose reduction as indicated by the patient's clinical condition
Ketamine 0.5–1 mg/kg repeated approximately every 30 minutes	A short period of apnoea may be seen in the first minute or two after administration. Be prepared to support ventilation for a short period
Ketamine 0.1–0.2 mg/kg/h	
Medetomidine 1–3 µg/kg bolus	Should provide effect of 30–40 minutes' duration. Be cautious in cardiovascularly unstable patients. Repeat dose once heart rate begins to rise towards resting rate. Concentration of volatile agent may need slight reduction to maintain 'level' of anaesthesia

21.5 Suggested adjuncts to potentiate or prolong anaesthesia.

Isoflurane is considered to have several benefits over halothane, including: lack of sensitization of the heart to the dysrhythmogenic effects of adrenaline; reduced myocardial depression; reduced tendency to decrease mean arterial pressure (MAP) due to vasodilation (which may be managed by fluid support); and less disruption of cerebral autoregulation. Recently the benefits of isoflurane for veterinary use have been shown to be more than theoretical, with a significant reduction in anaesthetic risk in patients anaesthetized with isoflurane compared to halothane (Brodbelt *et al.*, 2005). Isoflurane should, however, be used with caution in critically ill patients that have questionable intravascular volume status. The accompanying vasodilation can produce significant decreases in blood pressure which may be poorly responsive to the use of pressors.

Sevoflurane is gaining popularity for general anaesthesia due to a more rapid induction of anaesthesia (where an inhalational induction technique is used) and a modest reduction in recovery times (see the *BSAVA Manual of Canine and Feline Anaesthesia and Analgesia*). Its benefits above halothane are clear and similar to those of isoflurane. Currently there are insufficient studies describing the use of sevoflurane in critical patients to allow an informed opinion as to the advantages of its use.

Local anaesthetic techniques

A description of local anaesthetic techniques may be found in the *BSAVA Manual of Canine and Feline Anaesthesia and Analgesia,* and is outside the scope of this book. Local anaesthetic blocks may, like anaesthetic adjuncts, be especially useful in the critical patient to reduce doses of general anaesthetics and hence cardiovascular suppression. Newer agents, such as ropivacaine and levo-bupivacaine, have fewer intrinsic unwanted cardiac effects and long duration of action, and should be considered as part of anaesthesia in the critical patient when analgesia is required.

Supporting the sedated/anaesthetized intensive care unit patient

Specific considerations for monitoring during sedation and general anaesthesia of critical patients include cardiac rate and rhythm, respiratory status and fluid status.

Cardiac rate and rhythm

Use of a continuous waveform ECG to allow early detection of life-threatening dysrhythmias is strongly recommended. Specific therapy of individual dysrhythmias is described in Chapter 6. It should be remembered that the presence of a normal cardiac rhythm does not necessarily indicate that cardiac output is normal.

Fluid input, fluid loss and volume status

The rate and type of fluid support must take into account:

- Pre-existing cardiovascular function
- Type and rate of ongoing fluid loss
- Acid–base and electrolyte disturbances
- Rate and volume of intraoperative blood loss.

For normal intraoperative support, infusion of a balanced electrolyte solution with composition similar to that of extracellular fluid (e.g. lactated Ringer's solution) at a rate of 5–10 ml/kg/h is adequate. If the patient is hypoproteinaemic or if blood losses exceed 10% of blood volume, infusion of colloids (gelatins, hetastarch or dextrans) may be indicated to maintain intravascular volume (see Chapter 4). Acute severe blood losses (>15% of blood volume) or instances where the patient's PCV falls below 20% require the transfusion of fresh whole blood or packed red cells (see Chapter 14). Blood loss can be quantitatively evaluated by weighing swabs (1 ml of blood weighs 1.3 g) and by estimating losses from the suction reservoir if one is used.

Tissue and organ perfusion

Tissue perfusion can be assessed qualitatively by regular palpation of peripheral pulses and evaluation of mucous membrane colour and capillary refill time, although these are all notoriously subjective phenomena. Urine output is a valuable indicator of renal perfusion, and an indwelling catheter and closed collection system can be used throughout the perioperative period to monitor output. Mean arterial pressure should be maintained above 60–70 mmHg to ensure perfusion of vital organs.

Oxygenation and ventilation

Pulse oximetry

Pulse oximetry provides a continuous indication of the degree of saturation of arterial blood with oxygen. As accurate readings rely on the maintenance of peripheral perfusion and blood flow, changes in the status of these parameters will adversely affect accuracy. Pulse oximetry therefore provides an indicator of the presence of peripheral pulses and tissue perfusion, and an assessment of the patient's ability to oxygenate blood. It does not reflect arterial oxygen content or tissue oxygen delivery (see Chapter 7). False readings will be obtained in the presence of certain disease states, including carbon monoxide poisoning (smoke inhalation), methaemoglobinaemia (paracetamol poisoning) and conditions resulting in venous pulsatile flow (severe right-sided myocardial failure). Blood gas analysis represents the 'gold standard' for respiratory function monitoring, and more cost-effective machines are now becoming widely available.

Capnography

This is the most useful non-invasive estimation of the adequacy of ventilatory function in both the conscious and the anaesthetized animal. Measurement of expired carbon dioxide also provides an indication of the adequacy of cardiac output, and therefore estimations of ventilatory function based on capnography should be made in the light of cardiac functional status. The rapid response time of the capnogram is of use in alerting the anaesthetist to potential disasters, including:

- Cardiopulmonary arrest
- Patient disconnection from the breathing system
- Unrecognized oesophageal intubation
- Venous air embolism.

For the intubated patient, both mainstream and sidestream capnographs are available. Capnography may be performed in the sedated but unintubated veterinary patient using a sidestream analyser. A soft plastic, paediatric nasal oxygen administration set is easily held in place behind the animal's head (Figure 21.6). This is well tolerated by the animal, provides breath-by-breath information, and is the most accurate assessment of the effects of sedation on ventilatory function in the absence of blood gas analysis (see Chapter 7).

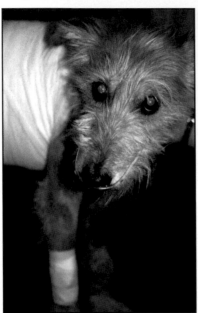

21.6 An intranasal cannula for administration of oxygen may also be used for sampling expired carbon dioxide for analysis by sidestream capnography in the conscious patient.

Body temperature

Maintenance of an adequate body temperature is mandatory to prevent a prolonged recovery and its attendant complications. Many critically ill patients rely heavily on ambient temperature to maintain core body temperature. Drugs involved in sedation and anaesthesia disrupt normal thermoregulatory mechanisms, and the respiration of cold dry gases significantly contributes to intraoperative heat loss, as do evaporative losses from exposed organs and tissues during major surgery. In the postoperative phase, muscle activity such as shivering increases endogenous heat production at the expense of an increased oxygen demand, which may not be tolerated by a compromised patient. Hypothermia produces a plethora of adverse effects that may be more significant in the critical patient (Figure 21.7). One of the most effective means of maintaining body temperature in the recumbent patient, the ICU patient or anaesthetized animals is the use of a hot air blanket (Bair Hugger). The advantages of hot air blankets include:

* Disposable blankets of variable sizes which are appropriate to veterinary patients
* Safe use without the possibility of burns or scalds
* Safety in the presence of electrical equipment
* They are also highly effective and well tolerated by the animal (Figure 21.8).

Adverse effects of hypothermia
Peripheral vasoconstriction and increased vascular resistance
Increased coagulability
Predisposition to dysrhythmias
Reduction in cerebral blood flow
Reduced effectiveness of analgesics
Derangements in substrate metabolism
Reduced ventilation and elimination of volatile agents

Methods of preventing/correcting hypothermia
Warm air blanket
Use of rebreathing systems (promotes inspiration of warm moist gases)
Use of heat and moisture exchangers (artificial nose)
High ambient temperatures in the operating theatre and recovery area
Patient insulation (e.g. foil wrap, water beds)
Avoidance of excessive preparation of surgical site
Expedient surgery
Warmed intravenous fluids
Postsurgical use of warmed isotonic enemas and urinary bladder lavage

21.7 Adverse effects of hypothermia and methods of supporting body temperature.

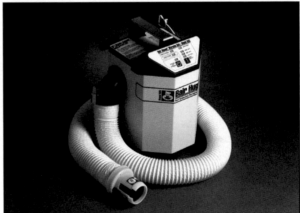

21.8 A Bair Hugger warm air blanket system. A safe and highly effective way of maintaining normothermia in both anaesthetized and debilitated animals.

Recovery from anaesthesia

The transitional phase from anaesthesia to recovery is critical and associated with high risk. When possible, support in terms of inspired oxygen, monitoring, intravenous fluids, body temperature management, analgesia and careful observation must continue until the additional effects of the anaesthetic agents are minimal.

References and further reading

Annane D (2005) ICU physicians should abandon the use of etomidate! *Intensive Care Medicine* **31**, 325–326

Brodbelt D, Brearley J, Young L, Wood J and Pfeiffer D (2005) Anaesthetic-related mortality risks in small animals in the UK. *Proceedings of the Association of Veterinary Anaesthetists*, Rimini Italy 20–23 April 2005

Heldmann E, Holt DE, Brockman DJ *et al.* (1999) Use of propofol to manage seizure activity after surgical treatment of portosystemic shunts. *Journal of Small Animal Practice* **40**, 590–594

Jackson MT and Ramos AS (2006) Etomidate – misused or misunderstood? *Anaesthesia* **61**, 190–191

Ko JC, Payton ME, White AG *et al.* (2006) Effects of intravenous diazepam or microdose medetomidine on propofol-induced sedation in dogs. *Journal of the American Animal Hospital Association* **42**, 18–27

Kong KL and Willatts SM (1995) Isoflurane sedation in pediatric intensive care. *Critical Care Medicine* **23**, 1308–1309

Kowaluk EA, Roberts MS and Polack AE (1982) Interactions between drugs and intravenous delivery systems. *American Journal of Hospital Pharmacy* **39**, 460–467

Meiser A, Sirtl C, Bellgardt M *et al.* (2003) Desflurane compared with propofol for postoperative sedation in the intensive care unit. *British Journal of Anaesthesia* **90**, 273–280

Perry SM, Whelan E, Shay S *et al.* (1991) Effect of i.v. anaesthesia with propofol on drug distribution and metabolism in the dog. *British Journal of Anaesthesia* **66**, 66–72

Ruiz-Ortega JA, Ugedo L, Pineda J *et al.* (1995) The stimulatory effect of clonidine through imidazoline receptors on locus coeruleus noradrenergic neurones is mediated by excitatory amino acids and modulated by serotonin. *Naunyn-Schmiedeberg's Archives of Pharmacology* **352**, 121–126

Schmeling WT, Kampine JP, Roerig DL *et al.* (1991) The effects of the stereoisomers of the alpha 2-adrenergic agonist medetomidine on systemic and coronary hemodynamics in conscious dogs. *Anesthesiology* **75**, 499–511

Seymour C and Duke-Novakovski T (2007) *BSAVA Manual of Canine and Feline Anaesthesia and Analgesia, 2nd edition.* BSAVA Publications, Gloucester

Shaham Y, Highfield D, Delfs J *et al.* (2000) Clonidine blocks stress-induced reinstatement of heroin seeking in rats: an effect independent of locus coeruleus noradrenergic neurons. *European Journal of Neuroscience* **12**, 292–302

22

Analgesia in the critical patient

Daniel Holden

Introduction

Pain is commonly identified in patients with critical illness. Conditions such as trauma, ischaemia, thrombosis, inflammation and ileus are all associated with pain, and many diagnostic and therapeutic procedures necessary in critically ill patients can cause pain or discomfort. Pre-existing chronic pain may worsen in the face of critical illness or injury. Both physiological and emotional stress can contribute to pain, but may also mask its clinical signs. It should be remembered that non-pharmacological management of pain plays a significant role in minimizing discomfort and distress in patients with severe disease or injury.

Recognition of pain

Responses to pain vary between species, breeds and individual animals. In debilitated, obtunded or heavily sedated patients, normal behavioural responses to nociceptive stimuli may be decreased or absent. Severe central nervous system (CNS) disease or sedation may limit ability to vocalize (more common as a sign of pain in dogs than in cats), and major trauma or weakness may limit movement responses. It has been hypothesized that some animals adopt a near-catatonic state in response to repeated or incessant pain. This may be misinterpreted as meaning that the animal is not in pain, with subsequent failure to provide analgesia when it is most needed. It may also be difficult to separate signs of pain from signs of the patient's underlying disease. Heart rate is an unreliable index of postoperative pain, and respiratory rate may be elevated by such factors as hypoxia, pyrexia, hyperthermia, or acid–base disturbances. If it is unclear whether an animal is experiencing pain, it is generally better to assume that it might be and to administer analgesia. Response to analgesic medications should be noted carefully to help guide further treatment decisions.

Left unmanaged, pain will have several clinically significant consequences:

- Reduced food intake will result in a negative protein–energy balance, resulting in weight loss, weakness and effects on wound healing
- Thoracic or cranial abdominal pain may result in hypoventilation and failure to expectorate
- Reduced patient movement may contribute to hypostasis, oedema, urinary and faecal retention and possibly vascular thrombosis

- Neuroendocrine stress responses may place increased demands on the cardiovascular and respiratory systems
- Prolonged stress responses to pain may precipitate immune dysfunction.

Management of pain

Nursing management
Although drugs form the mainstay of pain management in critical illness, the importance of constant and compassionate nursing care cannot be overemphasized. Regular contact, stroking and grooming not associated with clinical procedures will reassure nervous patients. Toys or blankets from home will provide familiar smells, and owner visits should be encouraged wherever possible. Cats should be provided with ample bedding or boxes in which to hide. Regular passive movement exercises and physiotherapy will assist in musculoskeletal blood flow and improve limb mobilization. Regular gentle cleaning of the nose, lips and oral mucosa with damp swabs prevents the build-up of secretions. Patients should be checked regularly to ensure that both skin and bedding are clean and dry.

Drug therapy
Analgesic therapy may be targeted at any of the main elements of the nociception pathways from peripheral receptors to the conscious perception of pain. A detailed discussion of the clinical pharmacology of acute pain is beyond the scope of this chapter, however most analgesic drugs act at one of the following levels:

- Stimulation and transduction at the level of peripheral nociceptors
- Transmission from the periphery to the dorsal horn of the spinal cord or cranial nerve nuclei
- Modulation within the spinal cord pathways
- Perception within the cerebrum.

Combination therapy (i.e. using more than one agent to target different elements of the nociceptive pathway) has many advantages. Not only will the analgesic effects be at least additive, but the combination or combinations may also allow reduction in doses of the agents used (so-called 'balanced analgesia'), thereby helping to reduce the frequency and severity of any unwanted side effects.

The main pharmacological classes of agents to consider are:

- Opioids
- Non-steroidal anti-inflammatory drugs (NSAIDs)
- Alpha-2 agonists
- Ketamine
- Nitrous oxide
- Local analgesics
- Other agents.

Opioids

Opioids are undeniably the drugs of choice for managing moderate to severe pain in dogs and cats. In humans, they reduce both the conscious sensation of pain and associated anxiety. Opioids may also mediate analgesia locally within damaged tissue. Opioid drugs fall under either Schedule II (pure agonists) or Schedule III (partial agonists) of the Misuse of Drugs Act 1971.

Of major importance to the intensive care and emergency clinician are the concurrent effects of any analgesic drug on cardiovascular and respiratory function. The cardiovascular effects of opioids depend on the species, the specific drug and the route of administration. Centrally mediated bradycardia may occur but is not usually clinically significant in patients that are already in pain, unless potent opioids such as fentanyl and its derivatives are given intravenously. Bradycardia associated with opioid administration in cats is more likely to result from an indirect calming effect. Hypotension may result from bradycardia and may also occur following rapid intravenous administration of morphine and pethidine (much more severely with the latter), probably as a result of histamine release.

Opioid-associated respiratory depression occurs as a result of reduced sensitivity of the respiratory centre to carbon dioxide. In contrast to humans, clinically significant respiratory depression is extremely uncommon in small animals unless potent opioids are used intraoperatively. Hypoventilation as a result of thoracic wall pain may, in fact, be improved by opioid analgesia. In contrast, exacerbation of respiratory depression by opioids in patients with hypoventilation following head injury may increase the risk of intracranial hypertension (developing as a result of carbon dioxide-induced cerebral vasodilation). Severely obtunded or comatose patients should probably not receive opioids until ventilation and/or intracranial pressure are controlled.

Much controversy exists over the clinical use of opioids in the management of pancreatic pain. Experimental studies have documented increases in pressure in the pancreatic ducts associated with the administration of morphine, methadone, fentanyl and also pethidine, a drug which has been credited with spasmolytic properties. However, the clinical significance of this effect is not clear and the author is not aware of any clinical studies in animals that demonstrate exacerbation of pancreatitis following administration of these drugs. If the clinician is concerned, buprenorphine may be preferred due to its minimal effect on ductal pressure; alternatively opioids may be given epidurally or other agents (e.g. ketamine) considered.

Morphine: Morphine is a powerful analgesic, which, despite its lack of a veterinary licence in the UK, is widely utilized due to its considerable efficacy and reliability. Systemic administration at doses of 0.1–0.4 mg/kg s.c. or i.m. produces analgesia of approximately 4 hours' duration. The duration of effect probably depends on both the dose used and the severity of the painful stimulus. Morphine is also effective orally (despite significant first-pass metabolism) and rectally. The time to onset of action is usually 5–10 minutes, even after intravenous injection. Analgesia is dose-dependent and doses higher than those recommended above may be required; in severe pain in dogs the author has occasionally needed to use morphine at doses as high as 4–5 mg/kg, titrated slowly up to a desired clinical effect. The poor lipid solubility of morphine makes it suitable for prolonged analgesia (up to 24 hours) when used epidurally. For the epidural route, the preservative-free preparation should be used at 0.1 mg/kg. Cats do not metabolize morphine as rapidly as dogs and a dosing interval of 4–6 hours is probably appropriate in this species. Vomiting seen after the use of morphine for premedication in healthy patients is much less common in painful critically ill patients. The incidence of vomiting can also be reduced by diluting the drug in saline and administering it slowly by the intravenous route.

Pethidine (meperidine): Pethidine is the only mu receptor agonist licensed as a sole agent for veterinary use in the UK. It is less potent than morphine but its onset of action is rapid, making it a potentially good choice for acute use in trauma. The duration of action is short, at 90–120 minutes, depending somewhat on the dose (2–5 mg/kg i.m.).

Fentanyl: Fentanyl is a very potent mu agonist, approximately 50 times more effective than morphine, but with a rapid onset and short duration of action. It is used primarily for intraoperative analgesia as part of a balanced anaesthetic protocol. Standard doses (5–20 µg/kg boluses i.v.) produce profound respiratory depression or apnoea in anaesthetized patients; provision for intermittent positive pressure ventilation (IPPV) must therefore be available. The short duration of action is mainly due to redistribution rather than elimination, therefore there is a risk of cumulative or prolonged respiratory depressant effects. Large doses may produce a profound bradycardia. Fentanyl may be used as a constant rate infusion (CRI) at 0.1–0.4 µg/kg/min in critically ill postoperative patients. Patients receiving a fentanyl CRI must be closely monitored (heart rate, blood pressure, respiratory rate) and facilities for IPPV must be available, however the level of analgesia can be titrated easily.

Fentanyl is also available as a transdermal patch (Durogesic®) intended for use in human patients suffering from chronic pain. The onset of analgesia is slow (up to 12 hours) but the patches can provide effective pain relief for up to 72 hours. All Schedule II regulations still apply. Recommended patch sizes are shown in Figure 22.1. Small dogs and cats may be dosed with a half patch, however the patch should not be cut in half; instead half the gel membrane

Patient weight	Dose of fentanyl	Total drug content
Small dogs (<5 kg) and cats	25 µg/h	2.5 mg
Dogs: 5–10 kg	25 µg/h	2.5 mg
Dogs: 10–20 kg	50 µg/h	5 mg
Dogs: 20–30 kg	75 µg/h	7.5 mg
Dogs: >30 kg	100 µg/h	10 mg

22.1 Recommended size of fentanyl patch for use in small animal patients.

should be covered with tape before the patch is applied. 'Half-patch dosing' is suggested for paediatric, geriatric and systemically ill cats and small dogs.

The patch may be placed either on the dorsal or lateral cervical area or the lateral thorax. If the neck is used, collars/leashes should not be placed over the patch. The thorax is an easy site to use and skin contact is maximized (especially in cats), but it can be difficult to bandage securely. Patches should NOT be placed at any site which may come into contact with a heating pad as this may increase the release of drug from the patch. The site should be closely clipped with at least a 1 cm margin around the patch. It should not be shaved because cuts, abrasions or wounds can alter drug absorption. After clipping, the site should be wiped with a damp swab to remove small hairs and skin debris; it should not be scrubbed or surgically prepared. The skin should be allowed to dry completely before application of the patch. The occlusive membrane is then removed from the patch, taking care not to expose the applier's skin to the gel surface. The patch is placed on the clipped area and held in place for 2–3 minutes to ensure adherence. A slightly padded bandage or transparent dressing is used with medical adhesive spray to assure adherence and to keep the patch dry. It should be checked every few hours to ensure proper placement and adherence. It is important that used patches are disposed of in a safe and effective manner and the disposal date and method are recorded. All patients wearing patches should have heart and respiratory rates monitored regularly.

Buprenorphine: Buprenorphine is classified as a partial agonist at mu opioid receptors, although partial agonist effects are probably not significant at doses currently used clinically (20–40 µg/kg i.v. or i.m. q6–8h). The drug has a slow onset of action (30–40 minutes for maximal receptor binding), which limits its usefulness in the acute setting, but duration of analgesia is good (6–8 hours) and analgesic potency in cats is comparable with that of morphine. Injectable buprenorphine can be administered orally in cats to provide analgesia at similar doses to those used parenterally.

Butorphanol: Butorphanol is a mu receptor antagonist and a kappa agonist. It possesses excellent sedative properties, particularly as part of a neurolept-analgesic combination, but its analgesic benefits are controversial and the author cannot currently recommend the drug for use as a 'front-line' analgesic. Its

effects are short in duration (<90 minutes). Butorphanol provides better visceral analgesia than somatic analgesia and its use should probably be limited to patients with acute visceral pain (enteritis, cystitis).

Non-steroidal anti-inflammatory drugs
NSAIDs are potent analgesics and provide significant opioid-sparing effects in both human and animal species. Analgesic efficacy is relatively uniform, and there is little to choose between the currently available agents in the UK in this regard. NSAIDs are capable of providing analgesia for up to 24 hours following a single administration. As such they play an important role in perioperative and acute analgesia.

NSAIDs act by inhibition of cyclo-oxygenase (COX) and in some instances 5-lipoxygenase. Different isoforms of COX exist, and the extent to which different forms are expressed varies between species; consequently safety and efficacy of a particular NSAID in one species cannot be assumed in another. Concerns over toxicity have, until recently, limited use of NSAIDs in cats. Rational use of NSAIDs has also been hampered by over-simplification of the COX-1/COX-2 relationship. Constitutive forms of COX-2 are recognized in cats although their significance remains to be fully elucidated, and pharmacokinetic data for these drugs in cats need to be established. Cats display much slower metabolism of many NSAIDs, resulting in longer half-lives and necessitating longer dosing intervals. Newer NSAIDs, such as carprofen and meloxicam, have been subjected to perioperative use studies and compare favourably with opioids.

NSAIDs produce potent anti-inflammatory, anti-pyretic and anti-endotoxic effects. However, the effects on COX isoforms may also mean that critically ill and hypotensive patients are at greater risk of developing side effects such as gastrointestinal irritation, ulceration and haemorrhage, and renal tubular injury. NSAIDs should generally be avoided in the following groups:

- Patients with current or recent haemodynamic instability
- Patients with gastrointestinal ulcerative disease
- Patients with acute or chronic renal failure
- Patients with haemostatic disorders or those receiving anticoagulants
- Patients receiving corticosteroids.

Carprofen: Carprofen is licensed in the UK in dogs for acute and chronic use and in cats for a single perioperative dose of 4 mg/kg. Reports of toxicity do exist; these are largely related to coexistent problems and prolonged usage. Idiosyncratic hepatotoxicity has been reported in dogs. Repeat administration in cats is hampered by the very variable kinetics noted in this species. Carprofen is a weak COX inhibitor, and its exact mechanisms of action are uncertain at present.

Meloxicam: Meloxicam is a COX-2 preferential NSAID licensed in the UK for perioperative use in the dog and cat as a single injectable dose of 0.2 mg/kg (dog) and 0.3 mg/kg (cat). Duration and intensity of analgesia are similar to those of carprofen. Considerable data exist to support successful longer-term 'off-label' use in cats via the oral route. The liquid preparation greatly facilitates administration in cats. Doses as low as one drop per cat per day have been used successfully.

Others: Other NSAIDs, such as ketoprofen, deracoxib, tepoxalin and tolfenamic acid, have undergone pharmacodynamic studies and have demonstrated similar analgesic efficacy in healthy patients. Anecdotal evidence suggests side effects are more likely with these agents than with carprofen or meloxicam. To date no studies of the efficacy of such drugs in critically ill or hypotensive patients exist. Older NSAIDs, such as aspirin, have little current use as analgesics due to their low safety margin. Other agents, such as paracetamol (a useful analgesic in dogs) and ibuprofen, are too toxic for routine use in cats.

Alpha-2 agonists
Medetomidine and, less commonly, xylazine are the most frequently used drugs in this category. These drugs have marked sedative and anaesthetic-sparing properties, as well as providing analgesia mediated via receptors located centrally and in the dorsal horn of the spinal cord. The cardiovascular and respiratory effects of these drugs are well known (see Chapter 21), and although often well tolerated in fit healthy patients, they are potentially hazardous in unstable or critically ill dogs or cats.

Low doses of medetomidine (0.5–2 µg/kg) may prove useful to provide additional sedation and analgesia in patients pretreated with an opioid. Medetomidine can also be used perioperatively to provide additional analgesia and sedation at infusion rates of 1–3 µg/kg/h. Mild bradycardia and peripheral vasoconstriction may develop, but in haemodynamically stable patients this is rarely significant.

Ketamine
Ketamine has enjoyed long-term use as an induction agent, especially in 'field' procedures and in unstable patients. More recently interest in its use in the intensive care unit (ICU) setting has increased. Ketamine acts as a non-competitive antagonist at NMDA (*N*-methyl-D-aspartate) receptors in the spinal cord. These receptors play a central role in the post-injury facilitation of nociception that occurs in the cord. This forms the basis of 'wind-up' and perception of pain at lower thresholds and intensities. Ketamine may therefore contribute significantly to longer-term postoperative analgesia as well as that experienced perioperatively.

Cardiovascular and respiratory side effects are minimal in healthy patients but may be more pronounced in patients already experiencing maximal sympathetic stimulation. Use of the drug at lower doses to provide analgesia is, however, a valuable strategy that creates minimal side effects. Infusions of 1–2 mg/kg/h i.v. combined with other sedatives and analgesics are extremely useful up to 24 hours postoperatively. Lower doses (0.2 mg/kg/h) minimize the risk of central effects. Ketamine appears to be particularly useful for surface and soft tissue pain in humans.

Ketamine is metabolized to an active metabolite (nor-ketamine), which requires elimination by the kidney. Care should be taken in animals with renal or hepatic dysfunction as this may increase the effects and rate of accumulation of the drug or its metabolites.

Ketamine has indirect sympathomimetic effects which include an increase in heart rate. This may be detrimental in patients with hypertrophic cardiomyopathy or ischaemic heart disease. Its use in patients with head trauma is controversial, as it may produce increases in cerebral blood flow, causing increases in intracranial pressure, although some experimental studies suggest that ketamine may have neuroprotective properties.

Other NMDA antagonists, such as amantidine, dextromethorphan and memantine, have been used to manage chronic pain in both dogs and cats.

Nitrous oxide
Due to its gaseous nature and very short duration of analgesic effect, the use of nitrous oxide is limited to the intraoperative period. The mode of analgesic action is uncertain; both NMDA antagonist and alpha-2 agonist effects have been postulated. Nitrous oxide has significant volatile agent-sparing properties in dogs and cats, but concerns relating to occupational exposure of personnel to nitrous oxide have led to a decline in its use. Its use also necessitates a reduction in fractional inspired oxygen concentration (F_iO_2) during anaesthesia, which may not be well tolerated by patients prone to hypoxia.

Local analgesic agents
Local analgesics are among the most versatile and useful agents at the ICU clinician's disposal. They may be used topically, locally or to provide analgesia of specific anatomical regions using peripheral nerve blockade or administration into the epidural or subarachnoid spaces. Systemic intravenous use of lidocaine can also provide significant analgesic benefits.

Lidocaine, prilocaine and proxymetacaine are all used topically for placement of various tubes and catheters (e.g. nasal, urinary) in critical patients. For placement of intravenous catheters, topical application of EMLA (eutectic mixture of local anaesthetics) cream, a 50:50 mixture of prilocaine and lidocaine, may prove useful. The cream should not be rubbed in and should be covered with a waterproof dressing for 40–45 minutes prior to the procedure to allow it to have its maximum effect.

Lidocaine is the most useful drug for local infiltration prior to tube placement, catheterization cut-down and similar procedures. Pain on injection can be minimized by warming the solution prior to use, and by the addition of 8.4% (1 mEq/ml) sodium bicarbonate at a ratio of 9:1 lidocaine:bicarbonate by volume. The time to onset of effect is usually 5–10 minutes.

Local nerve blockade may also be performed using lidocaine, but longer duration of action will be provided by bupivicaine 0.5% or ropivicaine 0.25%. These agents have a slower onset time (20–30 minutes) but a longer duration of effect (4–6 hours versus 1 hour for lidocaine). Administration of equal volumes of either drug with lidocaine will decrease latency.

Intravenous use: Lidocaine has well documented anaesthetic-sparing properties when used intravenously. It can be used alone or as part of a multiple drug infusion at doses of 0.5–2 mg/kg/h in dogs; however its use in critically ill cats is probably best avoided.

Lidocaine also possesses significant antioxidant and free radical scavenging properties which are potentially useful but not well understood at present.

Other analgesic drugs

Gabapentin is an anticonvulsant drug that has been used extensively for the management of chronic neuropathic pain in humans and small animals. Much anecdotal evidence exists to support its use, despite the mechanism of action remaining unclear. The reported dose is 3 mg/kg once daily.

Tramadol is often classed as an opioid, although it also has serotoninergic and monoaminergic properties. Numerous side effects have been reported in humans, but its use is increasing in dogs and anecdotal reports exist of its use in the cat. Reported doses are 1–4 mg/kg q8–12h.

Tricyclic antidepressants such as amitriptyline, imipramine and clomipramine have all been used to a greater or lesser extent in dogs and cats. Amitriptyline in particular has been used extensively in the management of feline idiopathic cystitis with promising results and few documented side effects with long-term usage.

Epidural analgesia

Use of the epidural route for administration of analgesic and local anaesthetic agents has increased in recent years as its benefits have become better recognized. The technique is particularly beneficial in animals with severe pain caudal to the diaphragm (e.g. peritonitis, pancreatitis, or severe trauma to the pelvic limbs) or for patients in which sedation or other central effects of systemic analgesia are undesirable. Depending on the agent and technique used, it is possible to achieve complete caudal anaesthesia with no loss of consciousness and to provide intense analgesia with minimal effects on motor function. This technique is therefore a valuable adjunct to general anaesthesia for surgery, as well as a useful method for providing analgesia in many critically ill patients. The benefits for the critically ill patient may go beyond the efficacy of the technique.

Drugs used for epidural administration

The most common agents used epidurally are:

- Opioids (most often morphine)
- Local analgesics
- Alpha-2 agonists.

Single preoperative injections of opioids may be usefully employed to provide a degree of postoperative analgesia for 12–24 hours following injection. If a longer duration of action is desired, insertion of an epidural catheter allows repeated or constant infusion of drug into the epidural space for several days. Morphine is the opioid used most commonly, as its low lipid solubility ensures analgesia at much lower concentrations than are needed in plasma, as well as prolonged effects and good distribution in the epidural space. More lipid-soluble agents (e.g. buprenorphine, fentanyl) provide more local and shorter-acting effects.

Local analgesics block small unmyelinated C and A-delta fibres (responsible for nociceptive transmission) much more effectively than the larger-diameter motor fibres. Typically, autonomic blockade is more widespread than sensory blockade, which in turn is greater than motor blockade. Autonomic blockade may occur when sympathetic nerve roots in the thoracolumbar (T1–L3) region are affected; this will reduce the neuroendocrine stress response to anaesthesia but may precipitate hypotension due to splanchnic vasodilation. Sympathetic blockade should be avoided at all costs and may increase morbidity and mortality in some critically ill patients. Ropivicaine produces less motor blockade than bupivicaine.

Doses of local analgesics for epidural use are:

- Lidocaine: 4 mg/kg (onset 5 minutes; duration 50–90 minutes)
- Bupivacaine: 1 mg/kg (onset 20 minutes; duration 120–360 minutes)
- Ropivacaine: 1 mg/kg (onset 7–20 minutes; duration 115–140 minutes).

Alpha-2 agonists may produce significant systemic effects (sedation, bradycardia) when given epidurally, despite producing useful analgesia. These drugs may therefore be poorly tolerated in unstable patients. Medetomidine may be administered epidurally at 2–10 µg/kg q4–8h. The technique for epidural injection is described in Figure 22.2 and illustrated in Figure 22.3.

1. The most common injection site used is the lumbosacral space. The dural sac terminates in most dogs at L6, but in cats the dural sac extends to S2 therefore inadvertent subdural injection is a risk. If cerebrospinal fluid (CSF) is obtained (suggesting the subdural space has been entered) the procedure should either be abandoned or the dose reduced by 50–65%.

2. The patient is placed in sternal recumbency with the hindlegs drawn cranially. Intravenous access is mandatory and, unless contraindicated, an isotonic crystalloid infusion should be administered at 10–20 ml/kg/h.

3. The area over the lumbosacral space is clipped and prepared aseptically.

4. The site for injection can be identified by drawing a line transversely across the cranial aspect of the ilial wings; this usually passes over the dorsal spinous process of L7 (which is shorter than L6) (Figure 22.3a).

5. If the patient is not anaesthetized or heavily sedated, the injection path should be infiltrated gradually down to the ligamentum flavum using 2% lidocaine injected with a 25 gauge needle or smaller.

6. A 22 gauge spinal needle (37–75 mm in length depending on patient size) is then inserted in the midline at the centre of the lumbosacral depression, at 90 degrees to the skin surface. The bevel of the needle should be directed cranially. A slight 'pop' or loss of resistance is encountered when the needle point enters the epidural space; the stylet should be withdrawn at this stage and the hub should be inspected for blood or CSF.

7. Correct placement of the needle should be ensured, either by checking for absence of resistance to a test injection of saline, or by placing a drop of fluid in the hub of the needle immediately prior to entering the epidural space; if the space is correctly entered the fluid will be sucked into the needle as epidural pressure is subatmospheric.

22.2 Technique for epidural injection. (continues) ▶

8. Injection of the drug should then follow slowly over 60 seconds. If unilateral effects are desired, placing the patient with the affected side down will assist with this to some extent.

9. Catheters may be placed epidurally to permit repeat injection or infusion of drugs. The technique is as previously described, except that a Tuohy (Figure 22.3c) or directional needle is used. The pre-measured catheter (inserted one to two vertebrae beyond the desired level of blockade) is inserted through the needle, which is then removed. The catheter is sutured to the skin and a microbiological in-line filter placed before attaching the hub to an injection cap. Catheters must be maintained in an aseptic fashion but correctly maintained catheters may be used for up to 2 weeks. The injection site should be evaluated twice daily for swelling or discharge.

22.2 (continued) Technique for epidural injection.

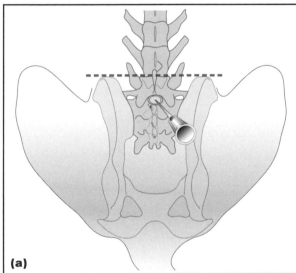

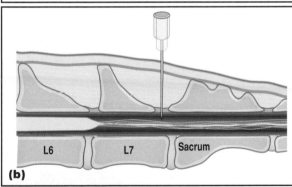

L6 L7 Sacrum

(b)

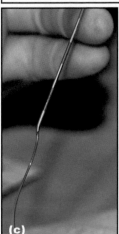

22.3 Anatomical landmarks for performing lumbo-sacral epidural anaesthesia and analgesia in dogs. **(a)** Dorsal view. **(b)** Lateral view. The lumbosacral space can be found caudal to a line drawn between the cranial borders of the ilia (marked with a dotted line). **(c)** Tuohy needle with epidural catheter; note the blunt curved end to the needle facilitating safe feeding of the catheter into the epidural space. (a,b Reproduced from *BSAVA Manual of Canine and Feline Anaesthesia and Analgesia, 2nd edition*; c, courtesy of L. Pelligand, Royal Veterinary College)

Complications of epidural analgesia

Complications arising from epidural analgesia may be due to the drugs used or to the procedure itself.
Complications of injection include:

* Failed technique
* Haemorrhage and haematoma formation
* Introduction of infection
* Excessive cranial spread of drug.

Excessive cranial spread of local analgesics within the epidural space may lead to hypotension and hypo-ventilation, as a result of splanchnic sympathetic block-ade and respiratory muscle paralysis. Patients with this complication may require ventilatory and haemo-dynamic support, using vasoactive agents if neces-sary. Inadvertent intravascular injection may cause CNS excitation, seizures and ultimately cardiotoxic effects (more likely with bupivicaine than ropivicaine or lidocaine). Aggressive management of seizures with anticonvulsants is recommended. Prolonged cardiac support may be necessary.

Complications of epidural opioid injection in humans typically include pruritus, delayed respiratory depres-sion and urinary retention, although these effects are uncommon in dogs and cats. All preparations contain-ing preservatives should ideally be avoided.
Contraindications to epidural analgesia include:

* Presence of bleeding disorders or receipt of anticoagulant drugs
* Severe hypotension or hypovolaemia
* Presence of infection (systemic sepsis or at the site of injection)
* Disruption of the normal anatomy, as this may complicate accurate injection.

Multiple drug constant rate infusions for perioperative analgesia

Many analgesics may be added to intravenous fluids for ease of administration and practice of multimodal analgesia. The dose rate is easily controlled and ti-trated and can be incorporated into the patient's cur-rent fluid regime. Analgesic drugs may be added to a separate bag of maintenance solution (e.g. glucose–saline) that is to be given at a slow unchanged rate. This fluid may be 'piggy-backed' on to the patient's other replacement fluid therapy. The most common analgesic drugs used in this way are shown in Figure 22.4. They may be used as sole agents or combined to increase the analgesic effect. The drug infusion may be delivered via a burette intravenous set so that, if reformulation is necessary, an entire bag is not wasted. When using this method of administration of analge-sia, care must be taken to ensure that the fluid ad-ministration rate is accurate, as inadvertent overdosing or underdosing may result from incorrect fluid flow rates. Therefore, these drug infusions are ideally ad-ministered using a fluid infusion pump or syringe pump. A volume of fluid equivalent to the volume of additives should be removed from the bag prior to addition of the analgesics to prevent excessive dilu-tion and to allow calculation of an accurate drug con-centration and infusion rate.

Drug	Dose
Morphine	Dog: 0.1 mg/kg/h Cat: 0.025–0.05 mg/kg/h
Fentanyl	0.1–0.4 µg/kg/min
Lidocaine (without adrenaline)	0.5–2 mg/kg/h Do not use in cats
Ketamine	0.2–2 mg/kg/h
Medetomidine	1 µg/kg/h

22.4 Doses of analgesic drugs used as constant rate infusions in the dog and cat.

References and further reading

Campoy L (2004) Epidural and spinal anaesthesia in the dog. *In Practice* **26**, 262–269

Flecknell P and Waterman-Pearson AE (eds) (2000) *Pain Management in Animals*. WB Saunders, Philadelphia

Hansen BD (2005) Analgesia and sedation in the critically ill. *Journal of Veterinary Emergency and Critical Care* **15**, 285–294

Robertson SA and Taylor PM (2004) Pain management in cats – past, present and future. Part 2. Treatment of pain – clinical pharmacology. *Journal of Feline Medicine and Surgery* **6**, 321–333

Robertson SA, Taylor PM and Sear JW (2003) Systemic uptake of buprenorphine by cats after oral mucosal administration. *Veterinary Record* **152**, 675–678

Solomon SB, Banks SM, Gerstenburger E *et al.* (2003) Sympathetic blockade in a canine model of gram-negative bacterial peritonitis. *Shock* **19**, 215–222

23

Nutritional support of the critical patient

Karyl J. Hurley and Kathryn E. Michel

Introduction

The provision of nutritional support to critical small animal patients is often postponed while the priorities of patient evaluation and stabilization are underway. However, studies in human clinical patients and experimental animal models demonstrate the benefits of early nutritional intervention, which include enhanced immune function, wound repair and response to therapy, more rapid recovery time and improved survival (Heyland, 1998). Once major fluid and electrolyte deficits have been addressed and the patient is haemodynamically stable, the clinician should consider whether nutritional support is indicated as part of the patient's treatment programme. After all, the goal of supporting cardiopulmonary function and vascular perfusion is to ensure adequate tissue oxygenation. The reason tissues require oxygen is to generate energy efficiently from the metabolism of nutrients.

This chapter provides an overview of the potential benefits of nutritional support for the critical patient; demonstrates how to assess whether a patient should be considered a candidate for nutritional support; illustrates methods of providing nutrition to patients unable or unwilling to nourish themselves and suggests methods for monitoring these patients to avoid or address complications.

Rationale for nutritional support

Any fasting animal must rely on its endogenous energy and nutrient stores until it is able to nourish itself again. A healthy animal deprived of food undergoes metabolic adaptations that improve its chances of survival by limiting the extent of tissue catabolism. The most critical of these adaptations are the ones that act to preserve endogenous proteins. Carbohydrate, fat and protein can all be utilized as sources of energy. Carbohydrate energy reserves are stored as glycogen in liver and muscle tissue, and fat is stored as triglycerides in adipose tissue. There are, however, no storage forms of protein. All endogenous proteins serve some functional purpose as structural proteins, enzymes, carrier proteins and so forth.

When an animal is deprived of food, glycogen is broken down to maintain blood glucose levels. Once the glycogen reserves have been depleted (within 24–48 hours) glucose must be synthesized from lactate, glycerol and certain amino acids in order to provide fuel for those tissues that preferentially or obligatorily use glucose for energy production. In the case of a simple fast in a healthy animal, metabolic adaptations over the course of days and weeks act to decrease tissue demands for glucose and thus spare amino acids.

Metabolic adaptations do not occur in the critical patient, however, even though these patients are often in a negative balance for both calories and nitrogen. The metabolic milieu of critical illness is very different from that of a simple fast. Mediators of the metabolic state (glucocorticoids, catecholamines, cytokines and other hormones) are released in response to tissue injury, infectious agents and inflammation. While some of the amino acids derived from the catabolism of endogenous proteins are either directly oxidized or converted to glucose, a significant portion are utilized for new protein synthesis. In the fasting critical patient it is not the lack of calories, but the lack of amino acids that is more likely to be life threatening. Amino acids are necessary for the synthesis of vital host defence proteins such as immunoglobulins, clotting factors and acute phase reactants.

Providing an exogenous source of amino acids, calories and other nutrients does not eliminate this catabolic response, but can blunt it to some extent and act to support the patient's response to disease and injury while preserving endogenous tissues. A recent study confirmed that providing caloric intake can have a significant, positive effect on patient outcome (Remillard et al., 2001). Another investigation in puppies with parvovirus showed that pups receiving early nutritional intervention responded faster with improved gastrointestinal tract barrier function, and had shorter recovery times (Mohr et al., 2003). Unfortunately, despite this evidence, a negative energy balance is common in our critical patients. Clearly nutritional supplementation should be a part of any critically ill patient's strategic therapeutic plan. In patients that have already experienced a significant degree of malnutrition, nutritional support may be essential for survival.

Nutritional assessment: who and when to feed

With the greater availability of tubes, catheters and nutrient formulae specifically tailored to veterinary patients, providing nutrition, even to the most critically ill dog or cat, has become increasingly feasible. Careful patient selection is required, as nutritional support may have disadvantages. These can include an increased risk of morbidity and even mortality, prolongation of hospitalization and additional cost of treatment. It is therefore important to reserve the more aggressive forms of intervention, such as tube feeding or parenteral nutrition, for those patients for whom lack of nutrition will be most likely to have a negative impact on their clinical outcome.

Traditionally, the tests and techniques for nutritional assessment have been directed at the identification of malnourished patients. These include body condition scoring, assessment of weight loss, measurement of serum proteins, functional tests such as intradermal skin tests and sophisticated body composition analysis (e.g. dual X-ray absorptiometry, bioelectrical impedance). While the severely malnourished individual is easily identified, the diagnostic accuracy of these techniques remains unknown in less obvious cases, as there is no universally accepted 'gold standard' of malnutrition against which these tests can be compared.

A system of subjective evaluation of a patient's history and physical examination has been developed for use in humans and has been shown to be accurate in predicting which patients are at risk of developing nutrition-associated complications such as infections or poor wound healing. Whilst this technique has not been validated in veterinary patients, it is a straightforward approach, organizing easily available information, with the objective of classifying the patient's nutritional status as normal, marginal (slightly malnourished) or severely malnourished (Figure 23.1).

Medical history
Changes in type of diet
Reduction in food intake on a voluntary and/or non-voluntary basis
Extent and time course of weight loss
Evidence of gastrointestinal disease
Effects of malnutrition on functional status
Underlying disease
Physical examination
Wasting of muscle mass
Wasting of adipose tissue
Presence of oedema or ascites
Evidence of micronutrient deficiencies
Ability to prehend, masticate and swallow normally
Evidence of physical trauma, in particular facial injuries
Evaluation of current intake
Calorie count
Estimation of caloric needs

23.1 Nutritional assessment.

Taking the history

A medical history should always include specific questions about the patient's diet and feeding behaviour. It is important to find out whether the current diet and food intake are normal or have changed. Particular attention should be paid to recent reductions in intake on both a voluntary and involuntary basis. Weight loss should be evaluated with respect to the extent of loss and the duration of time over which it has occurred. Loss of a particular amount of body mass over a 2-week period can be far more significant than the same loss over a 2-month period, since a greater proportion of the loss is likely to be lean tissue. Evidence of chronic gastrointestinal disease should be noted, as disorders causing malassimilation of dietary nutrients can lead to both protein–calorie malnutrition and specific micronutrient deficiencies, depending on the condition. A history may also reveal information about the impact of malnutrition on functional status, as revealed by weakness and exercise intolerance. Finally, knowledge of the underlying disease process helps to indicate whether continued deterioration or restoration of nutritional status is to be anticipated.

The physical examination

Several systems for scoring canine and feline body condition have been published. None of these systems is ideal for evaluation of the hospitalized patient, since they do not reflect the alterations in body composition seen in the acutely critical patient. As previously discussed, the critical patient is often in a state of accelerated catabolism, and lean tissue wasting outstrips adipose tissue breakdown in these circumstances. A more appropriate approach is to evaluate caloric and protein 'reserves' separately, by assessing adipose tissue and skeletal muscle mass, respectively.

In addition to assessment of body condition, other features of the physical examination that may indicate a state of malnutrition include oedema, ascites and skin and hair coat lesions that are specific for micronutrient deficiencies.

Selection of patients for nutritional support

Once a patient has been classified as being normal, mildly malnourished or obviously malnourished, it is necessary to decide whether that patient is a candidate for nutritional support (Figure 23.2). At this point, it is essential to have an accurate assessment of the patient's food intake. In cases where the patient appears to have a diminished appetite but is still voluntarily consuming food, it may be necessary to measure food intake for a day or two in order to determine if consumption is adequate. This assessment method requires the estimation of an 'ideal' caloric intake for the patient. Methods for the calculation of energy requirements of hospitalized patients will be discussed in the next section. Ideally, the patient should be consuming a diet balanced for all its nutritional needs.

Patients who were significantly malnourished before the onset of their current illness
Patients who are anticipated to be NPO (nil by mouth) for more than 3–5 days
Previously well nourished patients who develop or are likely to develop serious complications (e.g. septic peritonitis, open discharging skin wounds, aspiration pneumonia)

23.2 Selection of patients for nutritional support.

Often, palatable table foods are substituted for pet foods when animals are ill. If the patient refuses to take in at least 50% of its calories in the form of a pet food for more than a few days, efforts should be made to ensure that essential nutrients, such as protein and water-soluble vitamins, are being adequately supplied.

For the patient in which estimated food intake falls short of its ideal, it must be decided whether the lack of optimal nutrition will have an impact on clinical outcome. This is not always an easy judgement. Some general guidelines are listed in Figure 23.2. Patients assessed as obviously malnourished who have a serious illness should be considered automatic candidates for nutritional support if their voluntary food intake is below estimated goals. Normal or mildly malnourished critical patients, however, can also be at risk of malnutrition-associated complications, since their nutritional status can deteriorate rapidly in the face of suboptimal intake. It has been established that patients do better when nutritional support is initiated early on in their illness. The art of nutritional assessment is therefore to select patients that are likely to have a severe and complicated clinical course and prolonged partial or total anorexia. Furthermore, nutritional support should be initiated as soon as is clinically feasible.

Nutritional requirements of critical patients

Energy requirements
The calculation of energy requirements of critical patients is a subject of some controversy. Much of what has been published in the veterinary literature on this subject was based on human literature that is outdated and has been called into question. The daily energy requirement of an individual reflects the energy required for basic life processes (often referred to as resting energy requirement or RER), a small amount of energy used for the assimilation of nutrients, a variable amount of energy expended for body temperature regulation and the energy expended in physical activity. Generally, the more sick the patient, the more likely it is that RER will approximate that patient's total energy expenditure. The controversy involves the issue of how much the RER of critical illness differs from that of a well individual. It was previously thought that RER was often significantly elevated in critical illness, possibly to twice what would be expected under normal circumstances. This was the rationale for the IER (illness energy requirement) approach to estimating the energy requirements of hospitalized patients. That method involved multiplying RER by 'illness factors' ranging from 1.1 to 2.0. Clinical experience and measurements of the energy expenditure of actual patients using indirect calorimetry suggest that the RER of the majority of critical patients, both human and veterinary, is at most only modestly elevated (Chan, 2004). In addition, feeding excessive calories to critical patients may cause a number of untoward effects including gastrointestinal problems, electrolyte disturbances, hyperglycaemia, hepatic dysfunction and respiratory distress.

Consequently, the current recommendation for estimation of the caloric requirements of critical veterinary patients is to use one of the formulae for RER (Figure 23.3). The use of RER as a caloric goal is a reasonable and safe starting point, either for patients whose voluntary food intake is being assessed or for patients that will be nutritionally supported. The amount fed to a given patient can always be increased if that patient experiences weight loss.

Interspecific formulae

$RER = 70 \, (Wt_{kg})^{0.75}$

$RER = 30 \, (Wt_{kg}) + 70$

Feline formula

$RER = 40 \, (Wt_{kg})$

23.3 Calculation of RER for dogs and cats. The interspecific formulae tend to overestimate feline energy requirements.

Protein requirements
While it appears that most hospitalized patients do not have resting energy requirements that differ greatly from normal, their protein requirements can be significantly greater during critical illness. The amount of protein an animal requires in its diet is a reflection of amino acid needs for protein synthesis and replacement of degraded or lost amino acids. Cats also have an obligatory need for amino acids for energy production. The nature of the protein source will also affect the amount required in the diet, since some protein sources are limiting in one or more essential amino acids.

Ideally, the dietary source of protein for critical patients should be highly digestible and contain all of the essential amino acids in appropriate amounts. As a rule, animal sources of protein, in particular egg and milk proteins, meet these criteria. For patients receiving enteral nutrition, protein should comprise at least 20–30% of calories (2–3 g/kg body weight) for dogs and >30% of calories (3 g/kg body weight) for cats. There are veterinary products designed for the nutritional support of veterinary patients that meet these guidelines (Figures 23.4 and 23.5).

	Recovery Support	a/d	Maximum Calorie [a]
Energy density	1 kcal/ml	1.2 kcal/ml	2.1 kcal/ml
Protein	39%	33%	29%
Fat	55%	54%	66%
Carbohydrate	6%	13%	5%
Tube suitability	>8 Fr	>8 Fr	>8 Fr
Manufacturer	Royal Canin	Hill's Pet Nutrition, Inc.	Iams Company

23.4 Tube feeding diets for cats and dogs. Note that energy is given on an 'as fed' basis; protein, fat and carbohydrate are given on an 'energy' basis.
[a] Not currently available in the UK.

	Feline and Canine Liquid Convalescence Support
Energy density	1.5 kcal/ml
Protein	36%
Fat	45%
Carbohydrate	16%
Tube suitability	All types
Manufacturer	Royal Canin

23.5 Liquid diet for cats and dogs. Note that energy is given on an 'as fed' basis; protein, fat and carbohydrate are given on an 'energy' basis.

Some critical patients with renal or hepatic dysfunction may not tolerate this quantity of protein. These patients do not have decreased protein requirements; rather, they have impaired ability to eliminate nitrogen by-products of protein metabolism (e.g. urea and ammonia). Therefore feeding strategies for these patients should involve supportive therapies that improve the elimination of protein metabolic waste products (i.e. fluid diuresis for renal failure, oral lactulose for hepatic failure), thus allowing as much protein intake as possible.

Micronutrient requirements

In addition to water, calories and protein there are at least 25 other essential nutrients, including fatty acids, minerals and vitamins. The effect of critical illness on a patient's micronutrient requirements is unknown. Current recommendations are to provide amounts that meet at least normal adult maintenance requirements (Figure 23.6). Many patients have adequate endogenous stores of most of these nutrients to survive weeks or in some cases months of reduced food intake. A number of these nutrients, in particular the water-soluble vitamins, are, however, very labile and patients may become significantly depleted in a short period of time. Therefore, depending on a patient's nutritional status at the time of presentation, it may already be suffering from deficiencies of one or more B vitamins or electrolytes.

Most veterinary enteral products are nutritionally balanced, so barring problems with nutrient assimilation, deficiency states should not arise. Electrolyte deficiencies are generally secondary to excessive fluid losses as opposed to malnutrition, and are addressed in Chapter 5. In the case of severe protein–calorie malnutrition, extreme imbalances of potassium, phosphorus and magnesium may occur. This situation, known as 'refeeding syndrome', will be discussed in more detail in the section on complications of nutritional support.

In recent years there has been a good deal of investigation into the benefits of supplementation of specific nutrients such as glutamine, arginine, omega-3 fatty acids and zinc in critically ill human patients. A review of these nutrients is beyond the scope of this text; however, it is important to recognize that clinical trials in human patients have not consistently demonstrated benefits from their use. Moreover there is virtually no research on the safety and efficacy of these nutrients in critical small animal patients. Hence the evidence is currently not strong enough to make specific recommendations for the supplementation of these substances.

AAFCO nutrient profiles					
Nutrient	**Units/1000 kcal ME**	**Adult dog**		**Adult cat**	
		Minimum	**Maximum**	**Minimum**	**Maximum**
Protein	g	51.4		65	
Arginine	g	1.46		2.6	
Taurine	g			0.5	
Linoleic acid	g	2.9		1.25	
Arachidonic acid	g			0.05	
Phosphorus	g	1.4	4.6	1.25	
Potassium	g	1.7		1.5	
Zinc	mg	34	286	18.75	500
Vitamin A	IU	1429	71,429	1250	187,500
Vitamin D	IU	143	1429	125	2500
Vitamin E	IU	14	286	7.5	
Thiamin (vitamin B1)	mg	0.29		1.25	
Riboflavin (vitamin B2)	mg	0.63		1	
Pantothenic acid	mg	2.9		1.25	
Niacin (vitamin B3)	mg	3.3		15	
Pyridoxine (vitamin B6)	mg	0.29		1	
Folic acid	mg	0.05		0.2	
Vitamin B12	mg	0.006		0.005	

23.6 Micronutrient requirements of dogs and cats (ME, metabolizable energy).

Routes of nutritional support

Enteral nutrition

The age-old adage 'if the gut works, use it' still holds true. The intestinal epithelium requires glutamine and regular access to nutrients to maintain the health of enterocytes (including the height of the villi and the function of brush border enzymes) and to support other neuroendocrine exchanges between the pancreas, stomach and small intestine. The nourishment provided via enteral feeding, therefore, helps to protect against bacterial translocation, absorption of endotoxin and the development of sepsis in critically ill patients unwilling or unable to maintain their own nutrient intake. Fortunately, the enteral route is also more economical, easier to implement and associated with fewer complications than parenteral feeding. Methods of enteral feeding include coaxed feeding, chemical stimulation of appetite and infusion of nutrients via feeding tubes within the gastrointestinal tract, bypassing the oral cavity (Figure 23.7). Deciding which method to use is dependent upon several factors, including the animal's current nutritional status and general state of health, the estimated length of time that nutritional support will be required, the animal's tolerance of general anaesthesia, the experience of the clinician and the associated costs of the procedures.

Coaxed feeding

Coaxed feeding, depending on the patient, may be an easily applied method of nutritional support adequate for the partially anorexic patient. This method is directed at encouraging voluntary intake and does not imply force feeding. Force feeding should be avoided, as it increases the stress of an already compromised patient, increases the likelihood of aspiration and injury and more commonly results in the topical, rather than enteral, application of nutrients. Gently tempting the patient with small, frequent meals of a highly palatable diet consisting of wet, odiferous, warm food in a quiet environment may stimulate self-feeding. Home-prepared chicken, fish or red meats are often successful menu choices. If the patient does not voluntarily eat what is offered, gently syringing a soft or liquid diet into the corner of the mouth may stimulate the animal to eat on its own. If the animal does not express an interest in eating on its own after the first one or two attempts at coaxed feeding, other options should be considered.

Chemical stimulation of appetite

If an adequate intake is not attained, chemical stimulants such as diazepam (0.05–0.15 mg/kg i.v., i.m. or orally once daily) have been reported to increase the appetite and 'remind' a patient of the taste of food, encouraging them to eat voluntarily. Application of these drugs may result in the consumption of 25% of the daily requirement in responsive cats (Figure 23.8). However, this option is not without a degree of risk and should be reserved as a short-term 'kick-start' in patients likely to recover in a short time period rather than an option for the long-term anorexic or inappetent

Method	Advantages	Disadvantages
Coaxed feeding	Simple, less stressful	Not effective in many animals
Chemical stimulants	Simple, 'reminds' patients of the taste of foods	May induce sedation Short term (2–3 days)
Naso-oesophageal tube (3.5–5 Fr; cats) (3.5–8 Fr; dogs)	Easy to place, least invasive tube, low cost Requires minimal sedation, if any Use up to 1 week	Not well tolerated by some patients Must use an Elizabethan collar Requires liquid diet
Oesophagostomy tube (8–18 Fr)	No special equipment required Can be used long term	Requires brief general anaesthesia for placement Infection of wound may occur
Gastrostomy tube (14–20 Fr)	Easy to maintain, few complications Can be used for months	Requires general anaesthesia for placement Specialized equipment needed Tube must remain in place for a minimum of 14 days
Enterostomy tube (5–8 Fr)	Bypasses pancreas and dysfunctional upper gastrointestinal tract	Requires general anaesthesia for placement Liquid diet constantly infused Requires intensive care Tube must remain in place for a minimum of 14 days

23.7 Routes of enteral nutritional support.

Drug	Dose	Side effects
Diazepam	0.05–0.15 mg/kg i.v., i.m., or 1 mg orally q24h	Sedation, idiosyncratic hepatic necrosis
Oxazepam	5–10 mg orally q12h	Same as diazepam
Cyproheptadine	8 mg/m² or 2–4 mg/cat orally q12–24h 5–20 mg/dog orally q12–24h	Excitability, aggression, vomiting
Nandrolone	5 mg/kg i.m. weekly; dogs	Uncommon
Prednisolone	0.5–1 mg/kg q12–24h	PU/PD, decreased wound healing, may interfere with therapy for disease

23.8 Chemical stimulation of appetite (PU/PD: polyuria/polydipsia).

patient. The side effects of benzodiazepine appetite stimulants may include drowsiness, excessive sedation or, more seriously, idiosyncratic hepatic necrosis in cats (diazepam), limiting their usefulness. Cyproheptadine has fewer known side effects and, although it can cause excitement/agitation, may be more effective as an appetite stimulant. When using appetite stimulants, it is important that the animal's clinical response is accurately and honestly recorded with an ongoing assessment of calorie intake.

Tube feeding

In many critically ill animals, the best way to ensure that adequate nutritional intake is achieved is to place a feeding tube and deliver food and water according to the calculated requirements. Several types of feeding tubes have been described and will be reviewed here. In general, the more proximal the feeding tube, the more physiologically appropriate the feeding regimen and the less likelihood that a gastrointestinal upset will occur. The authors prefer the use of naso-oesophageal tubes for the short-term feeding of critically ill patients, and oesophagostomy or percutaneously placed gastrostomy tubes for periods longer than 7 days.

Naso-oesophageal tubes: These are the simplest, least invasive and most commonly used feeding tubes and are excellent choices for the short-term feeding of hospitalized patients. Owners will rarely opt to maintain these tubes in the home environment, but it can be done. Soft flexible polyvinyl feeding tubes are easily placed into the nostril with a topical anaesthetic and minimal sedation (Figures 23.9 and 23.10). They should terminate just short of the lower oesophageal sphincter rather than in the stomach, to avoid inducing gastro-oesophageal reflux. The largest tube diameter that fits snugly in the internal nares should be used to maximize the feeding capacity. Correct tube placement should be confirmed by radiographs. Naso-oesophageal feeding tubes are contraindicated in patients that have rhinitis or severe facial trauma involving the nares and nasal turbinates, those that are

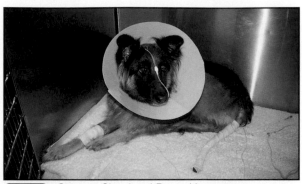

23.10 German Shepherd Dog with a naso-oesophageal tube. Once in place, the tube is secured to the external nares with 'superglue', or preferably a small suture passed retrograde through a 24 gauge needle. Two more sutures secure the tube to the dorsum of the nose and top of the head, out of the dog's direct line of vision. An Elizabethan collar prevents the dog from interfering with the tube.

experiencing protracted vomiting and/or regurgitation, those that are semi- or unconscious and those that have physical or functional abnormalities of the pharynx, larynx or oesophagus.

Once in place, these tubes may be used intermittently, dividing the total daily intake into small frequent meals or, less commonly, a liquid diet may be given as a continuous infusion. Complications that can arise with the use of these tubes may include rhinitis, vomiting or regurgitation. Aspiration of oesophageal contents is more likely if the animal is very weak or suffering neurological deficits and is fed in, or remains in, prolonged lateral recumbency.

Oesophagostomy tubes: Oesophagostomy tubes are variably sized tubes that are easily placed under light anaesthesia with minimal equipment requirements. Large-bore oesophagostomy tubes may be an ideal option for the general practice environment, as they are relatively simple to place and can be maintained and used for months. The only major associated complication (albeit rare) is the development of infection at the entry site, therefore meticulous care of the surgical wound is essential to maintain the tube. For this reason, oesophagostomy tubes are the preferred mode of support and pharyngostomy tubes, which have higher complication rates, are no longer recommended. Placement of an oesophagostomy tube is shown in Figure 23.11.

Gastrostomy tubes: Gastrostomy tubes have become invaluable for the long-term nutritional support of critically ill or recovering patients. Gastric feeding tubes may be placed surgically, endoscopically or by a 'blind' placement technique. Surgical placement of gastric feeding tubes is convenient when abdominal surgery is warranted for other purposes such as performing organ biopsies or removal of masses. These tubes may be 'pexed' in position and tightly sealed with omentum to prevent leakage. Balloon-tipped Foley catheters designed for use in the urinary tract should be avoided owing to the possibility of balloon rupture and displacement of the catheter, increasing the risk of peritoneal cavity contamination.

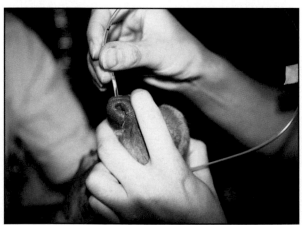

23.9 Placement of a nasogastric tube in a 5-month-old dog. A 5 Fr naso-oesophageal tube has been measured to the 9th rib space and marked with a piece of white tape, and a topical anaesthetic has been placed in the left nostril. To facilitate passage into the ventromedial nasal meatus, the nares are directed upwards.

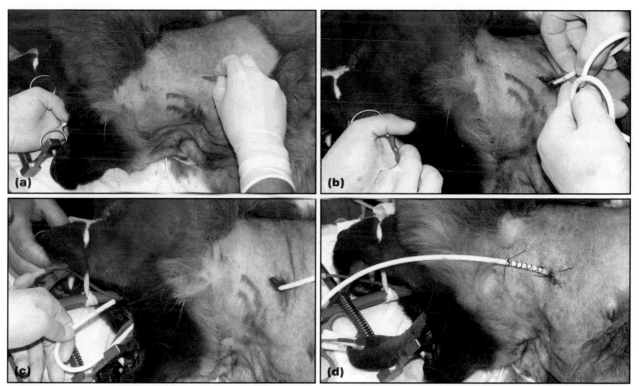

23.11 Oesophagostomy tube placement. **(a)** Forceps have been placed in the cervical oesophagus and their points are being used as a guide for the position of the skin incision. **(b)** The forceps are forced outwards through the incision to the external surface. The feeding tube is grasped with the forceps and drawn into the pharynx through the oesophagostomy incision. **(c)** The tube is redirected down the oesophagus. **(d)** The oesophagostomy tube in its final position. It should be capped off and sutured in place and the neck bandaged.

In the author's experience, an easier and less invasive means of gastric tube placement is by use of an endoscope (Figure 23.12). Tubes may be placed efficiently within 10–15 minutes under general anaesthesia, the limiting factors being accessibility of and experience with the endoscopic equipment. The most economical type of feeding tube is fashioned from a mushroom-tipped catheter in which only minor alterations are needed. The tip can be removed to add a feeding conduit and the widened catheter end is then cut to form two stents which are placed on either side of the positioned tube to anchor the tube in place and to prevent its inadvertent removal

(Figure 23.13). Once placed, the tube should be left in place for a minimum of 14 days prior to removal to allow a seal to form with the abdominal wall. The benefit of using this type of tube is that when the animal no longer requires nutritional support, the tube is simply pulled firmly and the stents slip off, allowing complete removal of the tube. The internal stent is usually small enough to be passed in the faeces and rarely if ever requires a second anaesthetic for endoscopic retrieval. The disadvantage of these tubes is that they may be inadvertently removed by a strong tug and so must remain carefully wrapped when not in use.

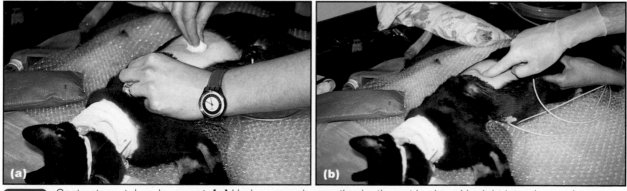

23.12 Gastrostomy tube placement. **(a)** Under general anaesthesia, the cat is placed in right lateral recumbency and an area (~10cm x 10cm) just behind the rib cage is clipped and surgically prepared. A mouth gag is used to protect the teeth from damaging the endoscope. The stomach is insufflated with air to move all other abdominal contents, specifically intestines and spleen, away from the body wall. **(b)** The site within the stomach where the tube will be anchored is chosen with the aid of an assistant, who wears sterile gloves and indents the surface of the prepared skin just caudal to the rib cage and directed cranially. (continues) ▶

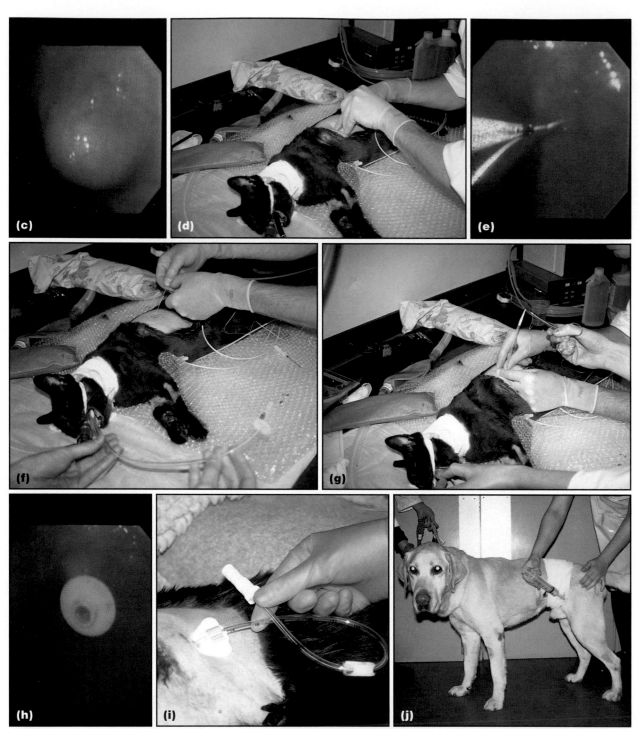

23.12 (continued) Gastrostomy tube placement. **(c)** This indentation can be seen by the endoscopist, who then directs the assistant to an area well away from the pyloric outflow tract into the fundus of the stomach where the tube is to be situated. **(d)** A small, ~2 mm incision is made in the skin just over the site, and a 19 gauge catheter (dogs and cats) is sharply introduced. **(e)** The catheter stylet is removed and a piece of suture material is passed into the stomach. Biopsy forceps are then used to retrieve the end of the suture, which is pulled into the endoscope as it is removed from the patient. The assistant must allow the suture to thread easily into the stomach, and the catheter can then be removed. **(f)** The suture now passes into the stomach via the body wall, extends up the oesophagus and out of the mouth. In human enteral feeding tubes such as this one (Fresenius), the tip is narrowed to pass through the body wall. When using a mushroom-tipped pezzar catheter, a small pipette tip is placed on to the end of the suture (tip threaded first!), and the suture is then fixed to the tube with multiple knots. **(g)** The assistant slowly retracts the suture, exiting the body wall until the tip of the pipette can be palpated. The stomach is held in place while the tube is pulled through the gastric mucosa and exits the body wall. A haemostat clamp can be used to grab hold of the pipette tip and exert an even upward pressure. Simply pulling the suture may result in breakage. **(h)** Once the tube has been pulled into place, it is important to go back and look in the stomach to verify that the tip is not stuck at the lower oesophageal sphincter and the tube is in an appropriate position, away from the pyloric outflow tract. **(i)** Flexible plastic fittings hold the feeding tube in place. Tight placement may result in pressure necrosis and increase the incidence of infection. The tube site is then wrapped in sterile material. **(j)** A percutaneously placed gastric tube in a 3-year-old Labrador with megaoesophagus.

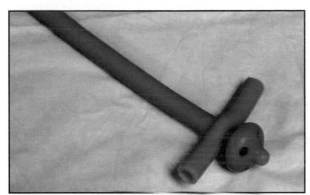

23.13 A relatively inexpensive feeding tube can be made from a mushroom-tipped catheter with minor alterations. The wide end of the catheter is cut to form two stents which are placed on either side of the body wall (internal stent shown) to anchor the tube in place and to prevent its inadvertent removal. (Reproduced from Battaglia (2006) with permission from Elsevier.)

A simpler, yet more expensive, system is the use of pre-packaged human enteral feeding tubes. The authors currently use a commercially available 15 Fr polyurethane tube (Fresenius). The advantages of these kits are that they contain all that is necessary to place the tube, they are suitable for use in cats and dogs, and they are difficult to remove inadvertently. The disadvantage is that a second anaesthetic is required to remove the solid plastic disc that keeps the tube anchored internally, preventing its removal. Once the external tube is cut away, this disc is not easily passed along the gastrointestinal tract and may result in a foreign body obstruction if not retrieved endoscopically. 'Blind' tube placement, without direct visualization of the site of internal insertion, is facilitated by the use of a long rigid stylet passed via the oesophagus and palpated through the stomach wall (Torrance, 1996). This may be a useful technique in the hands of some experienced practitioners when endoscopic or surgical placement is not possible, however, given the potential complications, the authors recommend oesophagostomy tube placement instead in most cases. Care must be taken not to lacerate the spleen or oesophagus during placement, and it is advisable to verify tube placement radiographically following the procedure.

Gastric feeding tubes may be used for periods up to 1 year if carefully maintained (Figure 23.14). Most patients tolerate the tubes quite well, although body wraps are advised to prevent the wound from becoming soiled. In the overly enthusiastic patient, an Elizabethan collar may be necessary to prevent the patient from chewing or removing the tube. Fortunately, complications are uncommon, but can include splenic laceration during placement as discussed above, infection or cellulitis at the site of exit from the body wall, vomiting due to slippage of the tube back into the gastric lumen, or peritonitis from contamination of the peritoneal cavity.

Low-profile enterostomy 'button' devices, which occupy the fistula between the gastrointestinal tract and the body wall, currently used in human medicine, are available for use in veterinary patients and may be left in place long term with minimal complications.

1. Don't use the tube for the first 24 hours. This will allow a primary seal to form between the stomach and body wall.
2. Start with small amounts of water, 5 ml/kg, to flush the tube.
3. Feed only one half of the calculated daily caloric requirement the first day. This is divided into small (20–30 ml) frequent (5–6) feedings.
4. The food is warmed to body temperature and injected into the stomach over several minutes. If the animal begins to retch or swallow, slow down or stop altogether and try again at the next feeding.
5. Aspirate the contents of the stomach with an empty syringe prior to each feeding. If gastric emptying is delayed and there is more than half the previous meal in the stomach, skip the feeding and consider motility modifiers such as metoclopramide.
6. ALWAYS FOLLOW BASIC TUBE ETIQUETTE: FLUSH before and after feedings with 5–10 ml of water, to clear debris and maintain tube patency.
7. On the second day of use, the feeding is increased to the calculated caloric intake if tolerated.
8. Change sterile bandage every 2–3 days after initial placement, check placement of tube and clean wound.

23.14 General guidelines for the use of gastrostomy tubes.

Enterostomy tubes: Placement of feeding tubes beyond the stomach is rarely indicated, but in cases of pancreatitis, diffuse gastric mucosal disease, protracted vomiting or delayed gastric emptying, an enterostomy tube may be life saving. Enterostomy tubes are most commonly placed surgically, or they may be introduced via a gastric tube and then directed through the pylorus with an endoscope. At surgery, a flexible, small-bore tube is threaded into the proximal jejunum or distal duodenum and secured with a purse string. The delivery end is exited through an abdominal stab incision and fixed to the abdominal wall (Simpson and Elwood, 1994). Feeding through an enterostomy tube must be carefully controlled since the diets are often concentrated in order to supply enough calories, and therefore may cause osmotic overload and diarrhoea. As with gastrostomy tubes, enterostomy tubes must remain in place for a minimum of 14 days to allow a seal to form with the abdominal wall. Continuous infusion of a dilute liquid diet is the preferred method of use, therefore the patient must remain hospitalized while the tube is in place, which limits its long-term employment.

Parenteral nutrition

Parenteral nutrition (PN) is nutrition delivered by the intravenous route. It can be life saving for patients who cannot tolerate enteral feeding. However, because there are numerous drawbacks associated with this form of nourishment, it should be reserved for patients with no other feeding option, and for whom the need for nourishment is felt to be a critical factor in their recovery. Generally, these are patients for whom enteral feeding is contraindicated or hazardous.

Special solutions are used for intravenous feeding; they must be mixed aseptically and in a specific order. PN is best delivered continuously (although this is not absolutely necessary); therefore 24-hour nursing care is desirable. Also, since many of the potential complications of PN (sepsis and various electrolyte disturbances) can be life threatening, careful monitoring of the patient is mandated. Therefore, a significant increase in the cost of care is an expected consequence of the intensive care and special supplies required to deliver PN to a patient.

Venous access

Ideally, a catheter should be dedicated for PN infusion alone, because of the increased risk of catheter sepsis associated with the infusion of a nutrient-rich solution. By dedicating a line to PN and observing strict aseptic care of the line and its connections, the potential for bacterial contamination is reduced. Central venous access is preferable to peripheral access, since PN solutions are hyperosmolar and associated with the development of thrombophlebitis. However, PN solutions can be diluted adequately to permit peripheral infusion as long as the patient is not at risk of fluid volume overload. PN solutions infused via peripheral catheters should not exceed 800 mOsm/l and if possible should be less than 600 mOsm/l. In addition, use of fine-bore polyurethane or silicone elastomer cannulae will greatly reduce the risk of thrombophlebitis.

Parenteral nutrition solutions

Basic PN is composed of a protein source (crystalline amino acid solution), a carbohydrate source (dextrose) and a fat source (lipid emulsion). Vitamins, electrolytes and trace minerals can also be added so that the resulting solution is complete and balanced, at least according to standards for healthy dogs and cats.

Because most veterinary patients receive PN for limited periods of time (often a week or less), the focus should be on providing protein, calories and the more labile vitamins (water-soluble vitamins). Electrolyte supplementation is managed as a component of fluid therapy rather than as part of PN.

Providing more complete nutrition to a patient parenterally is problematic due to compatibility problems between various nutrients and nutrient formulations, as well as expense. If the patient is not on a balanced enteral diet within a week of starting PN, fat-soluble vitamins are supplemented separately (intramuscularly or subcutaneously) on a weekly basis. The water-soluble vitamin folate should also be supplemented separately in long-term PN patients, as it is omitted from parenteral B-complex preparations. Parenteral trace mineral supplements are also available for use in these patients.

PN solutions should be made fresh daily and must be mixed in a specific order under aseptic conditions. Special PN compounding bags can be used, or solutions can be prepared in evacuated glass containers. In general, amino acid and dextrose solutions are mixed first and then electrolyte and mineral solutions are added. Great care must be taken when adding combinations of electrolytes, especially phosphorus and calcium, because precipitates can easily form. Next, multivitamins are added, and finally the lipid emulsion. The lipid emulsion is fragile and the suspended triglyceride particles can coalesce or even precipitate. Precipitation of lipid emulsions can be detected by visual inspection after the solution has been sitting for a while. There should not be any indication of separation or layering of the final solution. Risk of fat embolization can be eliminated by using an infusion set that contains a 1.2 micron filter to deliver PN solutions containing lipids.

Prescription formulation

Figure 23.15 shows a worksheet and a sample calculation for formulating PN. Because of the limited discussion of PN in this chapter the reader is encouraged to seek a more detailed review of this technique. There are several guidelines for formulating PN for small animals in the literature (Hill, 1994; Chan, 2005).

Day 1 goal: 50% RER
Day 2 goal: 100% RER

(see Figure 23.3 for RER formulae)

Protein calories: Dogs: 15–25% of RER
                         Cats: 25–35% of RER

Select % protein calories based on the patient's protein status and ability to tolerate dietary protein.

Non-protein calories: 30–70% from lipid
                             30–70% from dextrose

Dogs: provide 50% of non-protein calories from lipid and 50% from dextrose unless there is pre-existing hyperlipidaemia or hyperglycaemia.

Cats: provide 70% of non-protein calories from lipid and 30% from dextrose unless there is pre-existing hyperlipidaemia or hyperglycaemia. Cats are more likely to become hyperglycaemic, which is why more calories are provided as lipids as a rule.

Solutions:

1. Amino acids

   1 g of amino acids provides approximately 4 kcal.

   Use solutions containing 3.5–5% amino acids (350–500 mOsm/l).
   Use solutions without additional electrolytes to simplify management of electrolytes with fluid therapy.

2. Dextrose

   10% dextrose contains 500 mOsm/l and provides 0.34 kcal/ml.
   20% dextrose contains 1000 mOsm/l and provides 0.68 kcal/ml.

23.15 Worksheet for peripheral parenteral nutrition. (continues) ▶

3. Lipid emulsions

Use 20% lipid emulsions, which contain 268–340 mOsm/l and provide 2 kcal/ml.

4. Phosphorus

Use standard parenteral potassium phosphate solutions.

5. B vitamins

Use standard parenteral B complex solutions.

Example calculations: a 17.5 kg dog without hypoproteinaemia

RER = $70(17.5)^{0.75}$ = 600 kcal/day
Goal calories for day 1 = 0.5(600) = 300 kcal

1. **Amino acids**

   (0.15)(300 kcal) = 45 kcal from protein
   45 kcal ÷ 4 kcal/g = 11.25 g
   4.25% amino acid solution = 0.0425 g protein/ml
   therefore you need *265* ml 4.25% amino acid solution
   (x ml = 11.25 g ÷ 0.0425 g/ml)

2. **Non-protein calories**

   (0.85)(300 kcal) = 255 kcal from lipid and dextrose
   (a) 20% lipid emulsion to provide 50% non-protein calories =
   127.5 kcal
   20% lipid emulsion = 2.0 kcal/ml
   therefore you need *64* ml 20% lipid emulsion
   (x ml = 127.5 kcal ÷ 2.0 kcal/ml)
   (b) 20% dextrose to provide 50% non-protein calories = 127.5 kcal
   20% dextrose solution = 0.68 kcal/ml
   therefore you need *188* ml 20% dextrose solution
   (x ml = 127.5 kcal ÷ 0.68 kcal/ml)

3. **Potassium phosphate**

   dosed at 8 mM/1000 kcal delivered
   therefore you need *2.4* mM potassium phosphate
   (x mM = (8 mM)(300 kcal) ÷ (1000 kcal))

4. **Vitamin B complex**

   dosed at approximately 2 ml/l infused
   total infused for day 1 = 518 ml
   therefore *1.0* ml B complex should be sufficient

5. **Infusion rate**

   518 ml/24 hours = 22 ml/h
   The osmolarity of this solution is approximately 625 mOsm/l.

   Day 2 calculations
   Same as day 1, but substitute 600 kcal for 300 kcal.

23.15 (continued) Worksheet for peripheral parenteral nutrition.

Monitoring and treating the complications of nutritional support

The monitoring required in critically ill patients receiving nutritional support is typically no different from what might be expected for any critical patient: routine physical examinations; body temperature; heart rate and respiratory rate; twice daily weight measurements; and assessment of hydration status and general demeanour. Laboratory values frequently assessed include total protein, albumin, packed cell volume, electrolytes and blood urea nitrogen. Alterations in these parameters may indicate improved patient status due to correction and support of the underlying disease or, conversely, may signal early warnings of complications associated with nutritional support. In a study of anorexic cats, high creatinine kinase (CK) activity was found, exceeding an average of 250 times that of normally nourished cats (Fascetti *et al.*, 1997). In response to nutritional intervention, the CK activity decreased and eventually returned to normal. CK may prove to be a useful marker of nutritional status in the clinical setting.

Complications associated with enteral nutrition fall into the categories of mechanical, gastrointestinal or metabolic. Mechanical complications most commonly encountered include obstruction of the feeding tube, dislodgement of a tube, or infection/cellulitis at the site of tube entry. Obstruction of feeding tubes may be minimized by the use of foodstuffs of the appropriate consistency in relation to the tube size. Those tubes of 5 Fr diameter and smaller should only ever admit liquid diets, whereas larger sized tubes may admit thoroughly liquidized diets but still risk blockage if the diets are not properly diluted and the tubes are not flushed after feeding. Ideally, to minimize the chances of blockage and to prevent wear, tubes should be used solely for feeding purposes and not for the administration of medications. Should a tube become clogged and unresponsive to hydrostatic pressure, cola or, alternatively, pancreatic enzyme powder mixed in sodium bicarbonate can be left in the tube overnight to help dissolve the offending material. If neither is successful, the tube requires replacement.

Gastrointestinal complications are, unfortunately, common and typically manifest as nausea, vomiting and diarrhoea. These may be avoided by a slow introduction to feeding and by administering dilute solutions to avoid sudden intraluminal hypertonicity. The first day of feeding should begin with incremental amounts of water and half of the daily caloric requirements divided into five or six feedings. If feeding is tolerated well, the full calculated daily caloric requirements are given on the second day. Prior to each feeding via a gastrostomy tube, the tube is aspirated to ensure that the stomach has emptied from the previous meal. If not, the amount remaining is subtracted from the current feeding. Despite these precautions, diarrhoea may occur due to villous atrophy of prolonged anorexia, intolerance of the chosen diet, antibiotic-induced alterations in intestinal flora, or as a manifestation of the underlying illness. Treatment with motility-modifying drugs, the addition of fibre or a change to parenteral nutrition may be necessary.

Metabolic derangements resulting from enteral nutritional support are rare. The duration of illness and the severity and nature of the underlying disease may predispose some patients to glucose intolerance (and hence hyperglycaemia or glucosuria), hyperlipidaemia or electrolyte disturbances. These derangements are more commonly encountered in patients receiving PN. Correction of these abnormalities requires manipulation of the fluid regimen and dietary components, and appropriate therapy for the underlying disorder. Persistent hyperglycaemia may infrequently require the use of insulin. A phenomenon known as 'refeeding syndrome' has been described in which, upon initiation of nutritional support to malnourished patients, severe metabolic derangements occur, the most significant of which is hypophosphataemia. In one review, refeeding resulted in hypophosphataemia and haemolysis in cats within 12–72 hours (Justin and Hohenhous, 1995). Cats with diabetes mellitus or those with high liver enzyme activities, hyperbilirubinaemia and weight loss seem to be at increased risk. These patients should be closely monitored for the development of low serum phosphorus and subsequent haemolytic anaemia when initiating nutritional support (Justin and Hohenhous, 1995).

Complications of PN are more common than those of enteral support and are associated with the mechanics of administration, sepsis or metabolic derangements, the occurrence of which depends upon the components and proportions administered. Mechanical complications are frequent and include broken, chewed, obstructed or dislodged administration lines and catheters. They rarely have an effect on the patient, but do increase the possibility of sepsis. PN should be supplied via dedicated fluid lines to centrally placed catheters, the meticulous care of which is essential. To avoid contamination and potential sepsis, the ports must be tightly secured and wrapped with disinfectant-soaked swabs. The site of catheter placement should be inspected daily, gently scrubbed and wrapped aseptically. Patients receiving PN should be closely monitored for the development of fever, depression and leucocytosis, which signal probable sepsis. When these signs are recognized, the catheter is removed, the tip is cultured and aggressive fluid and broad-spectrum antibiotic therapy is instituted.

Metabolic derangements occur frequently in patients receiving PN but rarely result in clinical signs. Common abnormalities found include hyperglycaemia, glucosuria, azotaemia, lipaemia and electrolyte changes, such as hypokalaemia, hypomagnesaemia and hypophosphataemia. Cats and some dogs readily develop glucose intolerance and may require short-term insulin therapy. Azotaemia and lipaemia are likely to be a result of highly concentrated intravenous infusions of amino acids and lipid emulsions, which overwhelm the body's capacity for utilization or storage. Electrolyte disturbances occur most frequently in patients that are vomiting and are easily addressed with appropriate fluid therapy. Refeeding syndrome, manifested by hypophosphatemia and haemolysis (see above), is more common in patients receiving

PN than in those managed with enteral nutritional support. The key to minimizing metabolic abnormalities is early detection. Frequent haematological and biochemical profiles are indicated to allow prompt correction of fluid electrolyte concentrations. In addition, anti-emetics should be administered, infusion rates adjusted and proportions of components modified.

Conclusion

Nutritional support is rapidly and appropriately becoming a primary concern rather than an afterthought for our critically ill veterinary patients. As we become more experienced in the application of nutrition, we are increasingly aware of its benefits in shortening recovery time and decreasing morbidity and mortality experienced by our patients. The time and effort expended in stabilizing the critical patient is well spent if we do not allow that patient's nutritional status to become a limiting factor in its recovery.

References and further reading

Abood SK and Buffington CT (1992) Enteral feeding of dogs and cats: 51 cases (1989–1991). *Journal of the American Veterinary Medical Association* **201**, 610–622

Battaglia A (2006) *Small Animal Emergency and Critical Care for Veterinary Technicians, 2nd edition*. Elsevier, Philadelphia

Chan DL (2004) Nutritional requirements of the critically ill patient. *Clinical Techniques in Small Animal Practice* **1**, 1–5

Chan D (2005) Parenteral nutritional support. In: *Textbook of Veterinary Internal Medicine, 6th edn*, ed. SJ Ettinger and EC Feldman, pp. 586–591. Elsevier, Philadelphia

Fascetti AJ, Mauldin GE and Mauldin GN (1997) Correlation between serum creatinine kinase activities and anorexia in cats. *Journal of Veterinary Internal Medicine* **11**, 9–13

Heyland DK (1998) Nutritional support in the critically ill patient. A critical review of the evidence. *Critical Care Clinics* **14**, 423–440

Hill RC (1994) Critical care nutrition. In: *The Waltham Book of Clinical Nutrition of the Dog and Cat*, ed. JM Wills and KW Simpson, pp. 39–61. Elsevier Science, Oxford

Justin RB and Hohenhous AE (1995) Hypophosphatemia associated with enteral alimentation in cats. *Journal of Veterinary Internal Medicine* **9**, 228–233

Lippert AC (1992) The metabolic response to injury: enteral and parenteral nutritional support. In: *Veterinary Emergency and Critical Care Medicine*, ed. RJ Murtaugh and PM Kaplan, pp. 593–617. Mosby, Boston

Marks SL, Cook AK, Reader R *et al.* (1999) Effects of glutamine supplementation of an amino acid-based purified diet on intestinal mucosal integrity in cats with methotrexate-induced enteritis. *American Journal of Veterinary Research* **60**, 755–763

Michel KE (1997) Practice guidelines for gastrostomy tubes. *Compendium on Continuing Education for the Practicing Veterinarian* **19**, 306–309

Mohr A, Leisewitz A, Jacobson LS *et al.* (2003) Effect of early enteral nutrition on intestinal permeability, intestinal protein loss, and outcome in dogs with severe parvoviral enteritis. *Journal of Veterinary Internal Medicine* **17**, 791–798

Remillard RL, Darden DE, Michel KE *et al.* (2001) An investigation of the relationship between caloric intake and outcome in hospitalized dogs. *Veterinary Therapeutics* **2**, 301–310

Simpson KW and Elwood CM (1994) Techniques for enteral support. In: *The Waltham Book of Clinical Nutrition of the Dog and Cat*, ed. JM Wills and KW Simpson, pp. 63–74. Elsevier Science, Oxford

Tennant B (1996) Feeding the sick animal. In: *Manual of Companion Animal Nutrition and Feeding*, ed. N Kelly and J Wills, pp. 181–187. BSAVA, Cheltenham

Tennant G and Willoughby K (1993) The use of enteral nutrition in small animal medicine. *Compendium on Continuing Education for the Practicing Veterinarian* **15**, 1054–1068

Torrance AG (1996) Intensive care – nutritional support. In: *Manual of Companion Animal Nutrition and Feeding*, ed. N Kelly and J Wills, pp. 171–180. BSAVA, Cheltenham

24

Antibacterial therapy in the critical patient

Reid P. Groman and Dawn Merton-Boothe

Introduction

The management of serious bacterial infections is an integral part of intensive care medicine. Mortality from bacterial infections in critically ill patients remains high, and the emergence and spread of multiple-drug-resistant organisms is increasing (Ogeer-Gyles et al., 2005; Boothe, 2006). Critically ill patients are liable to develop infections due to their underlying disease(s) and numerous invasive procedures. Further, the critically ill patient often presents with pathophysiological changes that may profoundly affect drug disposition and response to therapy.

Therapy for critical patients with a documented focus of infection is multifaceted, including goal-directed fluid therapy, vasopressors or inotropes, nutritional support, oxygen administration and occasionally mechanical ventilation in addition to antimicrobial therapy. Bacterial infection promotes a complex series of host responses involving the kinin, complement and coagulation pathways, and the inflammatory response of the host is often responsible for the signs and symptoms of disease. Failure to contain or eradicate the microbe often results in further damage due to the progression of inflammation and infection. Thus, early initiation of appropriate antibiotic therapy is pivotal in ensuring a favourable outcome.

Considerations for empirical antibiotic selection and use

Antibiotics are directed against unique targets not present in mammalian cells (Greene, 2006a). The goal of therapy is to maximize chemotherapeutic activity against invading microbes whilst limiting toxicity to the host. Empirical antibiotic therapy is not, however, necessarily benign; indiscriminate use of broad-spectrum antibiotics is driving the development of in-hospital microbial resistance (Ogeer-Gyles et al., 2006) and inappropriate initial therapy in critically ill human patients is associated with a significant increase in mortality which is not necessarily reversed by changing the antibiotics once the bacterial susceptibility is known (Kollef et al., 1999; Kollef, 2000). In veterinary medicine, empirically selected antimicrobial therapy is often incorrect, requiring adjustments in close to 45% of critically ill patients. Moreover, 'common' pathogens such as Escherichia coli and Staphylococcus intermedius are no longer predictably sensitive to drugs that were once the

cornerstone of therapy (Boothe et al., 2006; Gurnee et al., 2006; Morris et al., 2006). Although, ideally, all antibiotic therapy should be culture-driven, invariably antimicrobials must be selected empirically, while awaiting culture and susceptibility data. In patients with bacterial infections, empirical therapy should be based on previous experience, knowledge of the pathogens that are most often recovered from the site of origin and history of prior antibiotic administration.

Hospital-acquired, or nosocomial, infections include almost all infections that are unassociated with the patient's original diagnosis (Greene, 2006b). Most infections that become clinically evident after 48 hours of hospitalization are considered hospital-acquired. Infections that are diagnosed after the patient's discharge from the hospital can be considered to have a nosocomial origin if the organisms were acquired during the hospital stay. Nosocomial pathogens vary from hospital to hospital, and temporally within intensive care units (ICUs). The organisms are typically (though not always) opportunistic, multiple-drug-resistant Gram-negative bacteria. An opportunistic microbe is one that usually has minimal pathogenic potential but causes morbidity in debilitated or otherwise immunocompromised hosts. The usual mechanism of infection with these bacteria is by colonization of the host's mucosal surfaces with resistant strains in patients rendered susceptible by antibiotic treatment, underlying disease and various medical procedures. Offending organisms often represent the normal flora of the alimentary canal.

Some nosocomial infections are caused by pathogens that are endemic to a particular hospital or ward. Thus, when selecting an antimicrobial in the ICU, it is not only important to take into account the site of infection and the most likely 'community-acquired' bacteria that may be involved, but also to consider the trends of antibiotic resistance observed in nosocomial infections within a particular hospital or clinic (Prescott et al., 2002).

Broad-spectrum antibiotic therapy is initially recommended for most critically ill patients with documented or suspected bacterial infections. The term 'broad spectrum' implies that antimicrobials have predictable efficacy against the most commonly encountered Gram-positive and Gram-negative pathogens. In veterinary medicine, this definition may be extended to include Mycoplasma and rickettsial species. Depending on the infection, extended anaerobic coverage may also be warranted, for example in patients with infectious endocarditis, osteomyelitis, pyothorax or a ruptured intestinal viscus. The time-honoured practice of covering for most possible pathogens is widely implemented and is appropriate until culture and susceptibility data are known. However, when culture and susceptibility information become available, antimicrobial therapy should be altered such that the patient is treated with the most effective narrow-spectrum agent. This basic tenet of pharmacotherapy is expected to reduce selective pressure for resistance to the more extended-spectrum antibiotics. For serious infections with nosocomial *Pseudomonas aeruginosa* or highly resistant *Enterococcus faecium*, the use of a cell wall active agent, such as a penicillin, *with* an aminoglycoside results in synergistic antibacterial activity. In such cases, combination therapy is maintained to optimize therapeutic success and reduce the emergence of superinfection and resistant strains. While some recent studies in human medicine suggest that monotherapy for *Pseudomonas* infections may be as effective as combination therapy, this has not yet been demonstrated in veterinary medicine.

The emergence of multiple-drug-resistant pathogens in critically ill patients represents a relatively new challenge for veterinary surgeons. 'Multiple-drug resistance' may be defined as resistance to three or more antibiotics to which the bacterium is normally considered susceptible. As the prevalence of these resistant pathogens increases, we might question whether currently selected regimens thought to be 'broad spectrum' (e.g. ampicillin/enrofloxacin, penicillin/gentamicin, ampicillin/sulbactam) remain appropriate 'first-line' choices for our critical patients. This is a particularly important question when we realize that the effectiveness of our initial antibiotic therapy is likely to influence mortality and morbidity in our patients. However, there is no uniformly effective single therapeutic regimen that can be applied to all critically ill dogs and cats, particularly for patients in referral facilities. In human intensive care, *initial* coverage for possible multiple-drug-resistant pathogens in the ICU can include vancomycin, third-generation cephalosporins and imipenem (a carbapenem). Widespread antibiotic utilization in humans is largely responsible for inducing resistance to every class of drugs presently in use, and there are very few new antibiotics in development. In view of this information, it is difficult to argue in favour of initially prescribing a third-generation cephalosporin, carbapenem or vancomycin for dogs and cats at this time in the absence of immunological incompetence, extended hospitalization with exposure to nosocomial pathogens, or compelling culture and susceptibility data. Similarly, there is limited evidence in veterinary medicine to endorse the policy in some human ICUs of empirically prescribing an antipseudomonal penicillin. The ever increasing and complex patterns of resistance in human ICUs mandate that antibiotics once considered the last line of defence (linezolid, quinupristin/dalfopristin, daptomycin) are prescribed prior to results of susceptibility testing in some patients. Avoidance of these agents at this time is a rational strategy to curtail the emergence of drug resistance in our patient population.

For *initial* antibiotic therapy the probability of microbial eradication is maximized by:

- Using more than one antibiotic
- Taking advantage of the pharmacodynamic properties of drugs that have been well evaluated in veterinary medicine
- Avoiding the urge to reach for 'bigger and better' drugs empirically.

Initial therapy with two antibiotics is generally expected to be superior to monotherapy for several reasons. First, the use of two drugs increases the likelihood that one of the drugs will be active against the pathogen. Second, dual therapy may attack the pathogen at two different sites, thereby decreasing the likelihood that resistance will develop. Even when antibiotic combinations are not synergistic, their effects may still be additive and thus enhance the likelihood of pathogen eradication. These benefits should be weighed against the possibility of enhanced toxicity with multiple agents.

The optimal pharmacodynamics for microbiological efficacy of certain antimicrobials should be exploited. For example, the efficacy of aminopenicillins or first-generation cephalosporins may be enhanced by more frequent administration, or administration as a constant rate infusion (CRI), while higher doses and less frequent administration of concentration-dependent antibiotics, such as the fluoroquinolones and aminoglycosides, are similarly associated with better microbiological outcomes (Estes, 1998).

A beta-lactam with a relatively short half-life, e.g. ampicillin, is appropriately administered every 6 hours (i.e. *no less than* three times daily) to ensure therapeutic drug levels at the site of infection, thus improving efficacy against many Gram-positive and anaerobic pathogens. Aminoglycosides or fluoroquinolones, administered in large single daily doses, are the present standard for treating severe Gram-negative infections (Marik, 1993). Both drug classes demonstrate antimicrobial synergy *in vitro* with beta-lactams; thus, the combination of a broad spectrum beta-lactam or beta-lactam/beta-lactamase agent plus an aminoglycoside or a fluoroquinolone is appropriate empirical initial therapy, pending culture and susceptibility reports. It is important to recognize that the fluoroquinolones are *not* a 'less nephrotoxic equivalent' to the aminoglycosides, and that the aminoglycosides have not been eclipsed by fluoroquinolones. While the fluoroquinolones are generally safer than aminoglycosides, the latter are predictably more effective for Gram-negative pathogens and less likely to contribute to antimicrobial resistance (Cooke *et al.*, 2002). Moreover, not all of the veterinary-approved fluoroquinolones are sufficiently similar in their pharmacology or spectrum of activity to be used interchangeably.

In certain situations, a less conventional drug may be chosen for initial therapy. For example, in the septic patient with a recent history of broad-spectrum antibiotic use, it is reasonable to assume infection with a multiple-drug-resistant pathogen. In such situations, the empirical use of a carbapenem, either alone or in conjunction with an aminoglycoside, is justified pending culture and susceptibility data. Similarly, if a patient's presentation is consistent with infection by a specific pathogen, e.g. a juvenile dog with suspected

Bordetella bronchiseptica pneumonia, treatment should include an antibiotic to which that pathogen is expected to be sensitive. In this example, a drug that might not otherwise be empirically selected for a hospitalized patient with pneumonia, e.g. azithromycin or doxycycline, would be appropriate. If the pathogen is suspected to be an anaerobe, predictable results have been obtained by administering metronidazole, ampicillin, clindamycin, chloramphenicol, or a second-generation cephalosporin. However, resistance among *Bacteroides fragilis* isolates to both ampicillin and clindamycin has increased in recent years, suggesting that therapy for anaerobic infections in the ICU should include metronidazole or a second-generation cephalosporin (Jang *et al.*, 1997).

Several strategies have been proposed to optimize therapeutic success and limit the development of resistance in hospitalized patients. First is the prompt implementation of narrow-spectrum, target-directed therapy based on culture and susceptibility results. With the exception of infections with *Pseudomonas aeruginosa* and *Enterococcus* spp., there is limited evidence that the use of more than one antimicrobial is superior to appropriate single-agent therapy, once the pathogen has been identified. Additional strategies for optimal antimicrobial use include re-evaluating each drug's antimicrobial spectrum, pharmacological characteristics and side effects, thus reducing the likelihood of selecting drug-resistant bacteria during therapy. In order to limit the development of resistance, the duration of antibiotic treatment should be limited to the shortest effective course of therapy (Dugan *et al.*, 2003). With the exception of immunosuppressed patients, or those with deep infections to which drug penetration may be limited, e.g. pyelonephritis, endocarditis and osteomyelitis, a 10-day course of an appropriate antibiotic(s) is frequently sufficient for the eradication of most aerobic pathogens without jeopardizing patient outcome.

Pathogen identification and susceptibility data

Drug selection is simplified once a pathogen is identified and susceptibility data are available (Jones, 2006). Properly collected samples should be obtained for culture before antimicrobial therapy is initiated. Avoidance of contamination, adequacy of sampling and preservation of viability are critical factors in specimen collection and handling. Bacterial culture may be performed on body fluids (cerebrospinal fluid (CSF), urine, blood, pleural, peritoneal or joint fluid), wounds, bronchial secretions, or aspirates and biopsy specimens of normally sterile organs. Both blood and urine should be submitted for culture in patients with suspected sepsis. As a general rule, the best samples for the microbiology laboratory are liquid specimens. Swabs should be avoided whenever possible, since these tend to dry out and swab fibres may be deleterious to some bacteria. When swab samples are obtained, they should be placed in an appropriate transport medium or a humidified transport chamber to prevent desiccation.

Urine and stool should be transported in sealed, sterile containers and refrigerated if not processed within 1 hour of collection. The results of a 'faecal culture' may be misleading as the identification of numerous *Escherichia coli* or other normal intestinal inhabitants is expected and generally represents normal floral colonization as opposed to polymicrobial infection. Faecal enteric panels, involving both faecal cultures and toxin assays, may document infection with one of four possible enteric pathogens, namely *Clostridium difficile*, *C. perfringens*, *Salmonella* and *Campylobacter* spp., although these pathogens may also be isolated from asymptomatic pets (Cave *et al.*, 2002). Other than urine and stool, most specimens, including blood and CSF, may be kept at room temperature if processing is delayed.

Fluid specimens that may harbour pathogenic anaerobic bacteria should be collected in a syringe, from which the air is immediately expressed and the end of the needle plugged with a rubber stopper. Alternatively the contents of the syringe may be placed in an anaerobic transport tube. Tissue specimens should be placed in designated anaerobic transport containers. Certain aerobic and facultatively anaerobic organisms will not grow on standard culture media, and if a particular pathogen is suspected, e.g. *Mycoplasma*, the laboratory should be contacted before the specimen is collected to ensure appropriate handling before transport.

Opportunistic fungal organisms are a frequent source of morbidity in human ICU patients, and are increasingly resistant to antifungal agents. Infections with saprophytic fungi, e.g. *Candida* and *Aspergillus* spp., may be under-recognized in veterinary patients. Although these organisms are ubiquitous and generally non-pathogenic, they may cause significant morbidity in immunocompromised patients with altered commensal flora due to underlying disease or prolonged antibiotic therapy. Some, though not all, filamentous fungal organisms will grow on standard bacterial growth media. Several weeks may be required for identification and susceptibility testing, however, and documentation of their presence does not distinguish infection from colonization.

In-house examination of Wright–Giemsa or Gram-stained slides of fluid samples or tissue impression smears should be performed when possible. Initial microscopic findings may allow preliminary suppositions about the pathogen well before culture and susceptibility data are available. The observation of a monomorphic population of Gram-positive cocci should prompt selection of drugs suitable for these organisms. If three or more bacterial forms are identified on cytology, sample contamination or anaerobic infection should be suspected and repeat sampling is warranted. Cytological preparations that reveal degenerate leucocytes and phagocytosed bacteria are consistent with infection, as opposed to colonization. This is an important distinction, since a culture result cannot distinguish between the two, and bacterial colonization, in contrast to active infection, does not require specific therapy.

Newer diagnostic methods show promise of permitting more rapid confirmation of bacterial infection.

For example, studies of polymerase chain reaction (PCR) technology have demonstrated encouraging results in clinical veterinary patients (Brown *et al.*, 2005), but are available at very few institutions. While turnaround time for results is typically quicker than traditional methods, it is not clear whether these rapid diagnostic techniques will be able to discriminate colonization from infection.

The time needed to grow, isolate and identify different organisms varies considerably. The most common aerobic pathogens grow rapidly, and preliminary reports can be expected from the laboratory within 24 hours. Anaerobes generally grow more slowly and plates are not examined for 48 hours. The disc-diffusion, or Kirby–Bauer, method is the most commonly applied technique for susceptibility testing in the clinical laboratory. This method is suited to screening large numbers of organisms but provides only semiquantitative information, and is not applicable to slow-growing or fastidious organisms. Quantitative susceptibility testing, or tube dilution, is usually performed by making two-fold dilutions of the test antibacterial agent in a liquid culture medium, inoculation with a standard number of microorganisms and incubation for 18–24 hours. The least amount of antibacterial that inhibits visible growth of the microorganism is the minimum inhibitory concentration (MIC). The MIC is not a measure of efficacy *per se*; it is simply an *in vitro* measurement of bacterial susceptibility.

In the USA, all veterinary and human microbiology laboratories utilize guidelines produced by the Clinical Laboratory Standards Institute (CLSI, previously the National Committee on Clinical Laboratory Standards (NCCLS)). CLSI interpretive results are based on the published breakpoint MIC. The breakpoint is the concentration of antibiotic that separates susceptible from resistant bacteria, and generally reflects the concentration of the drug that will be achieved in plasma following administration of the recommended dose. Once the MIC for a bacterial isolate is determined for a particular antibiotic, it is then compared to published breakpoints to determine whether the isolate is susceptible or resistant (or intermediately susceptible, in some cases). The spectrum of an antibiotic is essentially based on this breakpoint; without established breakpoints, MIC values are meaningless. If the majority of isolates of a given species are inhibited at concentrations below the breakpoint, the species is considered to be within the spectrum of the drug.

If CLSI protocols are employed, the breakpoint of a drug should be the same for any laboratory. Veterinary-specific breakpoints have been established for some but not all antibiotics. Otherwise, human interpretive criteria are applied, which may not always be relevant to our patients. If the MIC necessary to inhibit the organism is well below the breakpoint, this organism is considered susceptible (S). As the MIC approaches the breakpoint, the organism is considered to have intermediate (I) susceptibility. The organism is considered resistant (R) to the drug if the MIC equals or surpasses the breakpoint, since it is unlikely that effective concentrations of the drug will be achieved in plasma or tissue. Data that include MIC values (rather than simply an S, I or R designation) can be

particularly helpful in assessing the degree of susceptibility of an organism to a drug. Intermediate susceptibility implies that, although standard dosing may not be effective, in some circumstances higher doses might be efficacious. The further the MIC of the organism is from the breakpoint, the more likely it is that effective concentrations will be achieved in plasma. The distance between the MIC of the organism and the breakpoint becomes even more important when infections are located in tissues other than blood or urine, particularly in regions that are difficult to penetrate (prostate, eye, central nervous system (CNS)) or when host responses have a negative impact on antimicrobial efficacy. Examples include the presence of marked inflammatory debris, fibrosis, or an anaerobic environment.

The rate of kill for some antibiotics is closely related to the peak concentration achieved above breakpoint (concentration-dependent activity), while others have kill rates that correlate with the length of time drug concentrations are maintained above the breakpoint MIC (time-dependent activity). Penicillins, cephalosporins, macrolides and clindamycin are all characterized by time-dependent killing. Aminoglycosides and fluoroquinolones show concentration-dependent activity (Figure 24.1). Concentration-dependent antibiotics may be assessed by the ratio of peak serum antibiotic concentration (C_{max}) to MIC. It is generally accepted that antibiotic concentrations should be eight to ten times the MIC, although this may not always be possible for bacteria with a high breakpoint because of drug toxicity. For time-dependent drugs, plasma drug concentrations should remain above the MIC for the majority of the dosing interval. High peak serum concentrations do not appear to confer any additional benefit for time-dependent drugs. However, increasing the frequency of administration would be expected to enhance the efficacy of a time-dependent drug. Given this information, it is logical to suggest that time-dependent drugs with short half-lives may be more effectively administered as a CRI to ensure that the plasma concentration exceeds the MIC for the entire

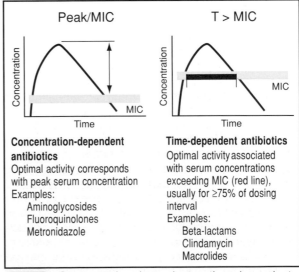

Concentration-dependent antibiotics
Optimal activity corresponds with peak serum concentration
Examples:
    Aminoglycosides
    Fluoroquinolones
    Metronidazole

Time-dependent antibiotics
Optimal activity associated with serum concentrations exceeding MIC (red line), usually for ≥75% of dosing interval
Examples:
    Beta-lactams
    Clindamycin
    Macrolides

24.1 Concentration-dependent vs time-dependent drugs: pharmacokinetic/pharmacodynamic profiles as predictors of bacterial eradication (MIC, minimum inhibitory concentration).

'interval'. However, studies in humans comparing the use of continuous infusion of beta-lactams with intermittent boluses reported similar microbiological and clinical outcomes. Comparable studies are lacking in veterinary medicine.

Some antimicrobials may still be effective if the plasma drug concentration drops below the MIC. These drugs exhibit a post-antibiotic effect (PAE), such that bacterial growth is inhibited after a brief exposure to the drug (Jernigan *et al.*, 1988). Thus, it is not necessary to maintain plasma drug concentrations above the MIC for the entire dosing interval. The impact of the PAE is most profound for concentration-dependent drugs, as it allows some of them to be administered at extended intervals, i.e. once daily for the aminoglycosides and fluoroquinolones (Figure 24.2). The PAE varies with each drug, and each organism. The duration of the PAE is in large part dependent on the magnitude of the peak plasma drug concentrations, and may be enhanced by combination antimicrobial therapy with a beta-lactam agent.

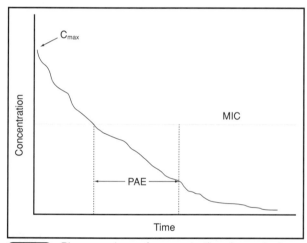

24.2 Pharmacology of concentration-dependent drugs: hypothetical serum drug levels following intravenous administration of an aminoglycoside or fluoroquinolone (C_{max}, maximum drug concentration; PAE, post-antibiotic effect; MIC, minimum inhibitory concentration).

The *in vitro* conditions under which susceptibility data are collected may vary considerably from those existing at the site of infection. Thus, MIC should be viewed as a rough guide to the likelihood of success or failure of treatment for that particular organism.

Reasons for therapeutic failure

Several factors can cause failure to respond to antimicrobial therapy. The most obvious cause is misdiagnosis; either identification of the wrong pathogen or treatment of a disorder that is not caused by a bacterial agent. In addition, the microbe may be resistant to the antibiotic or resistance may develop during the course of therapy, necessitating reassessment of *in vitro* susceptibility testing. Therefore, empirical changes may be made when culture reports are not available and the initially chosen antibiotic appears to be ineffective. The drug may be effective *in vitro* but

may not reach the site of infection in the host, or may be neutralized at the site of infection by ionization, binding to inflammatory debris, destruction by microbial enzymes and/or an anaerobic environment.

Surgical drainage or debridement may therefore be critical to successful antimicrobial therapy, especially for patients with closed-space infections or infections associated with foreign material. Notably, implanted materials have significant potential for incurring biofilm infection. Biofilms are antibiotic-resistant colonizations of bacteria that attach to surfaces and form a slime-like barrier that acts as a formidable defence mechanism, protecting the bacteria from eradication. The polysaccharide-containing biofilm matrix protects the bacteria and, thereby, increases resistance to humoral immunological responses, as well as to the phagocytic activity of neutrophils and tissue macrophages. Biofilms form rapidly on vascular catheters, urinary catheters and endotracheal tubes, necessitating not only aseptic technique at the time of placement, but vigilant hygiene and scheduled exchange or removal of these devices in critically ill patients.

Lastly, superinfection may contribute to therapeutic failure. Superinfection develops as resistant microorganisms proliferate and is more likely to occur following the use of broad-spectrum regimens, due to loss of commensal microbes which otherwise keep proliferating microorganisms in check.

Many causes of antimicrobial failure can be minimized by using the appropriate drug dose, interval and route of administration.

Changing patterns of resistance in selected species

The safety and efficacy of most antimicrobials has led to the false perception that antimicrobial prescriptions are at worst a neutral therapeutic choice and that antibiotics may help but will not harm the patient. However, the irrepressible increase in antimicrobial resistance over the past decade is in large part a result of widespread and inappropriate prescription of these agents (Lloyd *et al.*, 1999). The factors involved in antimicrobial resistance in the ICU appear at first to be quite complex but are, at their heart, relatively simple: *almost all antimicrobial resistance results from the convergence of two factors – poor infection control and selective pressure from antimicrobial agents.*

Unfortunately, multiple-drug-resistant opportunistic pathogens have become endemic to the veterinary hospital environment (Normand *et al.*, 2000; Guardabassi *et al.*, 2004). Resistance is growing for several reasons:

- The availability of medical advances (such as chemotherapy, mechanical ventilation, peritoneal or haemodialysis and organ transplantation) in veterinary medicine permits us to treat a greater number of critically ill patients. This likely correlates with immunological incompetence, decreased mobility and increased use of invasive devices which predispose to infections of the lungs, urinary tract and blood stream

- Antibiotics are often prescribed prophylactically, in *some* cases reducing the risk of specific infections at the price of increasing the risk that infections which do occur will be due to resistant organisms
- Severely ill patients tend to be clustered in the hospital. The relative crowding in these areas promotes the spread of bacteria among susceptible patients if appropriate infection control is not practised.

Gram-negative bacteria

Resistance is common among opportunistic Gram-negative bacteria, especially the Enterobacteriaceae (*Escherichia coli*, *Klebsiella*, *Proteus* and *Enterobacter*) and *Pseudomonas aeruginosa*. *P. aeruginosa* is one of the most resistant organisms encountered in the ICU, and infections with this organism are particularly problematic because of their intrinsic resistance to multiple classes of antibiotics and their ability to acquire adaptive resistance during therapy. Other non-fermenting Gram-negative bacteria, including nosocomial *Acinetobacter* and *Stenotrophomonas*, are often resistant to numerous antibiotics (Francey et al., 2000). Extended spectrum beta-lactamase (ESBL)-producing Gram-negative bacteria are a growing concern in human medicine. When producing these enzymes, organisms (most commonly *Escherichia coli* and *K. pneumoniae*) become highly efficient at inactivating the newer third-generation cephalosporins. Significantly, ESBL-producing bacteria are frequently also resistant to many classes of non-beta-lactam antibiotics, resulting in infections that are difficult to treat. At present, some ESBL-producing bacteria retain susceptibility to carbapenems, cefoxitin and cefotetan. Isolates are usually not capable of destroying clavulanic acid and thus should retain susceptibility to combinations with this drug. ESBL-producing bacteria have been isolated from veterinary patients, although thorough incidence and epidemiology studies are lacking. Clinical outcome data in humans indicate that ESBLs are clinically significant in terms of complication rates and mortality in critical illness, and the same is likely to hold true for veterinary patients.

Gram-positive bacteria

Staphylococci

While the focus of antibiotic resistance has traditionally been on enteric Gram-negative organisms, highly resistant Gram-positive cocci have emerged as an equally challenging concern (Boag et al., 2004; Weese et al., 2006). Methicillin-resistant *Staphylococcus* spp. (MRS) and multiple-drug-resistant *Enterococcus* spp. are present-day scourges in human ICUs, and have both been identified in dogs and cats (Pressel et al., 2005).

The incidence of methicillin-resistant *Staphylococcus aureus* (MRSA) infections in human ICU patients has dramatically increased in recent years. Compared with methicillin-sensitive *Staphylococcus aureus*, MRSA infections are associated with increased morbidity and mortality. MRSA is being increasingly isolated from companion animals, especially in conjunction with hospitalization and immunosuppression (Duquette and Nuttall, 2004; Middleton et al., 2005). Methicillin and oxacillin are members of a class of antibacterials known as the semi-synthetic penicillinase-resistant penicillins. Oxacillin is used as a surrogate in microbiology labs to test the susceptibility of bacteria to this entire class of antibacterials. Thus, if a staphylococcal organism is resistant to oxacillin, it is by definition resistant to methicillin. Moreover, methicillin (oxacillin) resistance implies resistance to *all* beta-lactam drugs, even if *in vitro* susceptibility data suggest otherwise. Addition of a beta-lactamase inhibitor will not overcome methicillin resistance. Among clinically infected animals, wounds are the most commonly reported sites of infection with MRSA, with fewer intravenous catheter site, urinary tract, skin and pulmonary infections (O'Mahony et al., 2005). As MRSA spreads, human physicians are left with an increasingly limited number of effective drugs. At the present time, not all MRSA infections are highly resistant, with some veterinary MRSA isolates retaining susceptibility to chloramphenicol and the potentiated sulphonamides. However, there is increasing resistance to clindamycin and the fluoroquinolones, once considered valuable in the management of staphylococcal infections. If they are selected, correct prescribing of fluoroquinolones is mandatory in this setting, as resistance among staphylococci to these drugs is facilitated by suboptimal dosing. Vancomycin has remained the most consistently effective approved drug for these infections in humans. However, this last line of defence is in itself a concern as vancomycin-resistant staphylococci have been identified in the UK, Asia and the USA. Other antibiotics currently used in the treatment of MRSA include linezolid, daptomycin and quinupristin/dalfopristin, none of which has been evaluated sufficiently in veterinary patients, therefore therapy with *any of these agents* cannot be advocated at this time, and is strongly discouraged.

Dogs are not considered a natural reservoir species for *Staphylococcus aureus*. Thus the most plausible explanation for colonization and/or infection of animals by this organism is transmission from humans. In one study, the most frequently occurring pattern of MRSA in small animals was indistinguishable from that of the human population in the same region. While much emphasis has been placed on the possibility of transmission of resistance from dogs or cats to humans, animals belonging to medical or veterinary personnel may be at more risk of being colonized with MRSA from contact with infected or colonized humans (Baptiste et al., 2005). Colonized pets may go on to develop infection or may serve as a source of spread of the organism to other animals or humans (Weese et al., 2006). The duration of asymptomatic carriage of MRSA by pets is not known at this time, posing a potential health risk to owners and veterinary staff. However, while humans may remain colonized for extended periods of time, it is unknown how long dogs and cats may remain colonized with MRSA. The need to treat animals colonized rather than infected with MRSA is debatable. Given the increasing emergence of multiple-drug-resistant isolates, it is essential to establish whether a patient is infected rather than colonized with MRSA before initiation of systemic antibiotic treatment.

S. aureus is not the only member of its genus that can be resistant to methicillin. Methicillin-resistant *Staphylococcus intermedius* (MRSI) and *Staphylococcus schleiferi* (MRSS) have both been isolated from humans and companion animals. Such resistance patterns appear to be more prevalent in hospital settings. To minimize transmission of resistant pathogens, practice protocols regarding hygiene of the staff and premises must be strictly implemented. Patients with methicillin-resistant infections should be isolated and handling should be minimal, using barrier precautions. Culture and susceptibility testing of affected tissue(s) is imperative, as the number of antimicrobial agents available for the treatment of MRS infections is often limited. Commercial laboratories should test *all* beta-lactam-resistant staphylococcal isolates for susceptibility to potentiated sulphonamides, chloramphenicol, clindamycin and tetracyclines. While awaiting the results of culture and susceptibility testing, chloramphenicol, potentiated sulphonamides or doxycycline may be prescribed for dogs with suspected MRSA infection.

Enterococci

Enterococci are commensal bacteria that inhabit the intestinal tract of dogs, cats, humans and other mammals (Devriese *et al.*, 1996; Simjee *et al.*, 2002). Pertubations in the host–commensal relationship, such as antibiotic treatment, host injury or diminished host immunity, allow these intestinal bacteria to cause infection in extraintestinal sites. Until recently pathogenic enterococcal infections were considered uncommon in veterinary medicine (Jackson *et al.*, 1994). However, antimicrobial-resistant *Enterococcus* spp. are now the second most common organisms recovered from nosocomial wound and urinary tract infections in human ICUs. Multiple-drug-resistant enterococcal infections are sporadically documented in dogs and cats, most commonly from surgical wounds and the genitourinary tract (Leener *et al.*, 2005). The majority of infection-derived clinical isolates belong to the species *E. faecalis*, while *E. faecium* exhibits a disproportionately greater resistance to multiple antibiotics.

One of the major reasons for the survival of these organisms is their intrinsic resistance to several commonly used antibiotics and, perhaps more important, their ability to acquire resistance to all currently available antibiotics. Pathogenic enterococci are inherently resistant to sulphonamides, cephalosporins and most fluoroquinolones. Enterococci with acquired resistance to macrolides, lincosamides and tetracyclines have been isolated from asymptomatic cats and dogs, raising concerns about selective pressure associated with the use of these agents.

When resistant enterococci are present in wound or body cavity infections, the organism may co-exist with other bacteria such as Gram-negative bacilli or anaerobes. Optimally, a single drug or combination of two drugs would be identified to eradicate both

bacteria, but this is not always easily accomplished. For practical purposes, it reasonable to direct *initial* treatment at the Gram-negative bacillus or anaerobe and not at the *Enterococcus*, while monitoring the patient closely for evidence of clinical improvement. Treatment of enterococcal infections is often frustrating, given the limited drug choices. If the isolate is sensitive to penicillin, ampicillin should be administered at the high end of the dose range, ideally in combination with an aminoglycoside. Each drug alone is poorly bactericidal against enterococci. Chloramphenicol is one of the few agents that retain *in vitro* activity against many strains of multiple-drug-resistant *E. faecium*. In veterinary medicine vancomycin is considered the *drug of last resort* in the treatment of multiple-drug-resistant enterococcal infections. Other recently approved agents with activity against vancomycin-resistant enterococci include the oxazolidondiones, ketolides and glycylcyclines. These agents are not routinely prescribed by veterinary surgeons, and susceptibility results are not commonly reported by most veterinary laboratories at this time.

General infection control measures

In addition to rational prescription of antimicrobials in the ICU, a major emphasis should be on adequate infection control procedures to prevent transmission among hospitalized patients. The importance of hand washing before and after handling an ICU patient cannot be overemphasized, since the hands of health care workers are considered to be the major source of transmission of pathogens. Careful attention to barrier precautions for preventing the nosocomial spread of resistant bacterial strains must also be stressed. Contaminated medical devices or environmental surfaces may also contribute to transmission, particularly of organisms that survive for prolonged periods on inanimate surfaces. As such, it is imperative that ICUs implement a thorough disinfection protocol and have in place a means of identifying patients infected with multiple-drug-resistant or nosocomial pathogens.

Pharmacological considerations for critical illness

Critically ill patients often present with complex physiological derangements that may affect antimicrobial distribution and elimination. The inflammatory response associated with sepsis/systemic inflammatory response syndrome (SIRS) may result in altered vascular permeability, decreased serum albumin levels, large fluid shifts and variable cardiac output, which in turn result in increased drug clearance. Unless these effects are offset by concomitant renal or hepatic impairment with subsequent drug accumulation, antibiotic levels may be too low for optimal efficacy. Most significant among the pathophysiological changes associated with severe bacterial infection are alterations in drug volume of distribution (Vd) and clearance.

An increase in Vd essentially corresponds to dilution of the antimicrobial in plasma and other extracellular fluids, and is of most relevance for the hydrophilic antimicrobials (beta-lactams and aminoglycosides). Causes of increases in Vd include vascular leak syndromes or decreased intravascular oncotic pressure associated with hypoproteinaemia. These processes may promote fluid extravasation and are responsible for oedema and loss of fluid into body cavities. Studies of the pharmacology of a variety of drugs suggest that higher doses (aminoglycosides and beta-lactams) or increased frequency of administration (beta-lactams) should be considered to ensure that therapeutic blood concentrations are reached in critically ill patients with oedema. Aggressive intravenous fluid therapy and parenteral nutrition may similarly contribute to the expansion of extracellular volume and cause dilution of antimicrobials in the extracellular compartment, potentially resulting in therapeutic failure. Both pleural and peritoneal transudative effusions may be responsible for a higher Vd for hydrophilic antimicrobials, but the precise impact of intracavitary drug dilution in patients with septic pleural or peritoneal exudates is less clear.

Impairment of renal and hepatic function results in prolongation of drug half-life, decreased clearance and drug accumulation. The effects of liver dysfunction on antibiotic concentrations are not well characterized. For most antibiotics, hepatic metabolism is limited and protein binding is low enough to make no difference to their effectiveness. However, patients with severe hepatic disease may require dose adjustments for antibiotics metabolized by the liver (chloramphenicol, sulphonamides, clindamycin, metronidazole, doxycycline, cefotaxime and erythromycin).

Renal excretion is the major route of elimination of most antibiotics. It is therefore not surprising that renal insufficiency can profoundly impact their disposition. With reduced renal clearance the parent drug and/or its metabolites may accumulate and cause toxicity. The Vd of some antibiotics is altered with renal insufficiency. Fluid retention characteristic of renal failure alters the Vd of drugs that are predominantly distributed to extracellular water.

In patients with renal dysfunction, protein binding of acidic drugs may be affected by accumulation of organic solutes, which displace acidic drugs from their albumin binding sites. While it is difficult to predict the absolute changes in protein binding in an individual patient, in patients with renal dysfunction therapeutic concentrations of many drugs may be achieved at lower doses than in normal animals. Acid–base derangements, fluid depletion and electrolyte changes may also be associated with renal failure. Administration of sodium- or potassium-containing antimicrobials, such as sodium ampicillin or potassium penicillin, may result rarely in sodium overload or potassium-induced cardiac or neuronal disturbances. Acidosis has been shown to increase ionic binding of aminoglycosides, increasing accumulation in the renal tubules, possibly enhancing nephrotoxicity.

In veterinary medicine there are no uniformly accepted formulae for dosage adjustments in renal failure. Ideally, therapeutic drug monitoring should be carried out in each patient, but this is only possible with some drugs, and in general it is impractical and cost-prohibitive. In hospitalized human patients, drug dosages are based on frequent estimates of creatinine clearance that take into account lean body weight, gender and age, amongst other factors. Similar formulae have not been validated in veterinary medicine. As a general rule, either drug dosages may be reduced while the interval is maintained, or the drug dose is maintained but the interval is extended. Interval extension is the preferred method for adjusting doses of aminoglycosides, which have a long PAE and ideally should have a low trough concentration. The dose-reduction method is preferred for adjusting doses of beta-lactams, in which maintaining plasma drug concentrations above MIC correlates with efficacy. Moreover, the beta-lactams are relatively non-toxic, even if accumulation occurs. To decide which method to use, determine whether antimicrobial efficacy and toxicity are related to peak, trough, or average plasma concentrations, and then select the method that balances efficacy against potential toxicity. The package insert on many human pharmaceuticals often provides guidelines for adjusting doses. With significant renal impairment, selection of an antibiotic that is metabolized by the liver and excreted in bile rather than eliminated by the kidneys, (e.g. doxycycline) should be considered.

In addition to the intrinsic pharmacokinetic and pharmacodynamic properties of the antibiotic, other factors can affect response to therapy, including host defence mechanisms, site of infection and underlying disease (Figure 24.3). Inadequate penetration of drug to the infection site is one of the principal factors related to failure of antibiotic therapy. When evidence of infection persists, removal of vascular and urinary catheters is recommended, given their propensity for biofilm development. Similarly, successful treatment of osteomyelitis is determined as much by adequate surgical debridement as it is by appropriate antibiotic selection. In meningitis, the ability of antibiotics to cross the blood–brain barrier is an important consideration. In other patients, the relative concentrations achieved in bronchial secretions and lung tissue may be of particular interest. For example, beta-lactams and aminoglycosides do not efficiently penetrate bronchial secretions; therefore, pulmonary infections may require higher drug doses. In contrast, macrolides, fluoroquinolones and doxycycline predictably cross the blood–bronchus barrier at recommended doses and thus achieve adequate concentrations in respiratory epithelial fluid.

Most bacterial infections are located extracellularly in the host, and can be reached by the majority of water-soluble drugs. However, some pathogenic organisms reside within the cell (*Brucella*, *Rhodococcus*, *Salmonella*, *Chlamydophila*, *Rickettsia* and *Bartonella* spp.) and as a result only lipid-soluble drugs are able to cross the cell wall and reach therapeutic levels at the site of infection. Antibiotics that predictably achieve high intracellular concentrations include macrolides, lincosamides and fluoroquinolones.

Infection	Common pathogens	Recommendations for empirical therapy	Comment
Bacterial pneumonia	*Bordetella bronchiseptica, Streptococcus* spp., *Escherichia coli, Pseudomonas aeruginosa, Klebsiella* spp., *Acinetobacter* spp., *Pasteurella multocida*	One of: 　Cefazolin (1st) 　Ampicillin 　Ticarcillin–clavulanate 　Amoxicillin–clavulanate AND one of: 　Amikacin 　Gentamicin 　Enrofloxacin Doxycyline or azithromycin for juvenile patients with *B. bronchiseptica* pneumonia	The importance of *Mycoplasma* in respiratory infections remains controversial. Whether antibiotics should be given by aerosol for respiratory infections remains uncertain
Intra-abdominal sepsis	*Bacteroides* spp., *Escherichia coli, Proteus* spp., *Enterobacter, Enterococcus* spp., *Pseudomonas* spp.	Cefoxitin (2nd) Imipenem–cilastatin Or one of: 　Ampicillin–sulbactam 　Amoxicillin–clavulanate 　Ticarcillin–clavulanate 　Piperacillin–tazobactam AND one of: 　Amikacin 　Gentamicin 　Cefotaxime (3rd)	Assume presence of facultative enteric Gram-negative bacteria and anaerobes. Peritoneal irrigation with antibiotic solutions is not recommended. Consider addition of metronidazole for obligate anaerobic pathogens
Infective endocarditis	*Streptococcus* spp., *Staphylococcus* spp., *Escherichia coli, Enterococcus* spp., *Klebsiella* spp., *Bartonella* spp.	One of: 　Ampicillin–sulbactam 　Amoxicillin–clavulanate 　Ticarcillin–clavulanate 　Cefazolin (1st) AND one of: 　Gentamicin 　Amikacin	Collect at least three sets of blood cultures over 24 hours. Diagnosis of *Bartonella* relies on positive serology or PCR
Bacterial meningitis	*Staphylococcus* spp., *Streptococcus* spp., *Pasteurella* spp., *Proteus* spp., *Nocardia* spp., *Actinomyces* spp.	One or more of: 　Ceftriaxone (3rd) 　Cefotaxime (3rd) 　Ampicillin 　Enrofloxacin 　Trimethoprim–sulfadiazine 　Clindamycin	Primary bacterial CNS infections are rare in companion animals. Consider protozoal aetiology in both dogs and cats. Adjunctive glucocorticoid administration remains controversial in veterinary medicine
Urinary tract infection Pyelonephritis Urosepsis	*Escherichia coli, Proteus* spp., *Enterobacter* spp., *Staphylococcus* spp., *Klebsiella* spp., *Enterococcus* spp., *Pseudomonas* spp.	One or more of: 　Ampicillin 　Ampicillin–sulbactam 　Enrofloxacin 　Cefazolin (1st) 　Amikacin	Primary urinary tract infections are uncommon in cats. In intact male dogs, always assume prostatic involvement. Use aminoglycosides with caution in patients with renal dysfunction
Surgical wound infections	*Staphylococcus* spp., *Escherichia coli, Pasteurella* spp., *Bacteroides fragilis, Enterococcus* spp., *Enterobacter* spp., *Klebsiella* spp.	One or more of: 　Ampicillin–sulbactam 　Amoxicillin–clavulanate 　Cefazolin (1st) 　Clindamycin 　Gentamicin 　Enrofloxacin	Consider adding cefoxitin or metronidazole if anaerobic infection suspected

24.3 Common bacterial pathogens and empirical antibiotic choices for selected syndromes in critical illness. Empirical antibiotic selection should always be accompanied by appropriate culture and susceptibility testing and the selection modified based on the results (1st, first-generation cephalosporin; 2nd, second-generation cephalosporin; 3rd, third-generation cephalosporin).

Specific drug classes

Commonly used antibiotics are listed in Figure 24.4.

Beta-lactams
The beta-lactams include the penicillins, cephalosporins, monobactams and carbapenems, which all contain an active beta-lactam ring in their chemical structure. The beta-lactams have a slow continuous kill characteristic,

and are thus classified as time-dependent drugs: their efficacy depends on the percentage of the dosage interval for which plasma and tissue drug concentrations remain above the MIC of the offending organism (T>MIC). The optimal length of time for which drug levels should exceed MIC is not known, but for most beta-lactam agents it is commonly recommended that plasma concentrations should exceed the MIC of the organism for >75% of the dosing interval.

Drug	Dosing	Notes
Ampicillin	22 mg/kg i.v. q6–8h	Administer slowly over 15 minutes. Incompatible with dopamine and sodium bicarbonate
Ampicillin–sulbactam	22 mg/kg i.v. q8h	Administer slowly over 15 minutes
Amoxicillin–clavulanate	20mg/kg i.v. q8h	Administer slowly over 5 minutes
Amikacin	15–18 mg/kg i.v. q24h	Dilute with 0.9% NaCl to a concentration of 5 mg/ml and administer over 20–30 minutes. Incompatible on mixing with many beta-lactams, heparin, potassium chloride and dexamethasone
Azithromycin	5–10 mg/kg i.v. q24h	Dilute to a concentration of 5 mg/ml and administer slowly over 1–2 hours
Aztreonam	30 mg/kg i.v. q8–12h	Extrapolated from human dose recommendations. Dilute to final concentration of 20 mg/ml and administer over 30–60 minutes. Contraindicated with renal impairment. Limited information in companion animals
Cefazolin	22 mg/kg i.v. q6–8h	Slow intravenous administration over 5 minutes
Cefepime	40 mg/kg i.v. q6h	Incompatible with ampicillin, heparin and potassium chloride. Reconstitute with 0.9% NaCl or 5% dextrose. Slow intravenous administration over 30 minutes
Cefotaxime	50 mg/kg i.v. q6–8h	Dilute to final concentration of 100 mg/ml and administer over 15–30 minutes
Cefotetan	30 mg/kg i.v. q8h	Reconstitute with sterile water. Intravenous administration over 15–30 minutes. Incompatible with aminoglycosides
Cefoxitin	30 mg/kg i.v. q6–8h	Reconstitute with sterile water. Dilute to final concentration of 100 mg/ml and administer slowly over 15–30 minutes
Ceftazidime	30 mg/kg i.v. q4–6h	Reconstitute to 100 mg/ml with sterile water, 5% dextrose or 0.9% NaCl. Infuse over 5–10 minutes. Incompatible with bicarbonate-containing fluids. Reduce dosing with renal impairment
Ceftriaxone	25–50 mg/kg i.v. q12–24h	No dosing adjustment necessary with renal or hepatic dysfunction. Reconstitute to a final concentration of 100 mg/ml and administer over 20–30 minutes. Incompatible with metronidazole and vancomycin
Cefuroxime	20–40 mg/kg i.v. q8h	Administer slowly over 5 minutes
Chloramphenicol	40–50 mg/kg i.v. q8h (dogs) 12.5–20 mg/kg i.v. q12h (cats)	Avoid long-term usage in cats
Clindamycin	10 mg/kg i.v. q12h	Given as slow infusion following dilution
Doxycycline	5–10 mg/kg i.v. q12h	Reconstitute with 0.9% NaCl to a final concentration of 1 mg/ml. Administer over 1 hour
Enrofloxacin	10–20 mg/kg i.v. q24h (dogs) 5 mg/kg i.v. q24h (cats)	Dilute 1:1 with 0.9% NaCl and infuse over 30 minutes
Gentamicin	6.6–8.8 mg/kg i.v. q24h	Dilute 1:1 with 0.9% NaCl and administer over 20–30 minutes. Do not mix with heparin or beta-lactams
Imipenem–cilastatin	5–10 mg/kg i.v. q6h	Contents of vials not for direct infusion. Reconstitute with 100 ml 5% dextrose or 0.9% NaCl. Transfer 10 ml from 100 ml bag of infusion solution to vial. Agitate and return resulting 10 ml to remaining 90 ml of solution. Administer over 30–60 minutes
Meropenem	22 mg/kg i.v. q12h	Reconstitute to 50 mg/ml with sterile water. Infuse over 20–30 minutes
Metronidazole	15 mg/kg i.v. q12h	Administer slowly over 15–30 minutes
Piperacillin–tazobactam	40 mg/kg i.v. q6h	Intravenous infusion over 30 minutes
Ticarcillin–clavulanate	50 mg/kg i.v. q6–8h	
Trimethoprim-sulfamethoxazole	15–30 mg/kg i.v. q12h	Each vial is diluted in 100 ml of 5% dextrose. Intravenous infusion over 60 minutes
Vancomycin	15 mg/kg i.v. q8h	Dilute in 5% dextrose to a maximum final concentration of 5 mg/ml. Administer over 1 hour

24.4 Parenteral antibiotics commonly used in emergency and critical care.

Penicillins were among the first antibiotics to be developed. They are typically well tolerated and *historically* were considered bactericidal against a broad range of pathogens. The spectrum of penicillin G often includes anaerobic rods (e.g. *Clostridium*, *Bacteroides*), spirochaetes (*Borrelia* and *Leptospira*), many streptococci and some enterococci. Few pathogenic staphylococci or Gram-negative aerobes remain susceptible to penicillin. Significant resistance has developed to aqueous penicillins, and they generally require administration every 6 hours. They are rarely prescribed to companion animals.

Historically, the spectrum of the aminopenicillins ampicillin and amoxicillin extends to include *some* Gram-negative rods, such as select isolates of *Escherichia coli, Proteus mirabilis* and *Salmonella*. However, resistance among *E. coli* isolates is increasing, highlighting the fact that just because a pathogen is reported to be 'within the spectrum' of a class of drugs, the organism may not, in fact, be susceptible in all cases. Aminopenicillins are typically more effective for enterococci than penicillin. Ampicillin is one of the few beta-lactams that is metabolized and excreted by the liver and thus achieves high concentrations in bile. About 50% of administered ampicillin is excreted unchanged in the urine. The addition of sulbactam (a beta lactamase inhibitor) extends the spectrum of ampicillin to include otherwise resistant strains of some Enterobacteriaceae and many anaerobes. Amoxicillin, also an aminopenicillin, has an identical spectrum of activity to ampicillin when used alone. The addition of clavulanic acid extends its Gram-negative spectrum. Amoxicillin is better absorbed following oral administration and has a longer duration of action when compared to ampicillin, and thus is appropriately prescribed for patients that both require and tolerate the transition to oral antibiotics. Amoxicillin–clavulanate is licensed for oral use in the USA and UK, and a human preparation is available for intravenous use in the UK.

The extended-spectrum penicillins (ticarcillin, piperacillin) are effective *in vitro* against *Pseudomonas aeruginosa* as well as enteric Gram-negative bacteria such as *E. coli, Klebsiella, Proteus* spp. and anaerobic organisms, including *Bacteroides fragilis*. However, the susceptibility of these penicillins to beta-lactamases markedly limits their utility for *in vivo* infections caused by Gram-negative enteric organisms. The addition of beta-lactamase inhibitors (clavulanic acid or tazobactam) to ticarcillin and piperacillin extends their spectrum to include many organisms rendered resistant by beta-lactamase production. However, the addition of a beta-lactamase inhibitor does *not* enhance efficacy against *Pseudomonas aeruginosa*. Thus, monotherapy with these agents is generally not advocated for treating pseudomonal infections. All penicillins may be combined with an aminoglycoside or fluoroquinolone for a synergistic effect when treating serious Gram-negative infections, most notably to optimize coverage for *P. aeruginosa*.

Cephalosporins are a broad group of beta-lactam antibiotics classified into 'generations' based on their spectrum of activity and susceptibility to beta-lactamase destruction. They are generally well tolerated and predominantly excreted by the kidneys. The cephalosporins are more resistant than the penicillins to beta-lactamase destruction. However, the recent emergence and spread of ESBL-producing organisms precludes the application of this generalization to all infections, particularly those caused by nosocomial Gram-negative pathogens. Enterococci and MRSA are resistant to cephalosporins.

The spectrum of the first-generation cephalosporins is similar to that of the aminopenicillins, with some enhanced coverage of Gram-negative pathogens. Two of the first-generation cephalosporins, cefazolin and cefalotin, have been used extensively in small animals. Cefalotin is no longer available in the USA. Cefazolin is frequently used to treat skin, bone and soft tissue infections with Gram-positive cocci, and remains the drug of choice for surgical prophylaxis for skin contamination. The first-generation cephalosporins are not predictably effective for anaerobic pathogens. Although first-generation cephalosporins have some activity against *E. coli, Klebsiella* and *Proteus*, their efficacy is most predictable for lower urinary tract infections caused by susceptible strains of these pathogens. While most cephalosporins attain high concentrations in urine, this is not necessarily true of urogenital tissues, i.e. they are not suitable agents for pyelonephritis.

The parenteral second-generation cephalosporins extend the Gram-negative spectrum of the first-generation compounds, although efficacy against Gram-positive and anaerobic organisms is often less. Cefoxitin and cefotetan, which are in the cephamycin group, have enhanced efficacy against anaerobic organisms, including *Bacteroides fragilis*. These drugs may be appropriate for treating hepatobiliary infections or septic peritonitis in which a mixed population of anaerobic bacteria and Gram-negative bacilli are observed.

Third-generation cephalosporins are generally more effective against Gram-negative bacteria than first- and second-generation cephalosporins. In addition, they are generally more resistant to degradation by beta-lactamases. With the exception of ceftazidime and cefoperazone, these agents have poor activity against *Pseudomonas aeruginosa*. In general, they have poor efficacy against anaerobes and are often less active than first-generation agents against Gram-positive organisms. Cefotaxime, ceftriaxone and ceftazidime are the most widely used parenteral third-generation cephalosporins. Because of its excellent Gram-negative spectrum, long serum half-life and high levels in both plasma and CSF, ceftriaxone is one of the drugs of choice for presumptive therapy of bacterial meningitis. The spectrum of each third-generation cephalosporin is sufficiently variable that each drug should be reviewed prior to use to assure the targeted organism is included in the spectrum. Ideally, the use of these agents should be guided by susceptibility testing.

Ceftiofur, a broad-spectrum third-generation cephalosporin primarily marketed for therapy of bovine respiratory disease, has received attention from small animal practitioners. Compared with other third-generation cephalosporins, it is significantly less costly and can be frozen in aliquots. Administered subcutaneously, ceftiofur is approved for the treatment of urinary tract infections caused by *E. coli* or *Proteus mirabilis* in dogs in the USA. At the labelled dose (2.2 mg/kg), ceftiofur achieves very high concentrations in urine for 24 hours, but the plasma half-life of ceftiofur and its metabolites is above *E. coli*'s MIC of 4.0 mg/l for only 3–4 hours. Thus, a higher dose and/or decreased dosing interval would be required to treat infections outside the urinary tract. Since no published studies have evaluated the efficacy or safety of ceftiofur at off-label dosages, its use in critical small animal patients is generally discouraged.

Cefovecin is a third-generation cephalosporin which has recently become available in the UK. It is highly protein bound and is licensed to be administered as a subcutaneous injection once every 2 weeks. Its use in critically ill veterinary patients has not yet been evaluated. As the pharmocokinetics of the drug in critically ill patients may be different, it is recommended that this drug should be used with caution in this population.

Cefepime is classified as a fourth-generation cephalosporin, unique from the other three generations in its extended spectrum of activity and its resistance to beta-lactamase hydrolysis. Its spectrum includes antipseudomonal activity comparable to ceftazidime and Gram-positive activity comparable to cefotaxime and ceftriaxone. *Enterococcus* spp. and MRSA strains are generally resistant *in vivo*. Its value in treating severe infections, alone or with other agents, is well established for resistant organisms in human ICUs. Cefepime is frequently active against nosocomial pathogens such as *Enterobacter* and *Acinetobacter*, and its use should therefore be restricted to the setting of nosocomial sepsis. There is limited information on the use of this drug in veterinary medicine (Gardner and Papich, 2001).

The carbapenems are beta-lactam antibiotics and include imipenem and meropenem (Bidgood and Papich, 2002). Imipenem is marketed in combination with the renal dipeptidase inhibitor cilastatin. Cilastatin prevents renal inactivation of imipenem, thus avoiding the accumulation of toxic metabolites while increasing the elimination half-life and urine levels of the drug. Imipenem is one of the broadest-spectrum antibiotics available. It has a short half-life after reconstitution, and must be diluted in a large volume of crystalloid prior to administration. Seizures and gastrointestinal distress are occasionally reported following administration, especially in patients with impaired renal function or incipient epilepsy. Meropenem is very similar to imipenem but does not require combination with a dipeptidase inhibitor, has a longer shelf-life after reconstitution, and is associated with less neurotoxicity. Meropenem is more soluble and therefore can be administered in a smaller volume of fluids (intravenously or subcutaneously) over a shorter period of time. The spectra of meropenem and imipenem are not identical, although coverage by both agents is excellent for most bacterial pathogens, including *Pseudomonas aeruginosa* and *Acinetobacter* spp. (Seol *et al.*, 2002). Whilst some anaerobes are susceptible to the carbapenems, these drugs are not active against MRSA or *Enterococcus faecium*. Imipenem and meropenem are rarely 'first-line' agents. Their use should always be dictated by culture and susceptibility data, but they can be used as empirical therapy for serious nosocomial infections thought to be caused by multiple pathogens or highly resistant Enterobacteriaceae, pending culture results.

Aztreonam is the only currently marketed monobactam. It has a significantly narrower spectrum than other beta-lactams. Specifically, its antibacterial spectrum is limited to Gram-negative aerobic bacteria. It is effective for most Enterobacteriaceae, including *Escherichia coli*, *Enterobacter*, *Klebsiella* spp., *Proteus* spp. and *Serratia* spp. It is generally very effective for *Pseudomonas aeruginosa*, but activity against *Acinetobacter* spp. is limited. About 60–70% of aztreonam is renally excreted. The drug is only available for intravenous administration, and it has an excellent safety profile. It is used for definitive treatment of nosocomial pneumonia and other serious infections in human ICU patients. Appropriately, most commercial veterinary laboratories do not provide susceptibility data for aztreonam at this time. Veterinary applications of aztreonam have not been defined and its administration is only justified in patients with infections caused by pathogens that are uniquely susceptible to this agent, or for patients that absolutely cannot tolerate aminoglycosides or other drugs appropriate for Gram-negative sepsis.

Aminoglycosides

The aminoglycosides remain important agents in the treatment of serious Gram-negative infections. They are rapidly bactericidal *in vitro* at low concentrations, and are predictably effective for most aerobic Gram-negative pathogens, including *Klebsiella*, *Serratia*, *Enterobacter* and most strains of *Acinetobacter* and *Pseudomonas aeruginosa* (Albarellos *et al.*, 2004). While tobramycin and netilmicin have been administered to cats and dogs, amikacin and gentamicin remain the most widely used aminoglycosides in veterinary medicine. Amikacin has the broadest Gram-negative spectrum, and may be more effective than gentamicin for *Pseudomonas aeruginosa* and *Escherichia coli* infections. Among Gram-positive organisms, gentamicin is often effective for many staphylococci. Enterococci are relatively resistant, but when gentamicin is combined with a penicillin or aminopenicillin, these organisms may be rendered susceptible. This synergistic effect occurs because the efficacy of the aminoglycoside appears to be enhanced by increased cell permeability induced by the beta-lactam, favouring movement of the aminoglycoside into the bacteria. Similar 'antimicrobial synergy' is also described for *Pseudomonas aeruginosa*. The aminoglycosides are not effective against anaerobes, or for pathogens in areas of low oxygen tension, such as abscesses or other hypoxic infected tissues. Aminoglycosides are highly water soluble and do not readily cross biological membranes; penetration into bronchial secretions, CSF and prostatic fluid is therefore poor. Therapeutic concentrations are generally achieved in non-exudative pleural and peritoneal effusions, bile, pulmonary parenchyma and synovial fluid. Inhalation therapy with gentamicin is reported to reduce the duration and severity of clinical signs associated with infectious tracheobronchitis in dogs, without producing detectable serum concentrations (Miller and MacKiernan, 2003). Aerosolization should never be used as the only means of treating serious respiratory infections such as pneumonia, but should be used alongside parenteral antimicrobial therapy. The role of nebulized aminoglycosides in veterinary patients with severe or ventilator-associated pneumonia remains unclear.

The aminoglycosides are administered systemically to well hydrated patients with stable renal function that are not receiving other nephroactive drugs. They are predominantly excreted by glomerular filtration, and historically nephrotoxicity is the major drawback to their use. Amikacin is reportedly less nephrotoxic than gentamicin. Nephrotoxicity is evidenced by non-oliguric renal insufficiency, and trough drug levels correlate with the development of toxicity. Administration of the total daily dose of aminoglycoside as a single daily dose (SDD) is associated with less nephrotoxicity than the same total amount given divided into multiple doses. SDD optimizes concentration-dependent bactericidal activity by maximizing peak plasma concentration (C_{max}) relative to the MIC of the pathogen. Since aminoglycosides are concentration-dependent drugs, SDD produces more rapid bacterial killing, less bacterial resistance and better clinical outcomes with less nephrotoxicity than conventional multiple daily dosing.

When the aminoglycosides are administered using SDD, their PAE effectively allows the patient to have daily drug-free intervals which ensure that trough levels are low enough to minimize toxicity, without compromising outcome. The PAE is extended by higher dosing. Daily examination of urine sediment for the presence of casts, with periodic evaluation for proteinuria and glucosuria using standard urine reagent strips, is an acceptable means to monitor for drug-induced tubular damage. Although some older reports describe an inexorable progression of aminoglycoside-induced renal injury, drug-induced renal lesions are frequently reversible if detected quickly, followed by prompt modification or discontinuation of therapy. When possible, systemic therapy with aminoglycosides should be limited to no more than 7 days. If it is necessary to treat for a longer period of time, therapeutic drug monitoring has been recommended. Although not borne out by studies in veterinary medicine, SDD may obviate the need for therapeutic drug monitoring due to reduced risk of toxicity and assured peak concentration-related efficacy. A reasonable monitoring strategy for SDD is to obtain a random trough concentration 2–4 hours prior to the next dose to ensure that there is adequate renal clearance and a sufficient 'drug-free' period. Trough serum concentrations correlate with nephrotoxicity, and should be <1.0 µg/ml and <2.5 µg/ml for gentamicin and amikacin, respectively. Trough serum concentrations >2.5 µg/ml are indicative (and not necessarily a cause) of renal dysfunction. Peak serum concentrations of gentamicin and amikacin should exceed the MIC by a factor of at least ten (C_{max}/MIC ≥10) in critically ill patients. Anticipated peak serum concentrations using SDD are 30–40 µg/ml for amikacin and 15–20 µg/ml for gentamicin. These peak serum concentrations are often achieved with SDD, but exceptions may occur when Vd is significantly altered in critical illness.

Other toxic effects associated with aminoglycosides include otovestibular toxicity and neuromuscular impairment. Otovestibular toxicity has been experimentally induced in both dogs and cats, but has not been reported following SDD in companion animals. Neuromuscular depression from aminoglycosides is rare. It is caused by reduced acetylcholine activity at postsynaptic membranes, and may be associated with respiratory depression. Weakness associated with neuromuscular blockade may be seen at doses just slightly higher than those recommended, but is likely to be of clinical consequence only when aminoglycosides are administered rapidly, in patients with neuromuscular disorders, e.g. myasthenia gravis, or in those receiving neuromuscular blocking agents. Injectable calcium and perhaps neostigmine may reverse the neuromuscular depression produced by the aminoglycosides. Neuromuscular toxicity has not been observed in neurologically normal human patients on SDD.

Fear of toxicity should not prevent the use of aminoglycosides when they are legitimately indicated, since toxicity is usually mild and reversible. In view of the favourable properties of SDD and alarming resistance patterns among Gram-negative pathogens to cephalosporins and fluoroquinolones, the aminoglycosides should be retained as a valuable part of our contemporary antibacterial arsenal.

Fluoroquinolones

In general, the veterinary-approved fluoroquinolones have excellent activity against many aerobic and facultative Gram-negative rods, fair activity against staphylococci, variable to poor activity against streptococci and minimal activity against obligate anaerobes. Chlamydiae, mycoplasmas, *Campylobacter* and some rickettsial species are also often susceptible to these drugs. In general, their high Vd corresponds to excellent penetration into most tissues, including skin, soft tissues, respiratory epithelium, bone, meninges, prostate and urine. High concentrations within phagocytes correspond with higher concentrations at inflammatory sites. The predicted therapeutic efficacy differs significantly among these agents such that they should not be used interchangeably in critical illness. The liberal use of fluoroquinolones in human medicine has contributed to several disturbing resistance patterns, including MRSA, ESBL-producing Gram-negative pathogens, fluoroquinolone-resistant *Pseudomonas aeruginosa* and vancomycin-resistant *Enterococcus faecium* (VRE). Similarly, the use of fluoroquinolones in small animals has been associated with increasing resistance among *P. aeruginosa*, *Staphylococcus intermedius* and *Escherichia coli*. Veterinary studies reveal that 26% of 'community-acquired' strains of *P. aeruginosa* were resistant *in vitro* to enrofloxacin, while only 8% were resistant to ciprofloxacin. More recent investigations show that resistance of *E. coli* to fluoroquinolone approximates 40%. Enrofloxacin is the only veterinary-approved fluoroquinolone available for parenteral administration. While it is commonly given intravenously, it is not labelled for this route of administration. Approximately 40% of enrofloxacin is metabolized to ciprofloxacin, and this active metabolite is further biotransformed to several additional compounds that are excreted primarily in the urine.

Although half-life varies among the fluoroquinolones, SDD of high doses of these agents can be used, allowing higher peak plasma levels to be achieved, resulting in maximal bacterial killing. All of the fluoroquinolones are bactericidal and exhibit a post-antibiotic effect (PAE). The PAE for the fluoroquinolones appears to be concentration-dependent, supporting high-dose, once-daily administration. The relationship between fluoroquinolone *use* and fluoroquinolone *resistance* is incontrovertible. *In vitro* studies indicate that the use of an inappropriately low dose of enrofloxacin in dogs can promote the development of resistant bacterial strains *in vivo* (Ganiere *et al.*, 2001). Increases in fluoroquinolone resistance may be a function of the relatively low dosages approved in clinical practice, which were designed to cure infection without considering resistance.

Possible toxicities include seizure activity (primarily observed following rapid intravenous administration), gastrointestinal distress and alterations in the cartilage of weightbearing bones of immature animals (Takizawa *et al.*, 1999). The specific mechanism responsible for fluoroquinolone-induced arthropathy and chondrotoxicity in juvenile animals has not been elucidated. At this time, the use of all fluoroquinolones in growing animals is discouraged unless no other therapeutic options exist. Partial, temporary or permanent blindness has been described in a small percentage of cats following therapy with enrofloxacin (Wiebe and Hamilton, 2002). Retinal degeneration is not unique to enrofloxacin, and retinal pathology may be seen with other fluoroquinolones. Administered at 2.5 mg/kg q12h, enrofloxacin has not been associated with any retinal changes and the manufacturers recommend not exceeding 5.0 mg/kg/day in cats. However, most susceptible isolates have MICs ≥0.25 µg/ml. As such, therapeutic concentrations of enrofloxacin are unlikely to be achieved at a total daily dose of 5.0 mg/kg in cats or dogs. Thus, it may not be possible to prescribe fluoroquinolones appropriately to critically ill cats without exceeding the recommendations imposed by the manufacturer.

Optimally, the fluoroquinolones are reserved for severe or recurrent genitourinary or systemic infections. When possible, their use in critical illness is based on results of culture and susceptibility data, and they are administered at the highest recommended dose. Enrofloxacin and other fluoroquinolones are widely used for empirical therapy given their broad range of antibacterial activity, once-daily administration, favourable side-effect profile and almost complete bioavailability following intravenous administration. However, continued clinical success can only be ensured if these agents are prescribed appropriately.

Metronidazole

Metronidazole is a bactericidal agent with a spectrum limited to anaerobic bacteria. It diffuses well into tissues and body fluids, including CSF, bile and abscesses. Effective tissue penetration and consistent bactericidal activity make metronidazole a drug of choice for severe anaerobic infections including intra-abdominal abscesses, endocarditis and osteomyelitis. Other antibacterial agents should be used in combination with metronidazole if additional facultative and aerobic pathogens are suspected. For example, a combination of metronidazole and a third-generation cephalosporin is an appropriate choice for intra-abdominal infections.

Seizures, vestibular syndromes and other neuropathies have been reported with high-dose and/or long-term use of metronidazole. While these untoward effects are generally self-limiting, complete recovery may take days to weeks. Metronidazole should be given with particular caution in patients with underlying neurological disorders. Diazepam may lessen the duration and severity of adverse neurological events.

Vancomycin

Vancomycin, a glycopeptide bactericidal antibiotic, has been in use in human medicine for over 40 years. Its spectrum is limited to Gram-positive cocci, including most isolates resistant to beta-lactams. While vancomycin has been considered the drug of last defence against Gram-positive multiple-drug-resistant bacteria in humans, the late 1980s saw a rise in vancomycin-resistant bacteria, including VRE and strains of *Staphylococcus aureus*. Colonization with VRE has been documented in dogs and cats, raising the spectre of transmission and subsequent illness in hospitalized patients (van Belkun *et al.*, 1996; Morley, 2004). However, reports of VRE infections are presently uncommon in veterinary medicine.

Vancomycin is administered intravenously and is cleared almost completely by glomerular filtration. Drug-associated renal impairment is reported but uncommon. Vancomycin can cause severe tissue damage if it is extravasated into subcutaneous tissues.

Vancomycin is occasionally used to treat severe, persistent staphylococcal infections and colitis associated with *Clostridium difficile*. In all situations, vancomycin should be considered a drug of absolute last resort, and should never be prescribed empirically. Consultation with a veterinary pharmacologist or infectious disease specialist is recommended before concluding that vancomycin is the most appropriate antimicrobial agent for any infection in dogs and cats.

Macrolides

The macrolides exhibit a broad spectrum of antimicrobial activity against many Gram-positive and Gram-negative bacteria. They are classified as bacteriostatic agents, but *in vitro* studies indicate that they are bactericidal against many pathogens. Macrolide antibiotics in general are used against susceptible organisms causing respiratory, urogenital, gastrointestinal and skin or soft tissue infections.

Erythromycin has activity against many Gram-positive cocci, *Campylobacter* spp., *Chlamydia* spp. and a variety of anaerobes. Its degradation products are motilin-like agonists which stimulate intestinal peristalsis, hence the use of low-dose erythromycin in patients with intestinal ileus. Erythromycin is widely distributed throughout the body. It achieves higher and more sustained concentrations in pulmonary tissues and secretions than comparable doses of beta-lactam antibiotics. However, it has disadvantages which include adverse gastrointestinal effects (vomiting and diarrhoea), short half-life and a requirement for frequent dosing intervals, therefore it is seldom used in the critical care setting.

Azithromycin, a macrolide derivative, is extensively distributed and persists within most tissues. Azithromycin has similar activity against Gram-positive organisms, and enhanced activity against Gram-negative organisms and Enterobacteriaceae, compared with erythromycin. Mean concentrations in tissues (lung, prostate, urinary tract, muscle and bone) exceed plasma concentrations 10–200-fold. Azithromycin accumulates in epithelial lining fluid and enters host defence cells, including alveolar macrophages. Azithromycin has been documented to accumulate to the greatest extent in neutrophils, when compared to other macrolides. This accumulation aids in the eradication of intracellular organisms. In the veterinary critical care setting, azithromycin has become a valuable addition to the traditional armamentarium for the treatment of respiratory tract infections, most notably in dogs with severe *Bordetella bronchiseptica* pneumonia. Azithromycin is among the drugs of choice for *Bordetella* infections in young dogs in which fluoroquinolones are contraindicated. Azithromycin is one of the drugs to which pathogenic *Bartonella* spp. are reportedly susceptible and it is also effective against *Borrelia* and mycobacteria. It has a long half-life that allows for once-daily dosing. Azithromycin is well tolerated when administered intravenously and is presently available in generic formulation.

Clindamycin

Clindamycin is the only parenteral lincosamide commonly used in veterinary medicine. The lincosamides are classified as bacteriostatic, but may be bactericidal *in vitro* against certain pathogens. Clindamycin has a broad spectrum of activity against Gram-positive and anaerobic bacteria, and is one of the drugs of choice for known or suspected anaerobic infections. Clindamycin has no clinically significant activity against facultative Gram-negative enteric bacteria. In veterinary medicine, it is considered the drug of choice for treatment of *Toxoplasma gondii* infection. Clindamycin, in combination with an antimicrobial with enhanced Gram-negative spectrum, is therefore appropriate for empirical therapy in patients with possible *Toxoplasma* infection. Clindamycin achieves particularly high concentrations in bone and has been recommended to treat osteomyelitis. Importantly, clindamycin achieves effective concentrations in walled-off abscesses, surpassing the concentrations achieved by penicillins or chloramphenicol. Clindamycin is one of several antimicrobials that are actively accumulated within phagocytic leucocytes, reaching concentrations 5–50-fold greater than plasma concentrations; thus, bacteria sequestered in white blood cells are not protected. Clindamycin also remains an effective therapy for some multiple-drug-resistant staphylococcal and enterococcal infections, and is considered a major component of therapy for both staphylococcal and streptococcal toxic shock syndrome (Naidoo *et al.*, 2005).

Chloramphenicol

Chloramphenicol is a broad-spectrum antibiotic that is effective against rickettsiae, chlamydiae, mycoplasmas, some spirochaetes, and most Gram-negative and Gram-positive aerobic and anaerobic bacteria. It is a preferred antibiotic for treating enteric *Salmonella* infections. Its spectrum generally does not include virulent Gram-negative pathogens such as *P. aeruginosa*. It is lipophilic and effectively penetrates the blood–brain barrier. In contrast to the majority of antibiotics used in critical illness chloramphenicol, like clindamycin, is classified as bacteriostatic. While bactericidal drugs are intuitively assumed to be more effective than bacteriostatic agents, the clinical importance of whether bactericidal action is better than bacteriostatic action has rarely been documented. The designation bactericidal or bacteriostatic is predominantly determined by *in vitro* studies, and is inconsistent against all bacteria for a particular agent.

Chloramphenicol is available for intravenous and oral administration. Although extremely rare, chloramphenicol exposure through aerosolization or oral intake is associated with idiosyncratic fatal bone marrow aplasia in humans. Contact with mucosal surfaces is required for this severe reaction. Oral veterinary preparations are film-coated, reducing the possibility of contact with active drug; therefore these already uncommon reactions are largely avoidable for caregivers. Drug-associated cytopenias are infrequently reported in veterinary medicine, and appear to be observed more commonly in cats than dogs. Routine haematological monitoring is recommended, especially when long-term therapy is instituted. Unlike the rare and idiosyncratic fatal reactions in people, in animals cell counts generally normalize when chloramphenicol is discontinued. Other adverse effects reported at various doses include anorexia, vomiting and diarrhoea.

Following concerns regarding potentially fatal toxicity, and the availability of 'safer' alternatives, the parenteral use of chloramphenicol was all but abandoned in human medicine until very recently. With the exception of certain exotic species and hindgut fermenters, its use had also diminished in veterinary medicine. However, current problematical organisms, notably multiple-drug-resistant enterococci and MRSA, often retain *in vitro* susceptibility to chloramphenicol, therefore it may serve as a viable treatment option for these infections. It is rarely, if ever, administered empirically to dogs or cats, only being prescribed based on culture and susceptibility data.

Potentiated sulphonamides

The potentiated sulphonamides (trimethoprim–sulfadiazine, trimethoprim–sulfamethoxazole) have been in widespread use since the late 1960s. They are bactericidal, and function by inhibiting sequential steps in folate synthesis (Trepanier, 2004). Their wide spectrum of activity and relatively low cost garnered global popularity for the treatment of skin, urinary tract and respiratory infections. However, increasing rates of resistance, an unfavourable incidence of adverse events in animals and the introduction of newer agents have led to decreased use of these drugs. The adverse pharmacological and idiosyncratic reactions to these agents include polyarthropathy, cytopenias, hepatic insufficiency, proteinuria, skin eruptions and keratoconjunctivitis sicca, and are particularly severe in dogs of Dobermann or Rottweiler lineage. The potentiated sulphonamides are frequently active against many Enterobacteriaceae, including *Escherichia coli*, *Klebsiella* spp. and *Proteus mirabilis*. Many isolates of *Staphylococcus* spp. remain susceptible, and the potentiated sulphonamides are among the drugs of choice for *Nocardia* infections. Opportunistic Gram-negative pathogens such as *Acinetobacter* spp., *Alcaligenes* spp. and *Burkholderia* (*Pseudomonas*) *cepacia*, typically resistant to several broad-spectrum classes of antibiotics, often remain susceptible. *Pseudomonas aeruginosa*, enterococci and strict anaerobes are inherently and uniformly resistant. Potentiated sulphonamides are effective for infections with *Toxoplasma gondii* and *Pneumocystis jaroveci* (formerly *P. carinii*). These agents are widely distributed, and may be especially useful for respiratory, prostate, CNS, complicated skin infections and osteomyelitis. Although the oral formulations are most familiar, trimethoprim–sulfadiazine is available for intravenous administration. As the potentiated sulphonamides are widely distributed and maintain efficacy against many multidrug-resistant staphylococci, their judicious use may serve as a model for appropriate use of broad-spectrum antibiotics in the setting of increasing resistance pressure.

Doxycycline

Doxycycline is a broad-spectrum, lipophilic antibiotic with excellent tissue penetration. Its concentrations in most tissues are generally equal to or greater than those in plasma. Unlike conventional tetracyclines, doxycycline is largely eliminated by non-renal mechanisms and is generally safe in patients with established or incipient renal disease. Doxycycline is effective against a broad range of Gram-positive, Gram-negative, aerobic and anaerobic bacteria, as well as *Brucella*, *Chlamydophila*, spirochaetes and *Rickettsia*. It is among the drugs of choice for Lyme disease and leptospirosis and is also an effective therapy for *Mycoplasma*, which may cause respiratory infections in dogs and cats. Many strains of *Bordetella bronchiseptica* remain susceptible to doxycycline, and *Bartonella* spp. may be treated with high-dose doxycycline.

As with other tetracyclines, doxycycline possesses anti-inflammatory effects independent of its antimicrobial properties. There is limited evidence that doxycycline causes tooth discoloration or inhibits bone growth in juvenile patients. While this problem is well documented with tetracycline (which is known to chelate divalent cations including calcium) it has not been substantiated for doxycycline. Doxycycline's tissue penetration, lipophilic nature and long serum half-life confers enhanced activity against some tetracycline-resistant organisms. Therefore tetracycline should not be viewed as a valid surrogate for doxycycline based on culture and susceptibility reports, particularly in the critically ill patient. Doxycycline may be administered intravenously once daily, or the total daily dose may be divided and given every 12 hours. Although doxycycline is generally well tolerated, gastrointestinal upset is occasionally seen. When given by mouth, pill-induced oesophageal ulceration is a well described adverse effect in both humans and pets, and may be prevented by giving water or food following drug administration.

References and further reading

Albarellos G, Montoya L, Ambros L *et al.* (2004) Multiple once-daily dose pharmacokinetics and renal safety of gentamicin in dogs. *Journal of Veterinary Pharmacology and Therapeutics* **27(1)**, 21–25

Baptiste KE, Williams K, Williams NJ *et al.* (2005) Methicillin-resistant staphylococci in companion animals. *Emerging Infectious Diseases* **11(12)**, 1942–1944

Bidgood T and Papich MG (2002) Plasma pharmacokinetics and tissue fluid concentrations of meropenem after intravenous and subcutaneous administration in dogs. *American Journal of Veterinary Research* **63(12)**, 1622–1628

Boag A, Loeffler A and Lloyd DH (2004) Methicillin-resistant *Staphylococcus aureus* isolates from companion animals. *Veterinary Record* **154(13)**, 411.

Boothe D (2006) Principles of antimicrobial therapy. *Veterinary Clinics of North America: Small Animal Practice* **36(5)**, 1003–1047

Boothe DM, Boeckh A, Simpson RB *et al.* (2006) Comparison of pharmacodynamic and pharmacokinetic indices of efficacy of five fluoroquinolones toward pathogens of dogs and cats. *Journal of Veterinary Internal Medicine* **20(6)**, 1297–1306

Brown A, Gorman R and Rankin SC (2005) A real-time 16S rRNA gene polymerase chain reaction assay to diagnose septic peritonitis. *Critical Care Medicine* **33(12 Suppl)**, A164

Cave NJ, Marks SL, Kass PH *et al.* (2002) Evaluation of a routine diagnostic fecal panel for dogs with diarrhea. *Journal of the American Veterinary Medical Association* **221(1)**, 52–59

Cooke CL, Singer RS, Jang SS *et al.* (2002) Enrofloxacin resistance in *Escherichia coli* isolated from dogs with urinary tract infections. *Journal of the American Veterinary Medical Association* **220(2)**, 190–192

Devriese LA, Ieven M, Goossens H *et al.* (1996) Presence of vancomycin-resistant enterococci in farm and pet animals. *Antimicrobial Agents and Chemotherapy* **40(10)**, 2285–2287

Dugan HA, MacLaren R and Jung R (2003) Duration of antimicrobial therapy for nosocomial pneumonia: possible strategies for minimizing antimicrobial use in intensive care units. *Journal of Clinical Pharmacy and Therapeutics* **28(2)**, 123–129

Duquette RA and Nuttall TJ (2004) Methicillin-resistant *Staphylococcus aureus* in dogs and cats: an emerging problem? *Journal of Small Animal Practice* **45(12)**, 591–597

Estes L (1998) Review of pharmacokinetics and pharmacodynamics of antimicrobial agents. *Mayo Clinic Proceedings* **73(11)**, 1114–1122

Francey T, Gaschen F, Nicolet J *et al.* (2000) The role of *Acinetobacter baumannii* as a nosocomial pathogen for dogs and cats in an intensive care unit. *Journal of Veterinary Internal Medicine* **14(2)**, 177–183

Ganiere JP, Medaille C, Limet A *et al.* (2001) Antimicrobial activity of enrofloxacin against *Staphylococcus intermedius* strains isolated from canine pyodermas. *Veterinary Dermatology* **12(3)**, 171–175

Gardner SY and Papich MG (2001) Comparison of cefepime pharmacokinetics in neonatal foals and adult dogs. *Journal of Veterinary Pharmacology and Therapeutics* **24(3)**, 187–192

Greene C (2006a) Antimicrobial chemotherapy. In: *Infectious Diseases of the Dog and Cat*, ed C Greene, pp. 274–301. Saunders Elsevier, Saint Louis

Greene C (2006b) Environmental factors in infectious disease. In: *Infectious Diseases of the Dog and Cat*, ed. C Greene, pp. 991-1000. Saunders Elsevier, St Louis

Guardabassi L, Schwarz S and Lloyd DH (2004) Pet animals as reservoirs of antimicrobial-resistant bacteria. *Journal of Antimicrobial Chemotherapy* **54(2)**, 321–332

Gurnee C, O'Shea K, Groman R *et al.* (2006) Molecular characterization of multidrug-resistant *E coli* infections at a veterinary teaching hospital. *Journal of Veterinary Internal Medicine* **20(3)**, 768

Jackson MW, Panciera DL and Hartmann F (1994) Administration of vancomycin for treatment of ascending bacterial cholangiohepatitis in a cat. *Journal of the American Veterinary Medical Association* **204(4)**, 602–605

Jang SS, Breher JE, Dabaco LA *et al.* (1997) Organisms isolated from dogs and cats with anaerobic infections and susceptibility to selected antimicrobial agents. *Journal of the American Veterinary Medical Association* **210(11)**, 1610–1614

Jernigan AD, Hatch RC, Wilson RC *et al.* (1988) Pharmacokinetics of gentamicin in cats given *Escherichia coli* endotoxin. *American Journal of Veterinary Research* **49(5)**, 603–607

Jones RL (2006) Laboratory Diagnosis of Bacterial Infections. In: *Infectious Diseases of the Dog and Cat*, ed. C Greene, pp. 267–273. Saunders Elsevier, St Louis

Kollef MH (2000) Inadequate antimicrobial treatment: an important determinant of outcome for hospitalized patients. *Clinical Infectious Diseases* **31** Suppl 4, S131–138

Kollef MH, Sherman G, Ward S *et al.* (1999) Inadequate antimicrobial treatment of infections: a risk factor for hospital mortality among critically ill patients. *Chest* **115(2)**, 462–474

Leener ED, Decostere A, DeGraef EM *et al.* (2005) Presence and mechanism of antimicrobial resistance among enterococci from cats and dogs. *Microbial Drug Resistance* **11(4)**, 395–403

Lloyd DH, Lamport AI and Noble WC (1999) Fluoroquinolone resistance in *Staphylococcus intermedius. Veterinary Dermatology* **10**, 249–251

Marik PE (1993) Aminoglycoside volume of distribution and illness severity in critically ill septic patients. *Anaesthesia and Intensive Care* **21(2)**, 172–173

Middleton JR, Fales WH, Luby CD *et al.* (2005) Surveillance of *Staphylococcus aureus* in veterinary teaching hospitals. *Journal of Clinical Microbiology* **43(6)**, 2916–2919

Miller CJM and McKiernan BC (2003) Gentamicin aerosolization for the treatment of infectious tracheobronchitis. *Journal of Veterinary Internal Medicine* **17(3)**, 386

Morley P (2004) Surveillance for methicillin-resistant *Staphylococcus aureus* and vancomycin-resistant *Enterococcus* in a veterinary hospital. In: *85th Conference of Research Workers in Animal Diseases*, Ames

Morris, DO, Rook KA, Shofer FS and Rankin SC (2006) Screening of *Staphylococcus aureus, Staphylococcus intermedius*, and *Staphylococcus schleiferi* isolates obtained from small companion animals for antimicrobial resistance: a retrospective review of 749 isolates (2003–04). *Veterinary Dermatology* **17(5)**, 332–337

Naidoo SL, Campbell DL, Miller LM *et al.* (2005) Necrotizing fasciitis: a review. *Journal of the American Animal Hospital Association* **41(2)**, 104–109

Normand EH, Gibson NR, Taylor DJ *et al.* (2000) Trends of antimicrobial resistance in bacterial isolates from a small animal referral hospital. *Veterinary Record* **146(6)**, 151–155

Ogeer-Gyles J, Mathews KA and Boerlin P (2005) Nosocomial infections and antimicrobial resistance in critical care medicine. *Journal of Veterinary Emergency and Critical Care* **16(1)**, 1–18

Ogeer-Gyles J, Mathews KA, Sears W *et al.* (2006) Development of antimicrobial drug resistance in rectal *Escherichia coli* isolates from dogs hospitalized in an intensive care unit. *Journal of the American Veterinary Medical Association* **229(5)**, 694–649

O'Mahony R, Abbott Y, Leonard FC *et al.* (2005) Methicillin-resistant *Staphylococcus aureus* (MRSA) isolated from animals and veterinary personnel in Ireland. *Veterinary Microbiology* **109(3-4)**, 285–296

Prescott JF, Hanna WJ, Reid-Smith R *et al.* (2002) Antimicrobial drug use and resistance in dogs. *Canadian Veterinary Journal* **43(2)**, 107–116

Pressel MA, Fox LE, Apley MD *et al.* (2005) Vancomycin for multi-drug resistant *Enterococcus faecium* cholangiohepatitis in a cat. *Journal of Feline Medicine and Surgery* **7(5)**, 317–321

Seol B, Naglic T, Madic J *et al.* (2002) In vitro antimicrobial susceptibility of 183 *Pseudomonas aeruginosa* strains isolated from dogs to selected antipseudomonal agents. *Journal of Veterinary Medicine. B, Infectious Diseases and Veterinary Public Health* **49(4)**, 188–192

Simjee S, White DG, McDermott PF *et al.* (2002) Characterization of Tn1546 in vancomycin-resistant *Enterococcus faecium* isolated from canine urinary tract infections: evidence of gene exchange between human and animal enterococci. *Journal of Clinical Microbiology* **40(12)**, 4659–4665

Takizawa T, Hashimoto K, Minami T *et al.* (1999) The comparative arthropathy of fluoroquinolones in dogs. *Human and Experimental Toxicology* **18(6)**, 392–399

Trepanier LA (2004) Idiosyncratic toxicity associated with potentiated sulfonamides in the dog. *Journal of Veterinary Pharmacology and Therapeutics* **27(3)**, 129–138

van Belkun A, van den Braak N, Thomassen R *et al.* (1996) Vancomycin-resistant enterococci in cats and dogs. *Lancet* **348(9033)**, 1038–1039

Weese JS (2005) Methicillin-resistant *Staphylococcus aureus:* an emerging pathogen in small animals. *Journal of the American Animal Hospital Association* **41(3)**, 150–157

Weese JS, Dick H, Willey BM *et al.* (2006) Suspected transmission of methicillin-resistant *Staphylococcus aureus* between domestic pets and humans in veterinary clinics and in the household. *Veterinary Microbiology* **115(1-3)**, 148–155

Wiebe V and Hamilton P (2002) Fluoroquinolone-induced retinal degeneration in cats. *Journal of the American Veterinary Medical Association* **221(11)**, 1568–1571

25

Imaging techniques for the critical patient

Frances Barr

Introduction

Imaging techniques should be used with care in critically ill patients, as manipulation and restraint of the patient may be a source of added stress, while existing injuries may inadvertently be exacerbated. It is therefore important to keep the number of procedures to a minimum by selecting the appropriate techniques for a given situation, and to carry out each examination carefully to minimize the need for repeat examinations. At all times, the patient should be handled gently, paying due regard to the existing clinical problem.

Plain radiography

Plain radiography is an invaluable imaging technique, which may be used to define the problem(s) in an individual patient and to monitor progress over a period of time. Detailed descriptions of radiographic positioning for different parts of the body are available elsewhere, but it may be useful to bear the following points in mind:

- If general anaesthesia is deemed inappropriate, then adequate positioning and restraint can usually be achieved using foam or plastic troughs, foam wedges and floppy sandbags. Manual restraint is only allowed under 'exceptional clinical circumstances' (Ionising Radiation Regulations, 1999) and is in fact rarely required
- In some clinical situations, it may be preferable to use a horizontal X-ray beam to obtain an orthogonal projection rather than repositioning the patient (e.g. in extreme dyspnoea, when lateral recumbency may not be tolerated; or in suspected spinal fracture/dislocation, when it is important to minimize patient manipulation). If a horizontal X-ray beam is used, due regard must be paid to radiation safety
- Ideally, select a fast film–screen combination so that exposure time may be kept to a minimum. This reduces the risk of movement blur impairing the sharpness of the image
- Examine the resulting images in a careful and systematic fashion, under appropriate viewing conditions, to minimize the risk of missing abnormalities. If manual processing is used, a final evaluation of the radiographs should not be made until they are dry.

Thorax

A minimum of two radiographic projections is required for complete evaluation of the thoracic cavity: dorsoventral and lateral. A dorsoventral projection is generally tolerated well by the patient and is usually preferred to a ventrodorsal projection in critical cases. Ventrodorsal positioning can lead to worsening of respiratory and cardiovascular function in unstable patients. A dorsoventral view may be the only projection taken before measures are instituted to stabilize the clinical condition of the patient. Substantial information can be obtained from this view alone regarding disease or injury of the thoracic wall, pleural space, heart or lungs.

A recumbent lateral projection may not be tolerated by an animal with dyspnoea, in which case an erect lateral projection can be achieved using a horizontal X-ray beam with the patient standing or in sternal recumbency. In some situations, it may be advisable to take radiographs with the animal in both right and left lateral recumbency. Small masses or areas of consolidation may be seen more clearly in the uppermost lung, where they are surrounded by air-filled alveoli, than in the lower lung, which tends to undergo partial collapse.

It is important to include the whole thoracic cavity on each radiograph, and the X-ray beam should be centred and collimated accordingly. The exposure should be made, wherever possible, at peak inspiration, so that the lungs are maximally aerated. Occasionally, an exposure may be made deliberately at end expiration to check that the lungs are able to deflate and there is no evidence of air trapping.

Abnormalities of the ribs, spine, sternum and soft tissues of the thoracic wall

It is important to check the soft tissues of the thoracic wall for swelling, emphysema or radio-opaque foreign material. The thoracic spine should be evaluated for evidence of fracture and/or dislocation and, if necessary, further radiographs should be taken centred on the thoracic spine. The sternum should also be assessed. It is important to bear in mind that congenital anomalies of the sternum are not uncommon in dogs and cats (e.g. pectus excavatum) and these must be differentiated from traumatic sternal disruption (Figure 25.1). Fractures of the ribs are not always easy to identify and a meticulous check should be made along the length of each rib on each radiograph. If several adjacent ribs have multiple fractures, it is wise to check the patient for evidence of 'flail chest'.

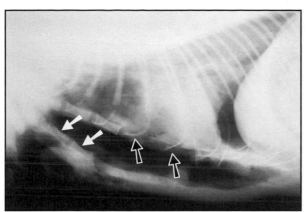

25.1 Lateral thoracic radiograph of a cat with dog bite injuries. Two sternal segments (white arrows) have been displaced ventrally and cranially, leaving a sternal defect (black arrows). There is extensive associated subcutaneous emphysema and a small pneumothorax.

Abnormalities of the diaphragm

Rupture of the diaphragm is most clearly demonstrated by the passage of abdominal viscera into the thoracic cavity. This results in an overall increase in radio-opacity in the thorax, and tubular structures containing gas or food/faecal material may be seen. There is often displacement of intrathoracic structures, together with a corresponding absence of some normal structures from the abdominal cavity (Figure 25.2). In some instances, the diagnosis is evident on plain radiography. In other cases, contrast radiography or ultrasonography may be needed to confirm the diagnosis. Barium can be administered orally and may highlight stomach or intestines within the thoracic cavity. Ultrasonography is particularly useful when a solid parenchymal organ such as the liver or spleen has moved into the thoracic cavity, or when free fluid is present. The outline of the diaphragm may become partially obscured by free thoracic fluid or adjacent intrathoracic masses.

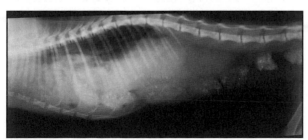

25.2 Lateral radiograph of the thorax and abdomen of a cat after a road traffic accident. Gas-filled small intestinal loops and part of the faeces-filled colon are visible in the ventral thorax, obscuring the cardiac outline and the ventral part of the diaphragmatic line. The radiographic diagnosis is traumatic rupture of the diaphragm.

Abnormalities of the pleural space

Pneumothorax: A small amount of free air in the thoracic cavity is most clearly seen on the recumbent or erect lateral radiograph. On the recumbent lateral projection, the heart apex appears raised from the sternum and, as the quantity of free air increases, the caudal lung lobes start to collapse and retract from

the thoracic spine and diaphragm. An erect lateral projection is particularly useful in unstable patients that will not tolerate lateral recumbency. On this view, the air accumulates in the dorsocaudal thorax, with retraction of the lung margins at this site (Figure 25.3). This projection may be useful in providing a semi-quantitative evaluation of the amount of free air. Collapse and retraction of the lung lobes are visible on the dorsoventral projection if moderate or large quantities of free air are present. If a tension pneumothorax is present, the ribs will be maximally spread and the diaphragm flattened. Intrathoracic structures may be displaced to one side if the problem is unilateral.

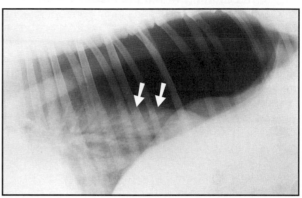

25.3 An erect lateral thoracic radiograph of a German Shepherd Dog with bilateral pneumothorax. Free air has accumulated in the dorsocaudal thorax and the edges of the retracted caudal lung lobes are visible (arrows).

It is important to recognize that collapsed or partially collapsed lung lobes will be of increased radio-opacity, even if they are otherwise normal. It is recommended that thoracic radiography is repeated, after drainage of free air and re-expansion of the lungs, to check for evidence of lung pathology (e.g. bullae, pulmonary haemorrhage).

Pleural fluid: A small amount of free fluid in the thoracic cavity is most clearly seen on the dorsoventral radiograph as a band of soft tissue separating the margins of the lung lobes from the thoracic wall and running between individual lung lobes (Figure 25.4).

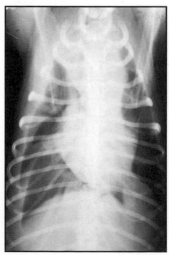

25.4
A dorsoventral thoracic radiograph of a dog with warfarin poisoning. A soft tissue opacity separates the lung lobes on the right from the thoracic wall. There is also marked widening of both the cranial and caudal mediastinum. The radiographic diagnosis is free pleural fluid on the right and mediastinal fluid, in this case blood.

On the recumbent lateral projection, fluid often lies in the ventral thorax, with partially retracted lung lobes apparently 'floating' on top. As the quantity of fluid increases, the caudal lung lobes become separated from the thoracic spine and diaphragm by fluid. Since most soft tissues and fluid have a similar radio-opacity, the presence of an intrathoracic mass may be masked by surrounding fluid. Ultrasonography is the imaging modality of choice in such instances as it will allow differentiation of fluid and soft tissue.

Abnormalities of the mediastinum and structures running within the mediastinum

Air may track within the mediastinum ('pneumomediastinum'; Figure 25.5), outlining the trachea, oesophagus, heart base and major vessels with abnormal clarity. This may be a consequence of dyspnoea or blunt thoracic trauma, but may also result from jugular venipuncture or penetrations of the pharynx, oesophagus or trachea.

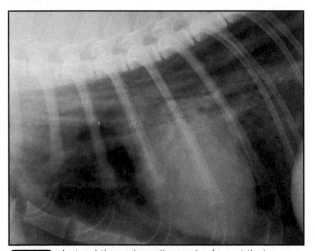

25.5 Lateral thoracic radiograph of a cat that was bitten by a dog. Air highlights structures running within the mediastinum, including blood vessels and the oesophagus. An overall streakiness is due to superimposition of subcutaneous emphysema.

Fluid within the mediastinum may result in radiographic widening of the mediastinum and 'reverse fissure' formation as fluid insinuates between the lobes of the lung at the hilus (Figure 25.4).

The lumen of the trachea should be carefully checked throughout its cervical and thoracic length. Foreign bodies are generally easily seen, as they are outlined by air. Localized narrowing of the lumen may be a consequence of a static lesion (e.g. a stricture, granuloma or neoplasm) or a dynamic lesion (e.g. tracheal collapse). Generalized narrowing of the lumen may be a result of tracheal hypoplasia, mucosal oedema or haemorrhage, or severe tracheal collapse. Tracheal penetrations result in extensive pneumomediastinum, subcutaneous emphysema and sometimes disruption of the visible tracheal outline. Intrathoracic tracheal rupture is typically associated with the formation of a thin-walled bullous structure in place of the normal tracheal walls (Figure 25.6).

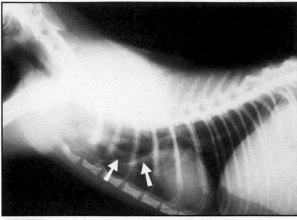

25.6 A lateral thoracic radiograph of a cat with inspiratory dyspnoea following a road traffic accident 11 days previously. No clear tracheal outline is visible between the lower cervical region and the 4th rib, and a thin-walled 'bullous' structure is apparent in this region (arrows). The radiographic diagnosis is tracheal rupture.

The oesophagus must also be carefully checked throughout its cervical and thoracic length. A little gas within the oesophagus is not unusual, especially in an animal with dyspnoea or under general anaesthesia, but large quantities of gas suggest either gas accumulation proximal to an oesophageal obstruction, or a motility disorder (e.g. megaoesophagus). Penetration of the oesophagus usually results in air and/or fluid within the mediastinum. Contrast studies may be required for a full evaluation of the oesophagus.

Abnormalities of the lungs

- Well defined soft tissue nodules or masses within the lung generally indicate primary or metastatic neoplasia, although granuloma or abscess formation may also be seen. Gas shadows within a mass can indicate cavitation, either within an abscess or necrotic tumour. Bullae or cysts usually contain air or air and fluid, and have thin, well defined walls.
- Flooding of the alveoli with blood, inflammatory or oedema fluid, or filling of the alveoli with neoplastic cells, result in areas of increased opacity within the lung. Small ill-defined areas which blur the normal pulmonary vascular pattern may coalesce to form large areas of opacity with air-filled bronchi running through them ('air bronchograms'; termed an 'alveolar' lung pattern) (Figure 25.7). The distribution of such changes may help narrow the list of differential diagnoses. For example, cardiogenic oedema in the dog often begins with a perihilar distribution, while aspiration pneumonia characteristically affects the ventral portions of the cranial and middle lobes.
- Collapse of a lung lobe may result in a similar radiographic appearance to alveolar filling. While lobar collapse (atelectasis) may be a consequence of disease processes, such as air or fluid in the pleural cavity or a space-occupying lesion, it may also be a consequence of

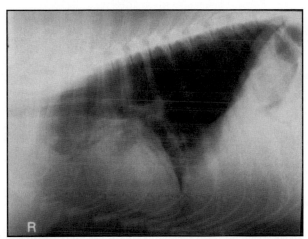

25.7 Right lateral thoracic radiograph of a young German Shepherd Dog with aspiration pneumonia. There is consolidation of the ventral parts of the cranial and middle lung lobes. Branching radiolucent tracts within the consolidated regions represent air bronchograms.

prolonged recumbency. If the increase in lung opacity is due to recumbency collapse, it is often associated with radiographic evidence of a loss of lung volume on that side (e.g. raising of the hemidiaphragm on that side and/or shifting of the heart to that side). This is important to remember when dealing with critically ill patients, which may spend much of their time recumbent.

- The walls of the major bronchi are usually visible radiographically as thin tapering radio-opaque lines and rings. The bronchial markings may become more prominent if the bronchial walls become thickened or calcified, or if there is peribronchial cellular infiltration. Some increase in bronchial markings is to be expected as the animal ages, but may also be associated with airway disease.

Abnormalities of the heart

The normal shape and size of the cardiac silhouette in the cat and dog are well established. In the dog, there is marked variation with breed and conformation. On a lateral radiograph, for example, a deep-chested dog normally has a narrow upright heart, while a barrel-chested dog normally has a rounded heart with marked sternal contact. There is far less variation among breeds of cat. Assessment of the shape and size of the cardiac silhouette should be made using lateral and dorsoventral radiographs, taking into account breed and conformation. Suboptimal positioning of the patient, and in particular rotation of the thorax on lateral and dorsoventral views, will change the appearance of the cardiac silhouette. Be wary, therefore, of interpreting changes in shape of the heart where there is rotation of the thorax.

- If the heart is smaller than normal, this may indicate hypovolaemia (e.g. blood loss, dehydration, Addison's disease).
- If the cardiac silhouette is larger than normal, this may indicate enlargement of one or more chambers of the heart. Changes in the shape of

the heart may help suggest which chambers or great vessels are involved. For example, an increase in the height of the heart on the lateral radiograph, with bulging of the dorsocaudal angle, indicates left chamber enlargement. An increase in the craniocaudal diameter of the heart is often seen with right chamber enlargement.
- A round, globular cardiac silhouette on both radiographic projections is often seen in association with pericardial fluid (Figure 25.8). Ultrasonography is the technique of choice for confirming the diagnosis and for searching for any underlying causes (Figure 25.9).

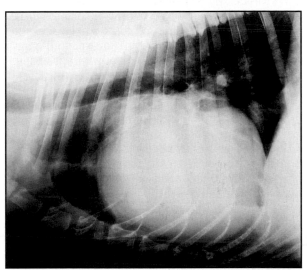

25.8 A lateral thoracic radiograph of a German Shepherd Dog with a pericardial effusion. The cardiac silhouette is generally enlarged, with an unusual globular shape.

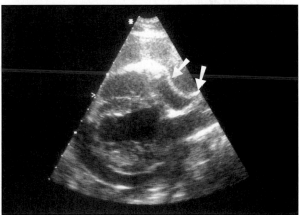

25.9 A long axis view taken during ultrasonographic examination of the heart of a Golden Retriever. The heart is seen contained within a sac of pericardial fluid. Note the collapse of the right atrial wall (arrows), indicating cardiac tamponade.

Abdomen

A minimum of two radiographic projections is necessary for complete evaluation of the abdominal cavity: ventrodorsal and lateral. A ventrodorsal projection is preferred to a dorsoventral projection, because the abdomen is stretched out and the hindlimbs are not superimposed on the area of interest. However, there may be situations (e.g. dyspnoea) where it is not desirable to turn the animal on to its back, in which case a dorsoventral projection of the abdomen may be used. In an unstable patient, it is often acceptable to take one radiograph of the abdomen (preferably in lateral recumbency) for an initial evaluation before taking measures to stabilize the clinical condition. If clinically appropriate, the animal should be starved for 12 hours prior to radiography and given the opportunity to defecate, so that food/faecal material does not obscure other structures in the abdomen.

It is important to include the whole abdominal cavity. In large-breed dogs, it may be necessary to take two separate radiographs centred on the cranial and caudal abdomen respectively. This may also be advisable in very narrow-waisted dogs when different exposures will be required for the thick cranial abdomen and the thin caudal abdomen. The exposure should ideally be made at the end of expiration, when abdominal thickness and respiratory movement are minimized. When the abdominal thickness exceeds 10 cm, the use of a grid will improve image quality by reducing the amount of scattered radiation reaching the film.

Abnormalities of the abdominal wall

The soft tissues of the abdominal wall should be checked for integrity, swelling, emphysema or radio-opaque foreign bodies. The lumbar spine should be assessed for evidence of trauma, bone proliferation or destruction. If necessary, further radiographs should be taken centred on this area.

Abnormalities of the abdominal cavity

- Detail in the abdominal cavity, allowing differentiation of the various soft tissue structures, is normally provided by fat. Consequently, poor abdominal detail may be seen in very young or very thin animals. However, the presence of free fluid in the abdominal cavity will also obscure detail; a small or moderate amount of fluid blurs fine detail, while larger quantities result in a homogeneous opacity throughout the abdomen, relieved only by gas/food/faecal material in the gastrointestinal tract.
- Peritonitis results in blurring of abdominal detail, either throughout the abdomen or in a localized area, due to the production of exudate (Figure 25.10). There may also be a mottled effect due to the formation of adhesions and pocketing of fluid. Intestinal loops in the area may be dilated and static due to paralytic ileus, corrugated due to irritation, or abnormally bunched due to adhesions.
- Free air in the abdominal cavity ('pneumoperitoneum'; Figure 25.11) may be seen as irregular accumulations of gas which cannot be localized within the bowel, sometimes accumulating between the liver and the diaphragm. If there is no penetrating wound of the abdominal wall, or recent laparotomy, a pneumoperitoneum is highly suggestive of perforation of the gastrointestinal tract.

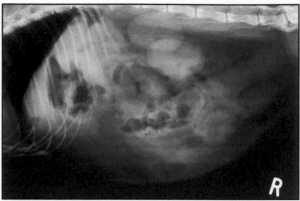

25.10 A lateral abdominal radiograph of a cat presented with vomiting and abdominal pain. There is a generalized loss of detail, which is particularly apparent in the mid-ventral abdomen. There are also small accumulations of free gas, especially evident craniodorsally. The diagnosis was peritonitis secondary to intestinal rupture.

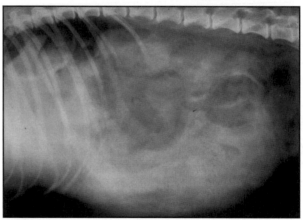

25.11 Lateral abdominal radiograph of a dog with a rupture of the gastrointestinal tract. There is a generalized lack of serosal detail consistent with peritonitis, and free air is visible in the dorsocranial abdomen.

Abnormalities of the gastrointestinal tract

- The stomach is a naturally distensible organ and so varies greatly in size. Excessive distension of the stomach may be an acute phenomenon (as part of the gastric dilatation–volvulus syndrome) or may be more chronic. Acute gastric distension is usually due to food or gas accumulation. When volvulus is present, transposition of the fundus and pylorus may be recognized, especially evident on the right lateral projection (see Figure 12.6), and soft tissue bands may be seen compartmentalizing the stomach. Chronic distension due to gastric outflow obstruction or motility disorders is usually associated with fluid and sometimes the collection of particulate 'gravel' in the pyloric region.
- The small intestine normally contains a mixture of gas and fluid. The diameter of small intestinal loops does not normally exceed the depth of a lumbar vertebral body. Undue fluid or gaseous distension of small intestinal loops may be seen in cases with generalized paralytic ileus (e.g. with infectious gastroenteritis, after a

laparotomy, due to hypokalaemia) or secondary to a mechanical obstruction. In cases of chronic partial intestinal obstruction, particulate material may accumulate proximal to the obstruction – a so-called 'gravel sign' (Figure 25.12). The cause of an obstructive process may be apparent on plain radiographs (e.g. radio-opaque foreign body), but in other cases contrast studies or ultrasonography may be required.

- The normal large intestine may contain gas or faecal material. If an enema has been given, or if the patient has diarrhoea, the contents may be fluid.
- Displacement of any part of the gastrointestinal tract may be useful evidence of other disease processes. For example, movement of sections of the gastrointestinal tract into the thoracic cavity or into the subcutaneous tissues indicates loss of integrity of the abdominal boundaries. A change in shape and size of the liver often results in gastric displacement. Any abdominal mass can push aside the small intestine. The descending colon may be displaced dorsally by an enlarged prostate and ventrally by enlarged sublumbar lymph nodes.
- The normal pancreas is not visible radiographically, but detection of a mass or evidence of a localized peritonitis in the right cranioventral abdomen should lead to the suspicion of pancreatic disease.

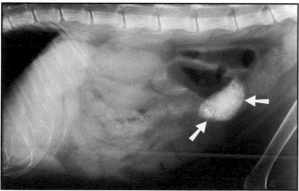

25.12 A lateral abdominal radiograph of a cat with a history of chronic vomiting. The radiograph shows a dense accumulation of mineral material (arrowed) superimposed on the faeces-filled colon. Dorsal to this are some distended gas-filled small intestinal loops. The diagnosis was a chronic partial obstruction of the distal small intestine, leading to 'gravel' accumulation.

Abnormalities of the liver and spleen

- Symmetrical hepatic enlargement results in extension of the ventral liver lobes well beyond the last rib, and often the tips of these lobes become rounded. The pyloric region of the stomach is pushed caudally and dorsally, resulting in an unusually horizontally positioned stomach. With focal asymmetrical enlargement, the normal triangular shape of the liver is lost.
- When the liver is unusually small, the ventral lobes lie well within the costal arch and lose their normal triangular shape. The stomach is

displaced cranially and becomes unusually upright. The spleen may also move cranially to lie within the costal arch. It should be remembered that the liver has a large functional reserve, and the radiographic detection of a small liver is not necessarily of clinical significance.

- The spleen is a very mobile organ, which is extraordinarily variable in both size and position. However, it is usually smooth in outline, with a triangular or elongated shape, and departures from this may be considered abnormal.

Abnormalities of the urogenital tract

- Renal enlargement may be smooth and symmetrical (e.g. hydronephrosis, amyloidosis) or irregular (e.g. renal neoplasia, polycystic disease). The accumulation of fluid between the kidney and its capsule may mimic renal enlargement. Reduction in renal size may be associated with renal dysplasia, hypoplasia or chronic parenchymal disease. Renal calculi may be recognized if they are radio-opaque. Further information about renal architecture and the ureters requires the use of contrast studies and/ or ultrasonography.
- The adrenal glands lie medial to the cranial pole of each kidney. In the dog, the presence of calcification or a mass in this region often indicates adrenal neoplasia. In the cat, adrenal calcification may be a normal finding.
- The bladder normally lies in the caudoventral abdomen, but is naturally very variable in size. Identification of a bladder shadow does not preclude a small tear in the bladder or urethra, and confirmation or exclusion of these possibilities requires the use of contrast studies (Figure 25.13). Radio-opaque calculi may be identified on plain radiographs, but for further information, proceed to contrast studies and/or ultrasonography.
- The prostate gland lies at the neck of the bladder in the male dog and cat. Enlargement of the prostate in the dog results in cranial displacement of the bladder and sometimes dorsal displacement of the rectum/descending colon. While a degree of enlargement is normal in entire dogs as they age, enlargement may also be associated with prostatic disease.
- The normal non-gravid uterus is not usually visible radiographically, except in very fat animals. Enlargement of the uterus may result in separation of the bladder from the descending colon by a soft tissue tubular structure and the identification of coiled, distended loops cranial to the bladder (Figure 25.14). Until fetal skeletal mineralization is detectable in the last trimester of pregnancy, it may be difficult to differentiate uterine enlargement due to pregnancy from that due to disease. Ultrasonography is helpful in this situation.

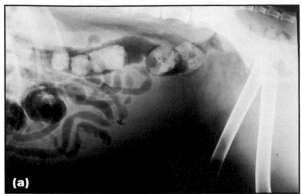

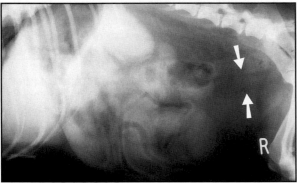

25.13 **(a)** Lateral abdominal radiograph of a cross-bred bitch with a traumatic bladder rupture. The plain radiograph shows a generalized loss of detail due to the presence of fluid in the abdominal cavity. **(b)** Water-soluble iodinated contrast medium has been introduced into the bladder and can be seen leaking into the peritoneal cavity (arrows).

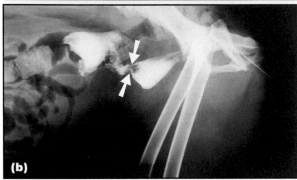

25.14 A lateral abdominal radiograph of a Jack Russell Terrier bitch with a closed pyometra. A distended, fluid-filled tubular viscus is visible in the mid-ventral abdomen. The uterine body and cervix lie between the bladder and descending colon (arrows).

Head

Accurate positioning of the patient is particularly important when undertaking radiography of the head and pharynx. Even slight rotation can result in confusion, since the anatomy of the area is relatively complex. It is, therefore, preferable to have the patient positioned under general anaesthesia. Occasionally, radiographs may be taken of a conscious patient, but it should be appreciated that positioning is likely to be suboptimal and all but gross lesions may be missed. This should therefore be reserved for initial evaluation of a critically injured and unstable patient. Once the patient has been stabilized, a complete radiographic examination under general anaesthesia should be considered.

Several specialized projections are described for different regions of the skull, such as the frontal sinuses, temporomandibular joints and tympanic bullae. It is necessary to plan the examination carefully so that all areas under suspicion, based on the clinical examination or standard radiographic projections, are fully evaluated. Non-screen film or film within flexible cassettes can be useful for intra-oral radiography of the maxilla/nasal chambers, the mandible and individual teeth.

- Check the soft tissues of the head for swelling, emphysema and radio-opaque foreign material.
- Evaluate the bony contours of the skull for disruption (usually traumatic), or bone destruction or proliferation (usually associated with neoplasia or infection).
- Check that the oro- and nasopharynx, the larynx and the cervical trachea are air filled and of a normal calibre.

Magnetic resonance imaging (MRI) or computed tomography (CT) may be indicated once the patient has been stabilized, in order to evaluate intracranial structures.

Spine

As with the head, accurate positioning of the spine is vital if the maximum amount of diagnostic information is to be gleaned from the radiographs. Therefore, general anaesthesia is usually required. If fracture/dislocation of the spine is suspected, survey radiographs may be taken with the animal conscious for a preliminary assessment of the site of the lesion and degree of damage. The patient may be kept in one position (lateral or sternal recumbency) and orthogonal views obtained by use of a horizontal and vertical X-ray beam.

The principles behind accurate positioning of the spine for radiography are:

- To keep the spine parallel to the cassette. This may involve padding areas that naturally sag (typically the neck and the lumbar region)
- To avoid any axial rotation
- To avoid bending of the spine to one side and undue flexion or extension. Specific stressed projections in hyperflexion or hyperextension may be used after the standard projections have been assessed, depending on the precise problem suspected.

A minimum of two projections is required for complete evaluation of the spine: lateral and ventrodorsal or dorsoventral. It is important to include only a small section of the spinal column on each radiograph, with accurate centring and collimation. This is because divergence of the X-ray beam towards the periphery of the X-ray film results in a slightly oblique projection of the vertebrae and intervertebral disc spaces, which is not ideal for interpretation. When patient positioning is suboptimal, there is likely to be rotation of the spine. Take care in such cases not to misinterpret asymmetrical positioning of transverse processes or articular facets as evidence of injury.

The radiographs should be checked for:

- The number and alignment of the vertebrae. Remember that a minor malalignment does not necessarily reflect minor spinal cord damage, as the displacement at the time of the injury may have been far greater (Figure 25.15)
- The shape of the vertebrae. Some changes in shape may be due to developmental anomalies (such as block vertebrae, hemivertebrae) while others may be associated with disease processes (e.g. compression fractures)
- Fractures of the vertebrae, including the dorsal spinous and transverse processes and the articular facets as well as the vertebral bodies
- Bone proliferation (e.g. associated with trauma, infection, neoplasia, nutritional disorders) or bone destruction (e.g. infection, neoplasia)
- Evidence of intervertebral disc disease (i.e. narrowing of the intervertebral disc space and/or intervertebral foramen; calcification of disc material with or without displacement).

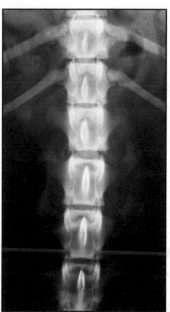

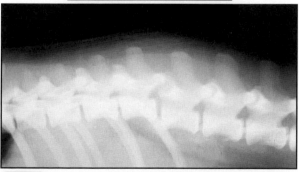

25.15 Radiographs of the thoracolumbar spine of a dog with a traumatic vertebral luxation. The ventrodorsal projection shows slight asymmetrical widening of the intervertebral disc space between L1 and L2 and slight malalignment of the dorsal spinous processes of L1 and L2. On the lateral projection, a subluxation is clearly visible, with widening of the facet joint and a step between the vertebral bodies at this site.

It may be necessary to proceed to contrast studies after studying the plain radiographs, in order to demonstrate the site and severity of any spinal cord compression. MRI or CT may be preferred to contrast studies where these modalities are available.

Contrast radiography

Contrast radiography is indicated in the following situations:

- When plain radiographs do not demonstrate a lesion, but the clinical examination and other diagnostic tests suggest that a lesion is present
- When plain radiographs do show a lesion, but further information is required in order to allow rational treatment to be instituted and an informed prognosis given.

It is important that a good plain radiographic examination precedes the contrast study. This ensures that the appropriate exposure factors are used for the contrast examination, confirms that the contrast technique is indeed necessary and appropriate, and that no lesions are visible on the plain radiographs which may subsequently be masked by contrast medium. Make sure that everything you may require is ready at the beginning of the procedure and that the examination is carried out carefully and thoroughly.

Detailed descriptions of recommended protocols for contrast examinations may be found in standard texts and may differ from the procedures given here, as a result of personal preference. It is very important to note the additional factors listed below.

Oesophageal contrast studies

- General anaesthesia is contraindicated because of the risk of regurgitation and inhalation. Drug-induced decreases in oesophageal motility will also preclude assessment of oesophageal function. In addition, the normal oesophagus may appear dilated during general anaesthesia.
- Oesophageal contrast studies are usually contraindicated in very dyspnoeic or collapsed patients because of the risk of aspiration.
- Some authorities argue that a water-soluble iodinated contrast medium should be used in preference to barium if an oesophageal perforation is suspected, as barium is inert and will persist in the thoracic cavity. If water-soluble iodinated contrast media are chosen, it should be remembered that they tend to be very bitter (so may not be accepted as readily as barium) and are also hypertonic (so that inadvertent inhalation may lead to pulmonary oedema).
- Liquid contrast medium is useful for outlining abnormalities of the oesophageal wall (e.g. ulceration, neoplasia, diverticula), intraluminal masses or foreign bodies, or for demonstrating a perforation.
- It may be useful to use contrast medium mixed with food to show a partial oesophageal obstruction or to fill a dilated oesophagus completely.

A procedure for oesophageal contrast studies is shown in Figure 25.16.

1. The patient should be conscious, not under general anaesthesia.
2. Administer orally 5–40 ml liquid barium sulphate, depending on the size of the patient and the site and nature of the lesion suspected. Alternatively, barium may be mixed with food and the animal allowed to eat this naturally. This technique may be used to demonstrate a partial oesophageal obstruction or to fill a distended oesophagus completely.
3. Take lateral radiographs of the neck and thorax 2–3 minutes after administration. A ventrodorsal or dorsoventral view is occasionally helpful. If contrast medium is retained, further radiographs may be useful to show its subsequent progress.

25.16 Procedure for oesophageal contrast studies.

Gastrointestinal contrast studies

These have now largely been superceded by ultra-sonography and endoscopy. However, they may still be useful for regions of the small intestine not accessible to endoscopy, and where ultrasonographic examination is inconclusive.

- Preparation of the patient is important in order to ensure that the stomach is empty and the colon contains minimal faecal material. Food and faeces will result in filling defects in the contrast column or pool, and thus mimic foreign bodies or masses.
- General anaesthesia should not be used, as it interferes with gastrointestinal motility and increases the risk of contrast inhalation.
- Water-soluble iodinated contrast media may be used in cases of suspected perforation. Arguments for and against their use are outlined in the section on oesophageal contrast studies. The hyperosmolarity of the iodinated contrast media tends to draw fluid into the lumen of the gastrointestinal tract, resulting in progressive dilution of the contrast and exacerbation of any existing dehydration.
- It is possible to evaluate the large intestine by following the barium through from the stomach. If a large intestinal lesion is specifically suspected, it may be quicker and more efficient to perform a barium enema instead, although endoscopy is usually the technique of choice in such situations.
- Normally, contrast begins to leave the stomach within 30 minutes but may be delayed up to 1 hour in nervous animals. Emptying of the stomach is usually complete within 4–6 hours. A delay in gastric emptying may occur in the presence of systemic illness (e.g. renal failure, peritonitis), with the administration of certain drugs (e.g. opioids) or due to gastric outflow obstruction. In most animals, the time between onset of gastric emptying and appearance of barium in the large intestine is between 30 minutes and 1 hour, although this is very variable. Delayed transit may result from systemic illness, or from paralytic or obstructive ileus.

- Check the contrast pool or column for persistent filling defects, which may represent foreign material or masses projecting into the lumen (Figure 25.17). Since an apparent defect may be caused by a peristaltic or segmental contraction, it is important to be able to demonstrate that an abnormality is consistently found on successive radiographs.
- Evaluate the walls of the gastrointestinal tract for persistent areas of thickening or irregularity.
- Check for evidence of perforation and consequent barium leakage.

A procedure for upper gastrointestinal contrast studies is given in Figure 25.18.

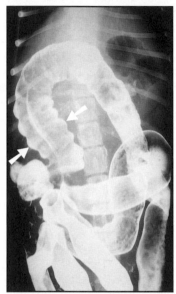

25.17 A ventrodorsal radiograph of the abdomen of a Golden Retriever taken 2 hours after oral administration of liquid barium. Distended small intestinal loops are visible in the caudal abdomen. In the right cranial abdomen, a corrugated section of intestine (arrows) with a streak of barium running centrally represents an ileocolic intussusception.

1. Starve the patient overnight, but allow access to water. Administer an enema or allow the animal an opportunity to evacuate the bowel naturally before beginning the procedure.
2. The patient should be conscious or sedated.
3. Administer 1–2 ml/kg liquid barium sulphate (the higher dose rate for smaller animals) either orally or by stomach tube.
4. Take a lateral projection immediately, centred on the cranial abdomen, followed by a ventrodorsal view of the same area.
5. If a gastric lesion is suspected, additional films should be taken at approximately 15 and 30 minutes. If anything suspicious is seen (e.g. a filling defect or an area of irregularity), the same view should be repeated as soon as possible to confirm or rule out the suspected problem. It can be useful in some cases to take four views of the stomach (right lateral recumbency, left lateral recumbency, ventrodorsal and dorsoventral) as the barium and any gas in the stomach will occupy different parts of the stomach in each view.
6. For the small intestine, radiographs should be taken at 30 minutes and thereafter at hourly intervals until a lesion is seen or passage of barium into the colon has been demonstrated and the stomach is empty.

25.18 Upper gastrointestinal contrast study.

Upper urinary tract contrast studies

- These studies are best carried out under general anaesthesia unless this is clinically contraindicated, as the intravenous administration of the contrast material may result in nausea or vomiting.
- A ventrodorsal projection of the abdomen immediately after injection of the contrast agent should show opacification of the renal parenchyma. A complete lack of opacification on this and subsequent radiographs may reflect disruption of the renal blood supply or a non-functional kidney. If the kidneys are opacified, then their size, shape and position should be evaluated.
- After about 5 minutes, excretion of the contrast agent should be apparent, with contrast visible in the renal pelvis and ureter on each side. 'Renal shut down' is a recognized but uncommon idiosyncratic reaction to the contrast medium, resulting in initial renal opacification but no visible excretion. Excretion usually begins a short while after administration of intravenous fluids and diuretics, and the animal should be treated for acute renal failure (see Chapter 8). Other reasons for delayed visualization of the renal pelvis include pelvic/ureteral dilation or obstruction, or severely impaired renal function (Figure 25.19).

- Once excretion of the contrast agent is apparent, any distension of, or filling defects within, the ureters can be seen. Loss of integrity of a ureter with consequent spillage of contrast medium into the retroperitoneal space may be seen. Occasionally, the ureters may be seen to be intact but displaced by a mass or haemorrhage within the retroperitoneal space.

A procedure for intravenous urography is given in Figure 25.20.

1. Except in an emergency, starve the patient overnight but allow access to water. Administer an enema and wait for evacuation of the bowels before premedication.
2. Use general anaesthesia unless clinically contraindicated.
3. If the distal ureters are to be examined, catheterize the bladder to empty it of urine and introduce air before administering the contrast medium.
4. Use water-soluble iodinated contrast medium with a high iodine concentration (ideally 300–450 mg/ml). Administer 1 ml/kg contrast medium rapidly intravenously, as a bolus.
5. For optimum delineation of the kidneys take a ventrodorsal view of the abdomen centred over the kidneys immediately after injection of the contrast medium. A ventrodorsal view 5 minutes later will show opacification of the renal pelvis and ureter on each side.
6. Further films centred on the areas of interest are taken as and when required, depending on the indications for the examination. Excretion normally continues for at least 1 hour, and bladder filling may be seen 10–15 minutes after the intravenous injection. If renal function is grossly impaired, opacification of the renal pelvis and ureter may not occur or may be delayed for several hours. For examination of the distal ureters and the vesico-ureteric junction, oblique views of the pelvic area may be helpful in addition to the standard lateral and ventrodorsal views.

25.20 Intravenous urography.

Lower urinary tract contrast studies

- It is preferable to ensure that the colon and rectum are empty before beginning lower urinary tract contrast procedures, as faecal material may compress and obscure the bladder and prostate. If possible, catheterize and empty the bladder once plain radiographs have been taken.
- A positive-contrast urethrogram (in the male) or vaginourethrogram (in the female) should allow evaluation of virtually the entire length of the urethra (Figure 25.21). Check for any irregularity of the urethral wall (e.g. due to neoplasia, inflammation or stricture formation), filling defects within the contrast column (e.g. due to calculi, blood clots, or masses), or leakage of contrast into the surrounding soft tissues (Figure 25.22). In the male dog, the path of the urethra through the prostate should be assessed, as an asymmetrical path is suggestive of focal prostatic disease (e.g. neoplasia, abscessation, cysts).

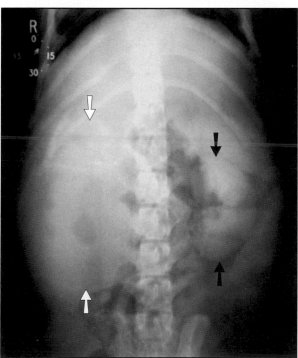

25.19 Ventrodorsal abdominal radiograph of a young Rottweiler taken 5 minutes after intravenous injection of a bolus of water-soluble iodinated contrast medium. The left kidney has opacified (black arrows) and contrast medium is visible in the left renal pelvis and ureter. There is a large soft tissue mass in the region of the right kidney (white arrows), but no excretion of contrast is apparent. The final diagnosis was an enlarged and non-functional right kidney due to a renal abscess.

- Cystography allows evaluation of the bladder wall and lumen. If bladder rupture is suspected, positive-contrast cystography is the preferred technique (Figure 25.23). Otherwise, double-contrast cystography allows accurate assessment of the wall for thickening and irregularity and of free structures within the lumen, such as calculi or blood clots.

Patient preparation

Encourage normal evacuation of the bowel or administer an enema. General anaesthesia is generally required except in very sick or placid animals. It is not necessary to catheterize and empty the bladder unless intending to proceed to cystography.

Urethrography

1. For a male dog, take a small balloon catheter and prefill the catheter with water-soluble iodinated contrast medium. Introduce the catheter into the distal penile urethra and gently inflate the balloon to hold it in place

2. Position the dog in lateral recumbency with both hindlegs drawn well forward

3. Inject 5–20 ml of contrast medium via the catheter. Ensure radiation safety by wearing appropriate protective clothing and standing as far as possible from the primary X-ray beam

4. Towards the end of the injection of contrast, take a lateral radiograph of the patient, including the caudal abdomen, pelvis and perineum

5. The technique in the male cat is similar, but it is not possible to use a balloon catheter. Instead introduce a plain catheter a couple of millimetres into the urethra and hold in place with a clamp across the prepuce. A volume of 2–3 ml of contrast medium is usually ample

6. In males and females, dogs and cats, an alternative approach is to introduce the catheter just as far as the bladder. Estimate the approximate expected length of the urethra. Begin injecting contrast medium and, at the same time, steadily withdraw the catheter. Make the X-ray exposure when you judge that the catheter has been withdrawn sufficiently so that the tip of the catheter lies just in the distal urethra

Vaginourethrography

1. For a bitch, prefill a balloon catheter with water-soluble iodinated contrast medium

2. Place the tip of the balloon catheter inside the vulva and inflate the balloon. Place tissue forceps to hold the vulva closed dorsal and ventral to the catheter, then gently pull the catheter back until the inflated balloon lies just inside the vulva

3. Inject contrast at a dose rate of approximately 1 ml/kg body weight. Ensure radiation safety by wearing appropriate protective clothing and standing as far as possible from the primary X-ray beam

4. Towards the end of the injection, take a lateral radiograph of the patient, including the caudal abdomen and pelvis

5. The technique is similar in the cat, except that it is necessary to use a plain catheter rather than a balloon type, held in place with a clamp across the vulva

6. The contrast will usually fill the vagina first and then the urethra. Therefore incomplete filling of the urethra may indicate an inadequate volume of contrast, leakage of contrast back around the catheter, or an animal at or around the time of oestrus

25.21 Retrograde urethrography and vaginourethrography.

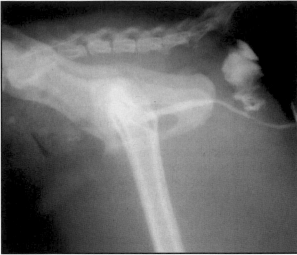

25.22 Lateral radiograph of the pelvic region of a cat during retrograde urethrography. Contrast is spilling into the soft tissues dorsal to the urethra due to rupture of the penile urethra. If the catheter had been introduced further into the urethra, the rupture might well have been missed.

1. Encourage normal evacuation of the bowel or administer an enema.
2. General anaesthesia is usually required except in very sick or placid animals.
3. Catheterize and empty the bladder.
4. (a) Positive-contrast cystography: Inject 10–50 ml water-soluble iodinated contrast medium through the urinary catheter – a high level of iodine is not essential for this technique. Withdraw the catheter.
   (b) Double-contrast cystography: Following a positive-contrast cystogram, aspirate as much of the contrast medium as possible. Roll the patient over so the residual contrast medium is spread over the bladder mucosa. Inject 30–200 ml of air according to the size of the animal. Inject the air until moderate resistance to injection is felt, or until distension of the bladder is felt on palpation of the caudal abdomen. Withdraw the catheter.
5. Take a lateral radiograph of the caudal abdomen as soon as possible after introduction of the contrast medium. Ventrodorsal and oblique views may be useful on occasion.

25.23 Cystography.

Spinal contrast studies

If available, MRI/CT may be preferred to spinal contrast studies.

- General anaesthesia is mandatory for such procedures.
- It is important that only non-ionic water-soluble iodinated contrast media are used. The ionic forms are too irritant for use around the spinal cord.
- Plan the procedure carefully before beginning, deciding on the preferred site of puncture and the required dose of contrast medium. These decisions will be influenced not only by the site of the suspected lesion, but the probable stability (or otherwise) of the vertebrae in the region.
- Once the contrast has been injected, follow its path from the site of injection to the region of interest, looking carefully for deviation or thinning of the contrast columns, which may

allow localization of any spinal cord compression and differentiation between extradural, intramedullary and extramedullary/intradural lesions (Figure 25.24). Once a lesion has been identified, it is important to take radiographs in at least two planes (usually lateral and ventrodorsal).

A procedure for spinal contrast studies is given in Figure 25.25.

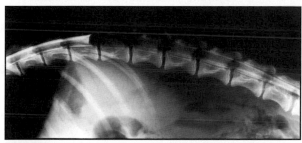

25.24 A lateral radiograph of the thoracolumbar spine of a young Springer Spaniel taken during cisternal myelography. The dorsal contrast column flares and stops abruptly at the caudal end of T13, outlining the cranial end of an extramedullary/intradural mass.

1. General anaesthesia is essential.
2. A water-soluble non-ionic iodinated contrast medium should be selected and warmed to approximately body temperature.
3. Dosage of the contrast medium will depend on both the size of the animal and the level of the suspected lesion. A dose rate of 0.3 ml/kg up to a maximum of 10 ml has been suggested, but this should be reduced if the suspected lesion is close to the site of injection.
4. (a) Cisternal puncture: Place the animal in lateral recumbency. Clip the site of puncture and prepare aseptically. With the head flexed and held steadily by an assistant, palpate the occipital crest and the two wings of the atlas. Place a sterile spinal needle, with the bevel facing caudally, perpendicular to the skin on the midline in the centre of the triangle formed by these landmarks (see Figure 9.3). Advance the needle slowly until a 'pop' is felt as the needle enters the cisterna magna. Withdraw the stylet and wait for the flow of CSF, which indicates correct needle placement. If the tap is bloody, then withdraw the needle and repeat the procedure with a clean needle.
   (b) Lumbar puncture: The animal may be placed in either lateral or ventral recumbency, and the site of puncture clipped and prepared aseptically. Palpate the dorsal spinous processes of the caudal lumbar vertebrae. Introduce a spinal needle in the midline, just in front of the dorsal spinous process of L6. Slowly advance the needle until it impinges on bone, then slowly 'walk' the tip of the needle forwards along the bone until it passes through the intervertebral space. The needle passes for a short distance, coming to a stop on the floor of the spinal canal. Often a twitch of the hindlimbs or tail is noted as the needle passes through the cauda equina. CSF is not invariably obtained, even if the needle is correctly located, so a test injection of contrast medium may be required to check the position of the needle tip.
5. Inject the required dose of contrast medium slowly, then withdraw the needle.
6. Following contrast medium injection, lateral radiographs are taken, starting at the site of the injection, and working progressively down (in the case of cisternal injection) or up (in the case of lumbar injection) the spinal column to follow the flow of contrast medium. If it fails to flow, then it may help to tilt the animal head up (if the contrast medium was given cisternally), or to apply traction to the spinal column. If a lesion is found, then a ventrodorsal view of the region should also be taken.

25.25 Myelography.

Ultrasonography

Diagnostic ultrasonography is an imaging technique that is a very useful complement to radiography. Ultrasonography is a safe non-invasive technique which produces cross-sectional images of the soft tissues of the body. Information regarding the internal architecture of organs may therefore be obtained. In addition, these images are continuously updated, so that movement of structures may be seen. Consequently, ultrasound examination is an extremely valuable imaging tool in critical patients. Furthermore, the patient can usually be allowed to adopt a comfortable position with minimal restraint during ultrasonographic examination. This is particularly helpful in critically ill and injured animals which may be in an unstable or fragile state.

Ultrasonography does, however, have limitations. The ultrasound beam is effectively blocked by bone or gas, so that the information gleaned from imaging skeletal structures, or gas-filled organs such as the lung or, on occasions, the gastrointestinal tract, is often minimal.

It may be useful to bear in mind the following principles when planning an ultrasonographic examination:

- Select the scanning site carefully by choosing an area of the body surface overlying the organ or tissue of interest, but avoiding intervening bone or gas
- Clip hair from the skin of the scanning site, clean the skin carefully and apply liberal quantities of acoustic gel to ensure good acoustic contact
- When a choice is available, select as high a frequency of sound as you can while still achieving an adequate depth of tissue penetration. In general, high-frequency sound (e.g. 7.5 MHz) will not penetrate as deeply, but will provide better image resolution than lower-frequency sound (e.g. 5 MHz)
- Once an image is obtained, optimize the detail by adjustment of gain controls, such that there is an even brightness throughout the depth of the image. Too dark an image will result in loss of visible detail, whereas too bright an image may obscure detail with background 'noise'
- Ensure that a thorough ultrasonographic examination is carried out, sweeping the sound beam through the entire area of interest, in at least two planes of section
- Colour-flow and spectral Doppler techniques may be useful in some cases in order to define blood flow (in terms of direction, nature and velocity) within the cardiac chambers and great vessels.

Thorax

The most common reason for ultrasonographic examination of the thoracic cavity is to evaluate the heart. While radiography enables an assessment of the shape and size of the cardiac silhouette only, ultrasonography will allow visualization of the separate chambers, great vessels and valves. For a full description of the recommended protocol for ultrasonographic examination of the heart and the abnormalities which may be found, see References and further reading. However, the following points may be helpful in assessing the critical patient:

- Pericardial fluid appears as an echolucent (black) band around the heart. It is important to evaluate the regions of the heart base and the right atrium carefully for evidence of hypoechoic (grey) masses, which when present are usually neoplastic and the underlying cause of the effusion. Collapse of the right atrial wall during systole is evidence of cardiac tamponade (see Figure 25.9) and is an indication for immediate drainage of the pericardial fluid
- The thickness of the myocardium should be assessed. The myocardium may be thickened as a physiological response to a cardiovascular abnormality (e.g. right ventricular hypertrophy in response to pulmonic stenosis) or as part of the primary disease process (e.g. hypertrophic cardiomyopathy)
- Chamber size should be evaluated. Ventricular dilation may be seen as a consequence of volume overload (e.g. a left-to-right shunting ventricular septal defect will result in pulmonary overcirculation and dilation of the left atrium and ventricle). Atrial dilation may occur in response to pressure or volume overload (e.g. reduced ventricular compliance as in hypertrophic or restrictive cardiomyopathy; atrioventricular valve insufficiency). A right parasternal short axis view of the base of the heart shows the left atrium adjacent to the aorta. An evaluation of the ratio of the diameters of the left atrium and aorta (normally around 1:1) gives a useful indication of atrial dilation (Figure 25.26). A left atrium to aortic ratio of greater than 1.5:1 is considered abnormal
- The leaflets of each of the major valves should be assessed. Thickening and irregularity of valve leaflets may be seen in congenital (valvular dysplasia) or acquired disease (endocardiosis, endocarditis). An abnormal motion may also sometimes be seen (e.g. rupture of chordae tendinae)
- Myocardial contractility may also be evaluated. It is useful to view overall myocardial movement on both long and short axis sections, in order to detect regions of myocardium with abnormal or reduced movements. M mode measurements may then be made in an attempt to quantify contractility – a number of different measurements may be made, but the potential limitations of each should be appreciated. For a full discussion of this complex area, see References and further reading. Myocardial activity may be reduced (e.g. due to myocardial disease) or increased (e.g. in association with atrioventricular valve incompetence).

The remaining structures in the thoracic cavity are not usually visualized in the normal animal, as they are obscured by air-filled lung. Thoracic ultrasonography is, however, an extremely useful way to confirm the presence of pleural effusion prior to thoracocentesis in dyspnoeic patients when radiography is considered too high a risk. Also, the presence of free thoracic fluid will act as an acoustic window, outlining and separating thoracic structures. If sufficient fluid is present, the great vessels may be followed in the mediastinum, partially collapsed lung lobes can be recognized and any solid masses lying within the fluid identified. The fluid itself usually appears echolucent (black), although the presence of particulate matter, gas bubbles or a highly cellular content may result in echoes swirling within the fluid.

Abdomen

The presence of free abdominal fluid, as in the thoracic cavity, enhances ultrasonographic visualization by outlining and separating structures. If only a small amount of free fluid is present, it will tend to accumulate in dependent parts of the abdomen and is most easily visualized between liver lobes or around the cranial pole of the bladder (Figure 25.27).

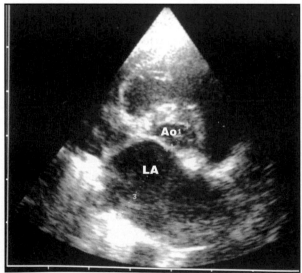

25.26 Right parasternal short axis view of the heart of a cat with marked dilation of the left atrium associated with cardiomyopathy. The left atrium (LA) to aortic (Ao) ratio is approximately 3:1.

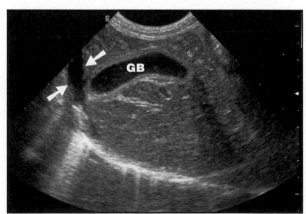

25.27 Sagittal image of the cranial abdomen of a dog showing a small volume of free abdominal fluid (arrows) lying between the liver and the diaphragm (GB, gall bladder).

Liver and spleen

It is preferable to fast the patient for 12 hours before imaging the liver, as a food-filled stomach will obscure part of the liver. It is acceptable to allow the patient to drink, as fluid within the stomach does not impair image quality and indeed may act as a useful landmark.

Evaluation of the hepatic and splenic parenchyma may reveal irregularity of the surface of the organ, and focal or diffuse disturbances of the parenchymal architecture (Figure 25.28). Such changes are usually indicative of disease, but are non-specific. For example, circumscribed nodules in the hepatic or splenic parenchyma may be neoplasia, hyperplasia, abscesses, infarcts, haematomas or granulomas. Equally, a normal ultrasonographic appearance does not preclude disease. Therefore, a fine needle aspirate or tissue core biopsy may be required for a definitive diagnosis.

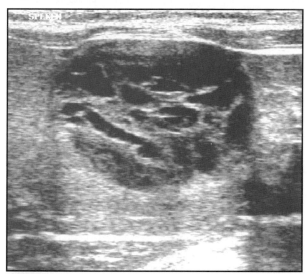

25.28 Ultrasonographic image of the spleen of a Labrador Retriever presented with pericardial effusion. A focal, loculated lesion bulges slightly from the surface of the spleen. The final diagnosis was haemangiosarcoma involving the right atrium and spleen.

The vascular supply can also be assessed. In the spleen, major vessels are only visible in the hilar region. In the liver, the caudal vena cava and portal veins can be identified, as well as their intrahepatic branches and tributaries. Thus venous congestion can be recognized, as well as intraluminal thrombi or neoplastic invasion. Vascular anomalies, such as portosystemic shunts and arteriovenous fistulation, may also be recognized by the presence of single or multiple tortuous anomalous vessels.

Within the liver, the gall bladder is readily seen, but the intrahepatic bile ducts are not usually visible. Distension of the common bile duct and subsequently the intrahepatic bile ducts can be detected in cases of obstructive jaundice.

The kidneys and adrenal glands

Ultrasonography provides a clear demonstration of the renal cortex, medulla and pelvis. Blurring or distortion of the normal architectural pattern indicates renal parenchymal disease but, once again, many of the changes seen are non-specific. In the critical patient, ultrasonography may be useful in differentiating between renal failure due to an acute renal insult or prerenal causes, when the kidney often appears ultrasonographically normal, and renal failure due to established underlying renal disease, when ultrasonographic changes can often be seen (Figure 25.29).

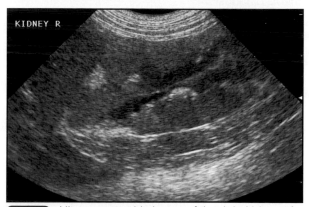

25.29 Ultrasonographic image of the right kidney of a 9-year-old Lhasa Apso, showing hyperechoic wedge-shaped cortical lesions consistent with infarction.

Dilation of the renal pelvis (e.g. due to ureteral obstruction, or ascending urinary tract infection) is readily detected. Dilation of the proximal ureter as it leaves the kidney and of the distal ureter as it approaches the bladder may be detected, but the middle section is often difficult to distinguish.

The adrenal glands may be identified medial to the cranial pole of each kidney in close apposition to the aorta (left adrenal) or caudal vena cava (right adrenal), providing the patient is not too obese. The adrenal glands are normally hypoechoic elongated structures. Enlargement of the gland, with loss of the normal elongated shape and even echotexture, may be seen with either adrenal hyperplasia or neoplasia. Remember to check the adjacent great vessels for evidence of invasion or thrombus formation if an adrenal mass is found.

The bladder and prostate

Ultrasonographic examination of the bladder allows careful evaluation of the wall for regions of thickening or irregularity or for discrete masses projecting into the lumen. It may be helpful in treatment planning to determine the precise location of any mass relative to the bladder neck and the points of entry of the ureters, as well as the size of the mass. It is difficult to differentiate between a polypoid or neoplastic mass and a blood clot adherent to the bladder wall. Sequential examinations over a period of time may be required to clarify the situation. Calculi, irrespective of their mineral composition, are seen as echogenic structures lying in the dependent part of the bladder. Hypoechoic masses floating freely within the lumen of the bladder are likely to be blood clots.

The prostate gland is located caudal to the bladder and may be predominantly intra-abdominal or intrapelvic in location. It should be smooth in outline, with an evenly granular hypoechoic appearance. Small fluid foci measuring <1 cm in diameter are considered normal findings. Larger fluid foci may represent intraprostatic cysts, haematocysts, abscesses or tumours with necrotic centres. Disturbance of the normal parenchymal architecture may occur as a result of either inflammatory or neoplastic disease. Therefore, fine needle aspiration of fluid foci and tissue core biopsy of disturbed parenchyma may be necessary for a definitive diagnosis.

The uterus

Ultrasonography is the imaging modality of choice for differentiation between uterine enlargement due to pregnancy and that due to disease. From 3–4 weeks of gestation onwards, fetal structures may be clearly recognized within the uterus, and fetal viability assessed in terms of generalized fetal movements and fetal cardiac activity. Cessation of fetal movements and subsequent loss of fetal structure is indicative of fetal death. In the absence of fetal structures, accumulation of fluid within the uterus is abnormal and usually indicates pyometritis.

The gastrointestinal tract and pancreas

The gastrointestinal tract is amenable to ultrasonographic examination provided it does not contain excessive gas. If a high-frequency transducer is used to obtain images of optimal quality, then a distinct layered appearance of the wall of the stomach and small intestine is seen. The alternating hyperechoic and hypoechoic layers correspond exactly to the histological layers of mucosa, submucosa, muscularis and serosa. The lumen may be collapsed, with a central hyperechoic streak representing residual mucus and ingesta, or may be fluid filled. In the normal animal, peristaltic and segmental contractions can be seen.

Gross thickening of the wall may be detected, either with retention of the normal layered structure (usually hypertrophy or inflammation) or loss of normal architecture (severe inflammation or neoplasia). If abnormal fluid distension of the stomach or small intestinal loops is seen, it is useful to determine whether peristaltic and segmental contractions remain, or whether they are reduced or absent. If fluid is present within the gastrointestinal lumen, then foreign material or intraluminal masses may become evident.

The pancreas is difficult to image ultrasonographically, partly because of its awkward location and partly because of its poorly defined margins. It lies in the right cranial quadrant of the abdomen, with the right limb closely apposed to the descending loop of the duodenum. In acute pancreatitis, the pancreas becomes enlarged, often with hypoechoic regions representing necrosis and haemorrhage. The adjacent duodenum may be dilated and static, with a thickened wall. Free abdominal fluid and increased echogenicity of fat may also be noted in this region.

Computed tomography and magnetic resonance imaging

Advanced imaging techniques are now increasingly widely available to veterinary surgeons, and therefore warrant consideration for the emergency or critically ill patient.

Computed tomography (CT) makes use of X-rays to produce detailed cross-sectional images of the patient. Initial images are usually acquired in the transverse plane, but may then be reconstructed to produce images in a variety of planes, with three-dimensional reconstruction also possible given appropriate software. The grey scale of the image can be manipulated by selection of window width and level, thus enhancing either bone or soft tissue detail. Scanning times with older equipment can be quite long, but modern helical and multi-channel technologies have greatly reduced scanning times, thus enabling imaging of not only the skull and spine, but also the thorax and abdomen. CT demonstrates bony structures particularly well, but soft tissue structures can also be seen. Administration of contrast medium intravenously allows blood vessels to be identified.

Magnetic resonance imaging (MRI) uses completely different principles; a combination of radiowaves and a powerful magnetic field allows acquisition of cross-sectional images with exquisite soft tissue detail (Figure 25.30). Image contrast will depend on the spin–echo pulse sequence selected, and the relaxation properties of individual tissues. Bony structures are generally not imaged as well as with CT, but some information can still be gained. Image acquisition times are generally longer than with CT, so MRI examination is usually confined to the skull or spine, where respiratory movement is not an issue.

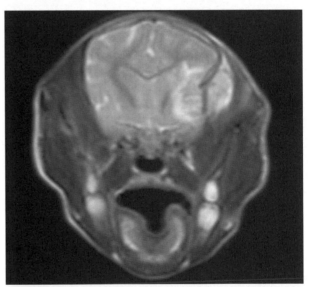

25.30 Transverse T2-weighted MR image of the cranium of a 9-week-old Jack Russell Terrier puppy that had been bitten on the head by another dog. A depressed cranial fracture is visible with an abnormal hyperintense signal from the adjacent brain parenchyma and temporal muscle indicating oedema and haemorrhage. Subdural haemorrhage is not present. (Courtesy of Ruth Dennis, Animal Health Trust)

The use of CT or MRI often necessitates referral of the patient to a centre with the relevant imaging equipment, or waiting for the next local visit of a mobile MRI/CT imaging unit. Furthermore, general anaesthesia is always essential for MRI, and often required for CT despite the shorter scanning times achieved with modern equipment. This means that MRI and CT are unlikely to be used in the initial evaluation of a critical and unstable patient except in a few specialist centres. However, either technique may provide valuable information once the patient has been stabilized.

References and further reading

Boon JA (1998) *Manual of Veterinary Echocardiography*. Williams and Wilkins, Baltimore

British Veterinary Association (2002) *Guidance Notes for the Safe Use of Ionising Radiations in Veterinary Practice*. British Veterinary Association, London

Burk RL and Feeney DA (2003) *Small Animal Radiology and Ultrasonography, 3rd edn.* WB Saunders, Philadelphia

Nyland TG and Mattoon JS (2001) *Small Animal Diagnostic Ultrasound.* Elsevier Health Sciences, Philadelphia

Suter PF (1984) *Thoracic Radiography of the Dog and Cat.* Wettswil, Switzerland

Thrall DE (2002) *Textbook of Veterinary Diagnostic Radiology, 4th edn.* WB Saunders, Philadelphia

26

Nursing care of the critical patient

Emily Savino, Elisa A. Petrollini and Dez Hughes

Introduction

Advanced veterinary nursing is an integral and essential part of the management of the critically ill patient. In addition to providing advanced traditional nursing care, most intensive monitoring should also be performed by the veterinary nurse. Indeed, the ability to detect early and subtle changes in an animal's clinical status is one of the hallmarks of a true critical care nurse. The critical care nurse must be able to assess several animals rapidly, identify the most unstable and prioritize care to the sickest patients first. In addition to triaging emergency patients effectively, the critical care nurse must become proficient at assessing hospitalized patients, observing them for changes in their physical condition and monitoring trends in specific parameters as requested by the clinician.

Effective patient assessment necessitates a full understanding of how to perform and interpret a clinical examination. It also demands in-depth familiarity with the specialized equipment used for monitoring critically ill patients, and some expertise in recognizing which abnormalities require urgent attention from a veterinary surgeon. In addition to monitoring, sophisticated therapeutic and supportive modalities, such as positive pressure ventilation and peritoneal dialysis, require very specialized knowledge regarding the application and complications of these techniques.

The workload inherent in the provision of critical care demands changes in the traditional role of the veterinary nurse as basic care and comfort provider. There is simply too much work for all treatments and monitoring to be performed by a veterinary surgeon. Critical care requires a team approach and the critical care nurse fills a unique role that greatly extends and supplements the capabilities of the veterinary surgeon. Critically ill patients require continuous 24-hour care; it is virtually impossible to perform critical care to a high standard without proficient, round the clock nursing coverage.

The major body systems are those that perform functions vital to the immediate survival of the animal, i.e. the cardiovascular, respiratory, central nervous and urinary systems. Changes in a major body system can have immediate and life-threatening consequences, therefore intensive monitoring of these particular systems is used to detect signs that may predict development of a problem before it becomes serious. The critically ill patient is sufficiently fragile that worsening of a problem affecting one major body system can rapidly progress to be fatal. Early recognition and action to prevent possible complications are fundamental parts of critical care. A convenient and helpful approach to critical care nursing is to consider the monitoring and nursing care applicable to each major body system. When examining a critically ill patient, the deleterious effects of stress on the animal cannot be overemphasized. The need to monitor these animals must be balanced against the recognition that manipulating some patients, especially those with severe respiratory compromise, can be fatal.

Examples of basic and advanced critical care nursing orders for treatment and monitoring of critically ill patients are given in Figures 26.1 and 26.2, and an example of a typical intensive care unit (ICU) treatment order sheet is given in Figure 26.3.

Rectal temperature every 4–12 hours

Mucous membrane colour, capillary refill time, pulse quality and heart rate every 2–12 hours

Respiratory rate and effort, auscultation of the lungs every 2–12 hours

Note urine output or palpate bladder every 2–6 hours

Note mentation and neurological status every 2–6 hours

Note the presence of vomiting, regurgitation or bowel movements every 4–8 hours

Assess comfort and adequacy of pain control every 2–4 hours

Turn from side to side if recumbent or stand and walk the patient every 4 hours

Lubricate eyes with artificial tears if the animal is sedated and unable to blink, every 2–4 hours

Offer water and/or food (specify food type and amount unless 'nil by mouth') and record volumes ingested

Check oxygen supplementation percentage every 2–4 hours

Check that intravenous fluids are of the type requested and are running at the correct rate every 2 hours

Check position, degree of tightness, adequacy of venous drainage and cleanliness of all bandages every 4–8 hours; replace if necessary

Heparinize and evaluate patency of all intravenous catheters every 4–6 hours

Packed cell volume, total solids, dipstick blood glucose and dipstick blood urea nitrogen estimation every 2–24 hours

---

26.1 Basic nursing monitoring orders applicable to most critically ill dogs and cats should include most of the above parameters. The frequency and interval of monitoring will depend on the severity of illness, the rate at which the patient's condition is changing and the type of disease.

Continuous or intermittent electrocardiography (ECG); note dysrhythmias
Blood pressure monitoring (direct or indirect) continuous or every 2–12 hours
Central venous pressure monitoring continuous or every 2–6 hours
Pulmonary artery or pulmonary capillary wedge pressure monitoring continuous or every 2 hours
Pulse oximetry continuous or every 2–12 hours
End-tidal capnography continuous or every 2–12 hours
Arterial blood gas analysis every 2–24 hours
Urine output quantitation via closed collection system every 2–4 hours
Intra-abdominal pressure monitoring every 2–6 hours
Electrolyte measurement every 4–24 hours
Colloid osmometry every 4–24 hours
Nebulize and coupage 10–20 minutes every 4–6 hours
Check and clean inner cannula of tracheostomy tube every 2–4 hours
Aspirate chest tubes every 2–4 hours, record volumes of air/fluid obtained
Record mechanical ventilator settings, airway pressures and tidal volume every 2 hours
Peritoneal dialysis: infuse dialysate, dwell and drain every 1–2 hours, record volumes and quality of fluid obtained

26.2 Advanced nursing monitoring and treatment orders applicable to critically ill dogs and cats could include many of the above parameters. The frequency and interval of monitoring will depend on the severity of illness, the rate at which the patient's condition is changing and the type of disease.

26.3

An example of a treatment sheet for a typical ICU patient. For this hospital, the convention is to place an X at the time a treatment or monitoring is ordered, and to circle the X once the treatment has been completed. (EDB, extended database (PCV, TS/TP, glucose, Azostick, serum electrolytes, venous blood gases); MDB, minimum database (PCV, TS/TP, glucose, Azostick))

Monitoring and nursing care of the cardiovascular system

Basic cardiovascular assessment involves evaluation of mucous membrane colour, capillary refill time (CRT) and vigour, pulse quality and heart rate. This is supplemented as appropriate by more advanced monitoring, which can include measurement of arterial blood pressure, central venous pressure and continuous electrocardiography, depending on the needs of the individual patient.

Mucous membranes and capillary refill time

The oral mucous membrane colour is usually easiest to assess and the best site to use for CRT is the gingiva above the canine tooth. A normal animal should have pink mucous membranes with a vigorous capillary refill that takes 1–1.25 seconds. Mucous membranes in normal cats are significantly paler than in dogs. Pale, white, grey or muddy mucous membranes usually indicate poor perfusion or anaemia. Red or injected membranes may be associated with excitement, fever or the systemic inflammatory response syndrome (SIRS) seen with sepsis, severe pancreatitis, metastatic neoplasia or other causes of severe and extensive tissue damage. Cyanosis (blue or purple colour) indicates severe and life-threatening arterial hypoxaemia necessitating immediate oxygen supplementation. Icterus may be due to increased red blood cell destruction, liver disease or obstructions to bile flow. Other rare abnormalities of mucous membrane colour include the brown membranes seen with paracetamol (acetaminophen) poisoning in cats and the cherry red colour caused by carbon monoxide poisoning. A slow CRT indicates a reduction in blood flow through the periphery and occurs most commonly with hypovolaemia and heart failure. A fast CRT can be seen in excited animals, with fever and SIRS, and following mild to moderate haemorrhage when the cardiovascular system can still compensate for the blood loss.

Pulses

Both femoral and dorsal pedal pulses should be carefully palpated. Pulse palpation is usually more difficult in cats than in dogs and accurate evaluation of pulse quality takes a great deal of practice. Femoral pulses are usually the easiest to feel; however, familiarity with where to feel a dorsal pedal pulse can be extremely helpful. The dorsal pedal pulse is palpated from the dorsal pedal artery on the craniomedial aspect of the proximal metatarsus (Figure 26.4). This pulse becomes non palpable (is 'lost') earlier than the femoral pulse in animals with poor perfusion. Absence of a dorsal pedal pulse can provide a rough estimate of blood pressure; patients with a non-palpable dorsal pedal pulse will typically have a systolic blood pressure that is below 80 mmHg. If the dorsal pedal pulse cannot be palpated, the animal should be evaluated for the presence of shock (see Chapter 3). Measurement and ongoing monitoring of arterial blood pressure may be important in these cases (see Chapter 3). Palpation of the dorsal pedal pulse is also useful in animals in which the femoral pulse is difficult to feel,

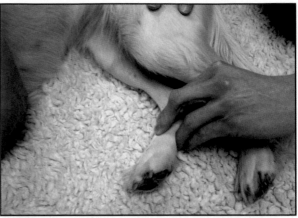

26.4 The dorsal pedal pulse is palpated on the craniomedial aspect of the hindleg below the hock. It can be a useful means of assessing the cardiovascular status of critically ill dogs. Inability to feel this pulse can indicate the presence of shock and hypotension.

such as obese or heavily muscled breeds. Fractious animals and animals with femoral or pelvic fractures will often tolerate palpation of a dorsal pedal pulse but not a femoral pulse.

Normal pulses are synchronous with the heartbeat and should not vary in strength. Asynchronous pulses or variations in pulse strength usually indicate the presence of a cardiac dysrhythmia and should be evaluated via an electrocardiogram (ECG).

Heart rate and rhythm

The vast majority of unstressed dogs have a heart rate of 80–120 beats per minute in the setting of an emergency clinic regardless of their body weight. The effect of body size on heart rate has been somewhat overemphasized. Normal heart rate in cats in a veterinary clinic usually varies from 170–200 beats per minute. Abnormal heart sounds, including murmurs, dysrhythmias, gallop rhythms or muffled heart sounds, should be noted and monitored.

Animals with abnormalities of heart rate or rhythm should be monitored with a continuous ECG. Adhesive patches (Figure 26.5) for the ECG leads are often tolerated much better than clips; however, the skin must be clipped, cleaned with alcohol, then dried to ensure good contact. The adhesive patches may desiccate over time and usually require replacing every day to maintain good skin contact. Specialized ECG leads are available to attach to the pads, or alternatively alligator clips can be attached directly to the contact button of the adhesive patch. After applying the skin contacts, it is often wise to let the animal settle in its cage before attaching the leads. Any abnormalities noted on the ECG should be recorded for review by a veterinary surgeon (see Chapter 6). In cases with cardiac disease or anuria that require fluid therapy, it is helpful to measure central venous pressure (CVP) to avoid fluid overload (see Chapter 4). Arterial blood pressure monitoring is also a vital part of ongoing monitoring of the critical patient with evidence of cardiovascular dysfunction (see Chapter 3). In addition, the respiratory rate and effort should be closely monitored.

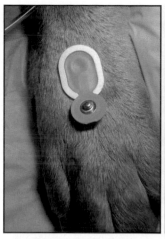
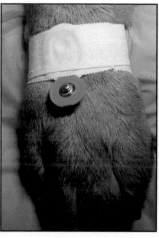
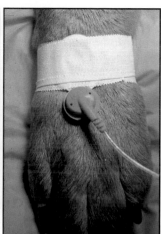

26.5 Adhesive patches are available for ECG lead attachment for continuous monitoring of critically ill patients. The skin is clipped and cleaned, then the adhesive patch is applied to the skin and taped in place. Specialized ECG leads can be obtained to attach to the patches.

Monitoring and nursing care of the respiratory system

All veterinary staff must remain acutely aware of the fragility of the dyspnoeic patient, and the risks of any procedures in these patients must be carefully weighed against the potential benefits. The stress of restraint for placement of an intravenous catheter can prove fatal, especially in dyspnoeic cats. Consequently, the physical examination and diagnostic tests may need to be performed in stages. Handling and manipulation of the patient should be kept to a minimum and the animal should be given ample time to rest between procedures. Most dyspnoeic cats will benefit from a period in a high concentration of supplemental oxygen in an oxygen cage or incubator prior to a complete evaluation.

Examination

Evaluation of the respiratory system usually includes determination of respiratory rate, evaluation of respiratory effort and auscultation of the lungs. A normal animal should have a respiratory rate of 15–30 breaths per minute and very little apparent chest movement, because the major contribution to a normal inspiration comes from diaphragmatic contraction. During normal inspiration, diaphragmatic contraction displaces abdominal viscera in a caudal direction and the abdominal wall moves out. Animals in respiratory distress exhibit postural adaptations to dyspnoea which include standing rather than sitting, abduction of the elbows, increased abdominal movement, extension of the neck and open-mouth breathing. Paradoxical abdominal movement can also occur as dyspnoea worsens. Increased intercostal movement draws the diaphragm and abdominal viscera cranially, and the abdominal wall moves inwards instead of outwards during inspiration. Some of the postural manifestations of dyspnoea vary between dogs and cats. Dogs prefer to stand with abducted elbows, while cats tend to sit in sternal recumbency. Constantly changing body position in cats implies a much worse degree of dyspnoea than it does in dogs. Lateral recumbency and open-mouth breathing caused by dyspnoea is a serious sign in a dog and often means impending death in a cat.

In a dyspnoeic animal the respiratory pattern can help localize the site of disease in the respiratory tract. This proves especially useful in two common situations. An upper airway obstruction is usually associated with a prolonged inspiratory time with inspiratory stridor or stertor and a short expiration. If possible without undue stress to the patient, body temperature should be measured as soon as possible in animals that might have an upper airway obstruction. The main thermoregulatory mechanism in the dog is panting, thus upper airway obstruction can be associated with dangerously high body temperatures. Small airway disease, such as feline asthma, typically has a longer expiratory than inspiratory phase, with increased abdominal effort. Most other causes of dyspnoea are associated with mixed respiratory patterns.

Pulmonary auscultation in the dyspnoeic patient is difficult to master, but is a skill that should be perfected by every critical care nurse. The easiest way to ensure a complete auscultation is to divide the chest into a noughts and crosses board, then auscultate each square (Figure 26.6). Lung sounds are normally slightly louder and coarser in the cranioventral lung fields compared to the caudodorsal fields. Lung sounds should be symmetrical when the same area is compared on both sides of the chest. Pleural space disease, such as pleural effusion or pneumothorax, causes muffling of lung sounds, whereas small airway or parenchymal

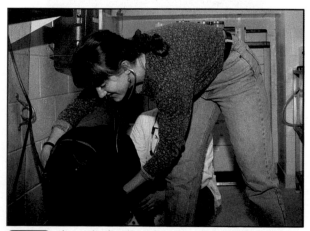

26.6 Auscultation is a vital part of monitoring the respiratory system.

disease usually makes them louder. On auscultation, a pneumothorax produces diminished breath sounds dorsally, whereas a pleural effusion more commonly causes diminished lung sounds ventrally. Auscultation of crackles may indicate pulmonary oedema caused by fluid overload, congestive heart failure or chronic pulmonary parenchymal disease such as pulmonary fibrosis.

Oxygen therapy

Oxygen therapy is often necessary in the patient with respiratory disease. Oxygen can be supplemented using an oxygen cage, oxygen mask or via an intranasal tube (see Chapter 7). An oxygen cage (Figure 26.7) allows the inspired oxygen concentration to be closely controlled (between room air and 100%) and is the least stressful method of oxygen administration. The inaccessibility of animals in an oxygen cage is often suggested as a drawback of this method of oxygen delivery; however, the reduced manipulation can be to their benefit. Opening the door to the cage should be avoided and the small access ports should be used whenever possible, to avoid rapid changes in oxygen concentration. Oxygen masks can be useful when a procedure must be performed on a dyspnoeic animal; however, many dyspnoeic animals will not tolerate a mask. In these cases, simply holding the oxygen tubing in front of the mouth and nose can suffice ('flow-by' oxygen, see Chapter 7). Intranasal oxygen delivery is convenient for longer-term supplementation of lower concentrations of oxygen. It requires the placement of an intranasal catheter or nasal prongs (see Chapter 7), which may not be tolerated by some animals. Placement can be greatly facilitated by instillation of local anaesthetic into the nostril 10 minutes prior to the procedure. Placement of an intranasal catheter is often

too stressful for a severely dyspnoeic animal, especially one that has just been presented to the veterinary surgeon as an emergency. Ideally, all methods of oxygen supplementation should include some form of humidification of the inspired gas. Humidification consists of the saturation of the inspired oxygen with water vapour, which helps to prevent damage to the airway mucosa by dry air.

When there is evidence of lung disease on clinical examination, lung function should be assessed using pulse oximetry or, ideally, arterial blood gas analysis. An arterial blood sample allows measurement of the arterial partial pressure of oxygen (P_aO_2), whereas pulse oximetry measures haemoglobin saturation (S_pO_2) (see Chapter 7). Pulse oximetry is non-invasive, requiring only that a light transmitting and receiving probe be placed on the animal. The tongue, ear, lip, toe or inguinal skin fold can all be used as sites for probe placement. Unfortunately, the accuracy of the pulse oximeter can be significantly affected by movement of the animal, inadequate clipping of the placement site, poor perfusion or pigmented mucous membranes or skin. Failure to achieve a good signal strength or waveform on the instrument display should lead one to question the accuracy of the results. Arterial blood gas samples are usually obtained from the femoral (Figure 26.8) or dorsal pedal artery and allow measurement of the partial pressure of oxygen, carbon dioxide and pH. If infrequent samples are anticipated, the samples can be obtained by puncture with a fine (25 or 26 gauge) needle. If repeated sampling is likely to be necessary, it is often safer and less stressful on the animal to place a catheter percutaneously into the dorsal pedal artery (see Chapter 2).

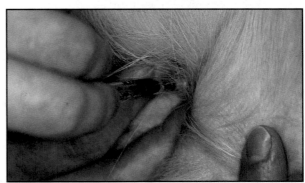

26.8 Samples of arterial blood are obtained by percutaneous puncture of the femoral (shown here) or dorsal pedal arteries. Specialized pre-heparinized syringes are available or alternatively standard 1 ml syringes can be flushed with heparin.

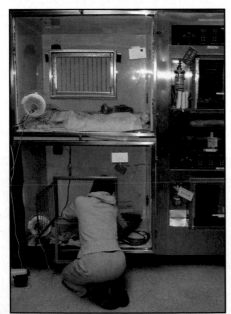

26.7 This oxygen cage can be adjusted to a specific temperature, percentage humidity and oxygen concentration based on patient requirements. To minimize stress to dyspnoeic patients, treatments may be completed through the pull-down window in the front of the cage, without causing a significant reduction in the oxygen concentration.

The goal of oxygen therapy is to maintain a P_aO_2 of at least 60 mmHg, which corresponds to S_pO_2 values greater than 90%. At partial pressures of oxygen below 60 mmHg, there is a rapid fall in haemoglobin saturation. It is therefore often better to aim for a P_aO_2 in the range of 70–80 mmHg to provide a margin of safety should the lung disease worsen. Ideally, the patient should receive the minimum inspired oxygen concentration required to maintain an adequate P_aO_2 or S_pO_2, to avoid the risks of oxygen toxicity caused by prolonged high inspired oxygen concentrations. If blood gas analysis or pulse oximetry is not available, the inspired concentration is titrated to the clinical response. In emergency patients, initially 100% oxygen should be given, then the concentration should be gradually reduced to the lowest level at which the animal breathes comfortably. Oxygen concentrations of >50% for more than 12 hours or >60% for 18 hours have been suggested to cause oxygen toxicity. Ideally, an inspired oxygen concentration of 40% is recommended for long-term therapy. Maintaining an adequate P_aO_2 is essential for life, so in animals with severe pulmonary parenchymal disease the guidelines for oxygen therapy may have to be exceeded in spite of the risk of oxygen toxicity.

Nebulization and coupage are used to facilitate the mobilization of respiratory secretions, usually in animals with pneumonia. Nebulization consists of the production of tiny droplets (ideally 3–7 μl) of water or saline, usually by an ultrasonic or oxygen-driven nebulizer (Figure 26.9). The mist of water droplets is infused into a closed cage every 4–6 hours and is inhaled to shower out in the small airways, moistening respiratory tract secretions and facilitating their movement out of the chest by the mucociliary escalator. Concurrently, the chest is patted firmly (coupaged) to stimulate coughing, which further assists airway clearance. In some circumstances, nebulization can be used to administer antibiotics or other respiratory medications.

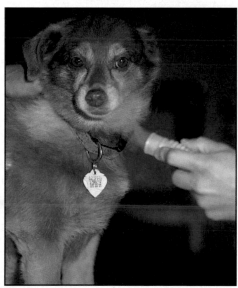

26.9 Nebulization consists of the generation of tiny droplets of water or saline, which are inhaled and then deposited in the airways, moistening airway secretions. Since the saline or water remains in the liquid phase, nebulization differs from humidification, which is the saturation of inspired gases with water vapour (gas phase).

Monitoring and nursing care of the neurological system

Since critical illness is often associated with significant muscle weakness and central nervous system (CNS) depression, nursing evaluation of the CNS often amounts to assessing whether the abnormalities of mental status and gait are appropriate for the other problems identified in the major body system assessment. Abnormalities of mental status include dullness/

depression, stupor and coma, hyperexcitability, hysteria and seizures. Depressed mentation is often associated with abnormalities of other body systems, such as hypoperfusion, renal failure and liver failure. When the degree of depression is greater than expected from the other disease processes present, this should raise the suspicion of primary CNS disease or CNS complications due to metabolic disorders, such as hepatic encephalopathy. In any patient with abnormal mental status the blood glucose concentration should be checked immediately; hypoglycaemia is a possible underlying cause that is easily and rapidly reversible, but which can cause irreversible neurological damage if left untreated. Seizures are a common emergency problem and can occur due to intracranial or extracranial causes. The body temperature of an animal presenting with seizures should be measured immediately, as hyperthermia due to muscle activity can occasionally be life threatening.

Precautionary measures are often instituted in animals with presumed brain disease or head trauma, to treat and avoid increases in intracranial pressure. Elevation of the head to an angle of approximately 30 degrees can be used to facilitate venous return and reduce intracranial pressure. It is important to place the entire animal on a board, rather than to try and elevate the head alone. Care should be taken to avoid occluding the jugular veins and jugular venepuncture should be avoided. Procedures that may result in coughing should also be avoided, as coughing can result in large increases in intracranial pressure. Neurological parameters monitored in the patient with neurological disease include the pupillary light response and pupil sizes, the palpebral or blink reflex, the menace reflex, the presence or absence of strabismus, and the general mental status. It should be noted that patients with head trauma or brain disease may lose their gag reflex and the ability to protect their airway. Animals that cannot protect their airway should be intubated and the cuff of the endotracheal tube should be inflated to prevent aspiration.

Spinal cord injury or disease is the other main category of neurological injury. There is only a limited number of underlying causes of acute onset paresis or paralysis of the hindlimbs or all four limbs (see Chapter 9). Intervertebral disc prolapse is by far the most common cause in emergency practice. Other causes include spinal fractures and luxations, tumours, fibrocartilaginous emboli and discospondylitis. In addition to causing paralysis of the limbs, cervical spinal cord injury can also impair the function of the phrenic and intercostal nerves, leading to inadequate ventilation; these patients may require mechanical ventilation. Arterial blood gas analysis and/or end-tidal capnography (see Chapter 7) allow the veterinary surgeon to monitor the partial pressure of carbon dioxide to determine whether artificial ventilation is needed. When spinal cord injury is present, progressive loss of neurological function is manifested as ataxia and loss of proprioception, followed by loss of voluntary motor activity, then extensor tone and, lastly, deep pain sensation. Deterioration in the patient's ambulatory status should be brought to the attention of a veterinary surgeon, as emergency surgical intervention may be necessary.

Monitoring and nursing care of the urinary system

Urine output is used as one of the most important indicators of renal function in the dynamic critically ill patient; however, clinicopathological tests such as blood urea nitrogen, creatinine and potassium concentration should also be monitored. In addition to intrinsic renal disease, urine output can fall due to prerenal or postrenal causes. The fall in urine output that accompanies prerenal problems (e.g. dehydration or hypoperfusion) is physiologically appropriate, as the body attempts to retain water and sodium. It should be associated with concentrated urine (high specific gravity) if renal function is normal. Postrenal azotaemia and subsequent decreases in urine output may occur with blockage of the urethra due to calculi or rupture of the bladder, urethra or ureter resulting in uroperitoneum. With urethral obstruction a large painful bladder can often be palpated and the patient may strain to urinate. Monitoring urine output is especially important in patients at risk for acute renal failure or in animals that have sustained abdominal or pelvic trauma which can be associated with rupture of the bladder or urethra. Indwelling urinary catheters with a sterile closed collection system may be placed to allow accurate measurement of urine output and sometimes to prevent urine scalding in the recumbent patient. Indiscriminate use should, however, be avoided as they are a potential route for bacterial infection and can also result in urethral trauma. If a catheter is necessary, it should be placed using sterile equipment and aseptic technique (see Chapter 8). In a female, hair should be clipped around the perineum followed by a full surgical scrub. The urinary catheter can be placed blind, by palpation of the urethral orifice with a sterile gloved finger, or the urethral meatus can be visualized using a speculum. In the male, an assistant should extrude the penis and the catheter should be placed without allowing the catheter to come into contact with the prepuce.

If acute changes are anticipated, urine output should be measured every 2–4 hours. Normal urine output is 0.5–2 ml/kg/h; however, the appropriate urine output in a critically ill animal can vary widely depending on the rate of fluid therapy being administered. If a reduction in urine output is detected, the bladder should be palpated and the catheter should be flushed with warm saline to ensure that there is no mechanical obstruction due to catheter kinking, blood clots or calculi. To avoid potential bacterial contamination, a system that allows the urine collection bag to be emptied without disconnecting the inflow line is preferred (Figure 26.10). In systems that necessitate disconnection of the tubing, care should be taken to prevent the ends coming into contact with foreign material. The collection bag should be kept below the patient to facilitate urine drainage, but ideally not on the floor. Any changes in the appearance or odour of the urine should be noted. If a urinary catheter is not placed, manual palpation of the bladder, noting its size, and/or weighing absorbent cage material before and after urination, are approximate methods of assessing urine production.

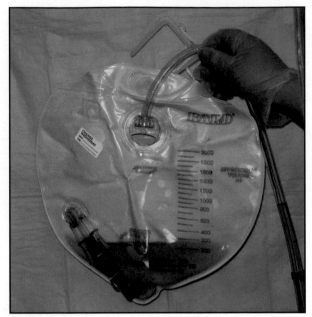

26.10 This urinary collection system includes an anti-reflux chamber which prevents urine from flowing backwards from the collection bag to the bladder even if the collection bag is full.

Pain detection and analgesia in the critical patient

Pain recognition

Assessment of pain can be difficult in critically ill animals, as many of them have abnormal mental status due to their underlying disease processes. Indicators of pain can be quite subtle and many animals do not exhibit obvious signs such as vocalization. It is especially difficult to recognize pain in cats, in which a crouched posture can sometimes be the only sign. In dogs, pain may be manifest as restlessness, reluctance to lie down, hypersalivation, hypertension, hyperthermia, inappetence, tachypnoea or tachycardia. Some stoical dogs may show only a worried facial expression, tremble or grimace with their lips drawn back. Dogs with severe abdominal pain may resent abdominal palpation, be reluctant to lie down, or assume the 'prayer position' by standing with their front legs extended and chest down, back arched and abdomen splinted.

Analgesia

Analgesic medications should be given as soon as possible, in adequate doses, because many analgesics are more effective when given before pain is severe. Furthermore, analgesics can sometimes effectively prevent pain but do not completely eliminate it once it has begun.

Many analgesic medications (see Chapter 22) used in critically ill animals can also result in sedation and dysphoria. This can complicate subsequent clinical evaluations and the interpretation of pain status in that animal. Analgesic drugs may also have deleterious effects on the cardiovascular, respiratory, renal and neurological systems and the side effects of analgesic medication must be weighed against humanitarian concerns for pain relief. Furthermore, sedation, which occurs with some pain medications, can mask serious deterioration in the status of the animal. Changes in behaviour, mental status or respiratory pattern are some of the earliest signs of problems in a critically ill patient and they can be extremely difficult to interpret following sedation. Consequently, the major body systems must be closely monitored following administration of pain medication and sedation.

Nursing care of the recumbent patient

The comfort and welfare of the critically ill animal should be paramount in the mind of all critical care personnel. Veterinary critical care entails supporting very sick animals and it is incumbent upon all veterinary surgeons and nurses to ensure that the level of discomfort is kept to a minimum. The level of discomfort that is considered acceptable must be assessed on an individual basis. Factors such as the likelihood of survival, the anticipated duration of survival and the expected quality of life following successful treatment may all impact on this assessment. The critical care nurse plays a vital role in the care of the critically ill patient, most of which are recumbent for at least some period during hospitalization. The care of the animal that cannot move around or clean itself is an important part of critical care nursing (Figure 26.11).

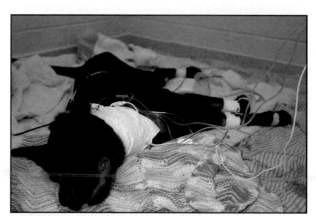

26.11 Patients that are recumbent for prolonged periods are at risk for pulmonary atelectasis, aspiration pneumonia, decubital ulcers and urine scalding. Important nursing strategies for these animals include frequent turning from side to side, physical therapy and limb massage to ensure good blood flow, and careful frequent cleaning of all excreta.

Respiratory care

The most important short-term effect of prolonged recumbency is impairment of respiratory function and subsequent hypoxia due to atelectasis, aspiration pneumonia and/or ventilation–perfusion mismatching. Atelectasis, or collapse of lung lobes, occurs when a patient lies in lateral recumbency for an extended period of time. Atelectasis tends to be most common in large-breed dogs. Frequent turning of the patient (every 4 hours) or maintaining the patient in a sternal position will avoid atelectasis and promote appropriate alveolar ventilation and perfusion. Aspiration pneumonia is a relatively common complication in the recumbent patient, especially if the animal is vomiting or regurgitating frequently. Regurgitation and aspiration can occasionally occur with no immediate clinical signs associated with the regurgitation episode, but later development of pneumonia; this is termed a silent aspiration episode.

Decubital ulcers

Recumbent patients are at risk of developing decubital ulceration. Although uncommon, decubital ulcers can occur if the patient is recumbent for a prolonged period of time (several days). Large, heavy dogs, or those with thin skin and minimal soft tissue coverage of their bones (e.g. Greyhounds), seem to be particularly at risk. Persistent localized pressure on the same area of the body impairs circulation, which eventually results in necrosis. Decubital ulcers extend through the skin and underlying subcutaneous tissue and even through muscle to bone in severe cases. They occur most commonly over the greater trochanter, ischial tuberosity and lateral aspect of the elbow. Healing of decubital ulcers is extremely slow and difficult, so prevention is far superior to cure. Frequent turning of the patient and provision of soft, clean bedding are the best ways to avoid decubital ulcers.

Hygiene

Close attention should be paid to the hygiene of recumbent patients. Bedding should be kept clean and dry and all faeces and urine should be removed promptly. Failure to keep the patient clean can result in urine scalding and perineal dermatitis, and can contaminate urinary and intravenous catheters. Fluid lines that become soiled with urine or faeces should be replaced. Clipping the hair from the perineal area and the use of topical medications can help to prevent perineal dermatitis. Urinary catheterization or manually expressing the bladder may be indicated for some patients.

Physical therapy

Many recumbent patients require physical therapy to maintain joint mobility; however, this should be kept to a minimum in the unstable critically ill patient. In patients with moderate to severe peripheral oedema, the legs should be warm compressed and gently massaged every 4–6 hours to improve circulation. If the patient is ambulatory, short walks may be appropriate.

Nursing care of intravenous catheters

Intravenous catheters are essential in the care of the critically ill patient to administer intravenous medication and fluid therapy (see Chapter 2). In addition, central venous catheters can be used to monitor central venous pressure, while arterial catheters are used directly to measure arterial blood pressure. Venous and arterial catheters can also be used for blood sampling, thus avoiding the risks and discomfort of serial vessel puncture. This is especially beneficial when frequent blood sampling is anticipated, such as might be needed for blood glucose monitoring in a diabetic animal. When obtaining blood samples from an indwelling arterial or venous catheter, the catheter port should be cleaned with alcohol, the catheter should be flushed and, using a syringe containing 0.5–1 ml heparinized saline to prevent clotting, an adequate pre-sample (2–6 ml of blood) is withdrawn. This avoids dilution of the test sample with flush solution remaining in the catheter. The test sample is then obtained and the pre-sample can be injected back into the animal via a venous catheter.

Intravenous access may be established via a peripheral vein, such as the cephalic or saphenous, or via a central vein, such as the jugular or medial femoral. Central venous access can also be established by placing a long catheter into the cephalic or saphenous vein. In very small patients, such as neonates, a needle inserted into the medullary cavity of a bone (usually the femur) can be used to administer fluids and medications (see Chapter 2). When placing catheters, all hair should be clipped from the site, which should be scrubbed using standard aseptic technique (Figure 26.12). Following placement, the catheter should be securely taped or sutured in place and covered by a wrap to keep the site clean and dry.

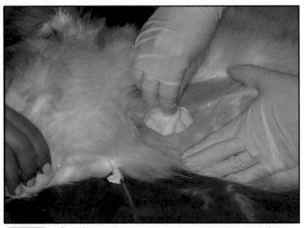

26.12 Careful catheter site preparation is one of the most important factors in preventing infections and thrombophlebitis. In this patient, the skin over the jugular vein has been clipped, and the area is being scrubbed for placement of a central venous catheter.

Catheter patency is maintained by flushing with heparinized saline (1 unit heparin per ml of 0.9% NaCl) every 6 hours. The catheter site should be evaluated frequently for any swelling, reddening or pain suggestive of phlebitis, and if the wrapping becomes dirty or wet it should be replaced immediately (Figure 26.13). If signs of local inflammation are seen or the animal develops an otherwise unexplained fever, the catheter should be removed.

Although routine removal and replacement of intravenous catheters every 72 hours has been advocated, studies have shown that removal of otherwise functional catheters in the absence of clinical signs of thrombophlebitis is probably unnecessary (Matthews *et al.*, 1996). Vascular access may become a limiting factor for care of critically ill dogs and cats, particularly those of small body size, or those that are

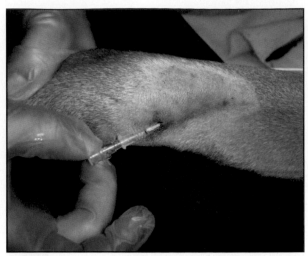

26.13 Intravenous catheter insertion sites must be examined daily for evidence of discharge, inflammation and discomfort. In this patient, the catheter insertion site was reddened and the vessel was hardened on palpation. The catheter was immediately removed.

hospitalized repeatedly or for prolonged periods of time. Clinical experience has confirmed that it is best to maintain catheters in place for the longest possible time, as long as they are patent, uninfected and not associated with thrombophlebitis. Peripheral catheters usually require changing more often than central venous catheters.

The size of the catheter selected will depend upon the size of the patient and the anticipated rate of fluid infusion. Flow through a catheter is proportional to the fourth power of the radius, i.e. halving the radius of the catheter will reduce the flow by 16 times. If rapid fluid administration is required in animals with systemic hypoperfusion or if blood products are to be given, the largest bore catheter possible should be used (e.g. an 18 gauge catheter or greater should be used in any dog over 20 kg). It is also best to place a second intravenous catheter in dogs heavier than 20 kg that require rapid intravascular volume expansion. This ensures that an adequate rate of fluids can be given and provides a backup if one catheter comes out or does not flow well. Blood products should ideally be administered through a separate catheter both because of their higher viscosity and because of the potential for interactions with other drugs or fluids especially those containing calcium.

The dorsal pedal artery is the most common site used for arterial access. In all but the smallest animals, a 22 gauge catheter is placed percutaneously into the artery. Paradoxically, placement of a dorsal pedal arterial catheter is often associated with fewer bleeding complications in high-risk animals than repeated arterial puncture using a needle. Arterial catheters are used to measure direct blood pressures and to obtain blood samples to measure arterial blood gases. Fluid therapy and medications should never be administered via an arterial line. There is a potential for rapid exsanguination if an arterial catheter becomes disconnected, so patients with these catheters must be kept under close supervision.

Patients with special nursing requirements

Chest tubes

Patients with chest tubes should be kept under close observation, because if the tube dislodges there is a risk that the patient may develop a pneumothorax and become acutely dyspnoeic. The tube should be secured by sutures and a chest bandage (Figure 26.14); an Elizabethan collar may also be required to reduce the risk of patient interference. Care must be taken not to bandage the chest too tightly as this may compromise ventilation. The chest tube bandage should be changed daily or sooner if it slips or becomes soiled. The chest tube insertion site should be examined daily for evidence of infection or inflammation.

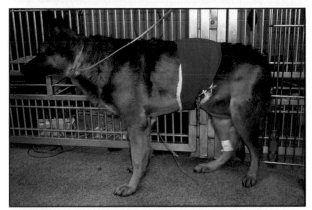

26.14 Chest tubes should be bandaged to prevent premature removal caused by the tube becoming caught in cage bars or on bedding. An Elizabethan collar is indicated if the patient attempts to remove its own chest tube.

The chest tube should generally be aspirated gently every 4–6 hours until negative pressure is achieved. The quantities of air and fluid obtained should be recorded. The characteristics of the fluid should be noted in the record and the clinician should be notified if the appearance of the fluid changes dramatically. Occasionally, depending on the patient's disease, the chest tube may need to be aspirated more or less frequently or a specific volume of fluid/air may be removed.

If a patient with a chest tube becomes tachypnoeic or dyspnoeic sooner than the allotted time for the next drainage, the tube should be aspirated immediately. Following aspiration of the chest tube, if negative pressure has been obtained but the patient's respiratory rate and effort are unchanged, the chest tube should be examined for kinks and the chest should be auscultated to determine if breath sounds are decreased. Additionally, other possible causes for changes in respiratory rate and effort should be considered. These may include worsening pain or progression of pulmonary parenchymal disease. Thoracic radiographs may be needed to confirm that the chest tube is still correctly in place and draining any fluid that is present, and to document possible progression of lung disease. If aspiration of the chest tube fails to yield negative pressure, the system should be examined for possible leaks. If a leak is not located, the clinician should be notified and continuous suction drainage may be necessary.

Tracheostomy tubes

Patients (especially cats) with tracheostomy tubes must be kept under close observation as there is the potential for the tube to become obstructed or dislodged at any time (Figure 26.15). Tracheostomy tubes should be evaluated every 2–4 hours, or more frequently if indicated, to confirm that there is unobstructed air movement. If the tracheostomy tube contains an inner cannula, the inner cannula should be removed aseptically and cleaned every 2–4 hours or as indicated to prevent occlusion of the airway with mucous plugs or airway secretions. Tracheostomy care trays are commercially available.

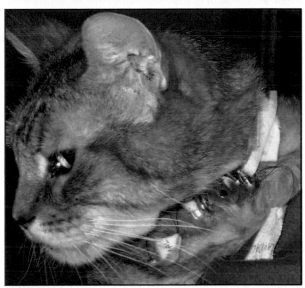

26.15 Cat with a tracheostomy tube placed to relieve airway obstruction caused by a laryngeal mass. The tracheostomy tube must be examined regularly for evidence of obstruction.

A sterile tracheostomy tube must be readily available in the event that the tracheostomy tube needs to be replaced on an emergency basis. The ability to provide flow-by oxygen supplementation should always be available and where possible patients should receive a period of preoxygenation (5–10 minutes of flow-by oxygen supplementation) before the tracheostomy tube is manipulated. Suction of the airway may need to be performed periodically with a suction catheter to remove secretions. However, this may contribute to tracheal mucosal injury and suction should only be carried out when there is a clinical indication of airway obstruction. Aseptic technique must be used during replacement of tubes or inner cannulas and during suction.

The area around the tracheostomy site should be kept clean and dry. Continuous or intermittent nebulization of saline or water should be performed to maintain airway humidification. Recumbent patients must be positioned in such a way that air flow through the tracheostomy site is unobstructed.

Wounds and wound management

Wounds should be examined several times daily for any evidence of infection, such as swelling or discharge. The wound and surrounding area should be kept clean and dry.

If drains are being used, the volume and characteristics of any fluid draining from a wound must be monitored and recorded in the record. The clinician should be notified if the appearance or quantity of the fluid from a drain changes dramatically. If a vacuum drain is used, a loose wrap should be placed over the insertion site and the drain should be attached to the animal to prevent unintentional drain removal.

Patients on mechanical ventilation

Basic and advanced nursing orders apply to any patient on a ventilator (see Figures 26.1 and 26.2). The degree of sedation/anaesthesia should be adjusted according to the clinician's orders. Some ventilator settings require that the patient is lightly sedated but still capable of generating a spontaneous breath. In other cases, it may be necessary for the patient to be more deeply anaesthetized with the ventilator initiating each breath at a set rate. In the lightly sedated patient, the depth of chest excursions, respiratory effort and temperature are closely monitored to determine if the patient is tolerating mechanical ventilation.

The patient's airway must be closely monitored. The endotracheal or tracheostomy tube may become totally or partially obstructed and may require suction or replacement. Suction of the airway and replacement of endotracheal tubes must be done aseptically. Sterile replacement endotracheal tubes should be readily available in case the endotracheal tube needs urgent replacement. A smaller size tube should be available in the event of inflammation and oedema of the airway. The cuff of the endotracheal tube should be deflated and the position of the tube changed every 4–6 hours to prevent pressure necrosis of the trachea.

The patient's chest should be auscultated frequently to monitor for a partially obstructed airway or pleural space complications, such as pneumothorax or pleural effusion. The patient's mouth should be cleaned gently every 4 hours with a dilute antiseptic solution. Suction of the oropharyngeal region may be required to remove mucus, using a Yankauer suction catheter. The tongue should be kept moist if possible. Artificial tears should be placed in both eyes every 4–8 hours as these patients do not blink normally and development of corneal ulceration is a concern. Ventilator tubing should be replaced every 24 hours.

References and further reading

Burrows CF (1982) Inadequate skin preparation as a cause of intravenous catheter-related infection in the dog. *Journal of the American Veterinary Medical Association* **180**, 747–749

Johnson JA and Murtaugh RJ (1997) Preventing and treating nosocomial infection. Part I. Urinary tract infections and pneumonia. *Compendium on Continuing Education for the Practicing Veterinarian* **19**, 581–586

Lees GF (1996) Use and misuse of indwelling catheters. *Veterinary Clinics of North America: Small Animal Practice* **26**, 499–504

Manning AM, Rush J and Ellis DR (1997) Physical therapy for critically ill veterinary patients. Part I. Chest physical therapy. *Compendium on Continuing Education for the Practicing Veterinarian* **19**, 675–688

Manning AM, Rush J and Ellis DR (1997) Physical therapy for critically ill veterinary patients. Part II. The musculoskeletal system. *Compendium on Continuing Education for the Practicing Veterinarian* **19**, 803–806

Matthews KA, Brooks MJ and Valliant AE (1996) A prospective study of intravenous catheter contamination. *Journal of Veterinary Emergency and Critical Care* **6**, 33–43

Nicoll SA and Remedios AM (1995) Recumbency in small animals: pathophysiology and management. *Compendium on Continuing Education for the Practicing Veterinarian* **17**, 1367–1374

Powell S and Petrollini E (1998) Emergency and first aid. In: *Comprehensive Review for Veterinary Technicians*, ed. MM Tighe and M Brown, pp. 327–337. Mosby Year Book, St Louis

Thelan LA, Urden LD, Lough ME and Stacy KM (1998) *Critical Care Nursing: Diagnosis and Management, 3rd edn.* Mosby Year Book, St Louis

Conversion tables

Biochemistry

	SI unit	Conversion	Non-SI unit
Alanine transferase	IU / l	x 1	IU / l
Albumin	g / l	x 0.1	g / dl
Alkaline phosphatase	IU / l	x 1	IU / l
Aspartate transaminase	IU / l	x 1	IU / l
Bilirubin	µmol / l	x 0.0584	mg / dl
Calcium	mmol / l	x 4	mg / dl
Carbon dioxide (total)	mmol / l	x 1	mEq / l
Cholesterol	mmol / l	x 38.61	mg / dl
Chloride	mmol / l	x 1	mEq / l
Cortisol	nmol / l	x 0.362	ng / ml
Creatine kinase	IU / l	x 1	IU / l
Creatinine	µmol / l	x 0.0113	mg / dl
Glucose	mmol / l	x 18.02	mg / dl
Insulin	pmol / l	x 0.1394	µIU / ml
Iron	µmol / l	x 5.587	µg / dl
Magnesium	mmol / l	x 2	mEq / l
Phosphorus	mmol / l	x 3.1	mg / dl
Potassium	mmol / l	x 1	mEq / l
Sodium	mmol / l	x 1	mEq / l
Total protein	g / l	x 0.1	g / dl
Thyroxine (T4) (free)	pmol / l	x 0.0775	ng / dl
Thyroxine (T4) (total)	nmol / l	x 0.0775	µg / dl
Tri-iodothyronine (T3)	nmol / l	x 65.1	ng / dl
Triglycerides	mmol / l	x 88.5	mg / dl
Urea	mmol / l	x 2.8	mg of urea nitrogen / dl

Temperature

	SI unit	Conversion	Conventional unit
	° C	(x 9/5) + 32	° F

Haematology

	SI unit	Conversion	Non-SI unit
Red blood cell count	10^{12} / l	x 1	10^6 / µl
Haemoglobin	g / l	x 0.1	g / dl
MCH	pg / cell	x 1	pg / cell
MCHC	g / l	x 0.1	g / dl
MCV	fl	x 1	µm³
Platelet count	10^9 / l	x 1	10^3 / µl
White blood cell count	10^9 / l	x 1	10^3 / µl

Hypodermic needles

	Metric	Non-metric
External diameter	0.8 mm	21 G
	0.6 mm	23 G
	0.5 mm	25 G
	0.4 mm	27 G
Needle length	12 mm	$\frac{1}{2}$ inch
	16 mm	$\frac{5}{8}$ inch
	25 mm	1 inch
	30 mm	$1\frac{1}{4}$ inch
	40 mm	$1\frac{1}{2}$ inch

Suture material sizes

Metric	USP
0.1	11/0
0.2	10/0
0.3	9/0
0.4	8/0
0.5	7/0
0.7	6/0
1	5/0
1.5	4/0
2	3/0
3	2/0
3.5	0
4	1
5	2
6	3

Index

Index

Index

Index

Index

Index

Index

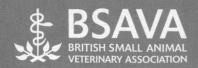

Clinical Pathology
biochemistry, cytology, haematology

BSAVA Manual of Canine and Feline
Clinical Pathology
2nd edition

Edited by Elizabeth Villiers and Laura Blackwood

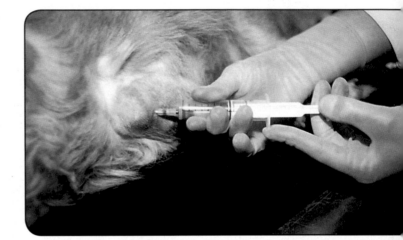

- Which tests to do, how to do them, and how to interpret results

- Features clinical case examples

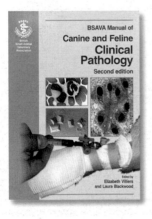

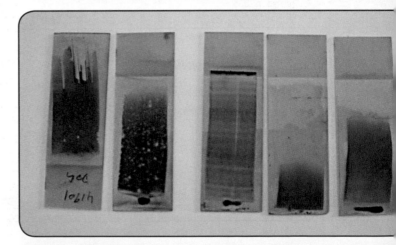

Member price: £50
Non-member price: £89

464 pages
ISBN   978 0 905214 79 5

BSAVA reserves the right to change these prices at any time

British Small Animal Veterinary Association
Woodrow House, 1 Telford Way, Waterwells Business Park, Quedgeley, Gloucester GL2 2AB

Tel: 01452 726700
Fax: 01452 726701
Email: customerservices@bsava.com
Web: www.bsava.com

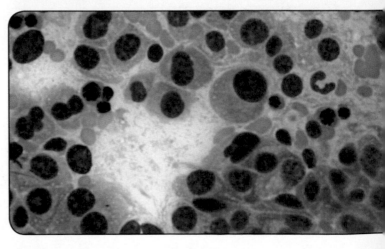